Visual Development, Diagnosis, and Treatment of the Pediatric Patient

Visual Development, Diagnosis, and Treatment of the Pediatric Patient

Robert H. Duckman, O.D., M.A., F.A.A.O.
Professor
Director, Services for Children with Special Needs
State University of New York
State College of Optometry
New York, New York

Lippincott Williams & Wilkins
a Wolters Kluwer business
Philadelphia · Baltimore · New York · London
Buenos Aires · Hong Kong · Sydney · Tokyo

Acquisitions Editor: Jonathan Pine
Managing Editor: Jean McGough
Project Manager: Jennifer Harper
Senior Manufacturing Manager: Benjamin Rivera
Marketing Manager: Adam Glazer
Creative Director: Risa Clow
Production Services: TechBooks
Printer: Edwards Brothers

Printed in the USA

Library of Congress Cataloging-in-Publication Data
Visual development, diagnosis, and treatment of the pediatric patient / [edited by] Robert H. Duckman.
    p. ; cm.
  Includes bibliographical references and index.
  ISBN 0-7817-5288-4
  1. Pediatric ophthalmology.   2. Vision disorders in children.   3. Vision.   I. Duckman, Robert H.
II. Title.
    [DNLM: 1. Vision.   2. Child.   3. Eye–growth & development.   4. Infant.   5. Vision
  Disorders–diagnosis.   6. Vision Disorders–therapy.   7. Visual Pathways–growth & development.
WW 600 V8336 2006]
  RE48.2.C5V52   2006
  618.92′0977–dc22

                              2006005861

                                            10 9 8 7 6 5 4

This book is dedicated to my wife Marla and my daughter Evynne, who tolerated me through a 7-day-a-week work schedule for the better part of 2 years. I could not have done it without their total love and support.

Contents

Preface

What we know about visual development of infants, toddlers and children is relatively new. It is only over the past thirty to forty years that we have come to realize how sophisticated and complex the visual function of these children is. There is still a lot that we do not understand, but over the past three or four decades, science has learned a lot about visual function from birth to adolescence. The motivation for writing this book was to provide myself with a textbook I could use for my Visual Development course. The book started out as a purely theoretical book. However, as the book evolved I decided that since I teach professional students who will become practicing optometrists, they would need to know the practical aspects of evaluating visual function in this population. I expanded the concept for the book to include practical or diagnostic aspects of the pediatric patient. As I was working on this second part of the book, I asked "What happens if they find anomalies?" They would need to treat them. And so I added the third part of the book which deals with treatment. This book is unique in that in one volume you can get theoretical aspects of visual development, testing protocols, and treatment modalities. This is extremely important because in increasing numbers, infants, toddlers and pediatric patients are being seen in private practices and the clinician needs to be ready.

It is extremely important that children receive visual evaluations by 6 months, at 2–3 years, and then as they enter school according to the American Academy of Pediatrics, the American Academy of Pediatric Ophthalmology, and the American Optometric Association. New initiatives are being mounted to ensure that visual problems are picked up as early as possible so intervention may take place as early as possible. InfantSee is a brand new program with more than 7000 participating optometrists who have pledged to see any child less than a year of age for a visual evaluation at no charge. Any infant whose parents want a visual evaluation for their child can get one independent of whether they can afford it or not. The objective is early identification of visual anomalies, e.g., strabismus, anisometropia, amblyopia, pathology, etc. so early intervention in the presence of the anomaly, can be most effective in restoring normal visual function. State legislatures are enacting laws mandating vision exams for all children before they can enter school. As more states adopt laws which mandate eye exams as a requirement to enter school, more and more children will be showing up in private eye care practices.

This book will provide the theoretical background of vision development, the basic clinical methods with which to test these very young children, guidelines toward management of visual anomalies in these patients, some information regarding *normal* childhood development, and a discussion of children with special needs.

While primarily written for eye care providers, this book should appeal to occupational, physical and speech therapists. There is a very ample supply of techniques to improve ocular tracking, ocular fixation and eye/hand coordination. And of course it is the ideal book for any visual development course.

Acknowledgments

would like to thank everyone who helped make this book a reality. First I would like to thank the contributing authors, all of whom made significant commitments of time and energy, for their efforts. I must acknowledge the efforts of SUNY, State College of Optometry's media center and library staffs, who consistently went out of their way to get me what I needed yesterday. There were many others who facilitated the completion of the book in small, but meaningful ways, and I thank them all.

Robert H. Duckman, O. D.

Contributors

Israel Abramov, Ph.D.
Professor
Applied Vision Institute, Psychology Department
Brooklyn College of the City University of New York
Brooklyn, New York

Amelia G. Bartolone, O.D., F.A.A.O.
Associate Clinical Professor
State University of New York
College of Optometry
New York, New York

Shoshana Bell-Craig, O.D.
Assistant Clinical Professor
State University of New York
College of Optometry
New York, New York

T. Rowan Candy, M.C.Optom., Ph.D.
Assistant Professor
Indiana University School of Optometry and
*   Cognitive Science Program*
Bloomington, Indiana

Ida Chung-Lock, O.D.
Chief of Pediatrics Service
Department of Clinical Sciences
State University of New York
College of Optometry
New York, New York

Karl Citek, O.D., Ph.D., F.A.A.O.
Associate Professor
Pacific University College of Optometry
Forest Grove, Oregon

Jay M. Cohen, O.D., F.A.A.O.
Professor of Optometry
Clinical Sciences Department
State University of New York
College of Optometry
New York, New York

Jojo W. Du, B.App.Sc., M.S.
State University of New York
College of Optometry
New York, New York

David E. FitzGerald, O.D.
Clinical Professor
State University of New York
College of Optometry
New York, New York

James Gordon, Ph.D.
Professor
Psychology Department
Hunter College of the City University of New York
New York, New York

Carl Gruning, O.D.
Clinical Professor
Department of Pediatric and Infants Clinic
Fairfield, Connecticut

Ralph E. Gundel, O.D., F.A.A.O.
Associate Clinical Professor
State University of New York
College of Optometry
New York, New York

M. H. Esther Han, O.D., F.C.O.V.D.
Assistant Clinical Professor
Department of Clinical Sciences
State University of New York
College of Optometry
New York, New York

Pamela Hooker, O.D.
Associate Clinical Professor
State University of New York
College of Optometry
New York, New York

Valerie M. Kattouf, O.D., F.A.A.O., F.C.O.V.D.
Associate Professor
Department of Pediatrics
Clinical Associate of Optometry and Visual Science
Illinois College of Optometry
University of Chicago
Optomology Department
Chicago, Illinois

Barry Kran, O.D., F.A.A.O.
Associate Professor of Optometry
Specialty and Advanced Care
New England College of Optometry
Boston, Massachusetts
Optometric Director, NE Eye Low Vision Clinic
*   at Perkins School for the Blind*
Chief, Individuals with Disabilities Service
Perkins School for the Blind
Watertown, Massachusetts

David P. Libassi, O.D., F.A.A.O.
Assistant Clinical Professor
State University of New York
College of Optometry
New York, New York

Richard London, M.A., O.D., F.A.A.O.
Professor
Pacific University College of Optometry
Forest Grove, Oregon

Stacy Lyons, O.D., F.A.A.O.
Associate Professor of Optometry
Specialty and Advanced Care
The New England College of Optometry
Chief
Pediatric Optometry Services
The New England Eye Institute
Boston, Massachusetts

David A. Maze, O.D.
Luckhardt and Maze, Ltd.
Westmont, Illinois
Consulting Optometrist
Easter Seals of DuPage
Addison, Illinois

Jordan R. Pola, Ph.D.
Distinguished Teaching Professor
Department of Vision Sciences
State University of New York
College of Optometry
New York, New York

Mark Rosenfield, M.C.Optom., Ph.D., F.A.A.O.
State University of New York
College of Optometry
New York, New York

Daniella Rutner, O.D., M.S.
Assistant Clinical Professor
State University of New York
College of Optometry
New York, New York

Melissa Suckow, O.D.
New England College of Optometry
Boston, Massachusetts

Jessica Yang, O.D.
Assistant Clinical Professor
State University of New York
College of Optometry
New York, New York

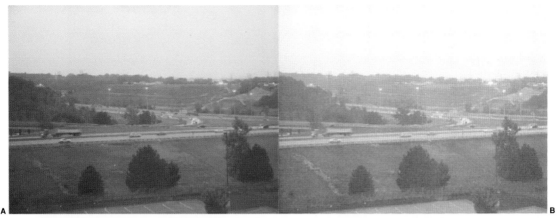

Color Figure 3.1a, b

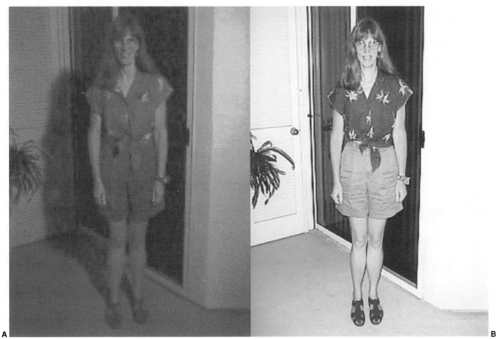

Color Figure 3.8a, b

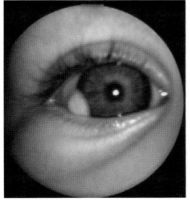

Color Figure 12.1

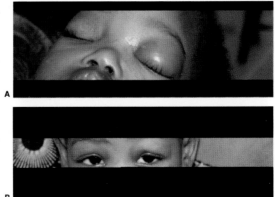

Color Figure 12.2a, b

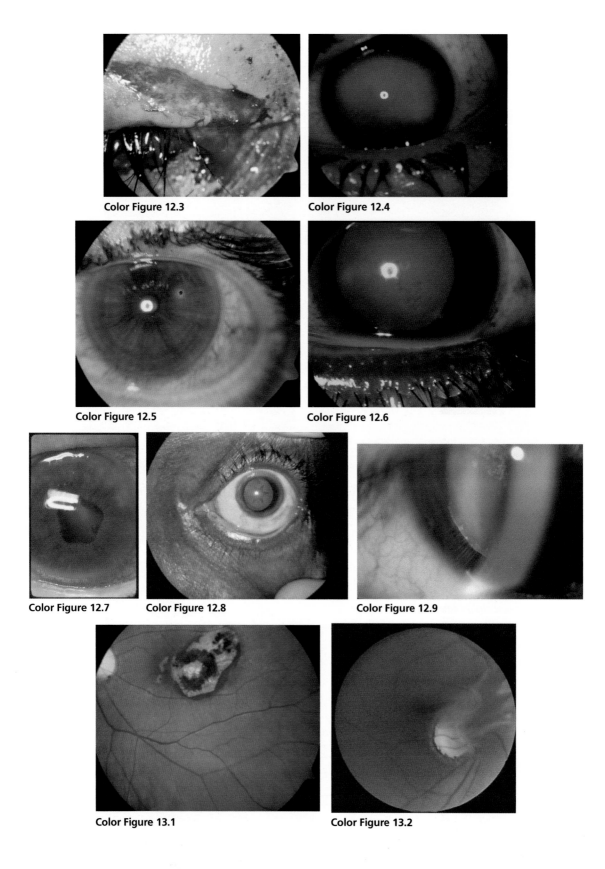

Color Figure 12.3

Color Figure 12.4

Color Figure 12.5

Color Figure 12.6

Color Figure 12.7

Color Figure 12.8

Color Figure 12.9

Color Figure 13.1

Color Figure 13.2

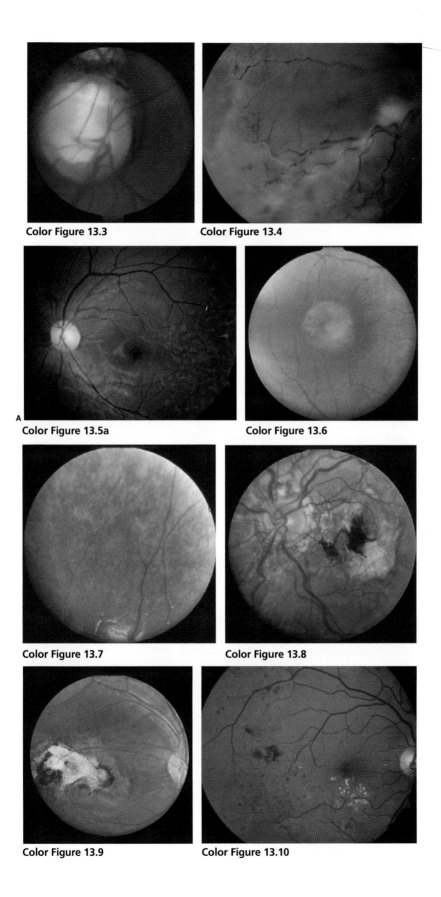

Color Figure 13.3

Color Figure 13.4

Color Figure 13.5a

Color Figure 13.6

Color Figure 13.7

Color Figure 13.8

Color Figure 13.9

Color Figure 13.10

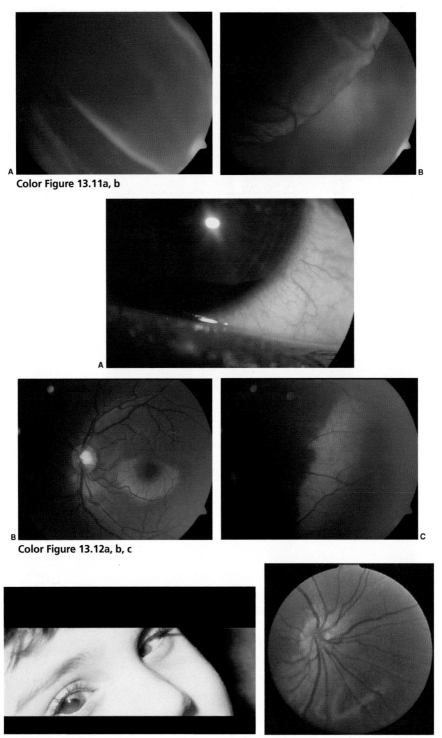

Color Figure 13.11a, b

A

B

Color Figure 13.12a, b, c

Color Figure 13.13

Color Figure 13.14

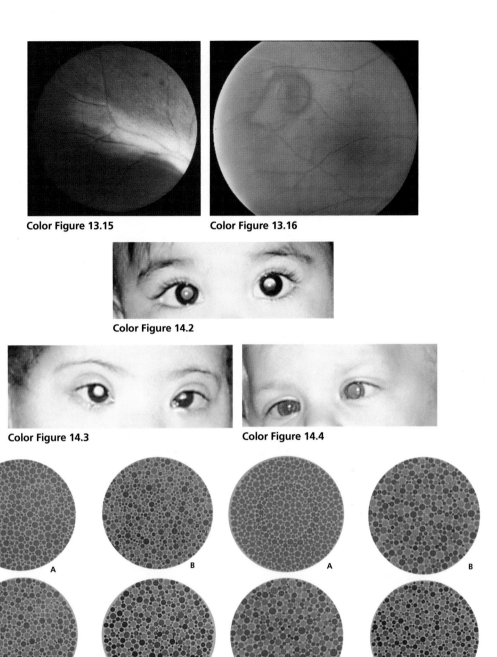

Color Figure 13.15

Color Figure 13.16

Color Figure 14.2

Color Figure 14.3

Color Figure 14.4

Color Figure 19.1

Color Figure 19.2

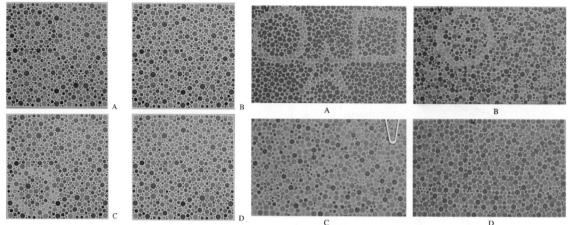

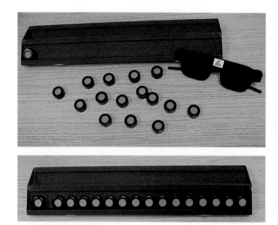

Color Figure 19.3

Color Figure 19.4

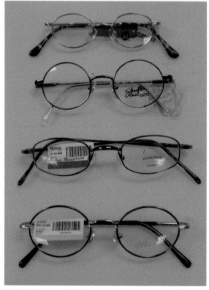

Color Figure 19.5

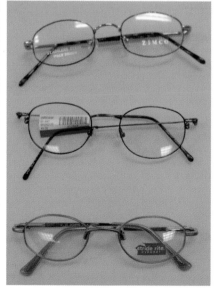

Color Figure 20.1

Color Figure 20.2

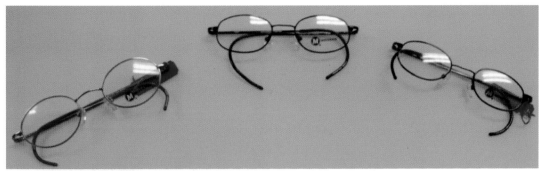

Color Figure 20.3

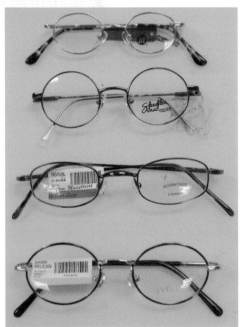

Color Figure 20.4

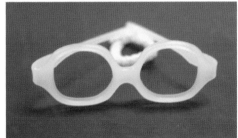

Color Figure 20.5

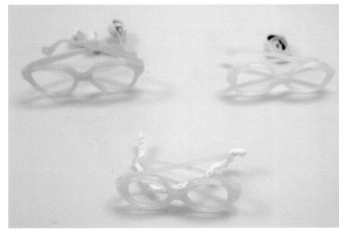

Color Figure 20.6

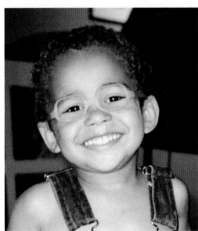

Color Figure 20.7

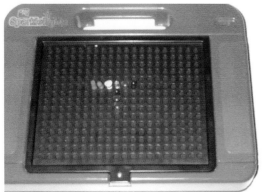

Color Figure 23.2

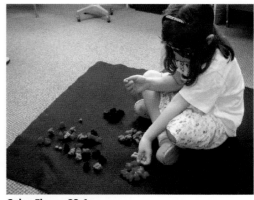

Color Figure 23.4

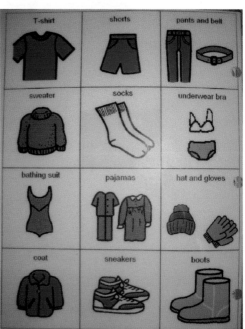

Color Figure 25.3

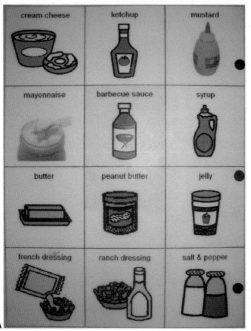

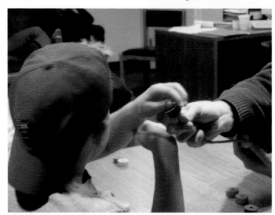

Color Figure 25.5a, b

Introduction

Robert H. Duckman, O.D.

A mere forty years ago, eye care professionals, when asked, would advise parents to have their children's eyes examined at about five years of age. It was believed at the time that children could not see well at birth and could not achieve 20/20 vision until about five years of age. Children were, for all intents and purposes, "personae non grata" in the eye doctor's office. The reason was relatively simple—there were very few practical tests which could assess what infants could or couldn't see and practitioners felt "incompetent" and "uncomfortable" around and intimidated by, these very small people. (I always find it ironic that my students, all of whom have mastered the examination of teenagers and adults, begin acting like neophytes again when faced with the younger patient.) So visual examinations were typically deferred until the time that children entered elementary school. By five years of age, the clinician could expect to be able to obtain some sort of acuity measurement, as well as assess ocular alignment, refraction and ocular health.

Around the end of the 1960's and the beginning of the 1970's, utilizing some of the observations made by Robert Fantz regarding infant visual preferences, experimental psychologists began probing the visual function of infants. As they collected data and published it, more and more interest was piqued in others to further probe visual function in this young population. Slowly these scientists began to realize that

infants were significantly more visually capable than anyone had ever imagined.

Psychometric measurements are necessary for scientific study, but much too time consuming and cumbersome to ever lend themselves to clinical utility. And so for a while, the techniques, which were developed within the laboratory to measure infant visual capabilities, remained in the laboratory. By the early 1980's, there was sufficient data collected to establish norms and to begin to "streamline" the laboratory procedures. With established norms for newborns and young infants, procedures could be abbreviated and threshold findings could still be achieved. As an example, a technique known as *forced-choice preferential looking (FPL)*, based on Fantz's observation that infants, when given a choice, will prefer to look at a patterned field rather than a homogenous field of equal luminance value. This is the premise upon which the FPL procedure is based. Thus the procedure was born. Early in its evolution, it was not known what infants of different ages were capable of seeing. So all ages had to be tested in a psychometric paradigm. This literally took years, but after enough data were collected, they were able to set up tables of norms for different aged infants and toddlers using this technique. These norms were based on thousands of babies and youngsters and tens of thousands of trials. When these data were compiled, age norms for this procedure were established.

Once the age norms were defined, investigators started trying to streamline the technique to make it faster and, therefore more clinically applicable. The technique was slowly transformed from a totally impractical laboratory paradigm to what it is today—the standard of a behavioral acuity measurement within a clinical setting where infants are evaluated.

Almost all aspects of infant visual function have been probed in a similar manner: Infant stereopsis, infant fusion, infant contrast sensitivity function, infant color vision, etc. The thing that has always fascinated me about research into the visual function of pre-verbal children is the incredible ingenuity of the experimental paradigms. The experimental psychologists have tweaked out the information they have needed, by finding some behavior which could be generalized, across the board, to all infants. They then "created" experimental designs which would allow them to get the information they wanted. They used these designs to get the needed visual information, and ultimately, the techniques were transformed into reliable clinical tools. As a result we now have a battery of clinical tools which can be used to evaluate infant visual function. Why is this so important? As infant vision research has evolved over the years, we have learned a lot that was previously unknown. One of the major things we have learned is that infants are hugely more competent and sophisticated visually than was previously believed. In fact, in many areas of visual functioning, infants can perform almost as well as the adult by six months of age or earlier. For example, it was believed that a newborn could not accommodate for near at birth and that accommodation was "locked" at five diopters. The newborn, then, could not see beyond eight inches. However, recent experimentation has clearly shown that newborns not only can, but do, accommodate. The accommodative responses of the newborn may not be as accurate as the adult, but they are definitely present. And by two to three months of age, these responses are approaching adult accuracy.

As we started to learn more about the precociousness of the infant's visual system, and as laboratory experimentation gave way to clinical techniques to assess visual function, clinicians started to evaluate children at younger and younger ages. As a result of the increased knowledge of the infant's visual capabilities and development of clinical tools to evaluate them, it has become more important to evaluate children's vision at earlier ages. As a result, it is now widely recommended that infants should have their first eye exam, not at *five years* of age, as usually recommended pre-1970, but at *six months* of age. The American Academy of Pediatrics (1), the American Association for Pediatric Ophthalmology and Strabismus (2), the American Academy of Ophthalmology (3), and the American Optometric Association (4) have all made position statements advising that a child's first visual examination should occur by six months of age. We know that the human infant has near adult visual function in many areas by six months of age.

We also know that if we can diagnose visual problems earlier, we can start *treating* them earlier. If we can intervene sufficiently early, we have a good chance of restoring normal visual function *before* irreversible loss, due to deprivation, occurs. We can intervene with strabismic amblyopia, much more easily at six months than we can, for example, at five years or fifteen years of age. If we can identify anisometropia at an early age, we can provide normal stimulation for the two eyes and prevent anisometropic refractive amblyopia. Often early identification of an ocular pathology can improve the outcome for the child from both a physical and functional perspective. As a result of the growth of the field of visual development, we now have tools to probe and intervene in order to improve/restore visual function and improve the child's quality of life throughout life.

Visual impairment can have a very significant impact on the child's development. Beyond the visual aspects, it can lead to anomalies of growth and development, posture, bonding, social interaction, head lifting, visual awareness and exploration, spatial concepts, balance and auditory orientation. As an example, if an infant is born with a visual impairment, its visual capabilities may be compromised so severely that eye contact with its parents is not possible. This significantly interferes with the process of parent/child bonding which will be delayed. As another example, the stimulus for an infant to lift its trunk and head while lying prone in the crib is the stimulation from objects outside the crib. It is also the stimulus to repeat this motor activity. If the visual impairment does not allow the infant sufficient resolution capabilities to "see" the objects in space, the child will lose interest and *NOT* lift head and torso. This will have significant impact on upper body muscle development. Vision drives development of other systems beyond the visual system, and therefore vision anomalies can impact many other areas of development.

The periods of infancy and toddlerhood seem to be the most "plastic" and malleable. Deprivation during these periods of time will have a much bigger impact than an equal deprivation in a seven-year old, a teenage child, or an adult. It is also a period of time during which loss in function as a result of deprivation can be most easily restored. The early diagnosis of visual problems can have a large impact on visual function, motor function, cognitive development and learning. The optometrist has the capability to step in and intervene when a visual anomaly is identified. This can have an enormous impact on the child and development.

And so this book is being written. I passionately believe that early diagnosis of visual problems, followed by early intervention is essential to achieve normal vision in infants and young children with visual anomalies. However, there are insufficient manpower resources today to handle the evaluation of *all* infants, in spite of the growing political and social demands to do so. If all parents of young babies sought eye examinations for their children, there would be a significant shortage of clinicians capable of attending to these children. The objective, then, must be to train more clinicians to be knowledgeable and comfortable in caring for the visual needs of young children. As a professor of Optometry at the State University of New York, State College of Optometry, I have taught a course in Visual Development for more than a dozen years. I have never found a text which satisfied all aspects of the material I teach in the course. As a result, I assign a little from one source and a little from another, until I have all the material covered. It has always proven to be very frustrating not to have a text I could assign for the course. Therefore I thought I should write a book which could serve as a text for a

visual development course. However, I am also a clinician at the college's clinical facility, the University Optometric Center, where I see infants and pediatric patients. I teach the students who are assigned to me what, why and how I do what I do with these young patients. I teach them about the importance of early intervention. But intervention with the infant is different than the intervention with the adult patient. There must be consideration of developmental factors as to when it is appropriate to apply lenses and how much medicine to prescribe. There must be modification based on the children and their parents. So in the clinical setting they learn the practical issues of infant visual examination. They learn how to assess the infant, what the clinical techniques are, and then they learn about intervention.

My objective in writing this book is threefold—and thus the book is broken into three main sections: first a theoretical discussion of visual development; second a portion to describe the clinical tools which are available to evaluate children's visual function; and third, a section on clinical techniques which may be used in the remediation of many of these problems. I've added a fourth section to look at normal and abnormal general development. What I hope everyone walks away with is a sufficient level of comfort to open their practices to the examination and visual care of the pediatric patient.

One thing that I have always been amazed by throughout my career and my work with children, but also in the observations I have made on my own daughter from birth on, is how much adults *underestimate* a child's capabilities, whether it be visual or cognitive or motoric. It is extraordinary and it seems to be nearly universal. Up until the early 1970's it had been fairly well accepted that children could not function well through vision, and that cognitively they could not understand a lot of the physical world around them. It is only in the past four decades that we have begun to understand how precocious the infant visual system really is and how much we had underestimated their capabilities. My daughter was able to demonstrate excellent saccadic fixations on some visual stimuli on her carriage when she was only three days old. She maintained attention and accurately saccaded at this very young age. This is not what I had learned in Optometry school. I learned that they did not have adult visual capability until around five years of age. And through the years it has been proven to be untrue in respect to so many things.

Throughout this book keep in mind *FUNC-TION*. Without an understanding of what function is, we can not know whether or not a difference between adult function and neonatal function is significant. With that in mind, I will point out that the *primary* function of vision is to gather photic spatial information from the environment we are in so that we may have the sensory information needed to direct *movement* through that environment. With vision, there are many other things which we are able to do and to direct. But, above all, vision provides the information needed to direct movement through space.

Vision is a process which allows us to understand the spatial layout of our environment. This process is developmental in nature. It has always intrigued me to think about what the neonate "sees" on that first day of life. If it were possible, I would gladly visit the body of a one-day old infant to experience what things look like. While what the baby sees may not yet have any cognitive meaning, does it "look" the same? We know that acuity is lower in the infant, but it is definitely present. Newborns can definitely maintain fixation and change fixation. At the very beginning, color vision, if present, is far from trichromatism. Form perception, again without the cognitive component, must be present. Through vision science we are learning some things about visual function and its development. We are getting nearer to the "truth" about the earliest visual experiences.

After birth, another question arises. It is a question that used to pit nature against nurture. In its oldest format, people would ask is it nature? or nurture? Early on people attempted to prove one or the other, genetics or environment, was "in control" of development. However, today we look more at the contribution from each. There are some things that are totally attributable to one or the other, but there are many others which involve significant contribution from both. Probably one of the best examples of nature and nurture co-contributing to development is seen in the immature fovea. At

birth the fovea is much larger and much more loosely packed with cones (immature cones) than the adult fovea. There are cells from the inner nuclear layer (INL) overlying the fovea at birth. In the first few months these INL cells migrate radially outward while the foveal cones migrate radially inward. It has been noted that no new foveal cones arise after birth and that during this migration connections between cells are not broken, and that reaching abilities remain accurate. Therefore "nature" is responsible for the migration of the cells, but "nurture" is responsible for "recalibrating" spatial value for each cone so that localization of objects remains accurate throughout this migratory process.

There is still so much we do not know about vision, but our knowledge is continually growing and expanding. It is my hope that the knowledge will grow and expand and that the clinician will embrace the visual care of infants and young children more universally.

Emphasizing the importance of early visual examination, are two initiatives which are underway. One is the trend for state legislative mandate, such as in Kentucky and Tennessee, for all children to have complete eye examinations before entering school. There are other states which are trying to enact similar legislation. The second initiative which premiered in June, 2005 is called "InfantSEE." This is a program involving approximately 6500 optometrists in the United States who, in order to encourage parents to get their baby's eyes examined early, are providing the initial eye and vision assessment within the first year of life, as a no cost public health service. InfantSEE will emphasize early diagnosis and intervention of amblyogenic and pathologic vision problems, such as for a) strabismus, b) anisometropia and c) ocular health anomalies. With the introduction of InfantSEE and with state legislated mandates for early eye examinations, the demand for eye care professionals who will see pediatric patients will increase as will the public's awareness that these exams are available and important. Early identification and early intervention of visual problems will diminish the prevalence of such clinical entities as refractive and strabismic amblyopia, anisometropic amblyopia and accommodative esotropia. Vision is a very important learning modality and that learning can be significantly impacted by uncorrected visual anomalies. As pointed out already, the most important thing is to identify these anomalies early and intervene as early as possible. Too often visual anomalies are not identified until significant, often irreversible damage, is done.

Only 39% of three-year olds are screened for vision problems in private pediatric practices (5). In addition, among children who do get a vision test, but fail it, half of their parents don't know this fact. Fewer than 40% of children in the crucial younger-than-four age group are evaluated for visual problems by pediatricians (5, 6). Ocular disorders are the leading cause of vision problems and combine to cause amblyopia in approximately 5% of the population (6–9). Vision disorders are the fourth most common disability in the United States and are the most prevalent handicapping condition in childhood (10). Facts like these are easy to list. What is more difficult is changing the statistics so that more children are being screened and/or evaluated at an early age. That way the problems can be picked up and intervened with at an age when it is still possible to restore normal visual function with intervention.

The eye care professional, whether it be optometrist or ophthalmologist, has the power to change and shape lives. By intervening with existing visual problems at an early enough age, the practitioner has the means of restoring normal function to an anomalous visual system and thus effect the entire organism. We learn throughout life that a very significant part of our learning occurs through vision (11). If the input is "damaged" so too will be the output. Children who are "caught" at an early enough age and who are intervened with can recover fully. Then these children can lead normal lives and not have compromised visual systems for their entire lives. All that from simple intervention at an early age. My hope, again, is that this book motivates people who are not comfortable working with children to get comfortable and start and for people who are comfortable working with children to expand their expertise. It is my hope that this book will fulfill those two goals.

REFERENCES

1. American Academy of Pediatrics, Committee on Practice and Ambulatory Medicine, Section on Ophthalmology. Eye examination and vision screening in infants, children and young adults. Pediatrics, 1996;98: 153–157.
2. American Association for Pediatric Ophthalmology and Strabismus: Eye care for the children of America. J Pediatric Ophthalmol Strabismus, 1991;28:64–67.
3. American Academy of Ophthalmology: Pediatric Eye Evaluation, Preferred Practice Pattern. San Francisco, American Academy of Ophthalmology, 1997.
4. Scheiman M, Amos C, Ciner E, et al. Pediatric Eye and Vision Examination: Optometric Clinical Practice Guideline. 1994, St. Louis, American Optometric Association, pp 1–45.
5. Wasserman R, Croft C, Brotherton S. Preschool vision screening in pediatric practice: a study from the pediatric research and office settings (PROS) Network. Pediatrics, 1992;89:834–838.
6. Granet D, Hoover A, Smith S, Brown D, Bartsch D, Brody B. A new objective digital computerized screening system. J Ped Ophthalmol and Strabismus, 1999; 36:251–256.
7. Simmons K. Preschool vision screening: rationale, methodology and outcome. Surv Ophthalmol, 1996; 41:3–30
8. Stayte M, Reeves B, Wortham C. Ocular and vision defects in preschool children. Br J Ophthalmol, 1993;77: 228–232.
9. Ehrlich M, Reinecke R, Simons K. Preschool vision screening for amblyopia and strabismus. Programs, methods, guidelines. Surv Ophthalmol, 1983;28: 145–163.
10. Ciner E, Dobson V, Schmidt P. A survey of vision screening policy of preschool children in the United States. Surv Ophthalmol, 1999;43:445–457.
11. Murphy J. Our myopic view of children's vision and the Rx for it. Rev of Optom, 1999;Sept:94–99.

PART 1

The Development of Vision

Development of the Visual System

1

T. Rowan Candy

Vision forms one of the sensory inputs that allow us to interact with our environment. For visual information to be integrated with information from our other senses, a representation of the visual environment needs to be created in a language that the brain can interpret. This is a language of electrical potentials. The chief role of the first stages of the visual system, therefore, is to convert an image of the world into interpretable electrical potentials.

The adult eye and visual system are able to achieve this goal. An image of the external world is formed on the retina and information contained in this image is converted into membrane voltages in approximately 120 million photoreceptors. The information from these photoreceptors is then transmitted in an orderly fashion into the visual cortex and beyond. To ensure that patients can enjoy this facility, the challenge for vision scientists and clinicians is to understand how a fully healthy system forms, how an abnormal system can arise, and how to treat or prevent abnormality.

The goal of this chapter is to provide our understanding of the development of the structures of the visual system. The discussion is split into two sections that represent the two major challenges: to build a transparent optical system capable of forming a continually focused image of the external world and to build a neural system that can transmit information reliably yet recalibrate constantly as a child grows. Recent research has shown that these systems are largely constructed according to a map and timetable defined by the transient expression of genes (1,2), with modulation and refinement guided by the local environment and ultimately neural activity (3,4).

BUILDING A TRANSPARENT OPTICAL SYSTEM

The optical components of the adult eye consist of the cornea, pupil, and lens to a first approximation. The aqueous and vitreous humors inflate the eye to maintain these components at the appropriate distances from the retinal image plane and support the needs of the structures that must remain transparent without clouding from blood vessels. The following section describes how this ultimately transparent and aligned optical system forms in humans. Most of this information has been gathered through light and electron microscopy studies of human tissue, which have been extensively reviewed in books (5–7). These reviews form the basis of the following section, together with information from Ozanic and Jakobiec (8).

The Embryonic Period (First 2 Months of Gestation)

The first 8 weeks of gestation forms the embryonic period during which fundamental ocular structures are forming. Abnormal events during this period (e.g., infection or trauma) will result in relatively major structural malformations of the eye and visual system.

The first evidence of the eyes appears in the human embryo at approximately 22 days of gestation, just 3 weeks after conception (9). The neural ectoderm, which goes on to form the nervous system, is rolling up to form a tube along the length of the embryo. At this point, the embryo is still less than 1 cm long. One end of this developing neural tube is destined to become the brain and already consists of three sections, the prosencephalon (forebrain), mesencephalon (midbrain), and rhombencephalon (hindbrain). The first evidence of the eyes appears in the internal wall of the rolling tube in the mesencephalon (between the soon-to-form telencephalon and diencephalon) (Fig. 1.1A). The evidence consists of a small section of the wall on each side of the head starting to bulge out toward the surface of the embryo. These evaginations (*optic primordia,* or *sulci*) continue to extend while the rest of the neural tube seals—the tube is complete at approximately 24 days. The evaginations extend to form a vesicle and stalk whose hollow center is continuous with the brain (Fig. 1.1B, Fig 1.2A). This optic vesicle forms parts of the eye, and the optic stalk forms the path for the later neural connections from the eye to the brain (Fig. 1.1C, Fig 1.2B).

The external layer of the embryo consists of surface ectoderm. As the optic stalk and vesicle extend, the proximity of the optic vesicle to the surface ectoderm causes the nearest section of surface ectoderm to thicken and start on a path to becoming the lens of the eye. This area of thickening forms on day 27 (8) and is called the *lens placode* (Fig. 1.1B). The fact that the surface ectoderm will only form the placode if the vesicle is present demonstrates the importance of local interactions between cells in normal development (10). The optic vesicle is said to *induce* the lens placode. The following day, the presence of the surface ectoderm starts to induce the closest section of the optic vesicle to form a thickened retinal disk (Fig. 1.1B). Abnormalities at this early point in gestation lead to relatively severe malformations such as anophthalmia or microophthalmia (see Chapters 12 and 13 on anterior and posterior chamber abnormalities).

Formation of the Optic Cup and Basic Optical Structures

The next step, at the end of the fourth week, is for the optic vesicle and lens placode to each fold back on themselves and invaginate toward the brain. The folding of the optic vesicle, which

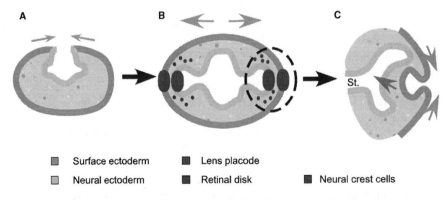

FIGURE 1.1. Early embryonic development of the human eye, showing the contributions of the surface and neural ectoderm. **A:** At 22 days, as the neural tube closes and the optic sulci form. **B:** At 4 weeks, after the optic vesicles have extended and the lens placodes and retinal disks are forming. **C:** At 5 weeks, as the optic vesicle invaginates at the end of the optic stalk (*St.*) and the lens vesicle forms.

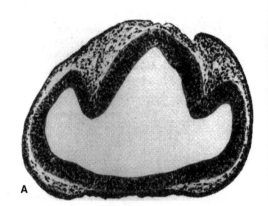

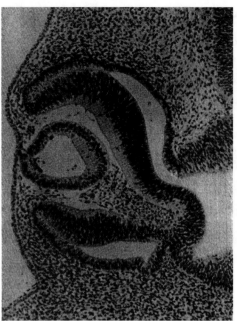

FIGURE 1.2. Tissue corresponding to the schematic diagrams in Figure 1.1A. **A:** A section through the forebrain of a 4-week-old human embryo showing the closed neural tube, optic vesicles, and future optic stalks (corresponding to Figure 1.1B before the formation of the lens placode and retinal disk). (From Hamilton WJ, Boyd JD, and Mossman HW. *Human Embryology: prenatal development of form and function*, 4th ed. Philadelphia: JB Lippincott; 1972.) **B:** A 5-week-old human embryo with optic cup and lens vesicle (corresponding to Figure 1.1C). (From Smelser GK. Embryology and morphology of the lens. *Invest Ophthalmol* 1965;44:398–410, with permission.)

starts a couple of days before that of the surface ectoderm, creates the formation of a two-layered cup—the optic cup—and the folding of the surface ectoderm creates the lens vesicle. This is a hollow ball of cells that will completely pinch off from the surface ectoderm at 33 days and lie in the mouth of the optic cup (Fig. 1.1C, Fig. 1.2B). This mouth will become the future pupil.

The other main optical component of the eye, the cornea, is formed from the surface ectoderm that sits over the lens vesicle and mouth of the optic cup after they have invaginated. Once the lens vesicle has disconnected, this tissue invaginates again to form the surface of the future eyelids and parts of the cornea (the continuous conjunctival sac) (Figs. 1.3 and 1.4B). The future margins of the eyelids start growing toward each other, finally meeting and fusing along the border. The corneal section of surface ectoderm forms the future corneal epithelium, which initially only consists of two layers of cells resting on a basement membrane.

The size of the future cornea has been shown in an avian model to depend on the size of the optic cup. A small cup implies a small but normal cornea (11)—another indication of local interactions.

Thus, in the fifth week of gestation, the future lens is already sitting behind the primitive cornea, in the mouth of the optic cup, and is

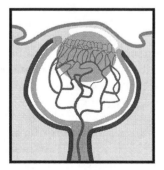

FIGURE 1.3. Schematic of the hyaloid vascular system at the end of the embryonic period.

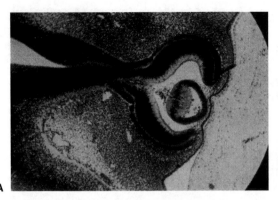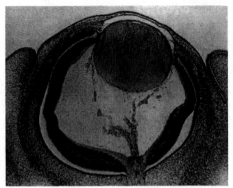

A   B

FIGURE 1.4. Light microscopy of human eyes at 5 (panel A) and 7 (panel B) weeks of gestation. (*Left-hand photo*: From Barber AN. *Embryology of the Human Eye*, Fig. 78. St. Louis: CV Mosby; 1955, with permission. *Right-hand photo*: From Smelser GK. Embryology and morphology of the lens. *Invest Ophthalmol* 1965;44:398–410, with permission.)

positioned to form an image on the developing retina. The basal lamina of the surface ecto-derm lies on the outside of the lens vesicle and later thickens to form the capsule around the mature lens.

During the fifth to seventh weeks, the hol-low vesicle of lens cells fills as it starts to take its mature form (induced by the proximity of the optic cup). The cells in the posterior wall, clos-est to the retina, start to elongate forward to fill in the hollow volume (Figs. 1.4 and 1.5). They continue forward until they meet the anterior cells at 45 days and the lens becomes solid. This is the embryonic lens nucleus. The nucleus is approximately spherical and the fibers within it are named the *primary lens fibers*. The optic cup then induces the cells from the anterior sur-face of the lens to migrate around to the vertical equator. The organelles in these cells begin to disintegrate and the cells elongate to form more fibers. The fiber tips extend over the primary lens fibers beneath the lens capsule, forward to the anterior pole and backward to the posterior pole of the lens. The tips of the fibers extend-ing from cells at the different locations around the equator all meet to form the clinically visible anterior and posterior sutures.

The first layer of secondary fibers is already in place in the seventh week of gestation and the further fibers are laid down sequentially in layers. Thus, depending on the timing of a problem during gestation (an infection such as rubella for instance), infants can be born with

congenital cataracts in isolated sections or lay-ers of the lens (see Chapter 12). Until 8 weeks of gestation, the diameter of the lens is greater in the anterior-posterior direction than across the equator parallel to the iris. The lens is then almost spherical at birth with a reversal occur-ring during childhood so that in adulthood it is elliptically elongated parallel to the iris plane.

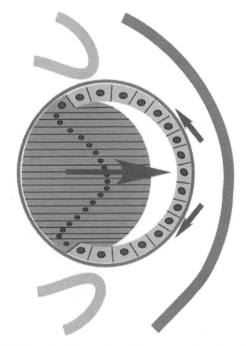

FIGURE 1.5. Schematic of the lens vesicle, showing the future capsule and formation of the primary lens fibers.

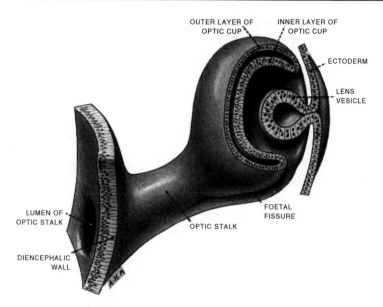

FIGURE 1.6. Schematic of the 5-week-old human embryo showing the lens vesicle pinching off from the surface ectoderm and the two-layered optic cup. The fetal fissure is seen along the base of the optic stalk and cup. (From Hamilton WJ, Boyd JD, and Mossman HW. *Human Embryology: prenatal development of form and function*, 4th ed. Philadelphia: JB Lippincott, 1972, with permission.)

The optical characteristics of the lens, therefore, must mature significantly over the first months or years after birth (see the discussion of emmetropisation in Chapter 4).

The optic cup is sitting behind the lens. One clinically important aspect of its development is its asymmetric invagination, which starts from the section that will form the inferior and nasal part of the eye. The most extreme invagination, including a part of the optic stalk, occurs there. The asymmetry results in the formation of a single, long embryonic fissure along the inferior nasal section of the cup and stalk (Fig. 1.6). The walls of the fissure should seal later in development, and a failure to do so results in a relatively rare condition seen in the clinic, coloboma.

The two walls of the cup are destined to become the retinal pigment epithelium and neural retina in the posterior part of the eye, and components of the iris and ciliary body in the anterior part of the eye. Another clinically important point that can be understood from the embryology of the posterior eye at this early point in gestation is that a retinal detachment, even in adults, occurs at the interface between the retinal pigment epithelium and the neural retina.

The tissue separates at the point where the apical sides of the layers had folded to meet each other in development.

Formation of Support Tissues

The other tissues of the eye that support the function of the neural retina, lens, and cornea are typically derived from a third type of embryologic tissue, mesoderm (as compared with the neural and surface ectoderms). This tissue in the head and neck region is somewhat different from that in the rest of the body, because no mesodermal somites are found in the head region. This tissue in and around the eye consists of some conventional mesoderm, but is mainly derived from neural crest cells that have migrated to the eye and, by day 26, surrounded the optic vesicle between it and the surface ectoderm (Fig. 1.1B). This combination of tissues is denoted as *ocular mesenchyme*. The neural crest cells also form components of the teeth, middle ear bones, meninges, and endocrine glands, and so abnormalities in the development of these cells can result in congenital malformation of a number of these tissues (12).

The primary contribution of mesenchyme to the anterior eye consists of three waves of neural crest cell migration into the anterior chamber during the seventh week of gestation. Disruption of these waves is thought to lead to a number of clinical disorders of the anterior chamber (13). The first wave enters between the surface ectoderm and lens to form the initially multilayered corneal and trabecular endothelium. Another wave migrates from the periphery between the developing corneal epithelium and endothelium, to form the keratocytes that will become the corneal stroma, and the third wave forms the iris stroma.

The mesenchyme gains access to the posterior section of the eye through the embryonic fissure along the side of the optic cup and stalk (Fig. 1.6). This mesenchyme has the role of filling the optic cup with vitreous and providing this early posterior chamber with a blood supply. The future transparency of the cornea, aqueous, lens, and vitreous is critically dependent on the nature and spacing of their contents. The vasculature is able to supply these structures without disrupting their future transparency or permanently blocking the optical path to the retina. There are two principal stages to the formation of the blood supply. The first, the hyaloid system, is only present during gestation and typically degenerates before birth. It does, in fact, temporarily block the optical path to the retina and, therefore, would not be an efficient system to maintain after birth.

The hyaloid system is supplied by the terminal portion of the ophthalmic artery (a branch of the internal carotid), which passes through the embryonic fissure into the optic stalk. It runs along the lumen of the invaginated stalk and into the optic cup through the future optic nerve head. This artery is called the *hyaloid artery*. It grows forward through the vitreous, sending branches to meet the posterior surface of the lens. These branches then form a network of capillaries over the posterior surface of the lens, known as the *posterior tunica vasculosa lentis*. They also pass further forward to connect with the annular vessel forming around the rim of the cup. The annular vessel principally forms from vessels approaching along the cup's outer surface (the ciliary arteries start to form around

the outside of the optic cup during the seventh and eighth weeks). The annular vessel, in turn, sends loops forward to supply the anterior surface of the lens. These loops form the anterior tunica vasculosa lentis. This hyaloid system is fully formed by the end of the second month of gestation. The blood in this network reaches the venous system via vessels starting to form in the choroid (Figs. 1.3 and 1.4).

The development of the vitreous also consists of two sequential stages. The primary vitreous develops during the fifth week of gestation. It is derived from mesenchyme migrating in through the embryonic fissure and ectodermal fibers connecting the sensory retina to the posterior side of the lens. As with the hyaloid vasculature, the primary vitreous also degenerates to be replaced by a more mature secondary system. In the case of the vitreous, this secondary system starts to form almost as soon as the primary version appears—the end of the sixth week. The secondary vitreous forms at the sensory retina as a compact fibrillar network that does not blend with the primary vitreous at all, but gradually detaches it from the retina pushing it toward the hyaloid artery running from the optic disc to the lens.

The embryonic fissure starts to close and seal around the posterior chamber containing the new hyaloid vessels and vitreous in the sixth week. The closure starts about halfway along the side of the optic cup and progresses anteriorly and posteriorly from there. The last notch at each end closes during the seventh week. As mentioned, the fissure failing to close completely results in a coloboma (see Chapter 13).

The outer layer of the optic cup itself starts to differentiate into the retinal pigment epithelium (RPE), which will ultimately provide support to the photoreceptors and neural retina. By the fifth week, the RPE consists of two to three layers of cells that by the end of the week stop mitotic division and show all stages of pigment granule formation (in a similar pattern to that of the epidermal melanocytes) (Fig. 1.4A). The layer becomes the mature one cell thick during the sixth week, with apical projections toward the future photoreceptor outer segments (Fig. 1.4B). The basal lamina, meanwhile, starts to develop into Bruch's membrane. The number and morphology of the RPE cells does not change after approximately 8 weeks, although generation of melanosomes to form pigment continues until week 27 (14). The RPE, therefore, grows in area through expansion of the cells rather than by cell division in the later stages of gestation and postnatal period.

The mesenchyme also starts to form structures around the outside of the optic cup during the second month. Outside the RPE, primitive vessels and stromal components of the choroid are visible in the mesenchyme during the fourth week of gestation. A vascular net of capillaries, derived from the dorsal and ventral ophthalmic arteries, becomes continuous over the whole cup in the fifth week. Formation of these vessels appears to depend on the development of pigment in the RPE. This net anastomoses with the annular vessel around the rim of the optic cup, and the hyaloid system within the cup. The connections with the vessels inside the cup are broken when the fissure seals, however. The blood passing through these capilliaries drains through a loose connection to two large plexuses, the supraorbital and the infraorbital venous plexuses. The first cells of the sclera are seen differentiating and condensing over the early choroid in the seventh week. They appear anterior to the equator of the cup first, then further forward toward the future limbus and more posteriorly, moving back toward the optic nerve.

The extraocular muscles that will move the eyes, to permit single binocular vision, first appear as small, dense condensations of mesenchyme tissue. The muscles that will be innervated by the third cranial nerve appear at 26 days, the lateral rectus that will be innervated by the sixth cranial nerve appears at 27 days, and the superior oblique that will be innervated by the fourth cranial nerve first appears at 29 days. The third and sixth cranial nerves grow from the brain into these condensations at about 31 days, and the fourth cranial nerve follows at 33 days. The fibrous trochlea is seen at the end of the embryonic period of gestation (8).

The Fetal Period (9 Weeks to Birth)

The fetal period of development stretches from 9 weeks of gestation until birth at around 38 weeks. This period is characterized by the development of the function of ocular tissues and, therefore, disruptions during this period more often result in abnormalities of function rather than gross structure.

Cornea

At 8 weeks, the primitive epithelium has been formed from surface ectoderm, the endothelium from the first wave of mesenchyme, and the stroma from a later wave. The epithelium consists of outer squamous and basal columnar cells that sit on a basal lamina. Behind that, the stroma consists of 15 layers of cells with rapidly appearing collagen fibrils. Peripherally, it is blended with condensing mesenchyme that has spread back around the outside of the optic cup forming the developing sclera. By the end of the third month, the endothelium has formed into a single layer of cells, as seen in the adult, and it rests on a basal lamina that forms the first evidence of Descemet's membrane. Hence, the only layer of the cornea missing at the beginning of the fourth month is Bowman's membrane. This final layer, which appears during the fifth month, is acellular from this first stage. These corneal layers become more specialized over the next months.

Many nerve endings are distributed in the corneal epithelium by midterm. Also present are neurotubules and vesicles indicating stimulus transduction (15).

The final transparency of the cornea depends on the patterning and spacing of collagen fibers. These fibers are laid down over some weeks, parallel to the corneal surface, and both thicken and lengthen as the cornea grows. The early embryonic cornea is translucent, rather than transparent, and only becomes transparent at the time that the corneal water content is controlled and balanced in the fetal period (during this period, as in adulthood, the corneal stroma is hydrophilic and a metabolic pump is needed to remove water). Zonulae occludens only appear in the endothelium during the fourth month, but they tightly seal the endothelium just at the onset of aqueous humor formation. Ehler et al. (16) found the diameter of unfixed human corneas to grow from 2 mm at 12 weeks of gestation to 4.2 mm at 16 weeks, to 9.3 mm at 35 weeks of gestation (the diameter then only increases by around 20% after birth). Collagen growth and replacement slow as the adult corneal diameter is reached.

Rapid growth of the cornea during the third month, relative to the rest of the eye, and the appearance of mesenchymal tissue in the limbal area both result in an increase in corneal curvature relative to that of the sclera (17). At birth, the optical power of the cornea is more than 50 D, significantly higher than that of the typical adult cornea (18–20). This has dramatic implications for the overall optical power of the neonatal eye (see the discussion of emmetropisation in Chapter 4).

Anterior Chamber

As development progresses into the fetal period, the space between the anterior section of the optic cup, the lens, and the cornea is filled with mesenchyme. The mesenchyme starts to form the structures of the future anterior chamber and angle. At this point, the vacuole forming the future chamber is much smaller than that found in adults and does not extend into the peripheral location of the future angle (Figs. 1.7 and 1.8). In fact, the structures that will drain the aqueous humor from the eye form in approximately the correct future location, but at this point are fully surrounded by mesenchyme. During the fourth month, the early trabecular meshwork consists of a triangular-shaped mass of undifferentiated mesenchymal cells with the anterior point forming between the corneal stroma and endothelium. The corneal endothelium, therefore, sits between the meshwork and the anterior chamber, unlike in the adult where the meshwork is open to drain aqueous from the anterior chamber (Fig. 1.7). Schlemm's canal starts to form as a loose collection of pieces that then coalesce over the next 3 months. It is complete in at least some quadrants in the seventh month and completely formed in the ninth month (21,22). During the second half of gestation, the cells of the trabecular meshwork and Schlemm's canal differentiate and form cavities to become more and more specialized for their role in draining and filtering the aqueous.

While the drainage system is maturing, the cells between the trabecular meshwork and ciliary body start to separate, allowing the anterior

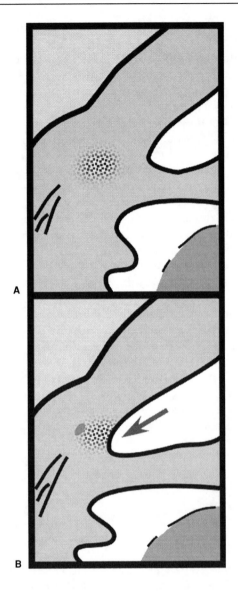

 Trabecular meshwork

 Schlemm's Canal

FIGURE 1.7. Schematic of development of the anterior chamber angle. **A:** The trabecular meshwork forms in the central tissue. **B:** The trabecular meshwork becomes exposed to the anterior chamber angle at around 7 months of gestation (based on a figure from Shields MB, Buckley E, Klintworth GK, et al. Axenfeld-Rieger syndrome. A spectrum of developmental disorders. *Surv Ophthalmo* 1985;29(6):387–409, with permission).

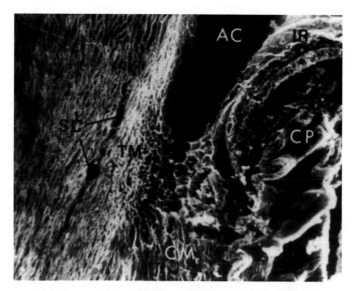

FIGURE 1.8. Human fetus at approximately 7 months. Scanning electron micrograph of the angle of the anterior chamber (*AC*). The apex of the angle is level with the middle portion of the area of Schlemm's canal (*SC*). CP, ciliary processes; TM, trabecular meshwork; IR, iris; CM, ciliary muscle. Magnification ×90. (From Anderson DR. The development of the trabecular meshwork and its abnormality in primary infantile glaucoma. *Trans Am Ophthalmol Soc* 1981;79:458–485, with permission.)

chamber angle to extend more peripherally. The ciliary muscle and ciliary body are initially found adjacent to the trabecular meshwork, but as the angle opens they move posteriorly to expose the angle structures to the aqueous humor (Figs. 1.7 and 1.8). The trabecular meshwork is uncovered at around 7 months, but the ciliary body and iris continue to slide backward for approximately a year after birth (23).

Kupfer and Ross (24) and Pandolfi and Astedt (25) measured aqueous outflow in fetal eyes. They found it to be 0.09 μL/min/Hg before 7 months and 0.3 μL/min/Hg at 8 months.

Infants with significantly reduced aqueous drainage develop congenital glaucoma (see Chapter 13). A number of studies have examined tissue from these eyes and noted that the ciliary body and iris lay further forward than in a typical eye. These structures overlap the posterior part of the trabecular meshwork, resembling the developing angle of an infant at 7 or 8 months of gestation. Evidence is mixed of cases where the abnormality appears to result from premature cessation of development of the angle, a disruption of differentiation of the

trabecular meshwork (26), or trabecular meshwork strands that are too thick and strong holding the angle shut (23). The trabecular meshwork and Schlemm's canal are present in these eyes and surgery to open the angle is usually successful. Similar anterior chamber malformations can be seen in other, more extensive anomalies and syndromes (12). These conditions can result in secondary glaucoma for similar reasons. Currently, numerous studies are exploring the role of abnormalities in neural crest cell migration and terminal induction in these conditions. As mentioned, many of the affected children have abnormalities of other adjacent structures that are derived from the same cells (27,28).

Ciliary Body and Iris

The posterior wall of the anterior chamber is formed by the iris and ciliary body. The anterior section of the optic cup forms the bulk of these structures. The outer pigmented layer of the cup forms the ciliary epithelium, anterior iris epithelium, and the iris sphincter and dilator muscles. The inner nonpigmented layer of the cup forms more ciliary epithelium and the posterior pigmented epithelium of the iris. By 12 weeks of gestation, the outer and inner layers of the optic cup are adhering to each other anteriorly, just behind the growing and advancing margin that will form the edge of the pupil and iris. This fused section of the optic cup starts to form 70 to 75 meridional ridges radiating out from the pupil. These are the precursors of the ciliary processes. The folding is thought to require the presence of the lens to induce differentiation. The next portion of the cup, on the peripheral side of the ciliary processes, forms a smooth section that will develop into the future pars plana.

Ozanics and Jakobiec (8) described the appearance of ciliary channels between the fourth and sixth month. These are enlargements of the intercellular spaces between the apposed apical surfaces of the pigmented and nonpigmented ciliary epithelial cells in the ciliary processes. They are presumed to correlate with the onset of aqueous secretion and form the primary reservoir for the aqueous humor. Intraocular pressure (IOP) has been studied in premature infants. Two studies found a similar mean IOP, of approximately 10 mmHg in babies at 25 to 37 weeks of gestation (29,30). The IOP continues to remain lower than adult levels throughout childhood.

The primitive ciliary muscle fibers are present late in the third month of gestation, in the mesenchyme between the region of the folding ciliary processes and the scleral condensations. This mesenchyme forms into orderly fibers and strands in the fourth month, the longitudinal fibers forming before the circular. The anterior ends of the fibers are attached to the developing scleral spur, although the tendons are not formed until 7.5 months (the ciliary muscle bundles will still increase in size and organization after birth). This muscle exerts its effect on the shape of the lens via the zonules. The formation of these fibers in the fourth month has been considered to be a tertiary stage of vitreous formation as they appear in the vitreous, but their protein is actually thought to be formed by the ciliary epithelium.

At the end of the third month, after the ciliary folds have formed, rapid growth ensues of

both walls of the optic cup between the folded region and the pupil margin. This region extends to form the epithelia of the iris. Unlike the retina and the ciliary body, both layers of the iris are pigmented. The pigmentation begins at midterm at the pupil margin and extends into the seventh month at the iris root. The third layer, the iris stroma, forms in the anterior chamber, over the surface of the iris epithelia. The mesenchyme cells line up against the epithelia without junctions or basal laminae leaving large intercellular gaps. Their alignment results in the formation of large crypts, which continue to develop along with pigment in the stroma after birth (31). Mund et al. (32) found mostly mature melanosomes in the human iris at term, whereas most of the chromatophores that give the individual their iris color appear to develop postnatally.

Construction of the mature iris also requires the generation of the sphincter and dilator muscles to control pupil size. These muscles are derived from the neural ectoderm even though they ultimately sit in the iris stroma. The sphincter first appears as infoldings in the anterior epithelial layer of the iris near the rim of the optic cup (this was the outer layer of the optic cup). Myofibrils appear in an unpigmented area in the fifth month and connective tissue septa and capillaries invade the muscle bundles in the sixth month, with cell-to-cell conduction likely in the seventh month. The fibers of the dilator muscle can be recognized in the sixth month. This muscle forms beside the sphincter at its peripheral edge and grows peripherally out to the iris root, where the iris connects to the ciliary body. The dilator muscle starts to function before the sphincter and very premature babies born at around 26 weeks may have a more dilated pupil than older infants. The pupils then respond to light at the end of seventh month (33,34).

Lens

Sitting behind the iris and ciliary body, the lens continues to grow in the fetal period. The cells of the anterior epithelium migrate around to the equator and form secondary fibers extending to the anterior and posterior poles. These fibers contribute to the formation of the Y sutures and form a fetal nucleus around the central embryonic nucleus. With these additional fibers, the lens gradually becomes more elliptical during the remaining months of gestation.

Posterior Chamber: Vitreous and Vasculature

The secondary vitreous is almost completely formed at the end of the third month of gestation. It compresses the remains of the primary vitreous and hyaloid vascular system into a cone with its apex at the optic disc and its base on the posterior surface of the lens. This cone is known as *Cloquet's canal.*

The hyaloid system starts to regress through apoptosis (programmed cell death) and the action of macrophages in the fourth month. The posterior tunica vasculosa lentis and complex of vessels around the hyaloid artery degenerate first and then the hylaoid artery itself (35). Bloodflow stops completely in the hyaloid artery in the seventh month. It detaches from the optic disc in the eighth month and disappears entirely in the nineth month, leaving the posterior chamber filled with the adultlike transparent secondary vitreous.

This process can be disrupted, resulting in a relatively rare congenital condition known as persistent hyperplastic primary vitreous (PHPV), which leaves excess material in Cloquet's canal. The material can block the visual axis of the eye and, hence, vision, and lead to a secondary glaucoma. The floaters routinely seen by adults are also thought to be remnants of the hyaloid vascular system.

The adultlike retinal blood supply that will nourish the inner two thirds of the retina is derived from the hyaloid system at the point where it leaves the optic nerve. Although the hyaloid system in the posterior chamber degenerates, the section passing through the neural visual system is incorporated into the central retinal artery and vein. These vessels emerge from near the hyaloid artery at the optic nerve head in the fourth month of gestation and start to grow to the periphery of the retina. The capillaries are estimated to grow 0.1 mm/d from the fourth to seventh month. They are thought to grow in response to the metabolic demands of the developing retina that is differentiating in a central to peripheral gradient. The capillaries reach the nasal ora serrata in the eighth month, and the temporal ora serrata in nineth month (36). In typical development, the avascular foveal zone reaches its adult size at approx 7 months of gestation. The mature pattern of capillaries is finally formed at approximately 3 months after birth. It can be dramatically disrupted as a result of an imbalance in oxygen supply after premature birth or low birthweight however (retinopathy of prematurity) (see Chapter 13).

Retinal Pigment Epithelium, Choroid, and Sclera

The RPE has finished mitotic division before the fetal period and, thus, the number of cells in the tissue is fixed. This stable population must stretch and realign to maintain a continuous layer over the increasing retinal area. In the fourth month, the RPE covers an area of approximately 240 mm^{26}, becoming 800 mm^{26} by around 2 years of age (8). The RPE cells lose all firm connection with the neural retina during this growth because retina cells are still migrating and immediate neighbor relationships between the RPE and photoreceptor layer are not maintained. The subretinal space develops while the two layers slide over each other. The cells of the RPE do follow the photoreceptors somewhat in their postnatal central migration, however (see next section on development of the retina (37)).

Outside the RPE, the development of the choroid consists of three waves of vascular development, described below, and differentiation of the stromal tissue. The loose stroma surrounds the blood vessels and is derived from mesenchyme. The choroid becomes pigmented around the seventh month of gestation, starting at the posterior pole and spreading to the anterior uvea. Its uveal melanocytes have the same origin as dermal melanocytes, unlike the RPE where the melanosomes have a neural origin. The choroid can fulfill its supply and support roles early in gestation and is already well differentiated at 5 months (5).

The sclera appears as a more dense condensation than the choroidal tissue. Its developing edge works back to the optic nerve and migrates between the axons to form the lamina cribrosa. The scleral fibres thicken over time, although the sclera is still rather thin at birth and some pigment may be seen through it.

Uveal Vasculature: Iris, Ciliary Body, and Choroid

In the embryonic period, the blood vessels of the eye consist of endothelial tubes sitting in mesenchyme, with no obvious distinction between arteries and veins. These vessels constitute the hyaloid system inside the optic cup, and a capillary network and primitive long posterior ciliary arteries over the optic cup in the layer of the future choroid. The outer network will form the future choriocapillaris and is supplied in the third month by the short posterior ciliary arteries carrying blood from the ophthalmic artery out through the sclera around the optic nerve head. During the third month, a second choroidal layer (i.e., a network of veins) develops between the choroidal capillary plexus and the condensing sclera. A few large trunks from this system emerge through the sclera to form the vortex veins. The third layer of choroidal vessels, between the other two, forms during the fourth month. This layer consists of arterial connections between the capillary and venous layers. By 5 months, all layers of the choroid are present and by the seventh month they are fully differentiated.

The long posterior ciliary arteries pass forward under the sclera to the anterior section of the uvea, the iris and ciliary body. They meet the anterior ciliary arteries, which pierce the sclera near the limbus, and are derived from the muscular and lacrimal branches of the ophthalmic artery. They appear in the fourth month. The long posterior ciliary arteries and the anterior ciliary arteries anastamose together to form the major circle of the iris in the sixth month. Three further sets of vessels are derived from this circle: the superficial branches of the iris, the intermediate vessels that sit deeper in the iris and run radially to the pupil margin, and the recurrent ciliary branches that run back to the ciliary body to supply each of the ciliary processes.

Extraocular Muscles

The last extraocular muscle to form, the levator palpebrae, separates from the dorsomedial aspect of the superior rectus at the end of the embryonic period, and grows laterally over the superior rectus toward the upper lid. It becomes complete and reaches its permanent position during the fourth month of gestation. The tendons of the other extraocular muscles fuse with the sclera near the equator at the end of the third month (8). The muscles gradually merge with the tendons in the fourth month.

Eyelids and Lacrimal System

The eyelids forming from the invaginating surface ectoderm grow toward each other over the cornea during the end of the embryonic period (Fig. 1.4B). They contact each other and fuse together early in the third month. The external skin then keratinizes and the glands of the lids appear before the lids split apart again in the fifth month. The first evidence of the orbicularis muscle appears in the 10th week, in the mesenchyme between the dermal and palpebral surfaces.

The developing lacrimal gland becomes visible at the end of the embryonic period, and the tendon of the levator palpebrae divides it during the fifth month. The nasolacrimal system becomes patent in the sixth month of gestation, but is not fully developed until 3 to 4 years after birth. A narrow or blocked nasolacrimal duct with the resulting tearing is a relatively common problem in young infants (see Chapter 12).

SUMMARY

The first evidence of the future eyes is present in the embryo at 3 weeks of gestation and the gross optical structures that will form an image of the external environment on the retina are present at only 4 months of gestation. Thus, significant developmental abnormalities of the optical visual system result from processes occurring relatively early in gestation.

Development of the eye is significantly slowed by the eighth month of pregnancy and postnatal development largely consists of only adjustment of the optical power of the eye (e.g., a relative flattening of the cornea) as the axial length of the eye increases during the early years after birth.

BUILDING A NEURAL VISUAL SYSTEM

The challenges involved in building the neural visual system include constructing mechanisms that can (a) encode the image formed on the retina, (b) reliably transmit information to higher stages of processing, and (c) provide the potential for the system to recalibrate as the individual grows (with increasing interpupillary distance, for example). Tracing the lineage of individual neurons in the retina or visual cortex or following the path of axons to their target structures, for example, has required complex experimental techniques such as labeling all cells born from repeated cell divisions or labeling the pathways from cells in the retina across their axonal synapses to their ultimate targets in the visual cortex. New techniques are being developed constantly and further understanding of the neuroscience underlying our visual experiences is accruing at a fast pace. Many of the techniques used to study the development of the neural visual system depend on animal models with short gestations and life cycles (e.g., mice and ferrets), while the similarity between species is relied on for interpretation in the context of human clinical conditions. The solutions to the challenges of building a neural visual system are not fully understood, but some general themes are emerging. These themes are described below using data gathered from a number of species.

The section is divided into three parts. The first addresses the formation of the principal neural structures in the early sensory visual pathway: the retina, the lateral geniculate nucleus (LGN), and the primary visual cortex, V1 (5–8). The second part covers the development of connections between these structures, via the optic nerve, chiasm, optic tract, and optic radiations. Here the fascinating question of how axons 'know' where to grow to will be addressed. The third part covers the formation of the precise set of synaptic connections within each structure.

Formation of the Principal Neural Structures

The process of cell birth in the retina, LGN, and visual cortex has been shown to have a number of stages in common, presumably related to their common derivation from neural ectoderm. In all cases, the most primitive cells divide many times to produce the large numbers of cells found in the mature tissue. Some cells leave this cycle of division and migrate from the place of *cell birth* to differentiate and mature in their final location, whereas other cells continue to divide to increase numbers. Interestingly, the time during gestation that the cells migrate from the cycle of division, after their *terminal* division, has a large effect on the type of cell that they are fated to form. Another common theme in the formation of these tissues is that many more cells are generated than are actually needed in the mature adult; the visual system will eliminate many cells during development (via apoptosis or programmed cell death).

The specific details of the development of the retina, LGN, and cortex are discussed below.

Retina

The inner layer of the optic cup goes on to form the neural retina. After the optic vesicle has invaginated to form the cup, this inner part consists of a continuous layer of homogenous neuroblasts that will form the different layers of the neural retina and the supportive Müller cells. These neuroblasts initially undergo rapid cycles of rhythmic mitotic division to increase their numbers. They have extensions that span the depth of the retina, from inner to outer surface (Fig. 1.9), while they cycle from stage 1 to 5. As they start to replicate, their nuclei move to the RPE side to replicate their DNA and then the vitreal side to divide into two daughter cells that will repeat the cycle. An internal or extrinsic signal finally tells the cells to stop their symmetric division and convert to asymmetric division, where they produce one cell that will stay in the cell cycle of division and another that will leave the cycle, migrate to its final retinal layer and differentiate to assume the characteristics of a mature cell (Fig. 1.9). The destination layer and type of cell formed depend on the time in gestation that this asymmetrical division occurs.

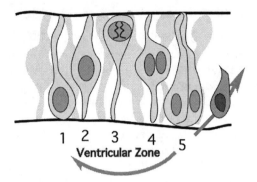

FIGURE 1.9. Schematic illustration of the cell cycle that takes place in the retina, lateral geniculate nucleus (LGN) and cortex during cell proliferation. The two cells formed at stage 5 either both pass through the cycle again or one cell migrates to its destination layer in the tissue.

A number of studies have shown that the cells still in the cell cycle can be transplanted to an eye of another gestational age and form the cells in the layer appropriate for that new age (38). In other words, these early cells are multipotent. It appears that they commit to their ultimate cell type right before their terminal asymmetric division. The cells actually undergoing terminal division, if transplanted to tissue of a different gestational age, form the cells appropriate for their original donor tissue rather than the recipient. Understanding this process obviously has significant implications for any future attempts to repair damaged or abnormal retina.

Cells start to divide and later convert from symmetric to asymmetric cell division in the central retina first, with each sequential stage progressing across the retina to the periphery over time. Early in gestation, the tissue consists of an outer nuclear proliferative layer and an inner marginal zone, near the vitreous, that is almost anuclear (Fig. 1.4A). In the fifth week of gestation, two layers of nuclei start to become visible in the posterior pole, as the inner and outer neuroblastic layers, which are separated by a relatively empty layer, the transient layer of Chevietz. By 8 weeks of gestation, the two layers of nuclei and transient layer are visible all the way to the equator of the eye (Fig. 1.10A).

The first cells to leave the cell cycle, migrate, and start to differentiate into their mature format are the ganglion cells, during the third month of gestation. They migrate to the primitive ganglion cell layer and start to seek connections around a week later, as revealed by the development of a nerve fiber layer and the conversion of the transient layer of Chevietz into a primitive *inner plexiform layer* (Fig. 1.10B). The cones, horizontal cells, and some types of amacrines start to appear soon after the ganglion cells, and the rest of the amacrines, the rods, and the bipolars follow later. Once again, these stages start first in the central retina and a gradual wave of terminal division and layer formation spreads from the center to the retinal periphery, taking until approximately 7 months of gestation. The ora serrata is established in the sixth month and matures in its scalloping even after birth (8). Thus, all of the cell division is basically over in humans before the baby is born, and postnatal growth of the eye only consists of rearrangement of retinal cells and not birth of new cells.

All of the layers of the adult retina can be seen, at least centrally, at midgestation (4.5 months), with evidence of synapses in the plexiform layers. Importantly, the outer segments of the photoreceptors are not present yet at this stage, so no influence of photoreceptor activity can have occurred on development at this point.

In addition to the cells migrating through the depth of the retina to their appropriate layer, some cells also migrate part of the distance across the retina, to form the appropriate local structure. The first evidence of a unique macula is evident at 11 or 12 weeks of gestation. The future fovea starts as a thickened area because of an accumulation of many ganglion cells. No inner retina exists over the fovea in the adult eye and so the ganglion cells need to migrate away from the fovea to form the foveal pit. The migration starts at approximately 7 months of gestation and continues until 11 to 15 months after birth (39). A second migration involves the immature foveal cones. At birth, their inner segments are about three times wider than those of the adult and their outer segments are around 10 times shorter (Fig. 1.10C). These wider cones logically form a less tightly packed array, and so another characteristic of late gestation and postnatal foveal development is a migration of the photoreceptors toward the center of the

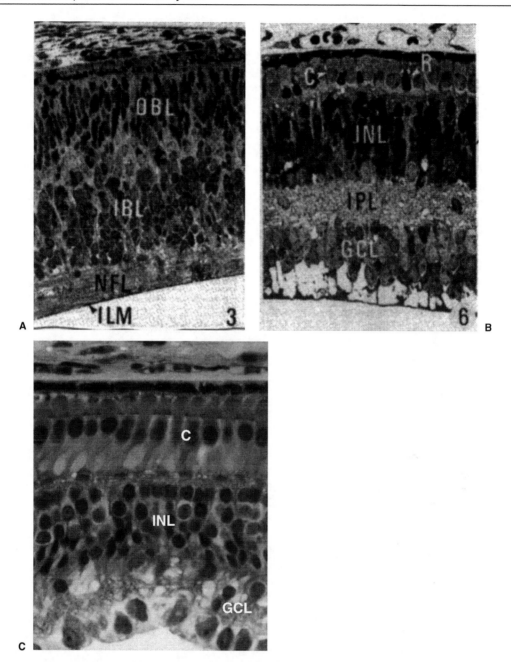

FIGURE 1.10. The developing human retina. **A:** The posterior pole at 8 weeks. The outer (*OBL*) and inner (*IBL*) neuroblastic layers, the early nerve fiber layer (*NFL*), and inner limiting-membrane (*ILM*) can all be seen. **B:** At 4 months. The main components are now all present [R-rods, C-cones, inner nuclear layer (*INL*), inner plexiform layer (*IPL*), and ganglion cell layer (*GCL*)]. (Panels A and B: From Hollenburg MJ, Spira AW. Early development of the human retina. *Can J Ophthalmol* 1972;7(4):472–491, with permission.) **C:** The neonatal foveal retina showing highly immature cones, and the absence of the later developing foveal pit. (From the human retina tissue collection of Anita Hendrickson.)

fovea. With this migration, the density of cone photoreceptors in the fovea increases and the size of the rod-free zone decreases until approximately 5 years after birth (39). Although the ganglion cells move peripherally and the photoreceptors move centrally, the cells all retain their original connections made with each other in the 10th to 15th week of gestation. The lengthening of these connections results in the formation of the fibers of Henle.

Beyond a rearrangement of cells in the fovea, the adult retina has gradients of cell density across its entire surface. One of the most studied examples of this is the gradient of retinal ganglion cell density, which is highest around the fovea and falls off with increasing eccentricity (40). The formation of this gradient and comparable ones of other cell types, is thought to result from the contributions of a number of processes. The retina grows 10 to 15 mm^2 per week throughout the fetal period (41), and then continues from a neonatal area of 590 mm^2 to 1250 mm^2 in the adult (42,43). Much of this growth occurs asymmetrically, with more expansion between that equator and ora serrata than at the posterior pole, acting to reduce the density of cells in the periphery somewhat. Another possible contribution might come from apoptosis. Taking the number of ganglion cell axons in the optic nerve as a representation of the ganglion cell population in the retina, Provis and Van Driel (41) counted a peak number of axons in the human nerve of 3.7 million at 16 weeks of gestation, with a rapid loss until 20 weeks, and then a slow further loss to 1.1 million at 30 weeks. They suggest that this apoptosis might help form the retinal cell density gradient. This represents a surprising and dramatic loss of more than half of the axons during gestation, which is also found in monkeys (44). In fact, it has been suggested that all ganglion cells are programmed to die unless they receive a signal from their environment telling them to continue.

Lateral Geniculate Nucleus

Neurogenesis in the LGN occurs in the same format as the retina (Fig. 1.9). The cells undergoing mitotic division also move through the

cell cycle, with their extensions reaching from the ventricular side through the depth of the LGN tissue. In humans, the cells are undergoing terminal division and migrating in the LGN by 9.5 weeks of gestation; at this point, however, these cells do not form the adultlike laminar structure of layers dedicated specifically to one eye or the other. This development appears to require an additional stimulus. Although the cells have migrated and are in place, a 12-week delay actually occurs before this lamination begins, but the layers do take the adult form by the 25th week of gestation (45).

Visual Cortex

The development of the primary visual cortex seems to follow a pattern that is characteristic of much of the cerebral cortex. The newborn cortex has six layers, as found in the adult, with cell birth lasting in humans from the sixth week until the fifth month of gestation. In fact, primates all generate their cortical neurons during the middle third of gestation (Fig. 1.11). Once again, the nuclei of the cells in the mitotic cell cycle move along extensions oriented from the ventricular zone across the tissue (Fig. 1.9). In the case of the cortex, the ventricular zone has a number of component layers all lying beneath the future cortical plate. These layers are transient and do not persist into maturity.

One of the transient layers formed beneath the cortical plate during gestation, the subplate, plays a particularly interesting role. Axons growing from subcortical structures (e.g., the LGN) that aim to innervate the cortex wait in this layer while the cortical plate becomes organized. The subplate is also proposed to have a significant influence on the later cortical organization of brainstem connections, and local cortico-cortical circuits (46). It appears in the middle third of gestation and degenerates in the last third to leave a few cells behind in the white matter. Abnormal degeneration of this tissue has been implicated in some forms of epilepsy (47).

Soon after corticogenesis has started, some post-mitotic cells leave the cell cycle and start to migrate to their destination layer. As in the retina and LGN, the cortical cells are also

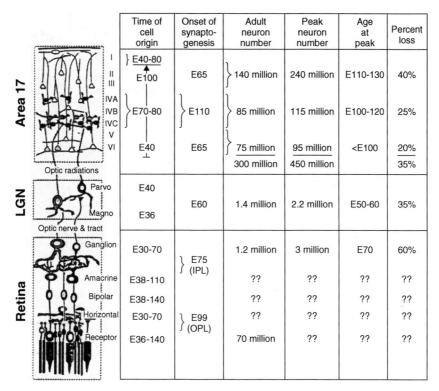

		Time of cell origin	Onset of synapto-genesis	Adult neuron number	Peak neuron number	Age at peak	Percent loss
Area 17	I	} E40-80					
	II	E100	E65	} 140 million	240 million	E110-130	40%
	III						
	IVA						
	IVB	} E70-80	} E110	} 85 million	115 million	E100-120	25%
	IVC						
	V						
	VI	E40	E65	{ 75 million	95 million	<E100	20%
				300 million	450 million		35%
LGN	Parvo	E40					
			E60	1.4 million	2.2 million	E50-60	35%
	Magno	E36					
Retina	Ganglion	E30-70	} E75 (IPL)	1.2 million	3 million	E70	60%
	Amacrine	E38-110		??	??	??	??
	Bipolar	E38-140		??	??	??	??
	Horizontal	E30-70	} E99 (OPL)	??	??	??	??
	Receptor	E36-140		70 million	??	??	??

FIGURE 1.11. The timing of events in development of the rhesus monkey neural visual system (Gestation length = 165 days). (From Lent R, ed. *The Visual System from Genesis to Maturity. An Overview.* Boston: Birkhäuser; 1992:9, with permission; copyright now owned by Springer.)

multipotent before their last cell division, the timing of which defines their future layer and cell fate (48,49). The cells migrate along glia up into the cortical plate. Those cells climbing along adjacent glia form adjacent radial columns that respond later to one region of space each. This patterning is common across the cortex for other areas too.

The layers through the depth of the cortex, from 1 to 6, are generated in an inside-out pattern. The innermost layer, layer 6, is formed first and then the cells destined for the other layers are obliged to climb along the glia through each of the previously formed layers. The only exception to this is a region at the top called the *marginal zone,* which will form the future layer 1. It is formed early in gestation with the ventricular zone. As each layer forms, the cells climb through the previous layers to lie just underneath this marginal zone. A number of congenital neurologic conditions are now considered to

be the result of abnormal neural migration into these layers of the cortex (e.g., lissencephaly) (50,51).

A significant loss of cells also occurs through programmed cell death in the cortex. It is a common theme across cortical areas. The monkey primary visual cortex contains 35% more neurons in midgestation than in adulthood (52).

Axon Growth and Guidance

Robinson and Dreher (53) took the period between conception and eye opening in 13 different species and calculated the percentage of that period at which various notable developmental events occurred. They noted that the retinal ganglion, LGN, and subcortical cells were all born at about 30% to 40% of the pre–eye-opening period across the species that they studied. Thus, it appears that the cells forming the structures of the sensory visual system are all born at approximately the same time. If the locations of these structures have all been pre-defined by the birth of these cells, how do the axons growing to take information from one structure to another know where to grow among the numerous millions of cells and axons? Robinson and Dreher note that the axons of the first-born retinal ganglion cells reach the LGN and superior colliculus at 40% to 45% of the pre–eye-opening period, and that the axons from the LGN reach the cortical subplate region between 50% and 60% of the period (Fig. 1.11).

Retinogeniculate Projection

The first challenge for axons growing from the retinal ganglion cells to the LGN is to find their way out of the eye. They must grow toward and exit through the optic stalk that will form the future optic nerve.

The adult human has approximately 1 million ganglion cell axons in each optic nerve. The axons, particularly the peripheral ones, have to seek the nerve head as they traverse the retina on the way to find their target. A number of studies have now demonstrated that axonal growth toward the nerve is guided by molecular cues that are expressed and laid down temporarily in the retinal tissue. In fact, axons change their behavior within minutes of their surface receptors being exposed to a guidance molecule (54,55).

The foremost tip of a growing axon that finds the pathway for the axon to travel is formed into a growth cone. This growth cone responds to and is guided by various molecular markers that attract or repel it (Fig. 1.12). For example, a molecular marker ring is thought to surround the expanding wave of ganglion cell birth on its peripheral side. This ring repels the growth cones from growing in the peripheral direction, thus encouraging them to head centrally across the retina from their cell bodies (56). Other markers (such as slit 1) are thought to attract the growing axon toward the nerve head, and yet others to encourage the growth cones to exit the eye (e.g., netrin 1 is laid down in a ring around the optic nerve head in mice) (57). Inhibitory molecules surrounding the length of the nerve are then thought to keep

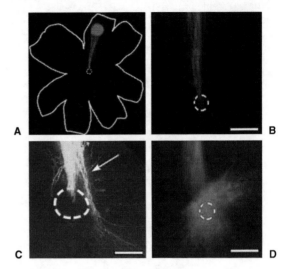

FIGURE 1.12. Axon pathfinding across the retina to the optic disc (*broken circle*). **A:** Retinal ganglion cells labeled in the periphery extend their axons to the disc in the typical, wildtype. **B:** Greater magnification of the axons traveling directly to the disc (all scale bars equal to 100 μm). **C:** In one form of mutant retina with abnormal guidance markers, some axons split off and fail to exit at the disc. **D:** In another mutant, the axons splay out at the disc and fail to pass through into the nerve. (From Oster SF, Sretavan DW. Connecting the eye to the brain: the molecular basis of ganglion cell axon guidance. *Br J Ophthalmol* 2003;87:639–645, with permission from the BMJ publishing group.)

the growing axons within the appropriate channel (e.g., sema5A; (58)). Studies are just starting to document the corresponding factors controlling formation of intrinsic circuits within the retina.

Once the growth cones of the retinal ganglion cell axons have been guided out of the eye and along the optic nerve, they hit a significant developmental challenge. The axons from the temporal retina need to be separated from those of the nasal retina at the optic chiasm so that they can grow appropriately to ipsilateral or contralateral visual cortex. This is the first instance where two growth cones at essentially the same point in space need to grow in fundamentally different directions, and identifying the retinal location of each cell body becomes critical. Studies starting to solve this guidance problem have been reviewed (2). It appears that this is an instance where guidance molecules interact with specific identifying receptors expressed on growth cones. This instance has been the focus of numerous studies because the outcome is so clear; the axons need to either cross the midline and enter the contralateral optic tract or deviate back into the ipsilateral one. The primary solution to this problem lies in the fact that the growth cones are capable of synthesizing their own proteins in temporary response to local cues in their external environment [e.g., the ratio between the amounts of cyclic adenosine monophosphate (cAMP) and cyclic guanosine monophosphate (cGMP) inside a growth cone determines whether that cone will be attracted or repelled by the guidance molecule netrin 1] (59). Thus, growth cones can behave in fundamentally different ways, depending on their internal cellular composition which, in turn, could act as a lasting identifier for their retinal location. In fact, logic suggests that it would be helpful if the growth cone were able to modify its behavior according to its external environment. The balance between being attracted to and repelled by a molecule could be important; otherwise, it might be feasible for a growth cone to grow toward an attractive marker at the optic nerve head, for example, and not be able to grow past it and leave the eye.

Recent studies have started to understand the role of these guidance cues in isolation in dishes (*in vitro*), using species that are relatively easy to work with. The challenge of understanding the system in the full developing animal (*in vivo*) is still poorly understood. The interactions between the numerous potential guidance cues all working simultaneously on millions of growing axons may well become central to our understanding of clinical conditions involving atypical axon growth (e.g., the abnormal chiasm in albinism; see Chapter 13).

Although the details of the guidance molecules in humans are not known, the fibers of the optic tract are seen to enter the human LGN as early as 7 to 8 weeks of gestation (60). Fibers from the contralateral eye are seen to arrive marginally before those of the ipsilateral eye in the monkey (61). A number of axons are thought to reach inappropriate targets and apoptosis is initiated to eliminate these surplus cells.

Geniculocortical Projection

Given that topographic maps of the visual field are found in both the LGN and the visual cortex, the growing axons from the LGN must, like ganglion cell axons, retain information regarding the spatial location of their cell body in the LGN.

Once again, the growth cones of axons from the LGN are thought to be guided along the path to the visual cortex by guidance molecules. Unlike in the LGN, however, the axons do not grow directly into their final destination tissue (cortical layer IV). As mentioned, these axons wait for a period of weeks in the transient subplate beneath the cortical plate (61–63). In some cases, the axons reach the subplate before their future postsynaptic cells in the cortex are even born. Robinson and Dreher (53) noted in a number of species that the axons waited in the subplate for 11% to 28% of the period from conception to eye opening. In humans, the presumed thalamic axons first make synapses in the subplate by 11 to 13 weeks of gestation (46,64) and synapses are noted in the cortical plate at 23 to 25 weeks, although the axons could have arrived there earlier (64). Thus, the human data are consistent with Robinson and Dreher's general scheme. What are the axons doing while they are 'waiting' in the subplate? This is still somewhat unclear, but this layer does include some of the earliest neurons, transmitters, and receptor systems in the telencephalon, implying that this waiting period may have a significant organizational role that is of clinical importance.

Synapse Formation

As growing axons arrive in the LGN from the retina, and in the visual cortex from the LGN, they initially form diffuse connections throughout their target tissue. They do form a coarse scale topographic map, perhaps defined by more molecular markers if the apparent basic strategies of axon guidance are maintained. In the adult, however, the system of synaptic connections formed by each axon in its target tissue is extremely precise. For example, in addition to topography, the connections in the LGN form eye-specific layers and the connections in visual cortex form eye-specific ocular dominance columns. How might this precise set of synapses be refined from the initially diffuse innervation?

Clinical evidence and experiments undertaken in animal models indicate that neural activity has a dramatic effect on the refinement of these connections (65,66). Very poor optical quality in one eye or a closed eyelid soon after birth results in abnormal neural signals passing up through the visual system and an abnormal refinement of synaptic connections that leads to a dramatic reduction in visual performance driven by the affected eye. Little if any effect is found on visual performance of the unaffected eye. Amblyopia is considered to be the human clinical manifestation of this process.

Many experiments and observations have now been made on the role of neural activity in the refinement of synapses. A theoretical framework now exists that has been shown to govern this synaptic refinement component of development in many neural structures, including those outside the visual system.

Hebb (67) proposed a theory of how this process might occur, long before direct experimental evidence was available to test his hypothesis. He proposed that 'when an axon of cell A is near enough to excite cell B and repeatedly or persistently takes part in firing it, some growth process or metabolic change takes place in one or both cells such that A's efficiency, as one of the cells firing B, is increased' (Fig. 1.13). What does this mean in the development of the visual system? In the context of an axon arriving in visual cortex from the LGN, it can be thought of as stating that, when the axon of an LGN cell

is near enough to excite a postsynaptic cortical cell and repeatedly takes part in making the cortical cell fire, the LGN cell will strengthen its connection with the cortical cell. In other words 'cells that fire together wire together.' So, a presynaptic cell that is very active and causes the postsynaptic cell to fire will have its synapse strengthened, and a cell that is not routinely involved in making the postsynaptic cell fire will lose its influence on the postsynaptic cell. The rules and implementation of these interactions are currently being studied in many branches of neuroscience and have significant implications for processes as distant from sensory vision as learning and memory acquisition. The sections below describe current understanding of Hebbian-like synaptic refinement in the developing LGN and visual cortex.

Retinogeniculate Projection

Although the first body of evidence for the importance of neural activity in synaptic refinement came from the visual cortex, a similar framework has been proposed more recently to govern the formation of eye-specific layers in the LGN. The immature LGN has diffuse connections from both eyes throughout its structure, but at approximately 22 weeks in the human a consistent and stereotypical series of cellular layers driven solely by one eye or the other develops (60,68) (Fig. 1.14). The progression from a diffuse to a layered structure has been observed in numerous species and, in all cases, this development is achieved before eye opening. How, then, can neural activity lead to coordinated refinement when a detailed visual scene is not being transduced to form action potentials? This question has been studied most extensively in the cat and ferret.

Elimination of neural activity from one eye [via action potential blockage using tetrodotoxin (TTX)] prevents the formation of the layers at the time when they should be forming in the LGN, before the eyes are open (69,70). Thus, action potentials are a key component in eye-specific layer formation. How can retinal topography and eye-specific layers be precisely laid out based on neural activity before the eyes are open?

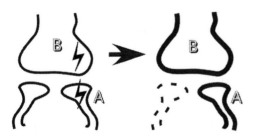

FIGURE 1.13. An illustration of the concept of synaptic competition. If pre- and postsynaptic cells (**A,B**) fire together routinely, over time they strengthen their synaptic connection.

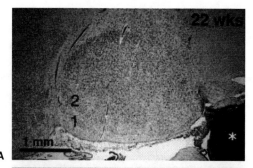

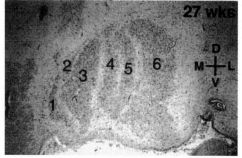

FIGURE 1.14. The appearance of layering starting at 22 weeks in human lateral geniculate nucleus (LGN). The layering initially forms in an orthogonal direction to the mature layout, but rotates with time. (From Hevner RF. Development of connections in the human visual system during fetal mid-gestation: a DiI-tracing study. *J Neuropathol Exp Neurol* 2000;59:385–392, with permission.)

Ganglion cells in the retina have been shown to generate *spontaneous* activity (in rat and ferret) during the period that eye-specific layers form, and this activity is sufficient to drive postsynaptic LGN cells (71). Thus, activity is at least present; for it to drive synaptic refinement that creates retinal topography and eye-specific layers, however, a Hebbian framework would require nearest neighbor synchrony and interocular asynchrony. Near retinal neighbors will 'wire together' and axons from the two eyes will not. Galli and Maffei (72), recording from single ganglion cells in ferrets, found spontaneous bursts of action potentials lasting around 5 seconds, with up to 2 minutes rest between them. Optical imaging and multielectrode recording techniques have permitted these bursts to be recorded from populations of these cells simultaneously, as reviewed by Shatz (73). When analyzed across the population, these bursts become waves traversing in different directions across the retina over time (74). In other words, the 5 seconds of activity are very slightly delayed between one cell and its neighbor and, across a population, these consistent delays lead to the creation of a wave of activity moving in one direction across the tissue. These waves provide nearest neighbor synchrony, consistent with the idea of activity representing topography, and the approximately 2-minute pauses between waves can generate the asynchrony between eyes. Hence, activity can actually instruct the LGN about which synapses should be strengthened and which should be weakened to construct the appropriate system. These waves have been documented while the eye-specific layers are forming, but they disappear shortly before eye opening. Hevner (60) noted the segregation of presynaptic axons into eye-specific layers in the human LGN at 20 weeks.

Once the process of synaptic refinement in the LGN is complete, the structure seems to remain stable. It is not affected by further visual experience the individual might have, so abnormal patterns of activity later in development and after eye opening do not dramatically restructure the LGN again. In fact, postnatal visual experience has little effect on synaptic refinement in the LGN. This importance of the timing of neural activity in refining synapses is represented in the concept of a *critical period* or *sensitive period* in development. The basic concept is that synapses in a structure are only susceptible to the influence of abnormal experience during a limited developmental time period. Before and after that period, the pattern of neural activity in the tissue does not change the progression of development significantly. Thus, in the LGN, the critical or sensitive period is before eye opening. In the visual cortex, however, in numerous species including cats, monkeys, and humans, the cortical critical period largely occurs after the eyes are open, which is important in the context of amblyopia.

Geniculocortical Projection

Many studies have been done of the postnatal refinement of synaptic connections in primary visual cortex, largely because of the relevance to clinical understanding of the condition amblyopia (75), but also because this process provides direct support for Hebbian-like competition between presynaptic axons for synaptic connections with postsynaptic cortical cells. Many reviews of this are found in the literature (76–78).

The mature primary visual cortex contains a number of overlapping coordinated systems of representation. For instance, the tissue is simultaneously organized based on retinal topography, ocular dominance, and stimulus orientation. The role of activity in refining synaptic connections has been studied most extensively in relation to the eye-specific segregation into ocular dominance columns. The segregation into columns takes place late in gestation and after eye opening in normal development of a number of species. Once again, the synaptic connections form initially throughout the tissue and then segregate into areas driven predominantly by one eye or the other. This time the segregation takes the form of columns that run perpendicular to the layered structure of the cortical plate.

Numerous studies have shown that competition between the eyes for cortical territory during a developmental critical period can heavily influence the mature structure of the tissue. If vision is blocked in one eye, as the result of a cataract or ptosis in humans, or a closed lid in animal models, axons from the unaffected eye form strong connections with the cortical neurons while the dramatically reduced neural activity in the affected eye leads to a loss of synapses driven by that eye in the cortex. Figure 1.15A shows the distribution of ocular dominance of cortical cells in a monkey that had one eye covered during the postnatal period. The cortical cells become driven by the uncovered eye.

Figure 1.15B, shows another clinically relevant manipulation. In this case, instead of closing one eye, surgery was performed on the extraocular muscles to turn one eye of a kitten (mimicking clinical strabismus). This surgery causes the images from the two eyes to be completely different; they no longer correspond with each other. This manipulation during the critical period results in an almost complete segregation of synapses from the two eyes in the

cortex. Postsynaptic cortical cells are driven by one eye or the other, rather than a proportion of binocular cells being driven by both eyes in the undisturbed animal. This result is consistent with poor correlation between activity in presynaptic axons from the two eyes that are now viewing different regions of the visual world. Thus, synapses from the two eyes will not be simultaneously strengthened on the same postsynaptic cell, and no binocular cells to support visual functions (e.g., stereopsis) will remain. The cells end up being dominated by input from one eye or the other.

Significant synaptic refinement of cortical circuitry exists in humans after birth. In fact, it has been shown that the peak number of synapses in the human visual cortex occurs at approximately 8 months after birth (79). Thus, significant cortical development exists that may be influenced by visual experience in human infant patients. The most critical period for cortical development in humans is thought to be until approximately 7 years of age at least in terms of the development of binocularity (80).

Is there any benefit to having this postnatal plasticity in the visual system? There is certainly a cost, in that pediatric patients with strabismus, anisometropia, or some forms of pathology are at risk for loss of cortical visual function. It can be argued, however, that this plasticity provides a basis for postnatal recalibration of the system as infants grow and their retinal neurons migrate. For instance, if a child is to have fine stereopsis, the visual system must carefully compare corresponding retinal points in the two eyes and assign a three-dimensional direction to retinal disparities. If the retinal location of photoreceptors is changing postnatally, and the interpupillary distance (PD) is increasing, both the visual direction of a photoreceptor and the three-dimensional location corresponding to a particular horizontal disparity will change. Thus, the visual system must be able to recalibrate with growth to correctly interpret the changing information.

SUMMARY

This chapter has provided a clinically and functionally oriented review of the development of

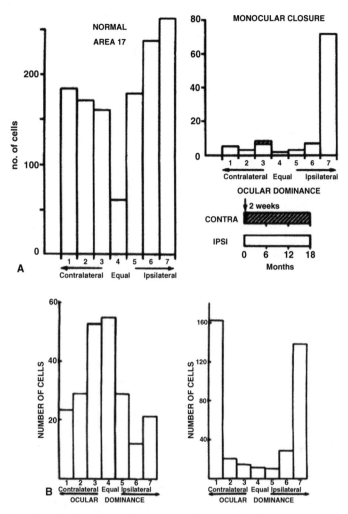

FIGURE 1.15. Examples of ocular dominance histograms showing the degree to which each cortical cell responds to each eye. Panel A: the left histogram shows data from a normal monkey for comparison with the right histogram showing data from a monkey that had one eye closed during the critical or sensitive period. After the monocular occlusion the majority of the cells respond to the uncovered, ipsilateral, eye. Panel B: the left histogram shows data from a normal cat for comparison with a strabismic cat on the right. In that case, there are many cells that respond to one eye or the other, but few cells that respond binocularly. (Panel A: From Hubel DH, Wiesel TN, LeVay S. Plasticity of ocular dominance columns in monkey striate cortex. *Philos Trans R Soc Lond B Biol Sci* 1977;278:377–409, with permission. Panel B: From Hubel DH, Wiesel TN. Binocular interaction in striate cortex of kittens reared with artificial squint. *J Physiol* 1965;28:1029–1040, with permission.)

the visual system for those interested in working pediatric patients (A summary of embryological chronology can be found in Table 1.1.) with Many of the cited references provide more detailed analyses of the development of individual components of the system, for those who would like to learn more.

Much of the recent work in this area has taken advantage of advances in genetics and molecular biology, frequently looking at the influence of gene expression and environmental interactions in animal models using genes that are homologous to those of humans (1,4). Our understanding of the genetic basis of congenital

TABLE 1.1 Chronological Survey of the Appearance of Ocular Structures* (Reproduced with permission from Ozanics and Jakobiec: Ocular anatomy, embryology, and teratology. Frederick A. Jakobiec, ed. Harper and Row, Philadelphia, 1982)

Age	Neuroectodermal	Uveal Components	Connective Tissue	Outflow Channels and Transparent Media
Embryonic period 1 month 1.5 to 8 mm	Optic primordium to optic fissure	Sinusoidal investment around optic cup. Hyaloid vessels in optic fissure		Lens placode
2 months 8 to 40 mm	Pigment epithelium with melanosomes. Inner and outer neuroblastic and Chievitz layers. Ganglion and müllerian cells. Optic nerve fibers in stalk	Choriocapillaris connects with primitive posterior ciliary arteries. Venous plexus. Collagen fibers in choroid	Corneal epithelium and endothelium. Collagen fibrils in stroma. Anterior scleral condensation	Lens vesicle, primary and secondary fibers, first suture. Primary vitreous; commencement of secondary vitreous
Fetal period 3 months 40 to 70 mm	Inner and outer plexiform layers. Immature cone synapses and synapses in inner plexiform layer	Choroid vascular layering. Bruch's membrane forming. Elastic fibers appear. Optic cup starts forward growth	Descemet's membrane. Corneal innervation. Sclera encircles the eye and has some elastic fibers	Lens diameter is 2 mm, has Y suture. Hyaloid vasculature regresses, Druault's bundle appears
4 months 70 to 120 mm	Retinal vessels grow into nerve fiber layer. Disc has a zone of vascularization. Bergmeister's papilla	Middle vascular layer in choroid. Ciliary folds elaborated and muscle anlage grows. Primordium of iris sphincter	Bowman's membrane commences. Corneal curvature different from that of sclera	Zonulx fibers form Hyaloid system atrophies except for pupillary membrane. Schlemm's canal appears
5 months 130 to 170 mm	Rod synapses. Horizontal cells differentiate. Pericytes around retinal capillaries. Lamina cribrosa and neural crest derived nerve sheaths	Choroid has chromatophores. Bruch's membrane completed. Ciliary epithelium with ciliary channels. Iris sphincter and stroma maturing	Bowman's membrane maturing. Scleral spur and anterior chamber extending to its level	Zonulx fibers attach around the primitive lens lamella
6 months 170 to 220 mm	Final arrangement of retinal cells. Macular differentiation commences. Definite ora serrata present	Choroid has recurrent arterial branches. Circular ciliary muscle and iris dilator fibers commence. Angle deepens. Diameter of pupil about 5 mm		Aqueous humor formation starts
7 months 220 to 260 mm	Photoreceptor outer segments differentiate. Avascular foveal area has appeared. Lamina cribrosa has mature structure	Uveal melanocytes are frequent. Circular fibers and a narrow pars plana in the ciliary body. Dilator extends to root of iris		Angle deepens and its tissue starts to rarefy. Cloquet's canal is outlined
8 months 260 to 300 mm	Two layers of ganglion cells cover macular indentation. Retinal capillaries reach ora nasally; equator temporally	In iris sphincter becomes functional. Nerve terminals demonstrable in stroma		Trabecular meshwork matures; the endothelium of Schlemm's canal has vacuoles. Outflow facility is measurable
9 months 300 to 500 mm or over	Retinal circulatory system is established, with capillaries reaching to the inner nuclear layer and extending to near the periphery. Myelination of optic nerve	Iris stromal melanosomes are frequent. Minor vascular circle is present. Pupillary membrane atrophies		Lens somewhat spherical; its diameter is from 4.5 mm to 6 mm

*The measurements in the literature vary greatly. An approximation is used for this table.

and pediatric visual system disorders is expanding rapidly with the advent of these techniques and approaches. Although we currently use many treatment interventions aimed at influencing neural activity during specific periods (e.g., glasses and patching) or surgically repairing malformation, we are just starting to understand the role of prevention in our care for these patients.

REFERENCES

1. Beebe DC. Homeobox genes and vertebrate eye development. *Invest Ophthalmol Vis Sci* 1994;35(7):2897–2900.
2. van Horck FP, Weinl C, Holt CE. Retinal axon guidance: novel mechanisms for steering. *Curr Opin Neurobiol* 2004;14(1): 61–66.
3. Katz LC, Shatz CJ. Synaptic activity and the construction of cortical circuits. *Science* 1996;274(5290):1133–1138.
4. Cline H. Sperry and Hebb: oil and vinegar? *Trends Neurosci* 2003;26(12):655–661.
5. Duke-Elder S, Cook C. Embryology. In: *Systems of Ophthalmology, Vol 3, Normal and Abnormal Development, Pt. 1.* St. Louis: CV Mosby; 1963.
6. Mann IC. *The Development of the Human Eye.* New York: Grune and Stratton; 1964.
7. Barishak YR. *Embryology of the Eye and its Adnexa,* 2nd revised ed. Basel: Karger; 2001.
8. Ozanics V, Jakobiec F. Prenatal development of the eye and its adnexae. In: Jakobiec F, ed. *Ocular Anatomy, Embyology and Teratology.* Philadelphia: Harper and Row; 1982:1–96.
9. O'Rahilly R. The timing and sequence of events in the development of the human eye and ear during the embryonic period proper. *Anat Embryol* 1983;168(1): 87–99.
10. Worgul BV. Lens. In: Jakobiec F, ed. *Ocular Anatomy, Embryology and Teratology.* Philadelphia: Harper and Row; 1982:355–389.
11. Hay E. Development of the vertebrate cornea. *Int Rev Cytol* 1980;63:263–322.
12. Shields MB, Buckley E, Klintworth GK, et al. Axenfeld-Rieger syndrome. A spectrum of developmental disorders. *Surv Ophthalmol* 1985;29(6):387–409.
13. Bahn CF, Falls HF, Varley GA, et al. Classification of corneal endothelial disorders based on neural crest origin. *Ophthalmology* 1984;91(6):558–563.
14. Hollenberg MJ, Spira AW. Human retinal development: ultrastructure of the outer retina. *Am J Anat* 1973;137(4):357–385.
15. Ozanics V, Rayborn M, Sagun D. Some aspects of corneal and scleral differentiation in the primate. *Exp Eye Res* 1976;22(4):305–327.
16. Ehlers N, Matthiessen ME, Andersen H. The prenatal growth of the human eye. *Acta Ophthalmologica* 1968;46(3):329–349.
17. Sevel D, Isaacs R. A re-evaluation of corneal development. *Tran Am Ophthalmol Soc* 1988;86:178–207.
18. Mandell RB. Corneal contour of the human infant. *Arch Ophthalmol* 1967;77(3): 345–348.
19. Inagaki Y. The rapid change of corneal curvature in the neonatal period and infancy. *Arch Ophthalmol* 1986;104(7):1026–1027.
20. Insler MS, Cooper HD, May SE, et al. Analysis of corneal thickness and corneal curvature in infants. *CLAO J* 1987;13(3):182–184.
21. Barishak YR. The development of the angle of the anterior chamber in vertebrate eyes. *Doc Ophthalmol* 1978;45(2):329–360.
22. Hamanaka T, Bill A, Ichinohasama R, et al. Aspects of the development of Schlemm's canal. *Exp Eye Res* 1992;55(3):479–488.
23. Anderson DR. The development of the trabecular meshwork and its abnormality in primary infantile glaucoma. *Trans Am Ophthalmol Soc* 1981;79:458–485.
24. Kupfer C, Ross K. The development of outflow facility in human eyes. *Investigative Ophthalmology* 1971;10(7): 513–517.
25. Pandolfi M, Astedt B. Outflow resistance in the foetal eye. *Acta Ophthalmol* 1971;49(2):344–350.
26. Arora R, Aggarwal HC, Sood NN. Observations on the histopathology of trabecular meshwork with reference to the pathogenesis of congenital glaucoma. *Glaucoma* 1990;12(4):112–116.
27. Kupfer C, Kaiser-Kupfer MI. Observations on the development of the anterior chamber angle with reference to the pathogenesis of congenital glaucomas. *Am J Ophthalmol* 1979;88(3 Pt 1):424–426.
28. Doran RM. Anterior segment malformations: aetiology and genetic implications. *Br J Ophthalmol* 1991;75(10): 579.
29. Tucker SM, Enzenauer RW, Levin AV, et al. Corneal diameter, axial length, and intraocular pressure in premature infants. *Ophthalmology* 1992;99(8): 1296–1300.
30. Spierer A, Huna R, Hirsh A, et al. Normal intraocular pressure in premature infants. *Am J Ophthalmol* 1994;117(6):801–803.
31. Spierer A, Isenberg SJ, Inkelis SH. Characteristics of the iris in 100 neonates. *J Pediatr Ophthalmol Strabismus* 1989;26(1):28–30.
32. Mund ML, Rodrigues MM, Fine BS. Light and electron microscopic observations on the pigmented layers of the developing human eye. *Am J Ophthalmol* 1972;73(2): 167–182.
33. Isenberg SJ, Molarte A, Vazquez M. The fixed and dilated pupils of premature neonates. *Am J Ophthalmol* 1990;110(2): 168–171
34. Robinson J, Fielder AR. Pupillary diameter and reaction to light in preterm neonates. *Arch Dis Child* 1990;65(1 Spec No):35–38.
35. Zhu M, Madigan MC, van Driel D, et al. The human hyaloid system: cell death and vascular regression. *Exp Eye Res* 2000;70(6): 767–776.
36. Michaelson IC. The mode of development of the vascular system of the retina with some observations on its significance for certain retinal diseases. *Trans Ophthalmol Soc UK* 1948;68:137–180.
37. Robinson SR, Hendrickson A. Shifting relationships between photoreceptors and pigment epithelial cells in monkey retina: implications for the development of retinal topography. *Vis Neurosci* 1995;12(4):767–778.
38. McConnell SK, Kaznowski CE. Cell cycle dependence of laminar determination in developing neocortex. *Science* 1991; 254(5029):282–285.

39. Yuodelis C, Hendrickson A. A qualitative and quantitative analysis of the human fovea during development. *Vision Res* 1986;26(6):847–855.

40. Wassle H, Grunert U, Rohrenbeck J, et al. Retinal ganglion cell density and cortical magnification factor in the primate. *Vision Res* 1990;30(11):1897–1911.

41. Provis JM, van Driel D. Retinal development in humans: the roles of differential growth rates, cell migration and naturally occurring cell death. *Aust NZ J Ophthalmol* 1985;13(2):125–133.

42. Wilmer HA, Scammon RE. Growth of the components of the human eyeball. I. Diagrams, calculations, computations and reference tables. *Arch Ophthalmol* 1950;43(4): 599–619.

43. Scammon RE, Wilmer HA. Growth of the components of the human eyeball. II. Comparison of the calculated volumes of the eyes of the newborn and of adults, and their components. *Arch Ophthalmol* 1950; 43(4):620–637.

44. Rakic P, Riley KP. Overproduction and elimination of retinal axons in the fetal rhesus monkey. *Science* 1983;219(4591):1441–1444.

45. Hitchcock PF, Hickey TL. Prenatal development of the human lateral geniculate nucleus. *J Comp Neurol* 1980;194(2):395–411.

46. Kostovic I, Rakic P. Developmental history of the transient subplate zone in the visual and somatosensory cortex of the macaque monkey and human brain. *J Comp Neurol* 1990;297(3):441–470.

47. Palamini A, Anderman F, Olier A, et al. Focal neuronal migration disorders and intractable partial epilepsy; Results of surgical treatment. *Ann Neurol* 1991;30: 750–757.

48. Rakic P. Neurons in rhesus monkey visual cortex: systematic relation between time of origin and eventual disposition. *Science* 1974;183(123):425–427.

49. Desai AR, McConnell SK. Progressive restriction in fate potential by neural progenitors during cerebral cortical development. *Development* 2000;127(13):2863–2872.

50. Dobyns WB, Truwit CL. Lissencephaly and other malformations of cortical development: 1995 update. *Neuropediatrics* 1995; 26(3):132–147.

51. Dobyns WB, Andermann E, Andermann F, et al. X-linked malformations of neuronal migration. *Neurology* 1996;47(2):331–339.

52. Williams RW, Ryder K, Rakic P. Emergence of cytoarchitectonic differences between areas 17 and 18 in the developing rhesus monkey. *Abstr Soc Neurosci* 1987;13: 1044.

53. Robinson SR, Dreher B. The visual pathways of eutherian mammals and marsupials develop according to a common timetable. *Brain Behav Evol* 1990;36(4): 177–195.

54. Sperry RW. Chemoaffinity in the orderly growth of nerve fiber patterns and connections. *Proc Natl Acad Sci U S A* 1963;50:703–709.

55. Campbell DS, Holt CE. Chemotropic responses of retinal growth cones mediated by rapid local protein synthesis and degradation [see comment]. *Neuron* 2001; 32(6):1013–1026.

56. Brittis PA, Canning DR, Silver J. Chondroitin sulfate as a regulator of neuronal patterning in the retina. *Science* 1992;255(5045):733–736.

57. Deiner MS, Kennedy TE, Fazeli A, et al. Netrin-1 and DCC mediate axon guidance locally at the optic disc: loss of function leads to optic nerve hypoplasia. *Neuron* 1997;19(3):575–589.

58. Oster SF, Deiner M, Birgbauer E, et al. Ganglion cell axon pathfinding in the retina and optic nerve. *Semin Cell Dev Biol* 2004;15(1):125–136.

59. Nishiyama M, Hoshino A, Tsai L, M, et al. Cyclic AMP/GMP-dependent modulation of Ca^{2+} channels sets the polarity of nerve growth-cone turning. *Nature* 2003;424(6943):990–995.

60. Hevner RF. Development of connections in the human visual system during fetal mid-gestation: a DiI-tracing study. *J Neuropathol Exp Neurol* 2000;59(5):385–392.

61. Rakic P. Prenatal development of the visual system in rhesus monkey. *Philos Trans R Soc Lond B Biol Sci* 1977;278(961):245–260.

62. Lund RD, Mustari MJ. Development of the geniculocortical pathway in rats. *J Comp Neurol* 1977;173(2):289–306.

63. Shatz CJ, Luskin MB. The relationship between the geniculocortical afferents and their cortical target cells during development of the cat's primary visual cortex. *J Neurosci* 1986;6(12):3655–3668.

64. Molliver ME, Kostovic I, van der Loos H. The development of synapses in cerebral cortex of the human fetus. *Brain Res* 1973; 50(2):403–407.

65. Hubel DH, Wiesel TN. Binocular interaction in striate cortex of kittens reared with artificial squint. *J Neurophysiol* 1965;28(6): 1041–1059.

66. Hubel DH, Wiesel TN, LeVay S. Plasticity of ocular dominance columns in monkey striate cortex. *Philos Trans R Soc Lond B Biol Sci* 1977;278(961):377–409.

67. Hebb DO. *The Organization of Behavior; A Neuropsychological Theory.* New York: Wiley; 1949.

68. Khan AA, Wadhwa S, Bijlani V. Development of human lateral geniculate nucleus: an electron microscopic study. *Int J Dev Neurosci* 1994;12(7):661–672.

69. Sretavan DW, Shatz CJ, Stryker MP. Modification of retinal ganglion cell axon morphology by prenatal infusion of tetro-dotoxin. *Nature* 1988;336(6198):468–471.

70. Shatz CJ, Stryker MP. Prenatal tetrodotoxin infusion blocks segregation of retinogeniculate afferents. *Science* 1988;242(4875):87–89.

71. Mooney R, Penn AA, Gallego R, et al. Thalamic relay of spontaneous retinal activity prior to vision. *Neuron* 1996;17(5):863–874.

72. Galli L, Maffei L. Spontaneous impulse activity of rat retinal ganglion cells in prenatal life. *Science* 1988;242(4875):90–91.

73. Shatz CJ. Form from function in visual system development. In: *The Harvey Lectures, Series 93.* New York: Wiley-Liss; 1999:17–34.

74. Meister M, Wong RO, Baylor DA, et al. Synchronous bursts of action potentials in ganglion cells of the developing mammalian retina. *Science* 1991;252(5008):939–943.

75. Kiorpes L, Kiper DC, O'Keefe LP, et al. Neuronal correlates of amblyopia in the visual cortex of macaque monkeys with experimental strabismus and anisometropia. *J Neurosci* 1998;18(16):6411–6424.

76. Mitchell DE, Timney B. Postnatal development of function in the mammalian visual system. In: *Handbook of Physiology. The Nervous System III. Vol. 3.* Washington, DC: American Physiological Society; 1984:501–555.

77. Sur M, Leamey CA. Development and plasticity of cortical areas and networks. *Nature Reviews Neuroscience* 2001;2(4):251–262.

78. Berardi N, Pizzorusso T, Ratto GM, Maffei L. Molecular basis of plasticity in the visual cortex. *Trends Neurosci* 2003;26(7):369–378.

79. Huttenlocher PR, de Courten C. The development of synapses in striate cortex of man. *Human Neurobiology* 1987;6(1):1–9.

80. Banks MS, Aslin RN, Letson RD. Sensitive period for the development of human binocular vision. *Science* 1975;190(4215): 675–677.

2 Visual Acuity in the Young Child

Robert H. Duckman

Ask the question: "Why does the clinician measure visual acuity in the adult?" The answer would be that, in the adult, visual acuity is a relatively simple and reliable clinical finding that should be a good indication of that person's visual function. If visual acuity were diminished, the clinician would take that finding as a sign that some interruption had occurred to normal acuity (e.g., refractive error, cataracts, retinal disease, or other ocular pathology). It could also indicate a dysfunction of ocular motility (e.g., nystagmus or eccentric fixation), central nervous system disease, and so forth. Ocular disease and visual acuity are usually highly correlated with one notable exception—glaucoma. Visual acuity is the foremost single test used to describe visual function of a human being. In the adult population, it determines whether people can qualify for a license to drive a car or fly a plane, be a police officer, or serve in the armed forces. It may not be the *best* gauge of a person's visual function, but visual acuity is surely the easiest and fastest means of determining if a person's visual function is in tact. This may not, however, be the case with infants. A series of developmental processes must occur before visual acuity can be considered to be 20/20. It has been demonstrated that infants under the age of 48 weeks post-conceptional age (PCA) with compromised visual cortices can demonstrate normal visual behaviors (1). In addition, the acquisition of visual acuity data is done by different methodologies than it is in the adult;

therefore, although it gives us data, it may not necessarily be comparable data, regarding visual acuity.

Clinically, the visual acuity finding is used to "guide" us through the examination. That is, if visual acuity is normal (Snellen VA 20/20), the clinician can infer that little refractive error exists, probably the macula areas are healthy, and no pathology is present that compromises the acuity of the person. Can the clinician make the same assumptions when measuring the infant's visual acuity? Not necessarily. Visual acuity development in the human infant follows the "law of improvement" (i.e., developmentally, the visual acuity starts out poorly and, over time, gets better). Much of the improvement results from *anatomic* and *physiologic* changes that occur in normal development (see Chapter 1). Decreased visual acuity in the infant, thus, does not give the clinician the same assurance that visual function is in some way disrupted. Rather, it must be considered within a developmental time table and the status of the infant during testing. If a testing procedure demands attention and the child is not sufficiently attentive, visual acuity values would be lower than they would be if the child were fully attentive. Subsequent visits, with the child in a more "cooperative" state, could yield more accurate and better acuity values. If during the examination the child is inattentive and uncooperative, it is often necessary to reschedule the child for another appointment.

Also, again remember that, depending on the child's age and the measuring instrument, it is *normal* to find infant acuity to be lower than that of an adult. In the evaluation of infant visual acuity, it is expected and common to find lower acuity values in the absence of any significant clinical findings. Then, with growth and maturation, the test results will approach adult levels of acuity, but at different times for different techniques and different individuals.

The infant is born with *expected* and *normal* lowered visual acuity. Visual acuity is expected to improve over the course of time. This chapter examines this development and how it proceeds. Normative data are important if we want to make any statement about an individual child's visual function. In the pediatric population, any visual acuity measurement must be considered within the context of two pieces of information:

1. What methodology was used to measure the visual acuity?
2. How old is the child?

For example, if an infant is shown to have 20/100 visual acuity, we cannot know if this is a normal finding or an abnormal finding until we have answered the two questions. If the child is 8 months old and the measurement is done with visual evoked potentials (VEP), the finding would be abnormal because the infant 6-months of age should be able to respond to checkerboard squares equivalent to 20/20 on a VEP. If, however, the child is 6 months old and the methodology used is forced choice preferential looking, this would be an expected and normal acuity value for the child at this age.

Before discussing the development of visual acuity, it is important to define the different types of visual acuities that can be measured. Basically, four types of acuity measurement are used, which will be discussed. Each is different and comparison between types may be inappropriate. For example, if a child has a spatial acuity of 30 cycles per degree (spatial separation equivalent to 20/20 acuity) and another child has a recognition acuity of 20/20, they should not be compared as if equivalent. They are not!

The four types of visual acuity that are generally considered are:

1. *Minimum visible* or *detection acuity* is being able to tell that a given visual stimulus is present or not, or what is the smallest stimulus an individual can detect. Detection acuity is not the best descriptor of visual acuity because it is stimulus bound (i.e., by changing the strength of the stimulus you can alter the visual acuity value). If, for example, you take a very small opening in an otherwise opaque background and put a light stimulus behind the hole and the person may or may not see it. If, however, the person does not see it, and you can increase illumination until the individual is able to tell that it is there, you will have changed the acuity by changing the stimulus. If modulating the stimulus can change the acuity, it may be an inaccurate way to quantify acuity.

2. *Minimum separable* or *resolution acuity* is a measure of a person's ability to detect separation of contours. The smaller the separation of the acuity prototype elements that the person can resolve, the better the resolution acuity (Fig. 2.1).

    Teller acuity cards (TAC) present square wave spatial frequency gratings on a gray background matched for mean luminance in a forced choice preferential looking (FPL) paradigm. The patient will be attracted to the striped stimulus as long as the contours between the black and white stripes can be seen. Once the width of the stripes falls below the child's threshold to resolve the detail, the infant will no longer be able to perceive the square wave gratings as a striped field. It will blend into a gray field that has been matched to the mean luminance of the gray background. Now, instead of seeing a striped stimulus on a gray background, the child will see a gray stimulus on a gray background. Once this happens, the preference the child had previously demonstrated for the striped stimulus, disappears. As long as the child is capable of *resolving* the stimulus detail and is attending to the task, the preference will be noted. The highest spatial frequency (narrowest

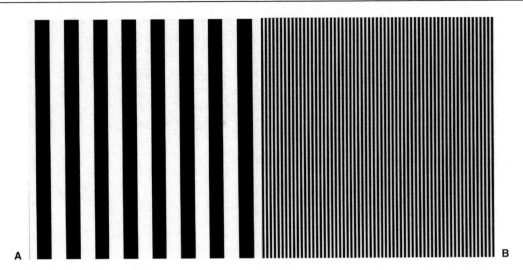

FIGURE 2.1. **A:** Spatial frequency square wave grating—higher spatial frequency. **B:** Spatial frequency square wave grating—lower spatial frequency.

line width) that produces a positive preference response will be the minimal separable visual acuity or spatial acuity. As with other types of acuity measures, minimal separable acuity starts out poorly and improves over time. Although most discussions of minimal separable visual acuities equate them to Snellen acuity equivalents on the basis of angular subtense, the minimal separable acuity is not synonymous with recognition acuity (see below).

3. *Vernier acuity* (hyperacuity) is a measure of the eye's ability to perceive that a disalignment exists between the elements of the stimulus when compared with a stimulus without such disalignment. The eye has a better ability to perceive the disalignment than to be able to resolve adjacent contours (resolution acuity) by a factor that changes over time and from 3 months on surpasses resolution acuity (2–4). Therefore, this is often referred to as *hyperacuity.* Hyperacuity can be measured via an FPL type paradigm where the infant will show a preference for the disaligned square wave grating stimulus over the aligned stimulus as long as the disalignment can be perceived (Fig. 2.2).

4. *Recognition acuity* is the type of acuity measurement normally used clinically on patients who are old enough to subjectively report what they see on the typical Snellen acuity letter chart, pictures, numbers, and

so forth. The age at which children can do this varies greatly, but starts at about 2 to 2.5 years of age. It involves being able to resolve the detail in the optotype and, on a cognitive level, to identify what the stimulus is. The differences between number or letter optotypes and pictures will be discussed in Chapter 10. Now, it is important to be aware that acuity values tend to be somewhat higher when picture optotypes are used than when letter or number optotypes are used. Recognition acuity, however, is the most universally used acuity measurement on patients who are old enough to respond to this type of testing.

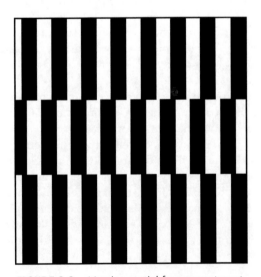

FIGURE 2.2. Vernier spatial frequency target.

Visual acuity values in infancy and early childhood are reflective of the acuity technique being used, the critical immaturities of the visual system (see Chapter 1), the child's developmental status, cognitive awareness, and attention to the visual input.

For decades clinicians and researchers have looked at the development of visual acuity. During that time, the base of knowledge has changed significantly because of increased understanding of visual development and the increasing sophistication of the experimental paradigms being used to measure function. Before the vision scientist can look at the development of visual acuity, an instrument or instruments must be available to measure that function. The development of these instruments started in the laboratory and, as soon as *practicable*, spread throughout the clinical community.

Teller and Movshon (4) described the "ancient history" of visual development as the early *1960s*. And if you examine the work on visual development before the 1960s, "you will not have far to travel." It is sparse and often the results are questionable. For example, before this time, the only real work on visual acuity in infants used optokinetic nystagmus (OKN) as the measuring tool. Aside from being a difficult observation to make in infants (observers often filmed a baby's eyes during the presentations so they could go back afterward to study whether the OKN was present), it has been shown that infants with considerable loss or total absence of visual cortex can demonstrate OKN (5–7). Daw (8) reported that "OKN is believed to be primarily a subcortical phenomenon, and needs a stimulus covering a substantial amount of the visual field." For an observer to elicit the OKN response, a child must *attend* to the drum and *accommodate* to its surface. The absence of a response might be nothing more than inattention. Thus, we are *unable* to draw definitive conclusions from either its presence or its absence.

In the early 1960s, Fantz (9–11) published his results of looking at an infant's pattern preferences using a procedure called "preferential looking" (PL). By 1962, Fantz et al. (12) published data on the early development of visual acuity by use of his PL technique and compared it with OKN responses by the same infants. The

acuity values that Fantz reported, at that time, closely reflect acuity values currently accepted for infants' spatial vision.

As recently as the early 1970s, if parents asked a pediatrician or eye care professional what their baby's vision was, the typical response would be something like "We will have to wait until around 5 years to know for sure. However, your baby fixes and follows" (meaning that the child could fixate and track a transilluminator or other visual stimulus). Indeed, many continue to evaluate an infant's early visual function on the basis of the "fix and follow" response. An ever increasing number of clinicians, however, attempt to quantify, either electrophysiologically or behaviorally, the visual acuity of the infant or toddler patient. This turning point for clinical evaluation of infants' visual acuity resulted from the work that Fantz published in the 1950s, 1960s, and 1970's. Fantz (13) noticed that infants had definite preferences when it came to looking at objects. His work clearly showed that these preferences were the natural predilection of the healthy, normal human infant. Infants, when given a choice, will show definite behavioral differences and prefer to look at objects with higher contrast, greater number of contours, and greater complexity over more simple patterns or homogenous backgrounds (13). In 1975, Fantz and Fagan (14) published findings showing that during the first 6 months of life, infants differentially prefer to look at objects of greater complexity over objects of simpler design. Later that same year, Fantz and Miranda (15) found that *neonates* show a differential preference for curved lines over straight lines. The other issue of interest is that these predilections were directly related to PCA and not chronological age. Fantz did an enormous amount of "observing" of infant visual behavior, and the message is that, given the choice to fixate a patterned field over an unpatterned, homogenous field matched for mean luminance, the infant will look at the patterned field. This is the basic premise of what has become the most utilized behavioral, clinical technique to evaluate visual function in infants today—forced choice preferential looking.

Forced choice preferential looking has evolved over approximately the past 35 years. It uses the premise that infants prefer to fixate "something" over nothing at all. When the "something" is a spatial frequency grating, the assumption is that if spatial frequency is paired with a homogenous gray field of *matched* luminance, as long as the child can resolve the stripes as stripes, the infant will prefer to fixate that target. When the spatial frequency falls below threshold and the infant's ability to resolve detail has been surpassed, the stripes will now appear gray and the preference previously seen for the pattern disappears.

The typical stimulus for FPL has almost always been square wave spatial frequency gratings. Spatial frequency gratings are described by the number of *cycles* (one black stripe and one white stripe per cycle) they subtend at the eye per degree of visual angle. The lower the number of cycles, the fewer the number of black and white stripes per degree of visual angle. The greater the number of cycles per degree of visual angle, the greater the number of stripes. Thus, high spatial frequencies are finer black and white lines than lower spatial frequencies lines, which are wider. A spatial frequency that is easy to remember is the spatial frequency of 30 cycles per degree (cpd). Thirty cycles per degree is equivalent to the resolution necessary to see 20/20 optotypes. It is unclear whether these acuity values are equivalent and they probably are not. In any case, it is not appropriate to express spatial acuity in Snellen equivalence (although it is done all the time), but rather they should be expressed in cpd.

From the early 1980s through the present time, much data has been collected assessing the visual acuity of infants by behavioral and electrophysiological procedures.

While researching material for this chapter and to offer an idea of the growth in interest in the area of infant vision, a search from 1960 to 1970 on infant visual acuity produced citations of just over one page (15). The same topic sampled from 1970 to 1980 produced 17 pages of citations (244).

FORCED CHOICE PREFERENTIAL LOOKING

As early as 1978, Dobson et al. (16) were exploring the utilization of the innate response of the infant to preferentially fixate a pattern over nothing at all in a behavioral paradigm to quantify "visual acuity," perhaps the beginning of FPL as a *clinical* tool. *Before* this, however, significant data were collected by psychometric means to establish the norms for this type of "acuity" measurement. In the psychometric procedure, the researchers would take *all* their spatial frequency slides, match them up with slides of equal luminance and randomly place all of them in pairs for presentation to the infants. Two people were required to run the paradigm—one to make the presentations to the infant and the "blind" observer who would watch to see where the child looked. The person controlling the presentations would record whether the "blind" observer was correct or incorrect. After *all* presentations were made, the psychometrists would go back and score the responses to see at which spatial frequency value the observer (infant) fell below 75% criterion level for correct responses. For example, if a child "saw" three quarters of the presentations at 4.9 cpd, but only half of the presentations at 6.5 cpd, then that child's threshold visual acuity would be 4.9 cpd. This paradigm involved a minimum of two people, sufficient time to make more than 100 presentations and a cooperative, attentive infant throughout the testing. Psychometric measurement could never be used clinically because it took too long, often requiring multiple visits to define threshold acuity. This was not a tenable *clinical* tool. It was an extremely difficult research procedure as well. In an attempt to make the FPL procedure easier and less time consuming, change came in the form of procedural "short cuts" (17–21).

In an attempt to streamline the procedure, Dobson et al. (22) attempted to define the "diagnostic stripe widths" (DSW) for infants at different ages. They wanted to find the age norms for FPL and what should be expected of a child by a certain age. Dobson et al. (22) obtained what they called "a preliminary estimate of the DSW." The study had a sample of 76 normal infants, of whom 69 infants (91%) completed testing. Dobson acknowledged that normative data would require a larger sample. The success with which the data were collected confirmed ages at which visual acuity levels should be attained. Dobson et al. defined the DSW as "the minimum stripe width to which infants with normal visual acuity will readily respond" at a given age. They evaluated children 4, 8, 12, and 16 weeks of age to find the minimal stripe width to which each age group would respond. This was one of the earliest attempts to take FPL out of the laboratory and into clinical use. With known values of what an infant should respond to by a given age, a clinician would be able to tell whether visual acuity for any child was normal for age. It *would not* provide a visual acuity threshold. The idea was that with norms for given ages, the clinician would take spatial frequency gratings of that child's diagnostic stripe width, show them a set of spatial frequency slides with their matched grays, and see whether the blind observer was correct 70% to 75% of the time. If so, the clinician could say that visual acuity development was *normal* for this child. The clinician would not know whether the infant could see better than his or her DSW, but would know that this child was where he or she was supposed to be for normal vision development. It was a much more practical thing to do clinically. In time, the following DSW were determined and utilized in the DSW procedure: The age norms for FPL DSW procedure are discussed below with the approximate Snellen equivalents (Table 2.1).

Dobson (21) discussed the slowness of behavioral techniques from the laboratory entering the clinical arena. She observed that OKN "is used widely by ophthalmologists as an informal, subjective estimate of an infant's visual status." The shortcomings of the OKN response limits it in the amount of information it can provide. On the other hand, the emergence of the FPL procedures, in the form of the diagnostic stripe width procedure, that had only recently been introduced into clinical settings,

promised a lot more. Dobson further observed that the procedure "appears to be effective in diagnosing infants with ophthalmic problems that would be expected to interfere with vision tested binocularly."

About the same time, Gwiazda et al. (23,24) started using their "fast" PL procedure to collect data on normal infants during the first year of life. Their babies ranged in age from 2 to 58 weeks of age. In the healthy, normal infant without visual problems, their technique measured visual acuity in less than 5 minutes—a vast improvement over the psychometric procedures discussed earlier. Although the data they were trying to gather replicated earlier experiments, the earlier data were collected with a much lengthier paradigm—the 60-trial method of constant stimuli. They were looking to see if the faster method produced similar results. They used gratings ranging from 1.5 to 18 cpd in approximately half octave steps. They measured acuity for horizontal, vertical, and right oblique gratings. They found that a *steady increase* in acuity occurred from 4 weeks to 1 year of age. Acuity for horizontal and vertical spatial frequency gratings increased from 20/1200 at 4 weeks to 20/50 for horizontal and 20/60 for vertical at 1 year of age.

In 1982, Mayer et al. (25) used a staircase PL presentation to evaluate visual acuity in children aged 11 days to 5 years, known to have an ophthalmologic disorder. In the *psychometric* PL measurement of acuity in infants, it was necessary to take all the spatial frequency slides with their matched grays, randomly present them in pairs, and go through all the stimuli before going back to see where the responses fell below the criterion level of 70%. With the staircase presentation, the stimuli were presented in pairs, except the pairs were ordered from lowest spatial frequency (widest stripes) to highest spatial frequency (thinnest stripes). The experimenter would then start at the beginning of "the staircase" (lowest spatial frequency) with stimulus pairs, and continue presenting them until the child stopped showing a preference for a stimulus 70% of the time. At that point, the experimenter would have a *threshold* visual acuity, and no trials would be given beyond that threshold level. This significantly decreased the amount of time for both testing and scoring these patients.

TABLE 2.1 Diagnostic Stripe Width from 1–9 Months

Age	Angular Subtense	Snellen Equivalent
1–2 Months	40′	20/800
3 Months	30′	20/600
4 Months	20′	20/400
6 Months	5′	20/100
9 Months	2.5′	20/50

Mayer et al. (25) noted that "acuity of infants and young children with normal eyes, obtained by the PL staircase procedure" agreed well with acuities obtained previously by the method of constant stimuli. This was a good indication that the faster methodology would yield visual acuities as accurate as the longer one.

The measurement of infant and toddler visual acuity by behavioral methods grew in popularity in the 1980s. FPL was a technique which provided the clinician with important information about an infant's visual function. As the technique became more popular, more and more data were available to define norms and streamline the procedure. With the advent of the commercially available Teller acuity cards in the mid 1980s, the clinical use of the technique came into its own. Slowly, more and more clinicians were embracing these cards as a crucial part of an infant visual examination. It had been noted early on that this was a technique that worked very well on infants up to about 10 to 12 months of age. As the infants become more interested in the world around them, their interest in black and white lines diminishes. Thus, the outside limit of successful measurement of acuity in infants was about 12 months. Of course, this is within a normal infant population. The FPL technique works successfully much longer when dealing with a population of multiply handicapped children (26). Developmentally disabled children will attend to the targets almost indefinitely. With normal children, however, FPL loses efficacy at about 1 year. From 1 to 2 years of age, an age during which a huge amount of development takes place and amblyopia often begins, it again becomes difficult to measure acuity. Thus, researchers started "playing around" with operant conditioning paradigms to measure behavioral visual acuity in the older infant and toddler. Dobson et al. (27) utilized the operant FPL (OFPL) to attempt behaviorally to measure acuity in children from 6 months to 3 years and to define diagnostic grating frequencies to use for screening visual acuity in this 6- to 36-month-old age group. To do so, however, they had to use an operant conditioning procedure to maintain the children's participation in the acuity measurement. Each child was trained to look at or point to a low spatial frequency grating. Each time they did

it correctly, a positive reinforcement (a mechanical toy would go off) was given. This continued for enough trials to be sure the child was responding to the stripes. Then, each child was tested to find what was termed the "diagnostic grating frequency" for children aged 12 months to 36 months. The results indicated a definable diagnostic grating frequency for all the age groups tested, except children 18 months of age. A chart of expected diagnostic grating frequencies was then published (Table 2.2).

The criterion used to define and establish the diagnostic frequency grating for each age was, for any given age, 90% of the children in that category had reach the acuity level and the frequency that was separated by one half to one octave from the next higher spatial frequency. Although not part of the discussed work, the authors chose to include data from an earlier work that evaluated infants aged 1 to 6 months with FPL.

Teller et al. (28) described the acuity card procedure as simplified and quick in the measurement of visual acuity by an FPL (behavioral) methodology. The general consensus of researchers working with FPL to evaluate visual acuity in infants has been that this procedure works well with infants and children, is fast and accurate, and is useful for both a normal population of children as well as children with visual and neurologic impairment (Fig. 2.3). They maintained that this procedure worked well in the laboratory, but now the possibility existed of using it as a clinical tool. The same group (29) also measured monocular acuities in normal infants using the TAC and found this method an accurate means of measuring monocular acuity during the first year of life. Preston et al.

TABLE 2.2 Diagnostic Grating Frequencies—Ages 1 Month to 36 Months

Age (months)	Procedure	Diagnostic Grating (cpd)
12	OFPL	4.6
18	OFPL	?
24	OFPL	6.9
30	OFPL	11.1
36	OFPL	11.1

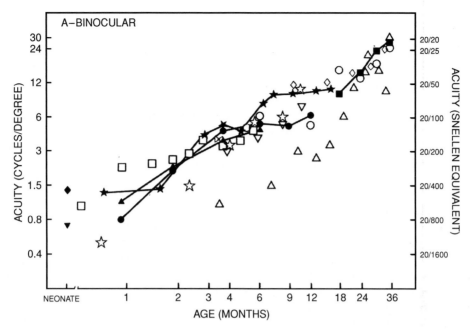

FIGURE 2.3. Development of behavioral visual acuity from 1–36+ months. Table 20.1, page 324 from *Early Visual Development: Normal and Abnormal,* edited by Kurt Simons, copyright 1993 by Oxford University Press, Inc. Used by permission of Oxford University Press, Inc.

(30) found that the acuity card procedure was effective in measuring acuity in eyes affected by some kind of ocular pathology (e.g., aphakia, ptosis, strabismus).

Although it is important to have a mechanism to test visual acuity in normal children, the more important issue is to identify children with visual acuity deficits. Once norms were established, the FPL technique could be used on a visually "abnormal" group of children. Several studies generated clear data that the FPL paradigm and the acuity card procedure were effective in identifying infants with abnormal visual acuity. One such study (31) looked at 397 infants and young children known to be normal and found a slow, but continuous development of visual acuity to grating acuity targets from 1 month to 5 years of age going from 1.8 cpd (20/330) at 0 to 2 months to 32 cpd (20/19) at 49 to 60 months. Then, they turned their attention to children with known monocular visual acuity deficits. They found that the FPL procedure was effective in identifying monocular grating acuity deficit. By this time, norms were established, and the acuity cards were commercially available and being widely used for clinical purposes. In addition, Mohn et al. (32) did

some clinical work with the TAC on a population of nonverbal infants and children, both neurologically normal and neurologically abnormal. They were successful in obtaining visual acuity estimates on most of their 842 binocular and 279 monocular tests. They concluded that their findings for the neurologically normal children agreed well with previous data. Children at risk for later neurologic involvement, but developing normally, demonstrated only a slight delay in the development of visual acuity. Those with severe neurologic defects, however, demonstrated low acuity for their age most of the time. The conclusion was that the TAC were effective in evaluating acuity in both normal and neurologically involved children.

Contrast sensitivity function (CSF), a more comprehensive descriptor of visual function than visual acuity, is typically measured with sine wave spatial frequency gratings, whereas visual acuity (spatial vision) had routinely been assessed with square wave gratings. Are the two comparable? In 1990, Jackson et al. (33) developed a set of acuity cards using sine wave gratings instead of the commonly used square wave gratings. They had 83 subjects with a mean age of 41.5 months (range 3–69 months). They compared their cards with the TAC and in 83% of their subjects the TAC acuity was identical to their sine wave acuity. They determined that the sine wave spatial cards can be used to measure FPL in children. TAC cards, however, are far more widely used to measure visual acuity in infants and young children and in developmentally handicapped children than are the sine wave spatial frequency grating cards.

The TAC procedure has been adopted as the best measure of "subjective" acuity in a preverbal population, and enjoys both laboratory and clinical popularity. Use of the procedure then started to generate some longitudinal data regarding visual acuity development. Hartmann et al. (34) used the procedure to look at visual acuity in a clinical population of more than 900 children. The patients were a cohort of children in an ophthalmologic practice. The data were not collected without bias and were used primarily to evaluate the result of interventions. Their conclusions were that the TAC procedure was "useful" in monitoring *treatment* regimens in preverbal pediatric ophthalmological patients. They found "the information provided by the acuity card assessments extremely helpful in quantifying the developmental and therapeutic changes in vision, previously monitored only qualitatively" (34).

Vital-Durand (35), acknowledging the increased utilization of TAC procedure in the clinical setting, wanted to test the linearity of visual resolution development. He performed grating acuity measurements on 11 normal children in the first year of life under "optimal" conditions. In doing this he found three things:

1. Grating acuity develops very regularly during the first year of life.
2. The two eyes never differ from each other by more than the smallest difference measurable (one half octave).
3. Binocular acuity was slightly better than monocular acuities

For FPL findings to have significance, they need to be reliable and they need to be repeatable. The question of interobserver reliability when using the TAC to measure visual acuity had to be determined so that visual acuities taken by different clinicians could be compared. This issue was explored by Mash et al. (36), who tested interobserver reliability for acuity and inter-ocular acuity difference in 342 infants and children. The children in this study had been treated in a neonatal intensive care unit for preterm birth or perinatal complications. The subjects were tested binocularly at term, and monocularly at eight different ages (corrected) with TAC. Testers were masked for location of the grating and size of the grating. They found that of the test–retest scores, 67% differed by no more than one half octave, and 87% agreed within one octave. Interocular acuity differences scores agreed within one half octave 54% of the time and 76% of the time were within one octave. Mash et al. (36) concluded that the TAC visual acuity measurement was reliable, but suggested that acuity estimates, which are critical to a patient's diagnosis and subsequent treatment, be confirmed by repeated measurement. Keep in mind that so much depends on a patient's state of arousal, attention, and physical health that these findings seem to be acceptable.

VISUALLY EVOKED POTENTIALS

While behavioral methods of collecting visual acuity data in infants progressed, electrophysiologic methods were also coming into their own. Technology was progressing and, although the hardware was very expensive, the experimenter or clinician who had it available could get an assessment of acuity quickly. Acknowledging the shortfall of assessing the "wiring" and not "perception," the VEP is a reliable tool that could easily be incorporated into an infant examination, given that the instrumentation was available. (The information obtained with VEP speaks to the intactness of the visual system from retina to visual cortex. It says nothing about the *perception* of what the child is *seeing*.) Sokol and Moskowitz (37) compared the responses of infants 3 months of age with patterned VEP and behavioral responses of FPL. VEP were obtained using phase alternated gratings of from 0.31 to 2.50 cpd. FPL data were collected using stationary square wave gratings with the method of constant stimuli or a staircase procedure. They used the same infants to compare their VEP acuities with their FPL acuities. Three important findings emerged:

1. It is possible to get recordable VEP for spatial patterns that are below threshold by behavioral measures. In infants 3 months of age, VEP values for acuity were at least two octaves higher than the behavioral acuities.

2. If different scoring criteria were used such that VEP and FPL group mean acuities were comparable, a significant correlation would be seen between them, but this was not the case.

3. Probably the most interesting finding was that if the VEP *latency* rather than the amplitude was compared to assess acuity, a significant correlation would be seen between electrophysiologic and behavioral findings.

When infant VEP is compared with preferential or forced-choice preferential looking, it is *always* true in normal development and over the first year of life (from about 3 months of age onward) that VEP data are significantly better than FPL data. The reasons have already been discussed, but what happens when the VEP data are compared with FPL data in which the stimuli have been presented as phase alternating gratings? Sokol et al. (38) asked that question. To find the answer, they tested normal infants at various ages and compared acuity findings using various rates of alternation, various ages, and various techniques. In all instances, independent of rate of alternation, VEP acuity was significantly higher than FPL acuity, and both values improved with age. With the passage of time, the VEP rate of development decelerates, whereas the FPL continues and the values of resolution acuity obtained with FPL and VEP approach one another.

Electrophysiologic methodologies have also been used to evaluate the visual function in infants, preverbal children, and developmentally disabled children. The technique measures, at the level of the visual cortex, the electrical potentials generated by the retinal ganglion cells, which travel along the optic pathways and arrive at the cortex. The cortical activity that is received can be recorded by use of an electrode placed just above the inion in the occipital area of the skull. A reference electrode is also needed. To measure a potential to a stimulus, the stimulus must be large enough to stimulate many cells in the visual cortex, which, when fired at the same time, produce a response. The typical stimulus pattern for a VEP is a phase-alternated checkerboard pattern (phase alternation is reversal of stimulus elements such that at any moment squares or stripes will be black and the next moment they will change to white, while the white ones become black). Black and white or colored (e.g., blue and red) squares would work. Spatial frequency gratings (stripes), which are phase-alternated, also work well. The phase alternation is important so the cells do not fatigue. By changing the size of the stimulus elements (i.e., size of the checkerboard squares), the clinician can watch to see where the response to the stimulation is lost and, thereby, determine the visual acuity. Stimulation at a relatively low rate (up to four cycles per second) will produce a transient VEP. Stimulation at higher rates of presentation (10 cycles/sec or greater), however, will produce responses that merge and persist for the duration of the process. These are referred to as steady-state VEPs (39). Patterned VEPs, detect minor visual pathway abnormalities with greater accuracy and sensitivity than do flash VEPs.

Amplitudes of VEPs range from 3 to 20 μV. Because of these small amplitudes, multiple potentials are averaged together to produce an accurate reading (39). One other type of VEP needs to be discussed—sweep VEP. The sweep VEP uses the same type of stimuli as the patterned VEP (i.e., stripes or checkerboard squares). The main difference is that during the "sweep" the stimulus changes size. Therefore, within a 10-second interval, for example, the observer is exposed to many differently sized stimuli going from lowest spatial frequency to highest spatial frequency. The tester would then look at the recordings to see where the "good" response was lost. The major advantage of the sweep VEP is that attention is needed only for a few seconds instead of several minutes to get a threshold acuity measure.

Several types of VEP (40) measurements exist and each has its advantages and disadvantages and each provides different information. The easiest VEP measurement to make is the flash VEP. It requires no attention; the person can actually be sleeping while the procedure is done. A stroboscopic light is placed near the infant's shut eyes, and the light strobes on and off. The light passes through the lids to the retina, causes electrical firing in the retina, which travels through the optic pathways to the visual cortex where firing is recorded by the VEP instrumentation. Because there is no pattern to the stimulus, nothing can be determined about the subject's visual acuity. What is learned is whether or not the visual pathways are intact. Of course, the beauty of the procedure is the speed with which it can be done, and the lack of attention needed from the child. The obvious disadvantage is that the information achieved by doing the test is limited.

Patterned VEP can obtain more information about visual status, but requires significantly greater attention and cooperation. Typically, phase-alternated checkerboard square patterns or stripes are used as targets for patterned VEP. A flash VEP can be performed on a sleeping child, but to successfully record a patterned VEP, the child must be awake, fixating the display, and tolerating the apparatus. This makes it more difficult, but by no means impossible, and it is much faster than the behavioral techniques.

Information obtained through *behavioral* techniques gives the best impression of the infant's *subjective* visual acuity. The behavioral response being sought requires the child to choose, on some cognitive level, that the patterned field is seen and preferred over the homogenous field. The child makes a cognitive decision to look at the pattern as long as the detail can be resolved. With continuing trials, the infant fatigues and the loss of response may mean that a threshold has been reached. It could also mean that the child has tired of the task.

The VEP, which takes significantly less time than FPL, may be more reliable, therefore, in the determination of the child's visual acuity. Especially with the utilization of sweep VEP, the time to reach threshold acuity is a matter of seconds. In a typical sweep VEP, a range of spatial frequency stimuli is presented on a CRT screen over a short period of time (typically 10 seconds). During these 10 seconds, the display goes from the lower spatial frequencies to the higher spatial frequencies with 12 reversals per second, for a total of 120 trials in 10 seconds (Fig. 2.4).

In young children, VEP are especially useful to (a) detect abnormalities of the sensory visual pathways and differentiate visual impairment from visual inattention; (b) to monitor very young patients with known pathology (e.g., retinopathy of prematurity) or children at risk for visual loss from some systemic condition (e.g., hydrocephalus); and (c) to confirm functional loss when visual system disorders are present (41).

The difference between "fix and follow" and 20/20 on a VEP or a FPL is significant. Even children with significant vision impairment can fix and follow a sufficiently strong stimulus such as a transilluminator light. It in no way assures

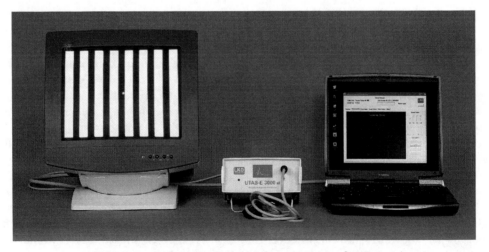

FIGURE 2.4. Sweep VEP apparatus (by permission of LKC Corp.).

that the child has normal visual function. The fix and follow, therefore, is not a means to describe definitively any type of visual function except perhaps detection. The VEP, being an electrophysiologic response to visual input, imparts specific information about the child's ability to resolve detail in a visual stimulus being presented. VEP, however, is not the full story either. VEP provides information about "wiring" of the visual pathways, but not perception. It provides knowledge that the information is getting from the stimulus to the retina, being transmitted through the visual pathways, and is being *received* at the level of the cortex. The VEP is the result of activity in the occipital cortex resulting from the reception of the activity generated in the retina and transduced to the cortex. The electrodes used in the VEP measure this activity at the level of the occipital cortex. The generation of a normal VEP response tells us, therefore, that the information regarding the resolution of detail of the stimulus is sustained in the cortex. It, however, says nothing about the processing of that information beyond occipital cortex. Nonetheless, it provides information on which to believe that the child can see the detail in the stimulus array. This procedure results in a minimal separable or spatial visual acuity measurement.

The work of Fantz (42,43) stirred a lot of curiosity, ultimately leading to the behavioral techniques that allow probing of the visual acuity of preverbal children as well as other visual skills, including binocularity, color perception, and contrast sensitivity function. In other places in this book, other behavioral techniques are described. In the discussion of visual acuity in infancy, however, the only behavioral technique of importance is what is now known as forced-choice preferential looking.

In studies supported by the National Institutes of Health, Fantz (42) explored both the infant's ability to resolve detail in a patterned stimulus and the preferences of the infant regarding the type of contours and form to which it would be attracted. He (42) showed that the infant would be attracted to and attend to the human face more than any other stimulus that could be introduced. Fantz found, in order of preference, that the infant is most strongly attracted to a real human face, then to a photo-

graph of a human face, then to a line drawing of a human face, and then even a discombobulated line drawing of a human face.

This work was done in the 1960s and 1970s when there were few answers to the question, "What can newborn babies see?" Fantz's work brought a lot of attention to this question, when he began demonstrating that infants show very real and consistent patterns of visual behavior. Ultimately, the preference that made clinical measurement of acuity in infants possible was that infants would universally prefer to look at "something" rather than nothing at all. This preference, which was demonstrated by Fantz and Miranda (44), Fantz and Fagan (15), Hershenson (45), and others gave birth to the FPL procedure.

OPTOKINETIC NYSTAGMUS

Before forced preferential looking paradigms were introduced and visually evoked potential technology emerged, the only way to quantify visual acuity of infants and toddlers was with optokinetic nystagmus (OKN) drums and canopies. OKN is an involuntary nystagmoid response that is triggered by a moving visual stimulus. The OKN can be elicited when an observer fixates on a moving target. In the case of OKN, that target is a series of black and white stripes. If the infant or toddler, can see the stripes (i.e., resolve the minimal separable detail of the stimulus), then the eye(s) will make a slow movement in the direction of rotation and then a rapid movement back, appearing nystagmoid in nature. This response is involuntary and was assumed to imply that the child was capable of seeing the stripes. By varying stripe width and fixation distance, the technique would give information about the child's visual acuity.

Several problems make the OKN procedure limited, at best, in determining the visual acuity of the infant. First, it is one thing to elicit a response. If a response is not elicited, however, it *does not* mean that the child does not have the ability to resolve the detail of the stimulus. OKN demands that the child fixate at and accommodate to the target. If the infant is "not in the mood," or is highly hyperopic or daydreaming, a response is not elicited. Another consideration is that the contrast resolution required to obtain a Snellen acuity is not the same phenomenon as the perception of vertical stripes moved on a horizontal plane (46). OKN is almost always vertical stripes rotated on a horizontal plane. Vertical stripes in a horizontal rotation, however, stimulate a much larger area of the retina than a Snellen equivalent letter. Another problem that must be considered is the movement of the stimulus in the elicitation of the OKN response. The movement must create interaction between the components of the visual system stimulated by movement and those that are involved in the resolution of detail.

Stripe widths for OKN drums are fixed. To change the angular subtense of the stripe width, the clinician, therefore, would have to move the target out from the child once the OKN was elicited at the starting distance and see at what distance the OKN response is lost. A relatively simple calculation would provide a resolution acuity at the point where the OKN stopped. As the target recedes, however, the angular subtense of the stripes and of the drum occupy less of the child's visual field and a loss in interest develops as this occurs. So does the loss of the response mean that the threshold of visual acuity has been reached or that the child is just no longer interested in the target and attends to something else. As mentioned earlier, the presence of a response indicates the child is "seeing" the target, but the absence of a response does not necessarily mean that the child cannot resolve the detail in the stimulus. Variations on a theme were used by Gorman et al. (47) with the construction of an OKN canopy where the child's head would be placed at the center of a circle such that no matter where the child fixated, the distance from the child to the stripes was equal. The stripes were than moved across the canopy and in front of the child while increasing in spatial frequency (stripes got progressively narrower) until the response was lost. The last stripe width that the child responded to with an OKN response would be defined as that child's visual acuity. The OKN canopy removed some of the variables from the OKN drum procedure, but many of the same factors were still at play regarding the attention and the movement of the target.

In 1983, Van Hof-van Duin and Mohn (48) showed that it was possible to elicit OKN responses from children who did not have a viable cortex or were cortically blind. This indicated that the underlying mechanism of OKN was mediated subcortically. Therefore, even in its presence, it may say nothing about cortical visual function. If OKN can be elicited in cortically blind children, it is important to incorporate that observation into our consideration of OKN as a clinical tool to evaluate visual function in nonverbal children.

Basically, what the clinician has, in the way of clinical tools to assess visual acuity in infants then, are VEP and several versions of FPL. Are the two comparable? In children during the first year of life, the VEP measures of acuity are about 200% better than acuities obtained with FPL. Two primary reasons exist for this: First, the responses are easier to elicit using the VEP because attention does not need to be maintained for as long as in FPL. It is possible to elicit a "flash" VEP (stroboscopic light as a target) while the baby is sleeping. Patterned VEP require higher levels of attention, but over a much shorter time course than FPL. Even with the streamlined FPL procedures of today, attention must be maintained for much longer to reach threshold acuity than VEP. Second, the VEP looks at the intactness of the wiring of the visual system (i.e., can light get from the retina to the cortex without consideration of processing). The FPL is a more cognitive task whereby the stimulus information gets to the cortex, but then the child, based on whether or not he or she can see the stimulus, makes a cognitive decision about visual preference. VEP tells about the integrity of the visual pathways and the FPL procedure more closely estimates what the child actually sees.

Remembering that visual acuity is very much dependent on age and the various testing paradigms, we now need to look at the development of visual acuity, over time, using the different measuring techniques. In all measuring methodologies, whether OKN, FPL or VEP, visual acuity improves from birth. This development is much slower in FPL than in VEP. According to Marg et al. (49), healthy infants were able to show VEP to stimuli with acuity resolution of 20/20 by 6 months of age. At the time, this fact was literally mystifying. Visual resolving power of the eye up to that point was believed to be 20/20, but not until 5 years of age. Marg et al.'s findings probably greatly contributed to the emergence of a new body of data that has led us to a new and much more comprehensive knowledge where visual function can be assessed and clinical visual findings can be ascertained at any age. With our new understanding, we can diagnose and treat earlier than ever before. And we have the means to monitor improvement in visual function affected by the intervention. As an example:

VERNIER ACUITY (HYPERACUITY)

Vernier acuity is of interest to visual developmental researchers because it is a "hyperacuity" based largely on cortical processing. Vernier stimuli have displacements that are smaller than the diameter and spacing of the retinal receptors. To detect such a stimulus "pooling" needs to occur across many receptors that occurs at higher stages of visual processing, needs to be performed. Vernier acuity is the ability to detect

CASE STUDY: J.D.

Patient **Visit 1**: This child was referred from the Brooklyn Infant Study Center regarding a suspected refractive error anomaly at age 4 months. Significant findings of the examination were:

VA (FPL/TAC):	OD	20/150(#2)	OS	20/1600 (#1, i.e., OS tested first)
Refraction:	OD	Plano	OS	−12.00 Sphere

Diagnosis: Anisometropia with OS amblyopia

Disposition: Monocular left eye contact lens (−8.00D) full time with monocular right eye patching for 2 hours per day with simple tracking and reaching activities. Child was to be followed in 4 weeks. Why the undercorrection of the myopic refractive error? It is very important to recognize that a child this age is operating primarily in "near" visual space and it is more important for the child to see clearly at near than at distance.

Patient **Visit 2:** Follow-up examination 4 weeks later. Per history, there was good compliance with contact lens wear, patching, and activities. Child was now 5 months of age.

VA (FPL/TAC):	OD 20/100(#2)	OS	20/400(#1)
Refraction:same as the previous visit:	OD Plano	OS	−12.00 D

Diagnosis and disposition were exactly the same: 2 hours of patching with activities; wear the contact lens full time. Return in 1 month.

Patient **Visit 3**: Follow-up examination 1 month later. Child was now 6 months of age. Compliance was reported to be excellent on contact lens wear, patching, and activities.

VA (FPL/TAC):	OD 20/100(#2)	OS	20/100 (#1)

Diagnosis: Anisometropia, but no longer amblyopia OD, because 20/100 is a normal visual acuity using TAC at age 6 months.

J.D. was initially evaluated by a group of developmental psychologists who were collecting data on *normal* visual development. In so doing, they identified J.D. with abnormal visual development at 4 months of age. The very early identification of the anomaly and the early intervention resulted in a different outcome than might have occurred if the anomaly was identified at 5 years of age, as the child entered school. This example is used to demonstrate how malleable an infant's visual system is, and that a minimal amount of intervention can produce important results at these early ages.

So, when is the infant able to see and when does an acuity value become problematic? Again, we have to search the data that have been collected over the past 30 years or so. To reiterate, variations in visual acuity are dependent on age of the child and the measurement technique. In all instances, visual acuity is better when measured electrophysiologically rather than behaviorally with square wave grating acuity cards (TAC) in the infant or toddler population.

a disalignment of two lines (8) (p. 39). In the adult, this measurement is about ten times better than grating acuity (spatial resolution acuity). Vernier acuity, however, does not start out superior to grating acuity and takes awhile to surpass it.

Shimojo et al. (50) assessed Vernier acuity in normal infants from 2 to 9 months of age in an FPL procedure with a "Vernier motion display." The motion in the stimulus is only seen if the Vernier offset is appreciated. In these normal children, they found Vernier acuity starts out worse than grating acuity, but surpasses it after 3 months of age. The authors demonstrated that, after 4 months of age, significant superiority of Vernier acuity over grating acuity, which is maintained. They suggested that the difference between Vernier acuity and grating acuity may be a reliable measure of the development of the central nervous system. Manny and Klein (51,52) measured Vernier acuity in infants 1 to 14 months of age using a dynamic three alternative tracking forced-choice paradigm. They showed that from birth through at least 11 months Vernier acuity improved continuously and was superior to grating acuity. They could not generalize in infants beyond 11 months of age because of poor attention to the stimulus display on the part of the older infants (>11 months). Shimojo and Held (53) studied a group of 22 infants longitudinally and measured both grating acuity (FPL) and Vernier acuity (motion-sound display). They found that grating acuity was superior to Vernier acuity at 11 to 12 weeks of age, but that the developmental rate of Vernier acuity is greater than for grating acuity to at least 20 weeks. They suggest that the infant visual system may be characterized by spatial undersampling. Hyperacuity is generally attributed to cortical mechanisms and runs a different time course than grating acuity (54). Linear offsets can produce VEP using a signal detection mechanism (55).

Vernier acuity, as tested by Shimojo et al. (51), was found to be better than grating acuity from 4 months of age onward. The superiority of Vernier acuity remains from that point on. The authors suggest Vernier (one form of hyperacuity) and stereoacuity (another form of hyperacuity) develop over the same time course and, therefore, may have a common neural mechanism. The age at which these two functions become superior coincides with the segregation of ocular dominance columns in the cortical layer IV (56).

In general, Vernier acuity has been shown to develop rapidly from the time of emergence. Brown (57) found that, at 9 weeks, Vernier acuity was 40 minutes of visual angle. After about 11 weeks Vernier acuity remained constant at approximately 17 minutes of visual angle. Vernier acuity emerged significantly earlier than the other hyperacuity, stereopsis, and stereopsis improves more quickly while Vernier acuity improves more slowly. Brown cites these observations to posit that these two hyperacuities are unlikely to have the same neural mechanism. Skoczenski and Norcia (58), using VEP to look at Vernier acuity, concluded, however, that VEP Vernier acuity remains "strikingly immature throughout the first year of life, as does behavioral Vernier acuity." Again, this difference may be attributable to the method of measurement much the way visual acuity varies using behavioral and electrophysiologic responses. Acuity is probably limited by retinal factors (58).

DEVELOPMENTAL ASPECTS OF VISUAL ACUITY

As mentioned earlier in this chapter, the normal development of visual acuity follows the "Law of Improvement." Simply stated, visual acuity starts out poorly and gets better over time. This is with the assumption that everything falls within normal limits. Early visual acuity is poor whether tested with electrophysiologic or behavioral methodologies. VEP measurements will typically give better visual acuity values than FPL measurements. Then, a gradual improvement in visual acuity develops until it reaches adult levels between 6 and 12 months, when VEP are used to measure the acuity, or about 3 to 5 years, when behavioral techniques are used. The early decreased visual acuity in the infant is usually attributable, at least (59,60), to the following:

1. Foveal cone immaturities: at birth, cones are very short and stumpy with small optical apertures.
2. Cortical immaturities.
3. Incomplete myelination of the optic pathways.

At birth, foveal cones are immature and sparsely populated as compared with the adult fovea. At 15 months, the cones are only half the length of an adult cone. The foveal cones are adult length at approximately 4 years. In addition, the cone density does not reach adult levels until about 45 months and the increase in cone density is a result of foveal cones migrating radially inward while amacrine, bipolar, horizontal, and ganglion cells are migrating radially outward from the fovea. Magoon and Robb (61) showed that myelination progresses from central peripheral to loci. The complete myelination of the optic nerve and the optic pathway takes more than 2 years, although most of it occurs in the first 24 months of life. Myelination of the subcortical pathways is complete by age 3 months, but that of the extrastriate areas by mid-childhood.

Methodologic differences primarily affect the time course over which visual acuity improves. The curve of acuity plotted against age looks similar for VEP and FPL data. The big difference is the time component. VEP data start out poorly and improve rapidly against time over the first year of life. FPL data improve as well, but much more gradually over 3 to 5 years. As seen in Table 2.2, which contains data compiled by Dobson et al. (27) using conditioned forced choice looking (CFPL) and TAC FPL, visual acuity starts out at about 0.8 cycles per degree and gradually and steadily improves to 30 cycles per degree at approximately 3 years of age or later.

Keep in mind that by the time the child is 2.5 to 3 years of age, better ways exist to assess visual acuity—methodologies that will provide the examiner with a recognition acuity rather than a minimal separable acuity. VEP data show that infant acuity reaches adult levels by 6 to 12 months, whereas behavioral data show that FPL infant acuity reaches adult levels between 3 and 5 years of age.

NATURE OR NURTURE

Is the development of vision controlled by environment or genetics? Once, two schools of thought existed regarding this question: one ascribed development to *nature* and one ascribed it to *nurture*. Nature was the school of nativism and nurture was the school of empiricism. People saw things as black or white (i.e., it was all nativism or all empiricism). Neither of these schools could satisfactorily explain everything. Today, it is not so much nature versus nurture as how much is nature and how much is nurture? Therefore, when we study visual development we want to look for the relative contribution of each. One of the first carefully controlled studies to look at this question was that of Brown and Yamamoto (62) (Fig. 2.5). They studied three groups of children:

1. Healthy full term infants
2. Healthy pre-term infants
3. Full-term infants with some health abnormality which was not ophthalmologic

The rationale was that if development of visual acuity was controlled by environment, then the healthy premature infants, with "extra" visual experience, should see better than their paired full-term healthy infant at *corrected* age. In other words, a child born 2 months prematurely, by chronological age 3 months will be a corrected age of 1 month, but will have 3 months of visual experience. So, this corrected aged 1-month-old child would see better than a healthy infant born at term at the age of 1 month. This did not happen, however.

Rather, the visual acuity development followed PCA and *not* chronological age. This supports the *nativistic* view that the development of acuity is genetically programmed. Brown and Yamamoto (62) found that visual acuity develops at the rate of 0.46 octaves per month between 34 and 44 weeks of gestational age. More recently Weinacht et al. (63) found that the additional visual experience which preterm babies have, does not influence the development of their visual acuity (nor binocular vision during the first months of life). Spierer et al. (64) showed that visual acuity (monocular and binocular) as measured with TAC was worse in premature infants than in full-term infants of the same chronological age. These studies all point to the genetic coding of visual acuity development.

This clearly downplays the role of environment in the progression of visual acuity development under normal conditions. If a child were raised in the dark or under some anomalous condition such as a strabismus, however, it is

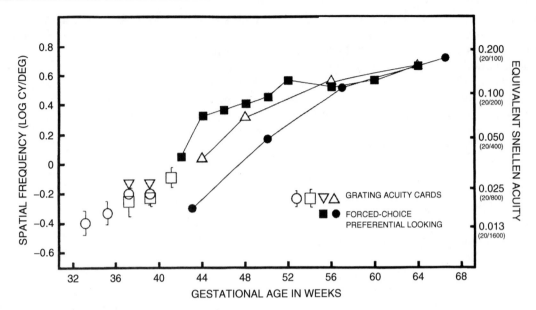

FIGURE 2.5. Development of visual acuity in premature births vs. full term births.

likely that environment would have a significant impact on visual acuity development.

SUMMARY

Visual acuity starts out poorly in the newborn infant and gradually improves over time. Measurement of the acuity indicates a steady increase in function over time until the infant reaches adult acuity. This development occurs much more rapidly when assessed with electrophysiologic methodologies (VEP) than when tested with behavioral methodologies. Behavioral results, however, are probably a more accurate reflection of what the infant is actually seeing. Normative data for both electrophysiologic and behavioral methodologies have been established so that it is now possible to test an infant or toddler rapidly in a clinical setting and determine whether visual acuity is normal.

REFERENCES

1. Dubowitz LM, Mushin J, De Vries L, et al. Visual function in the newborn infant: is it cortically mediated? *Lancet* 1986;1(8490):1139–1141.
2. Shimojo S, Birch EE, Gwiazda J, et al. Development of Vernier acuity in infants. *Vision Res* 1984;24(7):721–728.
3. Zanker J, Mohn G, Weber U, et al. The development of Vernier acuity in human infants. *Vision Res* 12(8):1557–1564.
4. Teller DY, Movshon JA. Visual development. *Vision Res* 1986;26(9):1483–1506.
5. Kagan K, Nakamura M, Furuya N, et al. Analysis of optokinetic nystagmus in patients with lesions on the left unilateral parietal lobe or the entire left hemisphere. *Acta Otolaryngol Suppl* 2001;545:166–169.
6. Morrone MC, Atkinson J, Cioni G, et al. Developmental changes in optokinetic mechanisms in the absence of unilateral cortical control. *Neuroreport* 1999;10–(13):2723–2729.
7. Van Hof-van Duin J, Mohn G. Optokinetic and spontaneous nystagmus in children with neurological disorders. *Behav Brain Res* 1983;10(1):163–175.
8. Daw NW. *Visual Development.* New York: Plenum Press; 1995:32.
9. Fantz RL. Pattern vision in newborn infants. *Science* 1963;140:296–297.
10. Fantz RL. Visual perception from birth as shown by pattern selectivity. *Ann N Y Acad Sci* 1965;118:793–814.
11. Schiffman HR. 1976. *Sensation and Perception.* New York: John Wiley and Sons; 1976:333–336.
12. Fantz R, Ord J, Udelf M. Maturation of pattern vision in infants during the first six months. *J Comp Physiol Psych* 1962;55:907–917.
13. Fantz, RL. The origin of form perception. *Sci Am* 1961;204:66–72.
14. Fantz RL, Fagan JF. Visual attention to size and number of pattern details by term and pre-term infants during the first six months. *Child Dev* 1975;16:3–18.
15. Fantz RL, Miranda SB. Newborn infant attention to form of contour. *Child Dev* 1975;46(1):224–228.
16. Dobson V, Teller DY, Lee CP, et al. A behavioral method for efficient screening of visual acuity in young infants. I. Preliminary laboratory development. *Invest Ophthalmol Vis Sci* 1978;17(12):1142–1150.
17. Fulton AB, Manning KA, Dobson V. A behavioral method for efficient screening of visual acuity in young infants. II. Clinical application. *Invest Ophthalmol Vis Sci* 1978;17(12):1151–1157.
18. Gwiazda J, Brill S, Held R. New methods for testing infant vision. *Sight Sav Rev* 1979;49(2):61–69.
19. Fulton AB, Manning KA, Dobson V. Infant vision testing

by a behavioral method. *Ophthalmology* 1979;86(3):431–439.

20. Atkinson J, Braddick O. New techniques for assessing vision in infants and young children. *Child Care Health Development* 1979;5(6):389–398.

21. Dobson V. Behavioral tests of visual acuity in infants. *Int Ophthalmol Clin* 1980;20(1):233–250.

22. Dobson V, Teller DY, Lee CP, et al. A behavioral method for efficient screening of visual acuity in young infants. I. Preliminary laboratory development. *Invest Ophthalmol Vis Sci* 1978;17(12):1142–1150.

23. Gwiazda J, Brill S, Mohindra I, et al. Preferential looking acuity in infants from two to fifty-eight weeks of age. *American Journal of Optometry and Physiological Optics* 1980;57(7):428–432.

24. Gwiazda J, Wolfe J, Brill S, et al. Quick assessment of PL acuity in infants. *Am J Optom Physiol Optics* 1980;57:420–427.

25. Mayer DL, Fulton AB, Hansen RM. Preferential looking acuity obtained with a staircase procedure in pediatric patients. *Invest Ophthalmol Vis Sci* 1982;23(4):538–543.

26. Duckman RH, Selenow A. Visual acuity in neurologically impaired children. *American Journal of Optometry and Physiological Optics* 1983;60(10):817–821.

27. Dobson V, Salem D, Mayer DL, et al. Visual acuity screening of children 6 months to 3 years of age. *Invest Ophthalmol Vis Sci* 1985;26(8):1057–1063.

28. Teller DY, McDonald MA, Preston K, et al. Assessment of visual acuity in infants and children: the acuity card procedure. *Dev Med Child Neurol* 1986;28(6):779–789.

29. McDonald M, Sebris SL, Mohn G, et al. Monocular acuity in normal infants: the acuity card procedure. *Am J Optom Physiol Opt* 1986;63(2):127–134.

30. Preston KL, McDonald M, Sebris SL, et al. Validation of the acuity card procedure for assessment of infants with ocular disorders. *Ophthalmology* 1987;94(6):644–653.

31. Birch EE, Hale LA. Criteria for monocular acuity deficit in infancy and early childhood. *Invest Ophthalmol Vis Sci* 1988;29(4):636–643.

32. Mohn G, van Hof-van Duin J, Fetter WP, et al. Acuity assessment of non-verbal infants and children: clinical experience with the acuity card procedure. *Dev Med Child Neurol* 1988;30(2):232–244.

33. Jackson GR, Jessup NS, Kavanaugh BL, et al. Measuring visual acuity in children using preferential looking and sine wave cards. *Optometry and Visual Science* 1990;67(8):590–594.

34. Hartmann EE, Ellis GS Jr, Morgan KS, et al. The acuity card procedure: longitudinal assessment. *J Pediatr Ophthalmol Strabismus* 1990;27(4):178–184.

35. Vital-Durand F. Acuity card procedure and the linearity of grating resolution development during the first year of human infants. *Behav Brain Res* 1992;49(1):99–106.

36. Mash C, Dobson V, Carpenter N. Interobserver agreement for measurement of grating acuity and interocular acuity differences with the Teller acuity card procedure. *Vision Res* 1995;(2):303–312.

37. Sokol S, Moskowitz A. Comparison of patterned VEPs and preferential looking behavior in three month old infants. *Invest Ophthalmol Vis Sci* 1985;26(3):359–365.

38. Sokol S, Moskowitz A, McCormack G, et al. Infant grating acuity is temporally tuned. *Vision Res* 1988;28(12):1357–1366.

39. Sokol S, Moskowitz A, McCormack G. Infant VEP and preferential looking acuity measured with phase alternating gratings. *Invest Ophthalmol Vis Sci* 1992;33(11):3156–3161.

40. www.acns.org/pdfs/Guideline%209B.pdf. Last accessed August 2004.

41. Taylor MJ, McCulloch DL. Visual evoked potentials in infants and children. *J Clin Neurophysiol* 1992;9(3):357–372.

42. Fantz RL. Pattern discrimination and selective attention. In: Kidd AH, Rivoire JL, eds. *Perceptual Development in Children.* New York: International Universities Press, 1966.

43. Fantz RL. Visual perception from birth as shown by pattern selectivity. *Ann NY Acad Sci* 1965;118(21):793–814.

44. Fantz RL, Miranda SB. Newborn infant attention to contour. *Child Dev* 1975;46(1):224–228.

45. Hershenson M. The development of the perception of form. *Psychol Bull* 1967; 67(5):326–336.

46. Campos EC, Chiesi C. Critical analysis of visual function evaluating techniques in newborn babies. *Int Ophthalmol* 1985;8(1):25–31.

47. Gorman JJ, Cogan DG, Gellis SS. A device for testing visual acuity in infants. The Sight-Saving Review, 1959;29(2):80–84.

48. Van Hof-van Duin J, Mohn G. Optokinetic and spontaneous nystagmus in children with neurological disorders. *Behav Brain Res* 1983;10(1):163–175.

49. Marg E, Freeman DN, Peltzman P, et al. Vision in human infants: evoked potential measurements. *Invest Ophthalmol* 1976;15(2):150–152.

50. Shimojo S, Birch EE, Gwiazda J, et al. Development of Vernier acuity in infants. *Vision Res* 1984;24(7):721–728.

51. Manny RE, Klein SA. The development of Vernier acuity in infants. *Curr Eye Res* 1984; 3(3):453–462.

52. Manny RE, Klein SA. A three alternative tracking paradigm to measure Vernier acuity of older infants. *Vision Res* 1985;25(9):1245–1252.

53. Shimojo S, Held R. Vernier acuity is less than grating acuity in 2- and 3-month olds. *Vision Res* 1987;27(1):77–86.

54. Zanker J, Mohn G, Weber U, et al. The development of Vernier acuity in human infants. *Vision Res* 1992;32(8):1557–1564.

55. Manny R. The visually evoked potential in response to Vernier offsets in infants. *Human Neurolbiology* 1988;6(4):273–279.

56. Shimojo S, Birch EE, Gwiazda J, et al. Development of Vernier acuity in infants. *Vision Res* 1984;24(7):721–728.

57. Brown AM. Vernier acuity in human infants: rapid emergence shown in longitudinal study. *Optom Vis Sci* 1997;74(9):732–740.

58. Skoczenski AM, Norcia AM. Development of VEP Vernier acuity and grating acuity in human infants. *Invest Ophthalmol Vis Sci* 1999;40(10):2411–2417.

59. Yuodelis C, Hendrickson A. A qualitative and quantitative analysis of the human fovea during development. *Vision Res* 1986;26:847–855.

60. Chandna A. Natural history of the development of visual acuity in infants. *Eye* 1991;5(Pt 1):20–26.

61. Magoon EH, Robb RM. Development of myelin in human optic nerve and tract. A light and electron microscopic study. *Arch Ophthalmol* 1981;99:655–659.

62. Brown AM, Yamamoto M. Visual acuity in newborn and pre-term infants measured with grating acuity cards. *Am J Ophthalmol* 1986;102(2):245–253.

63. Weinacht S, Kind C, Monting JS, et al. Visual development in pre-term and full term infants: a prospective masked study. *Invest Ophthalmol Vis Sci* 1999;40(2):346–353.

64. Spierer A, Royzman Z, Kuint J. Visual acuity in premature infants. *Ophthalmologica* 2004;218(6):397–401.

3 Contrast Sensitivity Function

Karl Citek

Scenes observed in everyday life are rich and complex with objects that differ in brightness, color, and size, as shown in Figure 3.1A. Tests of visual acuity (VA) assess only the patient's ability to see high contrast targets, which is an unrealistic representation of the normal visual environment. In addition, many patients with normal or near-normal VA complain of problems with their vision under everyday situations.

The ability to detect, discriminate, or recognize objects that vary slightly in relative luminance is referred to as *contrast sensitivity* (CS). Here, the object and background may appear as shades of gray, as in Figure 3.1B, which is identical to Figure 3.1A, but with the color information removed. In general, it is impossible to accurately predict a patient's CS responses based on VA, nor can VA alone properly explain difficulties in perceiving low contrast images or any other problems with visual function (1). In fact, as will be explained below, VA is merely one point on the contrast sensitivity function (CSF).

Other characteristics of real objects include dynamic changes, such as movement across the visual field, movement in depth, and flicker (2). Perception of an object and illusions caused by a misperception of objects also will depend on the observer's physiologic, psychological, and cognitive processing and responses. For example, a patient's retinal function can be compromised, as with color deficiency; the patient can have poor binocular vision, making depth perception difficult; the patient may not be able to attend to central and peripheral targets simultaneously; or, the patient's response threshold can be reduced or enhanced because of adaptation (e.g., when walking into a darkened movie theater from a sunny street).

Note, the factors listed above do not make up an all-inclusive list of possible contributions to overall visual function. Also, assessment of a patient's visual function would not be feasible if all possible combinations of factors are considered simultaneously. Consequently, clinical testing usually seeks to measure one aspect of visual function while keeping all other aspects constant, or, at least, in control. As examples, a typical color vision test incorporates targets of constant luminance and nearly similar size while varying color; an automated perimeter presents targets of constant size and varying luminance at different spatial locations; and a VA chart uses high contrast optotypes (i.e., black-and-white) of varying size.

This chapter explains some of the scientific and clinical foundations of CS, evaluates some of the procedures and devices used to assess CS, reviews the development of CS from infancy to adulthood, and discusses the individual factors that contribute to a patient's CS. Because this is such a broad topic area, we will not consider color contrast, temporal CS (i.e., flicker) (other than in the context of testing with visual evoked potentials), or any other combination of

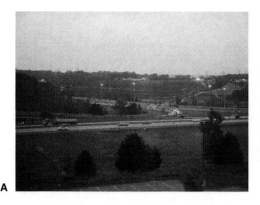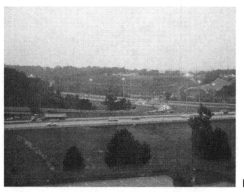

FIGURE 3.1. Landscape scene on an overcast, rainy morning with full color and luminance information **(A)**, and with luminance information only **(B)**. (See color well.)

multiple factors that incorporate contrast as a component.

DEFINITIONS AND NOMENCLATURE FOR CONTRAST SENSITIVITY TESTING

Most physiologic responses occur over ranges of amplitudes and in units of measure that are not familiar to the lay person. To fully appreciate the proper testing of CS, and to correctly interpret the resulting CSF, we need to define certain terms and concepts. Understandably, some of these terms are used synonymously and interchangeably in common language, but they have very specific definitions in the present context.

Luminance (L) is the physical amount of light emitted by a source or reflected from an illuminated object; the common unit of measure is candela per square meter, cd/m^2. *Brightness* is the perception of a luminous object by the human visual system, which can be affected by adaptation, aftereffects, and the presence or absence of other objects in the visual field.

Contrast (C) refers to the difference in luminance between an object (L_{max}) and its background (L_{min}), where the object is brighter than the background. The object itself may be small against the large, uniform background or, at the other extreme, it may be a single edge (not a repeating pattern) separating a light area from a dark area of visual space. Contrast is expressed as a ratio or percentage of this difference with respect to the object luminance,

$$C = (L_{max} - L_{min})/L_{max}$$

Modulation (M) is the term for the contrast of a repeating pattern, commonly referred to as a *grating*, where it is not apparent which part of the pattern is the "object" and which is the "background." An example is a series of light (L_{max}) and dark (L_{min}) stripes, as in the zebra in Figure 3.2. Modulation is calculated as the ratio of the difference of the luminances to the sum of the luminances,

$$M = (L_{max} - L_{min})/(L_{max} + L_{min}),$$

where the luminance is measured across the spatial extent of each component part of the pattern. Alternately, modulation can be expressed by the mathematically equivalent ratio of the difference between maximal and average luminances to the average luminance (L_{avg}),

$$M = (L_{max} - L_{avg})/L_{avg},$$

where

$$L_{avg} = (L_{max} + L_{min})/2$$

The stripes in the image in Fig. 3.2B have the same average luminance as the stripes in Fig. 3.2A, but with decreased modulation. Note, if the dark part of the target is totally black (i.e., $L_{min} = 0$), then both contrast and modulation will be 100%, regardless of the nature of the target or pattern. On the other hand, a grating with light and dark areas of similar luminance will have a modulation very different from the contrast calculated for a single object

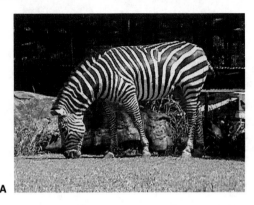 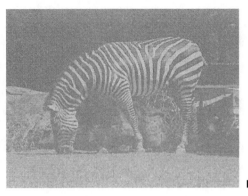

A   B

FIGURE 3.2. Zebra shown in high contrast **(A)** and low contrast **(B)**, with matched average luminance in the two images.

and background of the same respective luminances. For example, a grating with luminances of $L_{max} = 55$ cd/m^2 and $L_{min} = 45$ cd/m^2 has a modulation of 10%, whereas the comparable contrast of a single target and background with identical respective luminances is 18.1%. Most manufacturers of CS tests refer to their charts and instruments as presenting stimuli at certain "contrast" levels, but they correctly measure and report modulation values. In deference to this common usage, we will occasionally refer to targets as having high or low "contrast," even when the precise term is "modulation;" the reader should understand from the context of the discussion which concept is actually being considered.

Threshold is the minimal stimulus level needed to induce a physiologic or cognitive response. The person, however, does not always need to be cognitively aware of the stimulus for a response to occur. For example, very few persons who are not presbyopic are conscious of retinal image blur as they accommodate for targets at different distances under normal circumstances. *Sensitivity* is the reciprocal of threshold. For the CSF, points plotted on the abscissa represent the least possible sensitivity, corresponding to targets of 100% contrast (or modulation).

The *logarithm* of a number represents that value as a power of 10. For example, typical human photopic vision extends from about 1 to about 65,000 cd/m^2. Mathematically, it is much easier to characterize this range as 0 to 4.8 log units. For the CSF, because of the potentially large ranges of responses for both

spatial frequency and sensitivity, the data are commonly plotted on logarithmic scales on both axes, which results in the characteristic inverted-U shape of the function (see below).

Most spatial visual responses are properly specified by *angular* measures, such as degrees, minutes, or seconds of arc. Yet, the common expressions for eye movements and visual resolution are prism diopters and the Snellen fraction, respectively, both of which represent ratios of two *linear* distance measurements. Recall, one prism diopter is equivalent to a lateral displacement of one unit at a distance of 100 units, for example, a 1-cm shift at a 1-m distance. Likewise, the numerator of the Snellen fraction specifies the test distance, in feet or meters, and the denominator gives the reference distance at which the target subtends 5 arcmin; thus, we have the familiar designation of normal VA as 20/20 in English units and 6/6 in metric units.

The *spatial frequency* of a target indicates how many components of a repeating pattern, or grating, occur within a given area or space. For a series of stripes, one *cycle* represents one pair of light and dark stripes. The frequency is usually specified in cycles per degree (cpd). At a 20/20 acuity demand, each arm and gap of the letter "E" subtends 1 arcmin, with the entire letter subtending 5 arcmin. Thus, one cycle on the "E," that is, one arm and one gap, subtends 2 arcmin. Because there are 60 arcmin in one degree, the "E" has a spatial frequency of 30 cpd. To convert between cpd and the comparable Snellen demand, observe that the product of the spatial frequency and the denominator of the Snellen

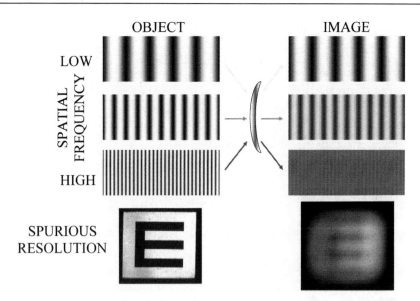

FIGURE 3.3. Demonstration of modulation transfer through a lens at different spatial frequencies. Low spatial frequencies are little affected by diffraction and aberrations, whereas high spatial frequencies can be totally obscured. Spurious resolution occurs when the optical system is sufficiently defocused to produce a phase shift of the image with respect to the object; thus, the imaged "E" appears to have four arms rather than three.

fraction is a constant: for 20-ft Snellen demand, use

$$600 = (\text{spatial frequency}) \times (\text{Snellen denominator}),$$

and for 6-m Snellen demand, use

$$180 = (\text{spatial frequency}) \times (\text{Snellen denominator})$$

In Fig. 3.2, the zebra's stripes are much narrower on the legs than on the neck. Therefore, the leg stripes have a higher spatial frequency. Also, in a complex presentation as in Fig. 3.2, different parts of the object may differ in *phase* and *orientation*. The stripes on the zebra's legs are roughly horizontal and those on the torso are roughly vertical, demonstrating a difference in orientation. The stripes on the front and back legs, while having similar orientation and frequency, do not line up exactly, thereby demonstrating a difference in phase.

Modulation transfer is the ability of an optical system to produce accurately an image of an object, calculated as the ratio of the image modulation to the object modulation for a given spa-

tial frequency. Because of diffraction, chromatic and monochromatic aberrations, and focus and power errors, the image will never be a perfect representation of the object. For low spatial frequencies, the image blur is hardly noticeable, whereas for high spatial frequencies, the image is almost fully obscured, as demonstrated in Fig. 3.3.

As an aberration or defocus increases, the resolving power of the system will be severely diminished, such that even middle (and, possibly, low) spatial frequency objects are imaged as a uniform gray. With sufficient defocus, however, the system may show *spurious resolution*, in which case the light and dark areas of the image exhibit a 180-degree phase shift (aka phase reversal) with respect to the object. Thus, for example, a person with uncorrected myopia of about 8 D might unexpectedly "see" a slightly blurry "E" at the top of a 20-ft letter chart; of course, that person will see the "E" with four arms rather than three!

Technically, a pattern of dark and light stripes is known as a *square wave* grating, where there is constant luminance across each stripe and a discrete change in luminance at the border between stripes. A *sine wave* (aka sinusoidal) grating, on the other hand, offers a continuous change in luminance from maximal to minimal, and back to maximal again, based on the trigonometric sine function. The vertical stripes at the top of Fig. 3.3 are sine wave gratings, whereas the horizontal arms of the "E" at the bottom of the figure form a square wave grating.

Mathematically, a sine wave is a more pure function than a square wave: the sine wave comprises only a single spatial frequency. Much like the timbre of a musical instrument, or the combination of several different instruments playing the same note, a square wave has a fundamental frequency that corresponds to a sine wave having identical maximal and minimal locations and several harmonics or overtones that are merely multiples of the fundamental frequency. See Cornsweet (3), Schwartz (4), and Palmer (5) for a more in-depth analysis of this concept. Suffice it to say that the harmonic frequencies of a square wave are odd multiples of its fundamental frequency, and that the harmonic frequencies have greatly reduced amplitudes with respect to the fundamental frequency. A square wave grating that provides a nominal spatial frequency at 10 cpd, therefore, also provides (dimmer) spatial frequen-cies at 30, 50, 70, and so forth cpd. Consider that 10 cpd corresponds to a Snellen demand of 20/60, and 30 cpd corresponds to 20/20. Even if an individual has 20/20 VA, which requires measurement with a target of high contrast, that person would not be able to detect the low-contrast 30-cpd harmonic frequency, nor any other higher-order frequency. Thus, a 10-cpd square wave grating will appear to be identical to a 10-cpd sine wave grating.

COMPONENTS OF THE CONTRAST SENSITIVITY FUNCTION

For any manner of simple lenses (e.g., spectacles) or complex lens systems (e.g., telescopes and cameras), the *modulation transfer function* (MTF) gives the modulation transfer for all possible spatial frequencies. For the human visual system, the comparable set of responses is referred to as the CSF. Here, however, neural and cortical processing and the optics of the eye contribute to the final outcome. (The ensuing discussion presumes that we are *not* dealing with the extreme limiting cases of total blindness nor severely compromised neural or cortical functioning.)

An idealized CSF is shown in Fig. 3.4 (solid line). Any target whose spatial frequency and

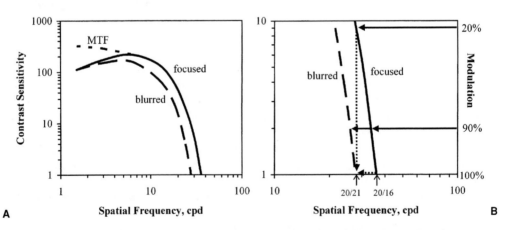

FIGURE 3.4. **A:** Idealized normal "focused" CSF (*solid line*) with 20/16 VA and predicted low-frequency sensitivity based on MTF, and "blurred" CSF (*long dashed line*) with 20/21 VA. **B:** Close-up of high spatial frequencies, demonstrating that slight blur has minimal effect on VA but significant effect on CS. (Adapted from Rabin J and Wicks J. Measuring resolution in the contrast domain: the Small Letter Contrast Test. *Optom Vis Sci* 1996;73:398–403.) In addition, there is little practical difference when assessing VA using a chart with 90% versus 100% modulation. CSF, contrast sensitivity function; VA, visual acuity; MTF, modulation transfer function.

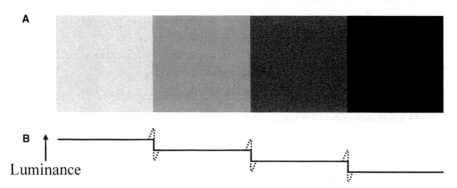

FIGURE 3.5.   Demonstration of Mach bands. **A:** Shaded squares of uniform luminance, positioned to give the perception of nonuniform shading. **B:** Luminance profile (*solid lines*) of the *shaded squares* and perceived brightness profile (*dashed lines*), indicating the apparent increase and decrease in brightness on either side of an edge, which is caused by lateral inhibition at the retinal ganglion cells.

contrast (or modulation) plot on or below the curve will be visible to the observer; targets that plot above the curve will not be seen. The CSF may be thought to be composed of two distinct segments, namely, responses to high and low spatial frequencies. Note that "high" and "low" are relative terms, and that a consistent or discrete delineation is not seen between them. Responses to high spatial frequencies depend primarily on the quality of the preretinal optics (i.e., of the eye and any auxiliary lens or optical medium). Responses to low spatial frequencies are mediated somewhat by neural (i.e., retinal and precortical) processing (4). In addition, the CSF can be either enhanced or diminished via further processing in the cortex, as described in various conditions below.

The high-frequency endpoint, or cut-off, of the CSF corresponds to the patient's VA, where target modulation must be at the maximum of 100% for the patient to report correctly seeing the target. In practice, most well-maintained charts and instruments used to assess VA provide targets with modulation of about 90%. As illustrated in Fig. 3.4B, this slight decrease in maximal modulation has little or no practical effect on the measured VA, even for a slightly defocused eye. Similarly, as suggested by Rabin and Wicks (6), a low degree of optical defocus (i.e., retinal image blur) will cause only a slight reduction in VA (about one line), but a significant reduction in CS, because of the steep slope of the CSF at the high spatial frequencies. In the condition illustrated in Fig. 3.4B, the same

size target that can be distinguished at only 20% modulation with the focused eye requires 100% modulation to be seen with the blurred eye.

At the other end of the CSF, the low-frequency drop-off results from lateral inhibition at the retinal ganglion cells (3,4). This is the same phenomenon that produces Mach bands, the apparent increase and decrease in brightness on either side of an edge separating a light surface from a dark surface, respectively, although both surfaces have uniform spatial luminances. Figure 3.5 demonstrates this phenomenon; cover everything but any single square to confirm that *no* variation exists in luminance across that square.

With foveal viewing, the adult CSF typically reaches a peak at 3 to 5 cpd, although considerable variability exists in absolute sensitivity, even across normal adult observers (7,8). Some individuals may erroneously refer to the high sensitivity at the center of the CSF as a "middle-frequency enhancement," suggesting that postretinal processing can exceed the modulation transfer limits of optical components governed at least by diffraction, not to mention spherical aberration, coma, chromatic aberration, and other higher-order aberrations that are present to some extent in every eye regardless of refractive error (2,3,9). As illustrated in Fig. 3.4, a theoretical diffraction-limited visual system would have significantly better sensitivity at low frequencies, rather than the drop-off that is actually observed.

CONTRAST SENSITIVITY TEST PARAMETERS

Clinical assessment of CS includes the full gamut of available subjective and objective techniques and procedures. As with testing of other aspects of visual function (e.g., VA, color vision, and flicker sensitivity), the ability of the patient to perform the test must be taken into account. For example, it would be useless to ask an infant to read aloud the letters on a standard acuity chart, although most adult patients know exactly what is expected of them and can perform the test easily and quickly.

Tests of CS can be grouped into several categories, and most tests will fall into multiple categories, depending on the nature of the stimuli and the procedure used to gather the data:

Subjective versus Objective

Subjective tests require an observer to make a decision in response to a stimulus, such as when a patient reads letters on a chart or reports the presence or orientation of a grating pattern. Subjective tests also are referred to as *psychophysical* tests, in that a stimulus must be processed and a response generated by the human observer.

An *objective* test allows measurement of a response without feedback or bias. Sometimes, such a test involves sophisticated instrumentation. For example, an infrared autorefractor will give a reading only if aligned properly but without concern for the patient's refractive or accommodative status, or even the patient's (in)ability to see the target of regard. Visual evoked potential (VEP), which measures the patient's cortical response to a flickering stimulus, is objective for both the patient and the clinician.

Note that the forced preferential looking (FPL) technique is subjective for the clinician, who tries to determine the direction of an infant's gaze without knowing the location of the stimulus. It is objective for the patient, because the patient does not need to give any physical indication (beyond a simple reflexive eye or head movement) that the patient can see the stimulus (10).

Symbols versus Sine Wave Gratings

All symbols or optotypes, such as letters, numbers, and line drawings (e.g., Lea symbols, Hiding Heidi) are based on square and rectangular waves. The most obvious depiction of a square wave is the letter "E," as described above. A rectangular wave has asymmetric light and dark stripes, such as the separation of opposite parts of the letter, "O," but the spatial frequency characteristics are consistent with those of sine and square waves (11). Thus, for brevity, any discussion of square waves will be understood to include rectangular waves. All other characters and pictures derive from the same mathematical principles. Other spatial distributions (e.g., sawtooth waves) have also been studied, but these offer no advantages over or differences with respect to square or sine waves (11).

Purists may argue that sine waves are the only proper stimuli for CS measurement, because they do not include the higher-order harmonic frequencies present in square waves. As suggested above, however, this is a moot point for the high spatial frequency part of the CSF, because no higher-order harmonics will be visible for any spatial frequency equal to or greater than one third of the patient's resolution limit. For spatial frequencies lower than one third of the resolution limit (e.g., <10 cpd, or larger than 20/60 demand, for 20/20 VA), the patient might only perceive the higher-order harmonics if the grating is presented with high modulation. For a grating whose fundamental frequency has low modulation, the modulation of the higher-order harmonics will be proportionately lower, again pushing them into the invisible region above the CSF.

Nonetheless, Campbell and Robson (11) reported higher sensitivity when testing with square waves versus sine waves. The increase in sensitivity, regardless of spatial frequency, was consistently about 27%, which corresponds to the higher amplitude of the component fundamental frequency of the square wave. That is, given sine and square wave gratings with the same maximum and minimum luminances, the fundamental frequency of the square wave has an amplitude $4/\pi$ ($=1.273$) times greater than the comparable sine wave. While this may seem significant, it is only about a 0.1 log unit increase in sensitivity, which is well within the test and response variability for most procedures (see below).

Printed versus Projected

All printed charts require full, even illumination to avoid a bright reflection ("hot spot") from one part of the chart, which constitutes an unwanted glare source, or a poorly lit (dark) area at another part. Most charts are provided with specific lighting instructions, and even a light meter for calibration purposes. Other charts are printed on translucent sheets and rear-illuminated by an accompanying light box; such set-ups are less susceptible to measurement variability with differences in room illumination. In any case, all printed charts should be replaced every few years, depending on the amount of usage and environmental conditions, because the background can yellow and the print can fade, thereby altering the nominal modulation. Near charts should be replaced or cleaned, if possible, on a more frequent basis, because the accumulation of oil and dirt from fingerprints will affect the integrity of the chart.

Projected charts include those intended for use with a standard projector as well as those displayed on computer monitors, televisions, and oscilloscopes. Room illumination should be at a minimum, to avoid unintentionally reducing the image contrast on the projector screen ("washing out") and to avoid hot spots from the glass surface of the display and excessive surround luminance (12). In addition, displays must be properly calibrated, adjusted, and maintained, and the display surface must be cleaned regularly to avoid buildup of dust and fingerprints (especially in a pediatric setting!).

Full versus Limited Contrast Sensitivity Function

A full CSF can only be measured if multiple spatial frequency targets each are presented at multiple contrasts. Because the shape of the CSF generally is invariant (10), the position of the CSF on the graph may be established with results from as few as four or five representative spatial frequencies. Most printed grating and standard projector charts follow this rule.

Most symbol charts fix one domain, either modulation (e.g., Bailey-Lovie chart) or spatial frequency (e.g., Pelli-Robson and Rabin charts), while varying the other. As such, only a single point on the CSF can be evaluated. Testing is fairly rapid and easy to conduct on patients familiar with standard VA testing, and the result, in conjunction with the VA, often provides a clinically adequate depiction of the patient's visual function. Nonetheless, many charts with variable spatial frequency and constant modulation on one chart are available in additional versions at different modulations, such that a full CSF can be assessed.

The clinician has the most control over the presentation of the frequency and modulation combinations when using a computer-based system. An example of a system that displays gratings is the B-VAT (Medtronic Solan), and one that displays letters is the AcuityMax software program (www.Science2020.com). Note, if more than four or five spatial frequencies are to be tested, then the test time will be significantly longer than normal.

Single Target versus Multiple Targets

Most clinical tests of CS present a series of single targets, either simultaneously (as on a full letter chart) or sequentially (as on a monitor, or a projected chart capable of isolating single targets). They require the patient to report for each target either that (a) the patient can correctly identify its orientation ("discrimination" of a grating); or (b) the patient can correctly identify its shape ("recognition" of a symbol).

To be able to evaluate subtle changes in CS, or variations across the CSF, a more painstaking task must be employed. A *forced-choice* preferential looking technique presents at least two options to the patient, only one of which has the characteristic(s) being tested; thus, this is a "detection" task. For example, in the FPL technique, one stimulus has a grating while the other has a luminance-matched gray patch. The stimuli can be presented simultaneously, as in FPL or with the Arden plates, or they can be presented sequentially over time, as on a computer display. Rather than identifying the target or any characteristic about it, the patient merely indicates which stimulus presentation contained the target. At the limits of visual function, the patient may not be cognitively aware of the presence of the target, but can still guess correctly. To avoid the undue influence of false–positive responses, multiple trials are conducted at each spatial frequency, usually following a *method of limits* or *staircase* paradigm. Consequently, the results will be precise, but testing at even only a limited number of spatial frequencies could take 5 minutes or longer (13,14), and as long as 15 to 20 minutes for a full evaluation (2).

CONTRAST SENSITIVITY TESTS

Sine Wave Gratings

Until the 1980s, CS testing was confined principally to research laboratories and clinics with expensive displays and electronic pattern generators that could produce the sine wave gratings thought to be necessary to properly test CS. In 1984, Ginsburg (7) introduced the Vistech printed chart for the clinical assessment of CS, as shown in Fig. 3.6A. This chart offers photographic reproductions of five different sinusoidal spatial frequency gratings, each at eight levels of modulation (the ninth pattern in each row is a uniform gray). Each grating is presented at one of three orientations, vertical or rotated left or right by 15°, and the patient is required to correctly identify the orientation to receive credit.

The B-VAT (Fig. 3.6B) provides gratings at similar orientations, vertical and rotated left or right by 14°, presented on the monitor individually and sequentially by the clinician. Again, the patient must identify the orientation of the presented target. Other computer- and monitor-based research instruments will often use a forced-choice technique, in which the subject must choose which of two (or more) presentations contain the stimulus. Nonetheless, all

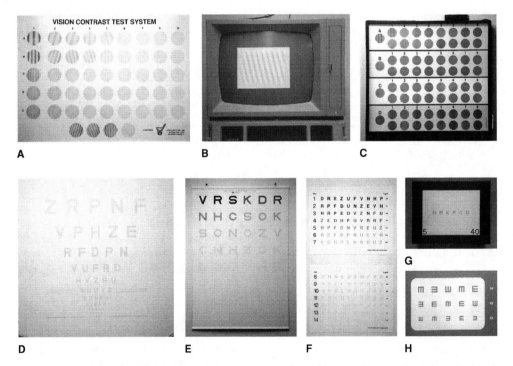

FIGURE 3.6. Potpourri of common contrast sensitivity (CS) charts and instruments (not depicted to scale): Vistech printed chart **(A)**; B-VAT computer display **(B)**; rear-illuminated Arden grating targets **(C)**; Bailey-Lovie printed chart **(D)**; Pelli-Robson printed chart **(E)**; Rabin Small Letter Contrast Test printed chart **(F)**; AcuityMax LCD display **(G)**; standard high-contrast projected chart with full room illumination **(H)**.

monitors should be properly calibrated and adjusted.

The Vistech chart (Lighthouse International) has been used extensively in clinical research of CS, most recently by Katz (15) and as part of a new FPL test that claims to be more efficient than others for pediatric patients (16). The chart has also been available as a projector slide and in a version calibrated for near testing. Similar charts include the Functional Acuity Contrast Test (successor to the Vistech chart; Stereo Optical Co.), the Optec vision screener (Stereo Optical Co.), and rear-illuminated charts such as Arden grating targets (Fig. 3.6C, Precision Vision). Arden grating targets use a different forced-choice technique, in that all gratings are vertical but paired with luminance-matched gray displays.

Aside from the expense and technical difficulty of creating precise sine wave targets, additional drawbacks of printed charts include (a) difficulty for the patient to correctly identify gratings in the presence of under- or uncorrected refractive error, especially uncorrected astigmatism(17); (b) difficulty for the clinician to use the test with children under about 5 years of age (14,18–20); (c) evaluator measurement variability (21); (d) poor test-retest reliability (22,23); and (e) poor correlation to other sine wave(24) or symbol CS tests (19). The problems with reliability could result from ceiling and floor effects, because a particular chart might not offer an adequate range of contrasts and spatial frequencies to properly assess a patient's visual function (23). The problems with correlation could likewise result from the limited number of targets available for presentation (19).

Symbols

The 1980s also saw the introduction of clinically practical letter charts for the assessment of low-contrast acuity. The Bailey-Lovie chart (Fig. 3.6D) contains letters of varying size and constant modulation (25), available at modulations of 1.25% to 25%, as well as high contrast (for standard VA testing) for distance and near. Charts for children with similar target parameters are available with Lea symbols and Hiding Heidi pictures. These, however, have

been found to be inadequate for the assessment of children with normal vision because of floor effects (26).

The Pelli-Robson chart (Fig. 3.6E) contains letters of varying modulation and constant size (27), nominally 1 cpd (20/600 demand). In the 1990s, Rabin and Wicks introduced the Small Letter Contrast Test (Fig 3.6F), which has a constant letter size of 24 cpd (20/25 demand) (6). This chart has since developed into the Rabin Contrast Sensitivity Test (Precision Vision), with a constant letter size of 12 cpd (20/50 demand). The main distinction between the Pelli-Robson and Rabin charts is that the former tests CS at a spatial frequency normally below the peak sensitivity (i.e., in the low frequency drop-off region), whereas the latter tests CS above the peak sensitivity (i.e., in the high-frequency region).

Computer-based charts also are available. For example, AcuityMax (Fig. 3.6G) allows for the display of any letter size at any of thirteen 0.1 log unit increments, from 100% (0.0 log unit) to 6.4% (1.2 log unit) modulation.

Finally, the clinician can turn any standard high-contrast projected chart into a low-contrast demand (Fig. 3.6H). A uniform, supplementary light source with variable power control and a light meter must be used to properly calibrate the test. However, this could prove more time-consuming and troublesome, and possibly less reliable (if not adjusted and calibrated properly), than a commercially available test.

Many of the physical limitations of symbol charts are identical to those for sine wave grating charts. Namely, proper lighting and monitor adjustment (if applicable), the presence of under- or uncorrected refractive error, and difficulty in conducting the test on very young patients.

Visual Evoked Potential

The VEP involves electrodes that are placed on the patient's scalp at the visual cortex. The electrodes register the minute electrical activity of the brain as it is stimulated. The patient views a flickering pattern, usually a checkerboard, presented on a monitor. If the variation in measured cortical activity is synchronized with the stimulus presentation, one can conclude that the patient "saw" the target. Otherwise, the response will be flat or random at best.

The measured responses will be sensitive to (a) the proper placement and attachment of the electrodes; (b) the size and flicker rate of the stimulus; and (c) under- or uncorrected refractive error, as well as any ocular media problems that would prevent the formation of a clear, focused retinal image.

The VEP has been used successfully to assess the visual function of infants as young as 1 week (28), and it has consistently demonstrated a better CS result than any psychophysical test (compare data plotted in Fig. 3.7A to Fig. 3.7B). Reasons for this difference may include (a) the nature of the stimulus—a flickering pattern presented in central and peripheral vision, compared with a stationary pattern viewed primarily with central vision during psychophysical tests; (b) the large number of presentations, over which the output signal is averaged; and (c) the presence of an appropriate response proves that the visual system is intact up to the visual cortex, but it does not assess higher-level visual processing, nor cognitive or motor processing, all of which are necessary for a successful result using a psychophysical test (10).

DEVELOPMENT OF CONTRAST SENSITIVITY IN HUMANS

Figure 3.7 shows representative data from studies that have tested infants' and children's vision using VEP (29), FPL (30,31), and a staircase psychophysical technique (32). Note that, although there are different ranges of responses for the different techniques, no doubt, with increasing age (a) CSF maintains its characteristic inverted-U shape; (b) CSF shifts upward on the graph (i.e., sensitivity to low contrast increases); and (c) CSF shifts rightward on the graph (i.e., sensitivity to high spatial frequency increases) (10). Data from other studies not presented in Fig. 3.7 offer similar findings (13,29,33,34), not only for human infants, but for macaque monkey infants as well (35).

Evidence indicates that CSF is not merely a single function but the combination of about half a dozen separate, smaller overlapping functions ("channels") that each respond to a selected subset of spatial frequencies (4). This corresponds somewhat to the magno- and parvocellular anatomic pathways of the visual system.

Additional evidence suggests that depressed CS at age 3 to 5 months, especially at 2.5 cpd

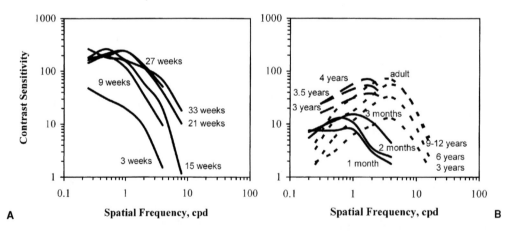

FIGURE 3.7. Development of contrast sensitivity function (CSF) in infants and children, measured with different techniques. **A:** Data for infants aged 3 to 33 weeks using sweep visual evoked potentials (VEP). (Adapted from Norcia AM, Tyler CW, Hamer RD. Development of contrast sensitivity in the human infant. *Vision Res* 1990;30:1475–1486.) **B:** Data for infants aged 1 to 3 months (From Banks MS, Salapatek P. *Invest Ophthalmol Vis Sci* 1978;17:361–365) and children aged 3, 3.5, and 4 years (From Atkinson J, French J, Braddick O. Contrast sensitivity of preschool children. *Br J Ophthalmol* 1981;65:525–529.) using preferential looking, and children 3, 6, and 9 to 12 years and adults using a staircase method (From Beazley LD, Illingworth DJ, Jahn A, et al. Contrast sensitivity in children and adults. *Br J Ophthalmol* 1980;64:863–866).

or greater, could result in the development of poor stereopsis (36). The prime culprit is hypothesized to be anisometropia and, possibly, uncorrected refractive error in general, which could lead to amblyopia as well (see below).

The one major point of controversy, as shown in the two sets of plots in Fig. 3.7, is the apparent better performance of infants with a VEP technique than with a psychophysical technique. Using VEP, Norcia et al. (33) found that 10-week-old infants have CS similar to adults for spatial frequencies below 1 cpd, and 8-month-old infants have a high-frequency cut-off at 16.3 cpd (about 20/37 equivalent) or more than half of the measured adult level (31.9 cpd, about 20/19 equivalent). On the other hand, psychophysical techniques suggest that CS does not reach adult levels until at least age 7 to 9 years (16,34,37,38), or even as late as adolescence (32,39).

CONDITIONS THAT AFFECT CONTRAST SENSITIVITY

Any condition or phenomenon that degrades the retinal image, whether exogenous or endogenous to the observer, has the potential of reducing that person's responsiveness to low-contrast stimuli. In general, an exogenous factor will cause only a temporary problem, just for as long as the factor is present; normal visual function will return once the cause of the image degradation is removed. In most cases, unless extreme retinal image degradation exists, only the sensitivity to high (and possibly some middle) frequencies will be reduced.

An endogenous factor, on the other hand, can lead to long-term or even permanent CS reduction. The natural demarcation line between the two types of factors is the cornea. The extent of the CS reduction depends on the location and severity of the condition. Some of the common causative conditions are summarized here.

Environmental Factors

Overall Luminance

Overall visual function might be thought to become immediately and progressively worse as ambient luminance decreases. In normal

subjects at mesopic levels, however, CSF only shifts downward on the graph, indicating a decrease in sensitivity to low contrast but no change in sensitivity to spatial frequency (40). Only when luminance reaches scotopic levels do we find a commensurate reduction in spatial resolution, consistent with the decreased acuity of the rods (41).

Atmospheric Conditions

Recall Fig. 3.1: any weather condition that induces light scatter (e.g., fog, haze, smoke, or smog) will reduce the quality of the retinal image, regardless of the ambient light level. The ability to detect low-contrast stimuli will be reduced, first for high spatial frequencies and then for all spatial frequencies as the weather deteriorates.

Glare Sources

Sources of light, or their images, that are close to an object of regard and bright enough to be seen will interfere with the retinal image, thus producing glare. Examples include direct or reflected sunlight during the day, direct or reflected car headlights at night, and street lighting at night. This will affect primarily high spatial frequencies, unless the glare is so strong that it is visually disabling.

Standard Light Sources

Many common light sources do not emit light evenly across the visible spectrum. Incandescent sources (e.g., standard light bulbs, candles, and lamps in romantic restaurants) provide most of their light output in the long wavelength ("red") portion of the spectrum but little output in the short wavelength ("blue") part. Thus, a red shirt or tablecloth will look deep red, but blue pants can appear almost black.

Fluorescent sources typically do not emit continuous spectra, but offer multiple line spectra at discrete wavelengths. In most cases, this is not a problem, unless the object being viewed reflects only parts of the spectrum at which the source has little output. Again, the object would appear reduced in brightness and likely altered in color appearance.

An extreme condition, but very common in public parking lots and urban street lighting, is the low-pressure sodium lamp. It emits a narrow-band spectrum at the yellow wavelengths, with no output in the red or blue. Thus, as shown in Fig. 3.8, anything that is not yellow will appear as a shade of gray; because white objects reflect all wavelengths, the walls in Fig. 3.8A take on a yellowish appearance. But the red blouse and shoes and blue wristband fade into obscurity.

Precorneal Optics

House Windows and Car Windshields

Windows and windshields that have small scratches, pits, or surface imperfections will cause diffraction of light at the surface, creating a blurred image even before the light enters the eye. Patients will often report seeing "halos" or multiple images of lights, especially at night. Windows and windshields dirty with fingerprints, smudges, or tarnish will cause light scatter, creating an image that has a "washed out" appearance. Rain on a windshield that is

allowed to accumulate before being wiped away will have a similar effect.

Spectacles, Goggles, and Safety Eyewear

Lenses without an antireflective coating on *both* surfaces can produce multiple surface reflections that act as sources of glare, as described above. This will occur under daytime and nighttime conditions. Lenses that have small scratches, pits, or surface imperfections, or lenses dirty with fingerprints, smudges, or tarnish, will create the same problems as described for windows and windshields above.

Lenses with an inappropriate tint density or spectral transmission curve for the given conditions are potentially dangerous. Driving with dark sun eyewear at night, or with a specialty tint (e.g., an orange ski goggle), during the day will make it difficult to see traffic signals, other vehicles, pedestrians, and other objects. A patient with color vision deficiencies should be warned against wearing certain color tints, because they can further distort the patient's limited perception of color.

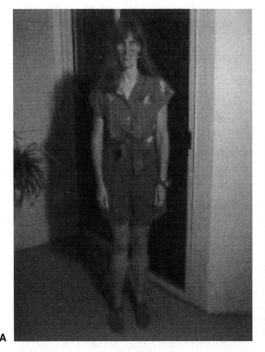
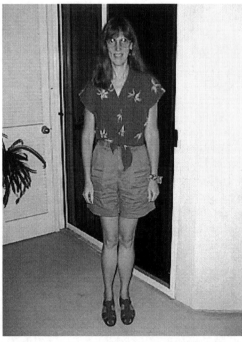

A   B

FIGURE 3.8. Nighttime scene photographed under narrow-bandpass low-pressure sodium lighting **(A)** and with flash ("full-spectrum") lighting **(B)**. (See color well.)

Contact Lenses

Surface imperfections (e.g., scratches on rigid, gas permeable contact lenses) rarely cause a direct problem, because the lens will usually have a sufficient tear film around it to mask minor imperfections; if the scratches are significant and noticeable when the lens is on the eye, then the lens is likely compromised beyond repair and should be replaced. On the other hand, surface deposits of proteins and other debris can easily build up on any lens that is not properly maintained and cause light scatter identical to that of a smudged window or spectacle lens.

With the recent availability of tinted contact lenses, the same issues of inappropriate tint density or spectral transmission curve apply as for spectacle lenses.

Ocular Optics

Cornea

Corneal edema, commonly caused by contact lens overwear, will cause glare and halos around lights, thus affecting primarily the CS of high spatial frequencies. The edema is usually managed with a change of the contact lens care regimen. Corneal microstriae following laser in situ keratomileusis (LASIK) surgery will reduce CS at high, and possibly, middle, spatial frequencies, and will improve over time as the microstriae fade (42). Nonetheless, if the LASIK flap or the photorefractive keratectomy (PRK) ablation zone is comparable in size to the pupil, especially at night, the discontinuity of the corneal surface will always act to scatter light, disrupt high spatial frequencies, and cause the patient to complain of halos around lights at night (43); this condition, however, will not resolve until the patient ages sufficiently so that the pupil no longer dilates to such a large size, or the patient adapts to the constant presence of the troublesome images. On the other hand, scarring caused by refractive surgery or keratoplasty can result in potential CS loss at all spatial frequencies, depending on the amount of scarring (44).

Aqueous Humor

Cells and flare in the aqueous caused by an active infection or inflammation produces light scatter and reduces CS of at least the high spatial frequencies.

Crystalline Lens

A lens with an early cataract will initially induce increased higher-order aberrations and light scatter, affecting VA and high spatial frequency CS (45). If left untreated, it will eventually become completely opaque and obscure vision completely. Treatment, of course, is to remove the cataractous lens before it becomes totally opaque and replace it with a plastic intraocular lens of either a monofocal or multifocal design. Recent research indicates that different monofocal lens designs have similar reductions of mesopic CS in the presence of glare (46), and that at least one multifocal intraocular lens will severely reduce high spatial frequency CS at distance under mesopic conditions, and all spatial frequency CS at near under all luminance conditions (47). In all cases, patients should be warned of the potential visual difficulties under different environmental conditions.

Vitreous Humor

Floaters, especially near the fovea, will scatter light within the eye and reduce CS of at least the high spatial frequencies.

Under- or Uncorrected Refractive Error

View Fig. 3.2 at about arm's-length with increasing powers of plus trial lenses to eventually overcompensate for the near distance by at least +2 D. The zebra in Fig. 3.2B will nearly fade into the background, whereas the stripes on the zebra's back in Fig. 3.2A will still be visible. Primarily the high and middle spatial frequencies will suffer from reduced CS. Because of differences in spherical aberration between myopic and nonmyopic eyes, however, those who are myopic possess an asymmetric sensitivity to positive and negative defocus, such that their reports of reduced accommodative responses can be explained by a myopic shift of the middle spatial frequencies (around 3 cpd), complete with "notches" in the CSF (see *Adaptation,* below) (17,48).

On the other hand, under controlled conditions, cylindrical myopic defocus (i.e., meridional blur) will primarily affect CS (at all spatial frequencies) when the cylinder axis is parallel to the grating. When the cylinder axis is at a 45° oblique angle to the grating, the cylinder will have the same overall effect as half the sphere power (i.e., the spherical equivalent), and when the cylinder axis is perpendicular to the grating, the cylinder induces no decrement in CS (17).

Neurologic

Central versus Peripheral Retina

For normal peripheral retina, the CSF is shifted to the left on the graph, such that the high-frequency cut-off, about 3 to 6 cpd, corresponds to the reduced acuity, about 20/200 to 20/100, respectively. Likewise, the peak sensitivity occurs at or below 1 cpd (41).

Adaptation

Each spatial frequency channel can be adapted independently of the other channels, such that CS will be reduced for that small range of spatial frequencies, resulting in a "notch" in the CSF. The adaptation, however, does not extend to those spatial frequencies if their orientation is different than the adapting stimulus. Persons with uncorrected myopia may display one or more such similar notches (17,48).

Pathologic

Optic Nerve

Any condition that affects retinal function will begin to take its first toll on CS at the middle and low spatial frequencies. For example, patients with retinitis pigmentosa may exhibit CS loss at low spatial frequencies as early as teenagers (49). Although CS reduction in patients with early glaucoma may be slight (50), eventually the entire function is reduced, even in areas with no apparent visual field loss (51).

It has been suggested that a dynamic CS test, using drifting stripe patterns and assessing optokinetic nystagmus simultaneously, is more sensitive a test than stationary CS for patients with glaucoma, optic neuritis, and optic atrophy (52). In addition, patients with multiple scle-

rosis were more likely to have recurrent optic neuritis within 10 years of the first episode and, consequently, have greater CS loss than patients who had no recurrent episodes (53).

Cortical or Systemic

In normal adults, CS measured binocularly is greater than CS measured monocularly (54,55). In normal infants between 3 and 36 months, however, monocular CS is similar to binocular CS at all ages except around 12 months, when it is significantly lower (56). Presumably, this is consistent with the different rates of development of the components of the infant's visual system. In other words, before 1 year of age, and up to 3 years of age, there should likely be *no* cause for alarm if, unlike in an adult, the binocular CS and monocular CS are similar.

Nonetheless, if monocular CS is ever significantly higher than binocular CS at any age, it is likely that the patient has amblyopia (57). The lack of development of the cortical binocular cells in patients who are amblyopic is borne out by the measurements of one-eyed subjects who had enucleation early in life. These subjects, never having experienced meaningful binocular vision, developed supernormal CS with the remaining eye, which had greater overall CS than the better eye of the binocular control group (58).

Other conditions in which CS loss has been demonstrated over some or all spatial frequencies include Duane syndrome (59), Down syndrome (60,61), and low birthweight (62). Patients with traumatic brain injury, although not necessarily exhibiting reduced CS, consistently achieved improvement in binocular CS with colored filters (63).

Premature children (64,65) and children with low vision (66), however, do not demonstrate CS reductions. Likewise, with regard to dyslexic patients, several recent studies report no consistent effects on CS compared with normal control subjects (67–69), with the exception of reduced low spatial frequency CS in the mixed (dysphoneidetic) subgroup (70).

Finally, drugs that act as central nervous system depressants have been shown to cause CS loss. This includes cases of direct exposure to alcohol (71) and antiepileptic drugs (72), and a case of prenatal exposure to an organic solvent (73).

CONCLUSION

Many environmental and organic factors affect an individual's CS. Reduced CS alone will likely never lead to a unique diagnosis, but it can be monitored if a particular condition or disease is suspected and it can be a predictor of subsequent vision loss (74). As laboratory and clinical research advance, we will be able to test more quickly and effectively the patient who has good visual acuity but still complains of difficulty with vision. Likewise, we will be able regularly to assess infants at an earlier age, to ensure that their visual system developmental milestones are being met, and that any potential problems are caught and treated early.

REFERENCES

1. Newacheck JS, Haegerstrom-Portnoy G, Adams AJ. Predicting visual acuity from detection thresholds. *Optometry and Vision Science* 1990;67:184–191.
2. Applegate RA, Hilmantel G, Thibos LN. Visual performance assessment. In: MacRae SM, Krueger RR, Applegate RA, eds. *Customized Corneal Ablation: The Quest for SuperVision.* Thorofare, NJ: Slack Incorporated; 2001: 81–92.
3. Cornsweet T. *Visual Perception.* New York: Academic Press, 1970.
4. Schwartz SH. *Visual Perception: A Clinical Orientation* 2nd ed. Stamford, CT: Appelton & Lange, 1999.
5. Palmer SE. *Vision Science: Photons to Phenomenology.* Cambridge, MA: MIT Press, 1999.
6. Rabin J, Wicks J. Measuring resolution in the contrast domain: the Small Letter Contrast Test. *Optom Vis Sci* 1996;73:398–403.
7. Ginsburg AP. A new contrast sensitivity vision test chart. *American Journal of Optometry and Physiological Optics* 1984;61:403–407.
8. Adams RJ, Courage ML. Monocular contrast sensitivity in 3- to 36-month-old human infants. *Optometry and Vision Science* 1996;73:546–551.
9. Brunette I, Bueno JM, Parent M, et al. Monochromatic aberrations as a function of age, from childhood to advanced age. *Invest Ophthalmol Vis Sci* 2003;44: 5438–5446.
10. Teller DY. First glances: The vision of infants. *Invest Ophthalmol Vis Sci* 1997;38:2183–2203.
11. Campbell FW, Robson JG. Application of Fourier analysis to the visibility of gratings. *J Physiol* 1968;197:561–566.
12. Cox MJ, Norman JH, Norman P. The effect of surround luminance on measurements of contrast sensitivity. *Ophthalmic Physiol Opt* 1999;19:401–414.
13. Adams RJ, Courage ML. Contrast sensitivity in 24- and 36-month-olds as assessed with the contrast sensitivity card procedure. *Optom Vis Sci* 1993;70:97–101.
14. Richman JE, Lyons S. A forced choice procedure for evaluation of contrast sensitivity function in preschool children. *Invest Ophthalmol Vis Sci* 1994;65:859–864.
15. Katz M. Contrast sensitivity through hybrid diffractive, Fresnel, and refractive prisms. *Optometry* 2004;75: 509–516.
16. Adams RJ, Courage ML. Using a single test to measure human contrast sensitivity from early childhood to maturity. *Vision Res* 2002;42:1205–1210.
17. Woods RL, Strang NC, Atchison DA. Measuring contrast sensitivity with inappropriate optical correction. *Ophthalmic Physiol Opt* 2000;20:442–451.
18. Rogers GL, Bremer DL, Leguire LE. Contrast sensitivity functions in normal children with the Vistech method. *J Pediatr Ophthalmol Strabismus* 1987;24:216–219.
19. Mantyjarvi MI, Autere MH, Silvennoinen AM, et al. Observations on the use of three different contrast sensitivity tests in children and young adults. *J Pediatr Ophthalmol Strabismus* 1989;26:113–119.
20. Westall CA, Woodhouse JM, Saunders K, et al. Problems measuring contrast sensitivity in children. *Ophthamic Physiol Opt* 1992;12:244–248.
21. Elliott DB, Whitaker D. Clinical contrast sensitivity chart evaluation. *Ophthalmic Physiol Opt* 1992;12:275–280.
22. Reeves BS, Wood JM, Hill AR. Vistech VCTS-6500 charts—within- and between-session reliability. *Optom Vis Sci* 1991;68:728–737.
23. Pesudovs K, Hazel CA, Doran RM, et al. The usefulness of Vistech and FACT contrast sensitivity charts for cataract and refractive surgery outcomes research. *Br J Ophthalmol* 2004;88:11–16.
24. Scialfa CT, Tyrrell RA, Garvey PM, et al. Age differences in Vistech near contrast sensitivity. *American Journal of Optometry and Physiological Optics* 1988;65:951–956.
25. Bailey IL, Lovie JE. New design principles for visual acuity letter charts. *American Journal of Optometry and Physiological Optics* 1976;53:740–745.
26. Leat SJ, Wegmann D. Clinical testing of contrast sensitivity in children: age-related norms and validity. *Optom Vis Sci* 2004;81:245–254.
27. Pelli DG, Robson JG, Wilkins AJ. The design of a new letter chart for measuring contrast sensitivity. *Clinical Vision Science* 1988;2:187–199.
28. Norcia AM, Tyler CW. Spatial frequency sweep VEP: visual acuity during the first year of life. *Vision Res* 1985;25:1399–1408.
29. Norcia AM, Tyler CW, Hamer RD. Development of contrast sensitivity in the human infant. *Vision Res* 1990;30:1475–1486.
30. Banks MS, Salapatek P. *Invest Ophthalmol Vis Sci* 1978;17: 361–365.
31. Atkinson J, French J, Braddick O. Contrast sensitivity function of preschool children. *Br J Ophthalmol* 1981;65:525–529.
32. Beazley LD, Illingworth DJ, Jahn A, et al. Contrast sensitivity in children and adults. *Br J Ophthalmol* 1980;64:863–866.
33. Norcia AM, Tyler CW, Hamer RD. High visual contrast sensitivity in the young human infant. *Invest Ophthalmol Vis Sci* 1988;29:44–49.
34. Gwiazda J, Bauer J, Thorn F, et al. Development of spatial contrast sensitivity from infancy to adulthood: Psychophysical data. *Optom Vis Sci* 1997;74:785–789.
35. Movshon JA, Kiorpes L. Analysis of the development of spatial contrast sensitivity in monkey and human

infants. *Journal of the Optical Society of America A*, 1988;5:2166–2172.

36. Schor CM. Development of stereopsis depends upon contrast sensitivity and spatial tuning. *Journal of the American Optometric Association*, 1985;56:628–635.

37. Scharre JE, Cotter SA, Block SS, et al. Normative contrast sensitivity data for young children. *Optom Vis Sci* 1990;67:826–832.

38. Ellemberg D, Lewis TL, Liu CH, et al. Development of spatial and temporal vision during childhood. *Vision Res* 1999;39:2325–2533.

39. Benedek G, Benedek K, Deri S, et al. The scotopic low-frequency spatial contrast sensitivity develops in children between the ages of 5 and 14 years. *Neurosci Lett* 2003;345:161–164.

40. Lew H, Seong G-J, Kim S-K, et al. Mesopic contrast sensitivity functions in amblyopic children. *Yonsei Medical Journal*, 2003;44:995–1000.

41. Levi DM, Klein SA, Yap YL. Positional uncertainty in peripheral and amblyopic vision. *Vision Res* 1987;27:581–597.

42. Quesnel NM, Lovasik JV, Ferremi C, et al. Laser in situ keratomileusis for myopia and the contrast sensitivity function. *Journal of Cataract and Refractive Surgery*, 2004;30:1209–1218.

43. Gauthier CA, Holden BA, Epstein D, et al. Assessment of high and low contrast visual acuity after photorefractive keratectomy for myopia. *Optom Vis Sci* 1998;75: 585–590.

44. Yagci A, Egrilmez S, Kaskaloglu M, et al. Quality of vision following clinically successful penetrating keratoplasty. *J Cataract Refract Surg* 2004;30:1287–1294.

45. Fujikado T, Kuroda T, Maeda N, et al. Light scattering and optical aberrations as objective parameters to predict visual deterioration in eyes with cataracts. *J Cataract Refract Surg* 2004;30:1198–1208.

46. Hayashi K, Hayashi H. Effect of a modified optic edge design on visual function: texture-edge versus round-anterior, slope-side edge. *J Cataract Refract Surg* 2004; 30:1668–1674.

47. Montes-Mico R, Espana E, Bueno I, et al. Visual performance with multifocal intraocular lenses: Mesopic contrast sensitivity under distance and near conditions. *Ophthalmology* 2004;111:85–96.

48. Radhakrishnan H, Pardhan S, Calver RI, et al. Effect of positive and negative defocus on contrast sensitivity in myopes and non-myopes. *Vision Res* 2004;44:1869–1878.

49. Hyvarinen L. Contrast sensitivity in visually impaired children. *Acta Ophthalmol Suppl* 1983;157:58–62.

50. Wood JM, Lovie-Kitchin JE. Evaluation of the efficacy of contrast sensitivity measures for the detection of early primary open-angle glaucoma. *Optom Vis Sci* 1992;69:175–181.

51. McKendrick AM, Badcock DR, Morgan WH. Psychophysical measurement of neural adaptation abnormalities in magnocellular and parvocellular pathways in glaucoma. *Invest Ophthalmol Vis Sci* 2004;45:1846–1853.

52. Abe H, Hasegawa S, Takagi M, et al. Contrast sensitivity for the stationary and drifting vertical stripe patterns in patients with optic nerve disorders. *Ophthalmologica* 1993;207:100–105.

53. Optic Neuritis Study Group. Visual function more than 10 years after optic neuritis: Experience of the optic neuritis treatment trial. *Am J Ophthalmol* 2004;137: 77–83.

54. Derefeldt G, Lennerstrand G, Lundh B. Age variations in normal human contrast sensitivity. *Acta Ophthalmologica (Copenhagen)* 1979;57:679–690.

55. Rabin J. Two eyes are better than one: binocular enhancement in the contrast domain. *Ophthalmic Physiol Opt* 1995;15:45–48.

56. Adams RJ, Courage ML. Monocular contrast sensitivity in 3- to 36-month-old human infants. *Optom Vis Sci* 1996;73:546–551.

57. McKee SP, Levi DM, Movshon JA. The pattern of visual deficits in amblyopia. *J Vision* 2003;3:380–405.

58. Nicholas JJ, Heywood CA, Cowey A. Contrast sensitivity in one-eyed subjects. *Vision Res* 1996;36:175–180.

59. Marshman WE, Dawson E, Neveu NM. Increased binocular enhancement of contrast sensitivity and reduced stereoacuity in Duane syndrome. *Invest Ophthalmol Vis Sci* 2001;42:2821–2825.

60. Courage ML, Adams RJ, Hall EJ. Contrast sensitivity in infants and children with Down syndrome. *Vision Res* 1997;37:1545–1555.

61. Suttle CA, Turner AM. Transient pattern visual evoked potentials in children with Down syndrome. *Ophthalmic Physiol Opt* 2004;24:91–99.

62. O'Connor AR, Stephenson TJ, Johnson A, et al. Visual function in low birthweight children. *Br J Ophthalmol* 2004;88:1149–1153.

63. Jackowski MM. Altered visual adaptation in patients with traumatic brain injury. In: Suchoff IB, Ciuffreda KJ, Kapoor N, eds. *Visual and Vestibular Consequences of Acquired Brain Injury*. Santa Ana, CA: Optometric Extension Program Foundation; 2001: 145–173.

64. Jackson TL, Ong GL, McIndoe MA, et al. Monocular chromatic contrast threshold and achromatic contrast sensitivity in children born prematurely. *Am J Ophthalmol* 2003;136:710–719.

65. Oliveira AG, Costa MF, Souza JM, et al. Contrast sensitivity threshold measured by sweep visual evoked potential in term and preterm infants at 3 and 10 months of age. *Braz J Med Biol Res* 2004;37:1389–1396.

66. Lovie-Kitchin JE, Bevan JD, Hein B. Reading performance in children with low vision. *Clinical and Experimental Optometry* 2001;84:148–154.

67. Victor JD, Conte MM, Burton L, et al. Visual evoked potentials in dyslexics and normals: failure to find a difference in transient or steady-state responses. *Vis Neurosci* 1993;10:939–946.

68. O'Brien BA, Mansfield JS, Legge GE. The effect of contrast on reading speed in dyslexia. *Vision Res* 2000;40:1921–1935.

69. Williams MJ, Stuart GW, Castles A, et al. Contrast sensitivity in subgroups of developmental dyslexia. *Vision Res* 2003;43:467–477.

70. Slaghuis WL, Ryan JF. Spatio-temporal contrast sensitivity, coherent motion, and visible persistence in developmental dyslexia. *Vision Res* 1999;39:651–668.

71. Pearson P, Timney B. Effects of moderate blood alcohol concentrations on spatial and temporal contrast sensitivity. *J Stud Alcohol* 1998;59:163–173.

72. Hilton EJ, Hosking SL, Betts T. The effect of antiepileptic drugs on visual performance. *Seizure* 2004;13:113–128.

73. Till C, Rovet JF, Koren G, et al. Assessment of visual functions following prenatal exposure to organic solvents. *Neurotoxicology* 2003;24:725–731.

74. Schneck ME, Haegerstrom-Portnoy G, Lott L, et al. Low contrast vision function predicts subsequent acuity loss in an aged population: the SKI study. *Vision Res* 2004;44:2317–2325.

Refractive Error

4

David E. FitzGerald

The development of the human refractive status from birth to the school-aged child has been the topic of theoretic models and research, particularly over the past 30 years. The resulting literature is voluminous and at times complex; consequently, it can be difficult for one unfamiliar with it to apply the knowledge to actual patient care. This chapter provides an overview of what is known about this dynamic aspect of human development in the interest of optometric patient care.

The concept of an emmetropization process has become the key model in understanding the early development of the human refractive status. In recognition of its importance, this chapter begins with a discussion of the process. This is followed by summarizing reports of the effects of optical interventions on emmetropization. The next section discusses in some detail the refractive status of premature infants, newborns, and provides an overview of refraction from infancy through the preschool years, and finally during the elementary school years. The last section focuses on developmental aspects of myopia, hyperopia, anisometropia, and astigmatism.

EMMETROPIZATION

Emmetropization is frequently discussed and infrequently defined by authors, which results in multiple meanings. The following definition is a reasonable standard, however:

"A process presumed to be operative in producing a greater frequency of occurrence of emmetropia and near emmetropia than would be expected in terms of chance distribution, as may be explained by postulating that a mechanism coordinates the formation and development of the various components of the human eye which contribute to the total refractive power" (1).

Thus, it is postulated that the desired result of the process is emmetropia: where parallel rays of light, emanating from an object at optical infinity, come to a point focus or near point on the retina of an eye, which is in a relaxed state of accommodation (2). In clinical terms, emmetropization is a process by which the refractive condition of the eye, regardless of whether it is initially hyperopia, myopia, or astigmatism, centers on a refractive range around low hyperopia to emmetropia (3,4). Sorsby et al. (3) defined these limits as $+0.50$ to $+1.00$ diopter (D) of hyperopia with a standard deviation (SD) of $±1.00$ D.

Some have proposed that emmetropization is a passive process, where nature and genetics are the guiding factors; others have viewed it as an active process, where nurture and the environment are the major influences. Further, evidence indicates that effectiveness of the process depends on four main elements: a healthy eye, a healthy environment, an operational refractive range, and an intact emmetropization mechanism (5–10).

Emmetropization as a Passive Process

Emmetropization as a passive process is a school of thought that suggests that nature and genetics are the key factors. Thus, the natural growth and development of most eyes are relatively predictable. Larsen (11–14), using ultrasound, tracked the changes in ocular growth over the first 13 years of life. Axial length, which was approximately 16.5 mm at birth, increased by 3.8 mm during the first 2 years of life. From 2 to 5 years of age the average increase was 1.2 mm. Most of this growth occurred in the vitreal chamber. Larsen noted that males tended, on average, to have a greater axial length, although at birth there appears to be little difference from females. But by 2 years of age, a differential of 0.3 mm existed, which tended to continue until puberty at which time the differential increased to 0.5 mm (11–14). During this same period, the crystalline lens flattens, the anterior chamber deepens, and the cornea flattens. All of these changes can contribute to the overall refraction of the eye (11–17).

The predictable programmed growth gives rise to the passive theory. In addition, genetic tendencies are cited as evidence supporting the passive theory. The likelihood of being myopic is directly correlated to the number of myopic parents. According to Gwiazda et al. (18), a 42% chance of being a myopic offspring exists if both parents are myopic, a 22.5% if one is myopic, and an 8% chance if neither is myopic. Ong and Ciuffreda (19) found a 60% chance of myopia if both parents had myopia, whereas Goss and Jackson (20) note a 57% chance. On the contrary, Zadnik et al. (21) found only a 12% prevalence. In addition, they noted that regardless of the number of parents with myopia, corneal curves were essentially 44.00 D (21). A number of other studies, including those of twins, have supported the hereditary aspects of myopia (22–26).

Emmetropization as an Active Process

Emmetropization as an active process is a theory that prepossesses that emmetropization is mediated by retinal blur (27,28). The visual system is able to compute the existence of a blur and then respond appropriately to compensate for it. A number of animal studies have been cited in support of the active process theory. Form deprivation and image degradation have been shown to have an intimate positive correlation to eye growth and subsequent refractive status (29,30).

Animal Studies

Convex and concave lenses, various levels of occlusion, and duration and timing of form deprivation have been methods used to create optical defocus in young primates. The lenses simulate a hyperopic or a myopic refractive condition. This causes the chick or monkey's eye to alter its anterior-posterior length to maintain image conjugacy. If the causative agent is removed within a specified period of time, the compensating adaptation will respond appropriately to meet the new demand for conjugacy (5,6,8,31,32). Smith et al. (33) note that relatively long periods of form deprivation can be offset by relatively short periods of normal viewing. In another monkey study, Smith and Hung (34) noted a positive correlation between varying degrees of form deprivation and the resulting axial myopia. This "graded phenomenon" can be initiated with lesser amounts of chronic defocus (34).

Human Studies

In humans, form deprivation can be caused by physical insult and substantial defocus. Eyes, which are compromised at birth or before being fully developed, are at risk for physical alteration and reduced function. Pathologic conditions (e.g., ptosis, lid alterations, corneal opacifications, glaucoma, cataracts, aphakia, vitreal abnormalities, retinal anomalies, and retinopathy of prematurity) have been cited in the literature (35–46). These compromising conditions frequently result in axial elongation and a relatively more myopic eye. Studies of identical twins with one of their four eyes having cataracts have documented this axial change (32,47,48).

These two seemingly competing theories may not be mutually independent and the emmetropization process may result as a summation and interaction of both. Saunders et al. (49) echo this by stating that the process is a result of the combination of the two theories.

Elements of Emmetropization

For emmetropization to be successfully completed, several prerequisite elements need to be present. Essential are healthy eyes, which are exposed to a visually healthy and stimulating environment. Further, the emmetropization mechanism must be intact, and lastly, the refractive status at particular ages of childhood must be within the limits of the process.

Healthy Eyes and Healthy Environment

Ocular pathologies and anomalies can compromise the eye and its refractive state. In animal studies, the greatest myopic shift occurred with early onset, essentially at birth, lid closure (6,50,51). The duration of occlusion appears to contribute to the gravity of the insult (52). Similarly, the alterations of the visual environment, whether it is done by restrictive stimuli, form deprivation, or optical defocus has a profound impact on the process. In form deprivation (myopia), which is a constant state of defocus, the eye seems to lack the ability to make appropriate ocular adjustments. This results in uncontrolled growth and an increase in refractive abnormalities (9). This process has both a local (eye level) control (39,53–57) and, to a degree, a higher level (brain), for the process is less accurate if the optic nerves are severed or accommodation is blocked (5,31,58). The former seems to have the greater influence on emmetropization, but the latter has been shown in chicks to have some regulating control.

Intact Emmetropization Mechanism

It is uncertain why some patients do not emmetropize or have an inhibitory response to the process. A proposed reason is that the emmetropization mechanism is compromised. In this regard, some predisposing conditions have been suggested.

Patients with amblyopia or strabismus have an altered emmetropization process (59–61). Abrahamsson et al. (59) and Lepard (60) found the deviating strabismic eye increased in hyperopia after the onset of the strabismus. An echobiometric (ultrasound) study of patients with strabismic amblyopia revealed ocular growth toward emmetropia in the fixing eye of those with hyperopia and ocular elongation in the nonfixing eye of those with myopia (62). Almeder et al. (63), in a longitudinal study of 686 children ages 3 months to 9 years, then proposed that anisometropia developed slowly and was the result of a microstrabismus. The concept of the existence of some higher level control of emmetropization can also be argued from the fact that patients with compromising mental (not including mental retardation) or neuromuscular conditions tend to have a higher incidence of higher refractive errors than the general population (64–66).

Evans et al. (38) suggest that an association exists between defective emmetropization and a faulty visual input or neural transmission. Patients with congenital achromatopsia tend to have higher refractive errors, which do not conform to the concept of emmetropization. In the patient who is achromatopsic, the hyperopia reduces, but the astigmatism noticeably increases. This emmetropization nonconformity would imply the existence of a faulty emmetropization mechanism. Evans (38) proceeds to make a correlation between myopia and early onset image degradation and a delay in retinal function, whereas hyperopia results in the failure of the normal retinal neural processing, such as in achromatopsia, Leber's amaurosis, albinism, and aniridia (38,67,68). Similar issues can be made about patients with other compromising conditions (e.g., Down syndrome and fragile X syndrome (69–71).

Limits of Refraction Status

Aurell and Norrsell (72), in a longitudinal study of children from 6 months to 4 years of age, found that, if a hyperopic refractive error of 4.00 D or more was evident at 6 months of age and strabismus resulted, emmetropization was compromised. Those children in the sample who did not develop a strabismus, however, did emmetropize.

Children whose refraction at 1 year of age was myopic in either meridian by 2.50 D or more tended not to emmetropize, whereas those with a lesser amount did (73). Smith et al. (9) note that the emmetropization process can offset moderate amounts of defocus; however, they proceed to speculate that a more moderate operational defocus range for emmetropization exists in the monkey than does in the chick. In the Ingram et al. and Atkinson et al. studies (73–76), their samples tend to have refractive limits. Although the emmetropization process occurs, true emmetropia is not always achieved. Ingram et al. (76) used the reduction of the more hyperopic meridian to +3.50 D or less as a criterion for emmetropization. However, 81% of their sample had +5.00 D or less as the more hyperopic meridian (76). In addition, in some of the studies, no statistics existed as to the end refractive states of each hyperopic dioptric level (76,77). In another Atkinson et al. (77) study, infants with more than 6.00 D of hyperopia in any meridian, 2.00 D of anisometropia, or 3.00 D of myopia were referred for immediate care. This would indicate the authors' concerns for proper care and the perception of outer refractive limits of emmetropization (77).

Children 6-months of age who became hyperopic were followed for a 3-year period. Children who had initially 4.00 D of hyperopia had a 21% chance of being strabismic. At 5.50 D, the incidence increased to 36%, and at the 6.00 D level it increased to 48%. Children who became strabismic had poorer accommodative skills and did not emmetropize when compared with nonstrabismic children (7). Again, this would raise the question of outer refractive limits, although interplay with strabismus existed.

In most studies cited above, refractive ranges between +5.00 D and −4.50 D encompass approximately 90% of the sample (78–81). Statistically, 67% of a sample within the first standard deviation (SD) will conform, whereas 95% of those within the second SD conform. If this concept is applied to emmetropization, it would seem logical that at some point a refractive error would be so great that it would be unlikely for an eye to conform to the process of emmetropization. Exceptions are known to occur, however.

The Effect of Optical Intervention on Emmetropization

Within operational limits, hyperopia decreases more when the initial refraction is higher; in general, this reduction is associated with not wearing glasses (74,75,82). Children who are hyperopic with poor accommodative skills tend not to emmetropize and are more inclined to become strabismic, whereas those with adequate accommodative skills tend to emmetropize and are binocularly aligned (82). Children with a greater degree of hyperopia are at a greater risk to become esotropic; thus, a dilemma exists in prescribing convex lenses to prevent the deviation as opposed to a possible interference with the emmetropization process.

A number of studies have dealt with this scenario, with mixed results. In some instances, the hyperopic prescription was routinely under corrected by 1.00 D to 2.00 D(74,75). Atkinson et al. (75) concluded that the use of a hyperopic prescription for infants did not impair emmetropization, but noted that the use of a full prescription might have a more deleterious effect on the process. It should be noted, however, that the difference in reduction of hyperopia between the treated group and the untreated group was 0.3 D (3.40 D to 3.10 D), and both groups had an overall reduction of hyperopia of 1.20 D between 9 months and 36 months of age. The Atkinson et al. (75) control group, however, had an initial refraction of 1.90 D of hyperopia, which reduced by 0.40 D during the same period of time. Ingram et al. (76) concluded that correcting children's eyes at an early age tended to leave children more hyperopic than their counterparts. Dobson et al. (83) found that patients with corrected accommodative esotropia remained more hyperopic than did the uncorrected aligned control group. The real issue here, however, maybe the accommodative skills and flexibility, such that children with poor accommodation tend to become strabismic and not emmetropize, whereas those with good accommodative skills tend to emmetropize and are binocularly aligned. Ingram et al. (7,76,82) note that possibly a congenital lesion may be the cause for accommodation and emmetropization being deficient in those children who become strabismic, regardless of spectacle wear, because their interpretation of blur is faulty.

As noted previously, the visual system needs to recognize the existence of blur. This raises the question of strabismus or refractive limits (or blur) to which the eye does not perceive the emmetropization signal. Ingram et al. (74) concluded that the patients who are hyperopic and strabismic who do not emmetropize, regardless of whether they have spectacles, might be the result of a congenital deficit in the system. Other factors can be the duration and amount of preexisting blur, although these were not directly addressed. In fact, if the deviating eyes in general tended (to a small degree) to become more hyperopic, that would also indicate a lack of an appropriate focus change. In this study, the control group who were not strabismic did emmetropize, although full-time spectacle wear impeded the process. A note was that the deviating eye became more hyperopic (74). Other studies have substantiated that the process can be impeded by early and constant wear of hyperopic prescriptions at 6 months of age. In each of these studies, however, the infant's refractive error was within expected limits of hyperopia (76,84).

Refractive Status of Infancy and Childhood Groups

Over the years, a number of investigators have performed cross-sectional and longitudinal studies of the refractive status of neonates, infants, toddlers, preschool, and school-aged children. They have used various methods to determine refractive error, resulting in some disparity of norms. Earlier investigators used an ophthalmoscope to assess the refraction of newborns. In some instances, no cycloplegic agents were used, whereas in others, the cycloplegic agent was administered to the patient or to both the patient and examiner (85). In the 20th century, retinoscopy, autorefraction, and photorefraction have become the methods of choice. Some investigators used cycloplegic agents in their studies, whereas others used a near retinoscopy method.

Premature Infants

Prematurity is defined as a gestation period of less than 37 weeks. Birthweights are categorized as low (LBW), less than 2500 g; very low (VLBW), less than 1500 g; and extremely low (ELBW), less than 1000 g (86). A positive correlation has been shown between prematurity or LBW, advanced stages of retinopathy of pre-

maturity (ROP), need for surgical intervention, and the severity of myopia (87–89). The incidence of myopia, high myopia, anisometropia, and astigmatism increases with the severity of ROP and conversely with increased birthweight (90–99). The following are a group of studies whose results vary because of the weight inclusion criterion, the presence of ROP, and whether surgical intervention was required.

Choi et al. (100) found an increase in myopia between 6 months of age and 3 years. They grouped their sample into no ROP (R-O), no cicatricial ROP with a history of ROP (R-1), and cicatricial ROP (R-2). The prevalence and severity of myopia and high myopia increased from R-O to R-2. Cryotherapy tended to increase the severity of the myopia. The R-1 group showed an increase in myopia between 6 months and 3 years of age. In general, between 3 and 6 years of age high myopia disappeared in the R-O group, whereas in the R-1 group, the rate doubled. The R-2 group had the highest prevalence of high myopia, which was present at 6 months (100). This group would tend to be the more premature neonate with the lower birthweights. Page et al. (93) summarizes this trend by saying that neonates weighing less than 751 g are 3.2 times more likely to develop myopia within the first year of life than those with birthweights between 751 and 1000 g and 10 times more likely than those with birthweights between 1001 and 1250 g. They continue to state that astigmatism and anisometropia were highly correlated to high myopia in the premature cohort. Interestingly, they also correlated the degree of ROP with the severity of myopia, by concluding that, for every increasing degree of ROP, the likelihood of myopia at 12 months of age doubled (93). Laws et al. (91) reported an increasing trend toward myopia, astigmatism, and anisometropia with increasing severity of ROP.

Quinn et al. (94) performed a multisite study of infants born less than 1251 g. Cycloplegic examinations were given at essentially 3, 12, and 24 months after birth (94). Refractive criteria were myopia ($\geq$0.25 D), high myopia ($\geq$5.00 D), astigmatism ($\geq$3.00 D), and anisometropia (>2.00 D). At the 3-month examination, the ELBW population had a greater incidence of myopia (31%), high myopia (4%), and anisometropia (73%). At the 12-month examination, the incidences increased to 36%, 9%, and 73%, respectively. Higher incidences of astigmatism were associated with myopia and high myopia. Anisometropia was also highly correlated to myopia. In general, no significant relationship was found between astigmatism and birthweight, and an overall astigmatic decrease was seen between the 3- and 12-month examination. This is in contrast to the increased incidence of myopia, high myopia, and anisometropia at the 12-month examination. Each of these refractive conditions tended to be relatively unchanged at the 24 month examination (94). Thus, from these data, it would appear that at 12 months the refractive status stabilized in their study population (Fig. 4.1). The effects of emmetropization are illustrated by the reduction in the number and amount of hyperopic refractive errors.

In contrast Holmstrom et al. (101) performed a study using a sample of preterm neonates (birthweight ≤1500 g) with and without ROP, who were followed from age 6 to 30 months. At 6 months of age, an 8% incidence of myopia was seen, which increased to 10% at 30 months. Infants who had cryotreatment had a 30% to 40% incidence. Astigmatism of greater than 1.00 D was present in 52% of the infants at 6 months and 26% at 30 months of age. Against the rule (ATR) had a greater incidence and the axis remained stable in 83% of the cases. Anisometropia was present in 6.5% of the infants at 6 months and in 8.4% at 30 months. In general, a positive correlation was found between severity of ROP and severity of refractive states and incidences (101).

Many of the studies mentioned above include infants with ROP, which can skew the data. The following is a study done on premature infants without ROP. Cycloplegic refractions were done on premature infants without ROP at birth, term, 6, 12, and 48 months of corrected age, and compared with a full-term cohort. Although the incidence of myopia was greater at term age, astigmatism and anisometropia were comparable to the full-term controls. At 6 months of corrected age, the preterm infants tended to have an increase in hyperopia that was not significantly different from the controls. The LBW babies tended to be more anisometropic until the 12-month examination. Between 12 months and 4 years, the mean spherical equivalent did not change

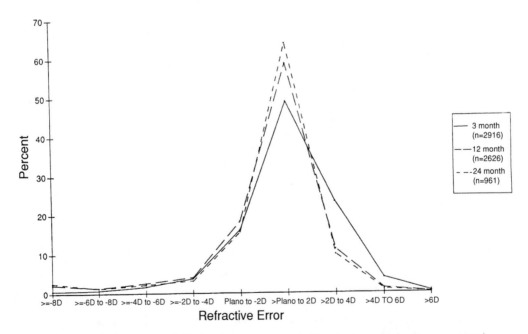

FIGURE 4.1. Refractive error of children born prematurely. Distribution of refractive errors at the three study examinations provided in 2.00 D steps from −8.00 D to +6.00 D. (From Quinn GE, Dobson V, Repka MX, et al. Development of myopia in infants with birth weights less than 1251 grams. *Ophthalmology* 1992;99:329–340, with permission.)

significantly, whereas the astigmatic error reduced. At 4 years of age, astigmatism of greater than 1.00 D was uncommon (96). The overall implication of this study is that at a 12-month adjusted age, the preterm, non-ROP infant tends to mirror its full-term counter part. Similar stable refractive findings of low hyperopia, matching full-term children, have been reported on the healthy eyes of prematurely born children between 6 months and 3.5 years (102).

Gallo and Lennerstrand (103) did follow-up examinations on Swedish children 5 to 10 years of age, who were born prematurely (>1501 g and >33 weeks gestation period). Data regarding the existence or level of ROP were not provided; thus, the criteria were simply birthweight and gestation period. They compared the premature cohort with a full-term control group, and concluded that prevalence of ocular abnormalities was much greater in the premature group as compared with the full-term children. The respective results of preterm to full-term were for myopia (6.3% s. 1.8%), anisometropia (5.9% vs. 1.5%), and strabismus (9.9% vs. 2.1%) (103).

Newborns

In 1925, Wibaut (104) published the refractive findings of 2398 newborns. The data were collected from several ophthalmologists; however, a standard protocol was not used, which resulted in interexaminer discrepancies. Regardless, more than 88% of the babies had a refractive error between emmetropia to 4.00 D of hyperopia, with a mode and medium of 2.00 D (104).

Most full-term newborns tend to have a hyperopic refraction of +2.00 D with a standard deviation of ±2.75 D, which conforms to a normal distribution resulting in a bell-shaped curve (105–107). Cook and Glasscock (108) performed cycloplegic refractions on 1000 newborns and found 73% of the eyes had hyperopia and 23% had myopia. The mean refraction was 2.07 D of hyperopia. Astigmatism was present in approximately 28% of each group. More than 86% of the eyes had a refractive range between +5.00 D to −5.00 D. The racial proportion of the sample was 370 white and 670 black newborns. The main difference between the two groups was the latter had more subjects with myopia between 3.00 and 5.00 D, otherwise their

distributions were similar (108). Black infants have a higher prevalence of high myopia than whites, but the latter are more likely to develop school-aged myopia (78). Mayer et al. (109) performed a cycloplegic cross-sectional study of 514 children from 1 through 48 months of age, of which 85% were white. The mean refraction of 64 eyes at 1 month of age was 2.20 D of hyperopia, with a 95% predictable range of 5.51 D of hyperopia to 1.12 D of myopia (109). Goldschmidt (85) performed cycloplegic retinoscopy on 356 Copenhagen neonates 2 to 10 days of age. Of the infants, 20% were emmetropic, 56% were myopic, and 24% were hyperopic. The mean refraction was +0.62 D with a SD of ±2.24 D. On average, the boys were a quarter diopter more hyperopic, but the SD findings between the genders were essentially the same (Fig. 4.2). Of the neonates, 97% had a refractive error between +5.00 to −4.00 D, with only one neonate being a hyperopic outlier (105).

Near-point retinoscopy (Mohindra technique) has been another method used to evaluate refractive status (110,111). In general, when compared with cycloplegic retinoscopy, the results tend to favor a relatively lesser amount of hyperopia, especially in the infant population and to a somewhat lesser extent in the preschoolers (78,112–114). Santonastaso (115) noted a 16% differential in finding more astigmatism using noncycloplegic versus cycloplegic retinoscopy.

Gwiazda et al. (18), using Mohindra near retinoscopy, found their newborn population to have a refractive range from 4.50 D of hyperopia to 4.50 D of myopia, with a mean refraction of low myopia (Fig. 4.3). Of the 144 eyes, 22% were emmetropic. Gwiazda et al. (18) noted that most of their findings of myopia occurred during the first 2 months of life. By 6 months, only a small degree of myopia persisted and by 1 year of age the average refraction was 0.50 D of hyperopia, which tended to remain stable for the next 7 years. Ingram and Barr (73) also found that the refractive state of the 1-year-old tended to remain during the toddler and preschool years.

In a cycloplegic retinoscopy study, however, a similar relative hyperopic shift was found during the first few weeks of life (116). During the period 2 weeks to 12 weeks, both myopic and

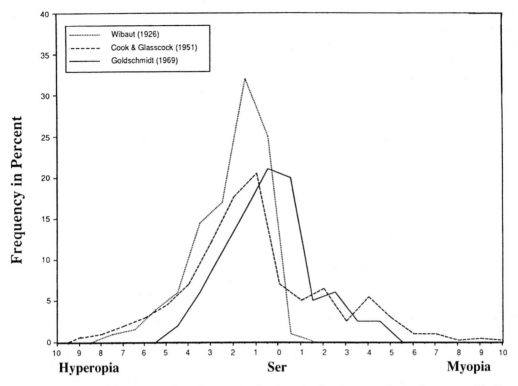

FIGURE 4.2. Refractive errors of newborns. Distribution of refractive errors in newborns provided in spherical equivalent refractions (SER). (From Baldwin WR. Refractive status of infants and children. In: Rosenbloom AA, Morgon MW, eds. *Principles and Practice of Pediatric Optometry*. Philadelphia: JB Lippincott; 1991:104–152, with permission.)

hyperopic newborns had a mean dioptric shift of +1.44 D and a mean spherical equivalent (MSE) range of refraction from +4.30 D to −1.83 D, of which most infants had a MSE of 2.60 D of hyperopia. From 12 to 26 weeks, no essential shift was noted, but from 26 weeks to 52 weeks a myopic shift of 0.76 D and a reduction of the refractive range were seen. These findings would conform to the concept of emmetropization. Anisometropia was present in 1.3% of the sample; in the one infant who had anisometropia persist, it did not develop until the child was 12 months of age. Astigmatism was greatest during the first 3 months of life and, in most instances, it decreased to insignificant clinical levels (116).

Infancy to School Years

The bell-shaped distribution of refractive errors at birth transition into an adultlike leptokurtic distribution by school age, with a mean refractive error of +0.50 D to +1.00 D and a SD of approximately ±1.00 D (3) (Fig. 4.4). Most

of emmetropization occurs within the first few years of life, with the greatest amount taking place within the first 2 years (49,75,117). Ingram (75) found a stable refraction after the first year of life, whereas in Hong Kong Chinese infants, the main reduction in MSE occurred by 40 weeks of age (118). Mayer et al. (109) followed children from 1 month to 48 months. By 18 months of age the MSE reduced by 1.00 D of hyperopia to between 1.00 and 1.25 D of hyperopia. The refraction remained at this level for the next 30 months (109) (Table 4.1). Ehrlich et al. (119) examined children from 8.5 months to 38.5 months of age using cycloplegic photorefraction. They divided the children into a myopic group and a control. At 8.5 months of age, the MSE for the former group was −0.53 D and the latter was +1.44 D. The former group had a yearly rate of change of +0.44 D, resulting in a final refractive MSE of +0.61 D, whereas the control group had no change in MSE at 38.5 months of age (119). Mohindra and Held (120) found emmetropization occurs during the first 4 to 5 years

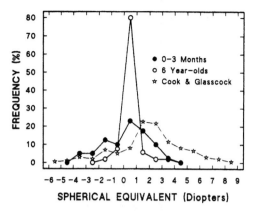

FIGURE 4.3. Distribution of newborns, infants, and 6 year olds refractive errors. Distribution of spherical equivalent refractions (SER) from studies of newborns by Cook RC, Glasscock RE. Refractive and ocular findings in the newborn. *Am J Ophthalmol* 1951; 34:1407–1413; and of infants at 0 to 3 months and 6-year-olds by Gwiazda J, Thorn F, Bauer J, et al. Emmetropization and the progression of manifest refraction in children followed from infancy to puberty. *Clinical Vision Science* 1993;8:337–344, with permission.)

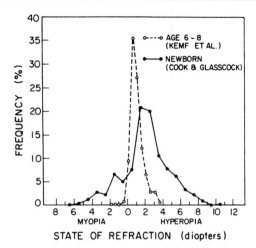

FIGURE 4.4. Emmetropization over time. Bell-shaped distribution of newborns spherical equivalent refractions (SER) to the leptokurtic distribution of SER in 6 to 8 year olds. (From Sivak JG, Bobier WR. Optical components of the eye: embryology and post-natal development. In: Rosenblum AA, Morgan MW, eds. *Practice of Pediatric Optometry*; Figure 2b. Philadelphia: JB Lippincott; 1990:40, with permission.)

TABLE 4.1 SER and Predictable Limits of Children From 1 to 48 Months

Age, Mo (No. of Patients)	Spherical Equivalent, Mean (SD), D*	95% Prediction Limits, D		99% Prediction Limits, D	
		Upper	Lower	Upper	Lower
1 (32)	2.20 (1.60)	5.51	−1.12	6.66	−2.27
1.5 (40)	2.08 (1.12)	4.36	−0.20	5.13	−0.98
2.5 (46)	2.44 (1.32)	5.13	−0.26	6.05	−1.17
4 (43)	2.03 (1.56)	5.21	−1.16	6.28	−2.23
6 (52)	1.79 (1.27)	4.39	−0.81	5.27	−1.69
9 (45)	1.32 (1.13)	3.63	−0.99	4.41	−1.77
12 (42)	1.57 (0.78)	3.16	−0.01	3.69	−0.55
18 (47)	1.23 (0.91)	3.09	−0.64	3.72	−1.27
24 (40)	1.19 (0.83)	2.89	−0.50	3.47	−1.08
30 (51)	1.25 (0.89)	3.07	−0.57	3.68	−1.19
36 (43)	1.00 (0.76)	2.56	−0.56	3.09	−1.09
48 (33)	1.13 (0.85)	2.89	−0.62	3.50	−1.23

*D indicates diopters

(From Mayer DL, Hansen RM, Moore BD, et al. Cycloplegic refractions in healthy children aged 1 through 48 months. *Arch Ophthalmol* 2001;119:1625–1628, with permission).

of life and results in a convergence of refractive errors on a low degree of hyperopia. In the Gwiazda et al. (18) longitudinal study, both newborn myopic and hyperopic children tended to achieve a hyperopic refractive state by 5 years of age, the former group were less hyperopic than the latter (Fig. 4.5). In cross-sectional data, Ehrlich had similar findings except for degree (Fig. 4.6). In general, the refractive state of children reaches an emmetropic plateau between 5 to 7 years of age (121).

School Years

Baldwin (78) believes that more than 80% of children between 5 and 7 years of age have a refractive error between +0.50 D to +3.00 D. Hyperopia greater than +5.00 D is present in less than 5% in this age group and less than 3% have myopia. A very low prevalence of myopia is found in 5 year olds (122,123). Less than 1% of Hirsch's (122) sample of 9552 school children had myopia greater than 1.00 D. He noted that it

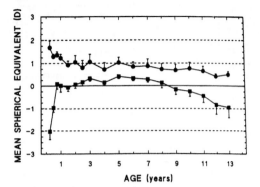

FIGURE 4.5. Refractive patterns from infancy to puberty. Longitudinal patterns mean spherical refractions (MSE) of children born myopic (■) and hyperopic (●). (From Gwiazda J, Thorn F, Bauer J, et al. Emmetropization and the progression of manifest refraction in children followed from infancy to puberty. *Clinical Vision Science* 1993;8:337–344, with permission.)

REDUCTION OF INFANT MYOPIA

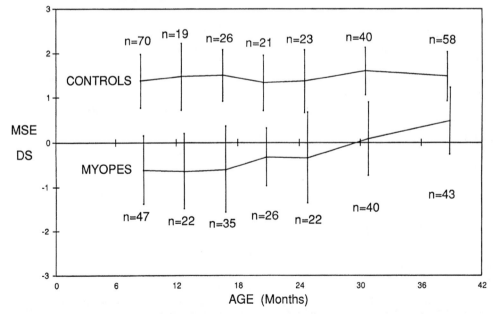

FIGURE 4.6. Refractive patterns from 8.5 to 38.5 months of age. Cross-sectional distribution of mean spherical refractions (MSE) in diopter spheres (DS) patterns in children born myopic and a control group of children. (From Ehrlich DL, Atkinson J, Braddick O, et al. Reduction of infant myopia: a longitudinal cycloplegic study. *Vision Res* 1995;35:1313–1324, with permission.)

is rare for a 5-year-old to have more than 1.00 D of myopia, except if the child had congenital or early onset high myopia (90). Native Americans and blacks tend to have a higher prevalence of hyperopia (121). During the elementary school years (5 to 14 years), a gradual reduction is noted of the MSE by approximately a 0.25 D to 0.50 D of hyperopia (79,122,123). During this period, however, school-aged myopia increases in incidence and is the major factor in refractive changes. It would appear that this shift would affect the MSE toward less hyperopia, although in most cases the refractive state of most children would be a relatively stable degree of hyperopia (105).

Hirsch (124) reported that 81% of 6-year-olds have less than 0.25 D of astigmatism and, at approximately 13 years of age, 72% have less than 0.25 D. Additionally, over this same period of time, an increase is seen of ATR from 3% to 11% (124), which may be associated with the increased incidence of myopia. Parssinen (125) found an association of increasing ATR and increasing myopia, which was not related to the initial degree of astigmatism. Thus, the onset and progression of school-aged myopia needs to be examined.

Baldwin (78) states that extreme errors are congenital or inherited. High ametropias, whether myopia or hyperopia, are most likely congenital. Congenital high myopia is found approximately two to three times more frequently than high hyperopia (113,137). High congenital myopia tends not to progress substantially (90,126).

DEVELOPMENTAL ASPECTS OF HYPEROPIA, MYOPIA, ANISOMETROPIA, AND ASTIGMATISM

Myopia

The lowest prevalence of myopia (1% to 2%) occurs at about 5 to 7 years of age (127). The criterion for myopia in most of the studies is between at least a 0.50 to 1 D (122,128–130). Myopia has the greatest prevalence in Jewish, Japanese, and Chinese races and ethnicities. Mutti et al. (131) found heredity to be the most significant risk factor for juvenile myopia. Excessive near work and greater academic success are also con-

tributory factors (131). Goss (132) found rates of progression were greater in children who had esophoria at near as compared with those myopic children whose near phoria was orthophoria to 6 Δexophoria (132). Additionally Asians, urban populations, near task oriented occupations, increased reading ability, higher education, and females have a higher prevalence of myopia (133,134). Others have found the prevalence of myopia to be 5% at 5 to 6 years of age and 25% in young adults (135). Myopia has been classified by the degree of myopia. Low myopia is considered to be less than 3.00 D; moderate is from 3.00 to 5.75 D, and high is above 6.00 D. It can also be categorized by age of onset into: congenital and school-aged or youth (136). Congenital or early onset can persist through infancy and follows a pattern of emmetropization or it can present as high myopia. The latter tends not to progress significantly (90,126).

Myopia Progression

Females tend to develop myopia at an earlier age and reach cessation at an earlier age than males. The difference seems to be about 2 years (80,81,122,137). Early onset of myopia tends to result in greater final myopia at cessation (138,139). Baldwin (78) believes that most children with high myopia develop myopia by 5 years of age. He believes that the average myopic progression per year is approximately −0.50 D and that if myopia commences before 9 years of age, the resultant endpoint will be at least 2.00 D and the MSE will be approximately 4.00 D of myopia. If onset is after 10 years of age, the resultant mean should be about 1.75 D of myopia with an outer limit of approximately 3.00 D, and myopia greater than −6.00 D, would be rare (78). The prevalence of myopia increases with school-aged and young adults (133).

In a Finnish study, 70% of children who became myopic before 11 years of age had 3.00 D to 5.75 D of myopia at 16. The other myopic children in the sample were divided between those who at 16 years of age had less than 3.00 D (12.5%) and 6.00 D or greater (17.5%). If myopia commenced between 11 and 15 years of age, 66.7% of the sample was less than 3.00 D myopic at 16 years of age, whereas 32.2% had between 3.00 and 5.75 D, and 1.1% had high myopia. Of the total sample of 214 children, 95.8% had myopia of less than 6.00 D at 16 years of age (138).

The reported prevalence of myopia in Taiwan school-aged children by 6 years of age is 12%, which increased to 56% by 12 years and 76% by 15 years, with a greater prevalence in both prevalence and degree for females. Lin (140) noted an association between early onset and morbidity. Studies have supported the concept of "the earlier the onset, the greater the myopia" (137,141–143).

Hirsch (128) tracked the refractive status of children 5 and 6 years of age for 8 years (children were then 13 to 14 years of age). Analysis of his data resulted in the following outcome predictions: (a) Children with hyperopia of +1.50 D or more at 5 to 6 years of age are likely to remain hyperopic at 13 to 14 years of age. (b) A number of children 5 to 6 years of age who are from +0.50 to +1.25 D hyperopic will be emmetropic at 13 to 14 years of age. (Note emmetropia to Hirsch was <−0.50 D to <+1.00 refraction). (c) A number of children 5 to 6 years of age whose refraction was plano to <+0.50 will become myopic by age 13 to 14 years. Those children 5 and 6-years of age became more myopic at age 13 to 14 years (128). Gwiazda (18) found myopia at birth or within the first few months of life to be a good predictor of future myopia. Although some of these infants emmetropized and even had their refractive states reach low hyperopia, they tended to revert to myopia during early school days (Fig. 4.5).

Langer (144) noted in his sample of 263 Canadian children, aged 5 to 15 years of age, that a child with greater than 0.50 D of myopia progressed in myopia in a linear fashion until the cessation of childhood myopia, which Goss and Winkler (137) found to be age 15 in girls and slightly less than 17 years in boys. Goss and Winkler (137) found that 90% of their myopic sample had a linear progression of their childhood myopia. They continue to conclude that refractive changes are greater in myopic children than hyperopic or emmetropic children (137).

Mäntyjärvi (143) tracked 1118 Scandinavian children, aged 7 to 15 years, using cycloplegic refractions for a period of 1 to 8 years. In the cross-sectional portion of the study, myopic children's mean yearly progression varied from −0.46 to −0.93 D, whereas the hyperopic average was −0.03 to −0.11 D. In the longitudinal portion, the mean yearly progression of the myopic children was −0.55 D, whereas the hyperopic children's mean progression was −0.21 D. She concluded that hyperopic children progress at a much slower rate than do myopic children of the same age (143).

A multicenter, longitudinal study found significant differences in prevalence of refractive states among ethnic groups (145). The sample consisted of Americans whose races were African (534), Asian (491), Hispanic (463), and Caucasian (1,035) from 5 to 17 years of age. In this study, myopia was defined as −0.75 D or more; hyperopia was +1.25 D or greater, and astigmatism was 1.00 D difference between the two principal meridians. Myopia was present in 9.2% of the sample, whereas hyperopia was present in 12.8% of the children, and astigmatism was present in 28.4% of the sample. Asians had the highest prevalence of myopia (18.5%), followed by Hispanics (13.2%), Africans (6.6%), and Caucasians (4.4%). Caucasians had the highest prevalence of hyperopia (19.3%), followed by Hispanics (12.7%), Africans (6.4%), and Asians (6.3%). Hispanics had the highest prevalence of astigmatism (36.9%), followed by Asians (33.6%), Caucasians (26.4%), and Africans (20%).

Hyperopia

Unlike myopia, hyperopia tends not to increase in the school-aged child. Interestingly, hyperopia, although having greater prevalence than any other childhood refractive conditions, tends to have fewer investigative studies, and probably receives less interest. As noted in the previous section, a child with hyperopia greater than +1.25 D at 6 years of age will very likely remain hyperopic throughout adolescence, as well as a number of their contemporaries who have a lesser degree of hyperopia (128). Zadnik et al. (79) found a hyperopic decrease of less than 0.25 D in their sample, and Mäntyjärvi (143) also noted a minimal reduction in hyperopia in children from age 7 to 15 years who remained hyperopic. Kempf et al. (146), using homatropine, did refractions on Washington, DC school children from age 6 to more than 12 years. They noted an overall shift toward less hyperopia with age, but most of the children remained hyperopic, with a median refraction at the older age category of slightly greater than 0.50 D of hyperopia.

The initial cross-sectional results of the Orinda longitudinal study of myopia were published in 1993. The study sample was mainly Caucasian and essentially equally divided among first, third, and sixth grades, as well as by gender. Autorefraction refractive findings were obtained 25 minutes after installation of tropicamide. The study concluded that, on average during the 6-year period between 6 and 12 years of age, a minimal decrease in hyperopia occurs, from +0.73 D to +0.50 D (79).

Accommodative Esotropia

In accommodative esotropia, the course of hyperopia has been shown to increase between the ages of 3 and 6 years by approximately 1.00 D (147). Others have reported an increase in hyperopia up to 7 years of age (148–152). The hyperopia tends to gradually decrease from 7 years to puberty; however, the average overall total degree of change is less than 1.00 D. Many of these studies fail to adequately identify or exclude subjects with residual strabismus, questionable or poor binocularity, and amblyopia nor its depth. Thus, a mean reduction in hyperopia may be represented more by the fixing eye changing, whereas the nonfixing eye remains stable. Greater hyperopic errors are more likely to remain unchanged.

Congenital Conditions

High hyperopia is defined as a hyperopic refractive error greater than 5.00 D (152) and is associated with a number of congenital or early onset anomalies. Among these are microphthalmia, cornea plana, foveal hypoplasias, Leber's congenital amaurosis, and optic atrophy (154). In these instances, emmetropization is compromised, resulting in high hyperopia. Syndromes such as fragile X, Down, and Rubinstein-Taybi are associated with hyperopia (69–71,154). As with congenital high myopia, congenital high hyperopia tends not to progress. In each of these high refractive conditions, some inherent defect seems to exist (78). Risk factors for high hyperopia include heredity (154).

Anisometropia

Chinese infants have a rapid reduction of anisometropia with a low incidence by 9 months of life. In Edwards' study (118), no infant had anisometropia of 2 D or astigmatic anisometropia of 1 D. In another study, only 1.3% of British infants had anisometropia greater than 1 D at 1 year of age (116). Other researchers have found a greater prevalence of anisometropia. A total of 310 anisometropic children were tracked once a year for a 3-year period between the ages of 1 and 4 years. The prevalence at each dioptric criterion of (1.00, 1.50, and ≥2.00) was relatively unchanged at 11%, 5%, and 2%, respectively, over the period of the study. No consistent pattern was noted within each category, such that some children would lose or maintain the anisometropia whereas others would develop it (155). Ingram and Barr (73) found a similar pattern of inconsistency in their children between the ages of 1 and 3.5. The Abrahamsson et al. study (156) on infantile anisometropia of 3.00 D or more, found three distinct anisometropic patterns: (a) an increase in anisometropia resulting in amblyopia; (b) a mean decrease in anisometropia of 3.00 D resulting in no amblyopia; and (c) a mean decease of 1.2 D resulting in amblyopia, strabismus, or both. They concluded that if at 1 year of age the hyperopic anisometropia is 3.00 D or more, a 90% chance existed that it would be present at 10 years and a 60% chance the child would have amblyopia. In addition, they note that persistent substantial anisometropia in the absence of amblyopia or strabismus is rare (156).

During the school years, deficiencies in binocularity (e.g., convergence insufficiency) can contribute to the development of anisometropia. Flom and Bedell (157) found a prevalence of 3.4% in children from age 5 to 12 years and Hirsch (158) found 6% prevalence in the teenagers he studied.

Almeder et al. (63) add the concept that anisometropia is the result of an esotropic microstrabismus, in which the fixing eye continues to emmetropize while the process ceases in the nonfixing eye, which may increase in hyperopia over time. This concept has been demonstrated by other studies (59,60,72). Burtolo et al. (62) tracked the refraction of fixing and nonfixing eyes in patients with strabismus. Their findings indicated a reduction in hyperopia (increase in axial length) in that the nonfixing eye lagged behind that of the fixing eye, whereas in myopic patients the opposite result occurred. Exodeviations tend to be alternating and this may contribute to an isometropic refraction (63).

Astigmatism

Astigmatism is common in the newborn, in infants, and during early childhood. Most studies agree astigmatism decreases more rapidly over the first 2 years of life, although the rate can vary from study to study (83,159–162). The age of highest incidence varies from study to study, but occurs within the first year of life. Mohindra (161), using near retinoscopy, found 1 D or more present in approximately 30% of newborns (1 to 10 weeks) studied, which increased to a peak incidence of approximately 57% between 11 to 20 weeks, of which more than half of the infants had 2.00 D or more of astigmatism. Between 20 and 50 weeks, a pattern was seen of decreasing degrees of significant astigmatism (>2.00 D), and an overall reduced incidence of significant astigmatism.

Tracked were 28 eyes of children between 3 and 6 months with 2 D or more of astigmatism. At 50 weeks, half (14 eyes), had no astigmatism, 7 had a reduction of 1 D or more of astigmatism, and the 7 maintained their 2.50 to 4.00 D of astigmatism. Mohindra noted that once the astigmatism was lost, it rarely reappeared, whereas only 30% of eyes with significant astigmatism lost it after the child was 1 year of age. Fulton et al. (163) found the highest incidence in infants 30 to 50 weeks of age. Howland et al. (164), using noncycloplegic photorefraction, and Gwiazda et al. (160), using near retinoscopy, both found a higher incidence of astigmatism and at the earlier age of birth to 6 months. Lyle et al. (165), who collated various studies, made a schematic progression trend curve of astigmatism form birth to 5 years of age. The initial degree of astigmatism was between 2.00 and 2.50 D at 6 months, which decreased to 1.00 D at 18 months and was less than 0.50 at 24 months (Fig. 4.7).

Mutti et al. (166) found a progressive reduction of astigmatism over the first 3 years of life from 41.6% at age 3 months to 4.1% at 36 months. They found the reduction of astigmatism and the emmetropization of the spherical refraction to be independent variables (166). Wood et al. (116) noted the gradual reduction of astigmatism over time, with more rapid reduction occurring with astigmatism greater than 1.50 D. Saunders et al. (49) suggest that the rate of emmetropization is a direct correlation

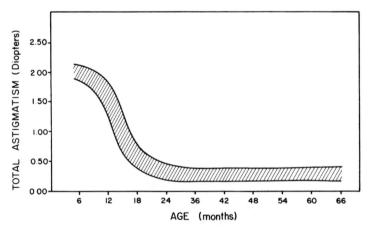

FIGURE 4.7. Astigmatism in children less than 6 years of age. A collation of studies illustrating the total amount of astigmatism in children less than 6 years of age. (From Lyle WM. Astigmatism. In: Grosvenor T, Flom MC, eds. *Refractive Anomalies*. Boston: Butterworth-Heinemann; 1991:146–173, with permission.)

to the initial refractive status (i.e. the greater the error, the greater the amount of emmetropization over the same period of time). Using linear regression, Mohindra and Held (120) suggest that, essentially, 3.00 D of astigmatism at birth should be reduced to 1.00 D between 129 and 256 weeks. The risk of amblyopia, however, would be greatly increased if significant astigmatism is not treated after the age of 2 years (167).

Using cycloplegic retinoscopy, Edwards (118) found 24% of Chinese infants 10 weeks of age had 2 D or more of astigmatism, which decreased to 2% by 37 weeks. Although the degree of astigmatism was similar to that of Caucasian infants, the axes were overwhelming with the rule (WTR) (118,168,169). In another study of Chinese infants, Chan and Edwards (170) also noted a rapid decrease of astigmatism, which stabilized within the first year of life. In the Hong Kong children, WTR astigmatism remaining at 1 year of age is less likely to emmetropize (118). Some believe the Mongoloid lid anatomy to be the etiology of WTR in these children (118,171). A high prevalence of WTR astigmatism exists and persists in the North American Indians (172–175), which has implications for other cultures with Indian lineage such as Mexican and South American children.

In Spain, using noncycloplegic retinoscopy, Montes-Mico (176) did a cross-sectional study of astigmatism in which he found a gradual reduction of astigmatism of 1.00 D or more from an incidence of 44.3% in children at 2 years of age to 5.2% at age 12 years.

Ingram et al. (177), in their randomized study of infants 6 months of age who were randomly chosen to wear or not wear a 2.00 D under correction for hyperopia, found that the reduction of hyperopia in the normal sample was not associated with the changes in astigmatism. The degree of astigmatism decreased significantly in both the normal and the strabismic groups, but to a lesser degree in the latter group (177).

Ingram and Barr (73) found that children whose refraction at 1 year of age was myopic in either meridian by 2.50 D or more tended not to emmetropize, whereas those with a lesser amount did. Ehrlich et al. (119), however, found a more liberal time limit. They studied the reduction of astigmatism in myopic children from age 8.5 months to 38.5 months in which the

more myopic meridian had to be no greater than 3.50 D. Their control group consisted of astigmatic children who had no greater than 3.50 D of hyperopia in its most ametropic meridian. The myopic group emmetropized to low hyperopia by 3 years of age. Both groups showed significant reduction in astigmatism with age significant emmetropization of meridians for both WTR and against the rule astigmatism (ATR). The control group remained with more overall hyperopia as compared with the myopic group. Thus, both myopic and hyperopic children, regardless of axis orientation, emmetropized not only in cylinder but also in sphere (119). However, the refractive error limits criteria of this study should be noted.

Although most researchers agree on the rapid reduction of astigmatism, their studies are not all in agreement about the orientation of the cylinder. WTR and ATR astigmatism are the major orientations of astigmatism. As noted previously, Ehrlich found significant reduction of astigmatism over time regardless of whether the child had WTR or ATR (120); however, a higher prevalence was noted of WTR at 9 months of age (81%), as compared with 17% ATR. Interestingly, Fulton et al. (163) found the axis orientation percentages to be similar but in favor of ATR. The studies of Mohindra et al. (120,161) also had substantially greater number of children with ATR astigmatism. Mutti et al. (166) found 37% of the infants 3 months of age had WTR, whereas 2% had ATR. At 36 months, however, a reversal of dominate orientation was seen, such that 3.2% had ATR and 0.9% had WTR. Oblique astigmatism also reduces with age, and has been reported to decline from 1% to 4% at 1 year of age to less than 1.00 D in 1% of children at 20 months of age (116,117). Persistence of ATR has been linked to the development of myopia (18,128,136), although generally WTR is more likely to persist (124,178,179) through 6 years of age. Dodson et al. (95) found that children less than 3.6 years of age who had ATR had a 2.5 times greater chance of having ATR at 5.6 years when compared with children who had WTR. Hirsch (124) noted the ratio of WTR to ATR was 5:1 at 6 years of age and 2:11 at 12 years of age. Woodruff (178) found a higher prevalence of WTR in children 3 to 6 years of age, whereas Lyle (165) found the higher prevalence existed in those 5 to 10 years of age.

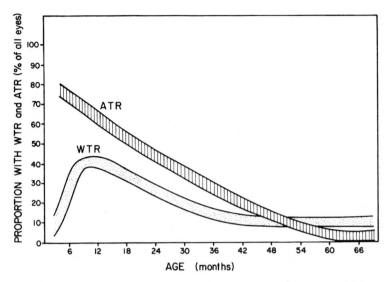

FIGURE 4.8. Against the rule versus (ATR) with the rule (WTR) in children less than 6 years of age. A collation of studies illustrating astigmatic axis patterns in children less than 6 years of age. (Lyle WM. Astigmatism. In: Grosvenor T, Flom MC, eds. *Refractive Anomalies*. Boston: Butterworth-Heinemann; 1991:146–173, with permission.)

Lyle (165) collated the results of a number of studies. The incidence of ATR was greatest at more than 6 months and had a steady downward trend to approximately 3% incidence at 5 years of age. WTR incidence was approximately 10% at more than 6 months, peaked to 40% at 9 months, and then had a steady decline to 10% at 48 months of age. The ATR and WTR slopes intersected at 54 months (165) (Fig. 4.8). Dobson et al. (180) summarized their cycloplegic refractive study by noting that astigmatism decreased with age and that up to 3.5 years of age ATR was the predominate form of astigmatism, whereas by 5.5 years of age WTR predominated (180).

SUMMARY

In most full-term developmentally normal children, a significant refractive error is not uncommon. The spherical refraction is distributed in a bell-shaped curve around a mean of low moderate hyperopia (80). During the first couple of years of life, the process of emmetropization has a dramatic effect on the initial ametropia. The interaction of both the passive and active components of the process on a healthy, uncompromised eye exposed to a stimulating environment results in a marked decline in the refractive error, such that by school age (5–7 years), the mean refractive state is markedly skewed in a leptokurtic manner to low hyperopia (18,110,146). Although most elementary school-aged children remain hyperopic, some will start to develop juvenile myopia. In general, it is believed that the earlier the onset of myopia, the greater the final myopia (138,139). For those who present with school-aged myopia, the process tends to be somewhat progressive with a cessation in the early to late teens (128). During the school days, "true" hyperopic children tend to have a stable refractive state with little alteration. Astigmatism follows a similar emmetropization pattern, in that it is common in the newborn to have a cylindric refractive error, which declines to an insignificant level during the first couple of years of life (110,159). By school age (5 to 7 years), the prevalence of significant amounts of astigmatism is between 2% and 4% (124,160).

REFERENCES

1. Hofstetter HW, Griffin JR, Berman MS, et al. *Dictionary of Visual Science and Related Clinical Terms*, 5th ed. Boston: Butterworth Heinemann, 2000;172.

2. Grosvenor T. *Primary Care Optometry*. Boston: Butterworth-Heineman, 1996;17.
3. Sorsby A, Sheridan M, Leary GA, et al. Visual acuity and ocular refraction of young men. *BMJ* 1960;1:1394.
4. Lam SR, LaRoche GR, De Becker I, et al. The range and variability of ophthalmological parameters in normal children aged 4.5 to 5.5 years. *J Pediatr Ophthalmol Strabismus* 1996;33:251–256.
5. Troilo D, Wallman J. The regulation of eye growth and refractive state: an experimental study of emmetropization. *Vision Res* 1991;31:1237–1250.
6. Wiesel TN, Raviola E. Myopia and eye enlargement after neonatal lid fusion in monkeys. *Nature* 1977;266:66–68.
7. Ingram RM, Gill LE, Goldacre MJ. Emmetropisation and accommodation in hypermetropic children before they show signs of squint: a preliminary analysis. *Bulletin de lla Societe Belge d Ophtalmologie* 1994;253:41–56.
8. Norton TT, Siegwart JT Jr. Animal models of emmetropization: matching axial length to focal plane. *Journal of the American Optometric Association* 1995;66:405–414.
9. Smith EL III, Hung LF, Harwerth RS. Effects of optically induced blur on the refractive status of young monkeys. *Vision Res* 1994;34:293–301.
10. Smith EL III. Spectacle lenses and emmetropization: the role of optical defocus in regulating ocular development. *Optom Vis Sci* 1998;75:388–398.
11. Larsen JS. The sagittal growth of the eye. IV. Ultrasonic measurement of the axial length of the eye from birth to puberty. *Acta Ophthalmol* 1971;49:872–886.
12. Larsen JS. The sagittal growth of the eye. III. Ultrasonic measurement of the posterior segment (axial length of the vitreous) from birth to puberty. *Acta Ophthalmol* 1971;49:441–453.
13. Larsen JS. The sagittal growth of the eye. II. Ultrasonic measurement of the axial diameter of the lens and anterior segment from birth to puberty. *Acta Ophthalmol* 1971;49:427–440.
14. Larsen JS. The sagittal growth of the eye. I. Ultrasonic measurement of the depth of the anterior chamber from birth to puberty. *Acta Ophthalmol* 1971;49:239–262.
15. Sorsby A. Biology of the eye as an optical system. In: Duane TD, ed. *Clinical Ophthalmology*. Philadelphia: Harper & Row, 1979;1–17.
16. Mark HH. Emmetropisation: physical aspects of a statistical phenomenon. *Ann Ophthalmol* 1972;4:393–401.
17. Gernet H, Oblrich H. Excess of the human refraction curve. In: Deeney AH, Sarin LK, Meyer D, eds. *Ophthalmic Ultrasound*. St. Louis: CV Mosby; 1969:42–148.
18. Gwiazda J, Thorn F, Bauer J, et al. Emmetropization and the progression of manifest refraction in children followed from infancy to puberty. *Clinical Vision Science* 1993;8:337–344.
19. Ong E, Ciuffreda KJ. *Accommodation, Nearwork and Myopia*. Santa Ana, CA: Optometric Extension Program, 1997.
20. Goss DA, Jackson TW. Clinical findings before the onset of myopia in youth: 4. Parental history of myopia. *Optom Vis Sci* 1996c;73:279–282.
21. Zadnik K, Satariano WA, Mutti DO, et al. The effect of parental history of myopia on children's eye size. *JAMA* 1994;271:1323–1327.
22. Wold KC. Hereditary myopia. *Arch Ophthalmol* 1949;42:225–237.
23. Teikari JM, O'Donnell, Kapiro J, et al. Impact of heredity in myopia. *Hum Hered* 1991;41:151–156.
24. Curtin BJ. *The Myopias*. Philadelphia: Harper & Row, 1985.
25. Sorsby A, Sheridan M, Leary GA. Refraction and its components in twins. Medical Research Council Special Report Series. No. 303. London: HMSO, 1962.
26. Lin LLK, Chen CJ. Twin study on myopia. *Acta Geneticae Medicae et Gemellologicae* 1987;36:535–540.
27. Troilo D. Neonatal eye growth and emmetropisation a literature review. *Eye* 1992;6:154–160.
28. Brown NP, Koretz JF, Bron AJ. The development and maintenance of emmetropia. *Eye* 1999;13:83–92.
29. Smith EL III, Harwerth RS, Crawford ML, et al. Observations on the effect of form deprivation on the refractive status of the monkey. *Invest Ophthalmol Vis Sci* 1987;28:1236–1245.
30. Ni J, Smith EL III. Effects of chronic defocus on the kitten's refractive status. *Vision Res* 1989;29:929–938.
31. Troilo D. Neonatal eye growth and emmetropisation: a literature review. *Eye* 1992;6:154–160.
32. Yackle K, FitzGerald DE. Emmetropization: an overview. *J Behav Optom* 1999;2:38–43.
33. Smith EL III, Hung LF, Kee CS, et al. Effects of brief periods of unrestricted vision on the development of form-deprivation myopia in monkeys. *Invest Ophthalmol Vis Sci* 2002;43:291–299.
34. Smith EL III, Hung LF. Form-deprivation myopia in monkeys is a graded phenomenon. *Vision Res* 2000;40:371–381.
35. Calossi A. Increase of ocular axial length in infantile traumatic cataract. *Optom Vis Sci* 1994;7:386–391.
36. Lorenz B, Worle J, Friedl N, et al. Ocular growth in infant aphakia. *Ophthalmic Pediatrics and Genetics* 1993;14:177–188.
37. Toulemont PJ, Urvoy M, Coscas G, et al. Association of congenital microcoria with myopia and glaucoma. *Ophthalmology* 1995;102:193–197.
38. Evans NM, Fielder AR, Majer DL. Ametropia in congenital cone deficiency—achromatopsia: a defect of emmetropization. *Clinical Vision Science* 1989;4:129–136.
39. Daw NJ. *Visual Development*. New York: Plenum Press, 1995.
40. Gee SS, Tabbara KF. Increase in ocular axial length in patients with corneal opacification. *Ophthalmology* 1988;95:1276–1278.
41. Hoyt CS, Stone RD, Fromer C, et al. Monocular axial myopia associated with neonatal eyelid closure in human infant. *Am J Ophthalmol* 1981;91: 197–200.
42. O'Leary DJ, Millodot M. Eyelid closure causes myopia in humans. *Experentia* 1979;35:1478–1479.
43. Robb RM. Refractive errors associated with hemangiomas of the eyelids and orbit in infancy. *Am J Ophthalmol* 1977;83:52–58.
44. Miller-Meeks MJ, Bennett SR, Keech RV, et al. Myopia induced by vitreous hemorrhage. *Am J Ophthalmol* 1990;109:199–203.
45. Lue CL, Hansen RM, Reisner DS, et al. The course of myopia in children with mild retinopathy of prematurity. *Vision Res* 1995;35:1329–1335.
46. Fledelius HC. Pre-term delivery and subsequent ocular development. *Acta Ophththalmol Scand* 1996;74:301–305.
47. Hooker PJ, FitzGerald DE, Rutner D, et al. Monocular deprivation in an identical twin. *Optometry* 2005; 76:579–587.
48. Johnson CA, Post RB, Chalupa LM, et al. Monocular

deprivation in humans: a study of identical twins. *Invest Ophthalmol Vis Sci* 1982;23:135–138.

49. Saunders KJ, Woodhouse JM, Westall CA. Emmetropisation in humans infancy: rate of change is related to initial error. *Vision Res* 1995;35:1325–1328.

50. Greene PR, Guyton DL. Time course of rhesus lid-suture myopia. *Exp Eye Res* 1986;2:529–534.

51. Raviola E, Wiesel TN. An animal model of myopia. *N Eng J Med* 1985;312:1609–1615.

52. Thorn F, Doty RW, Gramiak R. Effect of eyelid suture on development of ocular dimensions in macaques. *Curr Eye Res* 1981/82;1:727–733.

53. Christensen AM, Wallman J. Evidence that increased scleral growth underlies visual deprivation myopia in chicks. *Invest Ophthalomol Vis Sci* 1991;32:2143–2150.

54. Rada JA, Thoft RA, Hassell JR. Increased aggrecan (cartilage proteoglycan) production in the sclera of myopic chicks. *Dev Biol* 1991;147:303–312.

55. Stone RA, Lin T, Laties AM, et al. Retinal dopamine and form-deprivation myopia. *Proc Natl Acad USA* 1989;86:704–706.

56. Stone RA, Laties AM, Raviola E, et al. Increase in retinal vasoactive intestinal peptide after eye lid fusion in primates. *Proc Natl Acad USA* 1988;85:257–260.

57. Wallman J. Retinal factors in myopia and emmetropization: In: Grosvenor T, Flom MC, eds. *Refractive Anomalies*. Boston: Butterworth-Heinemann; 1991:270–280.

58. Wallman J, Adams J. Developmental aspects of experimental myopia in chicks. *Vision Res* 1987;27:1139–1163.

59. Abrahamsson M, Fabian G, Sjostrand J. Refraction changes in children developing convergent or divergent strabismus. *Br J Ophthalmol* 1992;76:723–727.

60. Lepard CW. Comparative changes in the error of refraction between fixing and amblyopic eyes during growth and development. *Am J Ophthalmol* 1975;80:485–490.

61. Kiorpes L, Wallman J. Does experimentally-induced amblyopia cause hyperopia in monkeys? *Vision Res* 1995;35:1289–1298.

62. Burtolo C, Ciurlo C, Polizzi A, et al. Echobiometric study of ocular growth in patients with amblyopia. *J Pediatr Ophthalmol Strabismus* 2002;39:209–214.

63. Almeder LM, Peck LB, Howland HC. Prevalence of anisometropia in volunteer laboratory and school screening populations. *Invest Ophthalmol Vis Sci* 1990;31:2448–2455.

64. van der Pol BA. Causes of visual impairment in children. *Doc Ophthalmol* 1986;61:223–228.

65. Hill AE, McKendrick O, Poole JJ, et al. The Liverpool visual assessment team: 10 years experience. *Child Care Health Development* 1986;21:37–51.

66. Maino D. *Diagnosis and Management of Special Populations.* St. Louis: CV Mosby, 1995.

67. Wagner R, Caputo AR, Nelson LB, et al. High hypermetropia in Leber's congenital amaurosis. *Arch Ophthalmol* 1985;103:1507–1509.

68. Nathan J, Kiely PM, Crewther SG, et al. Disease-associated visual image degradation and spherical refractive errors in children. *American Journal of Optometry and Physiological Optics* 1985;62:680–688.

69. Woodhouse JM, Pakeman VH, Cregg M, et al. Refractive errors in young children with Down syndrome. *Optom Vis Sci* 1997;74:844–851.

70. Maino D, Schlange D, Maino J, et al. Ocular anomalies in fragile X syndrome. *Journal of the American Optometric Association* 1990;61:316–323.

71. Storm RL, Pebenito R, Ferretti R. Ophthalmologic findings in the fragile X syndrome. *Arch Ophthalmol* 1987;105:1099–1102.

72. Aurell E, Norrsell K. A longitudinal study of children with a family history of strabismus: factors determining the incidence of strabismus. *Br J Ophthalmol* 1990;74:589–594.

73. Ingram RM, Barr A. Changes in refraction between the ages of 1 and 31/2 years. *Br J Ophthalmol* 1979;63:339–342.

74. Ingram RM, Gill LE, Lambert TW. Effect of spectacles on change of spherical hypermetropia in infants who did, and did not, have strabismus. *Br J Ophthalmol* 2000;84:324–326.

75. Atkinson J, Anker S, Bobier W, et al. Normal emmetropization in infants with spectacle correction for hyperopia. *Invest Ophthalmol Vis Sci* 2000;41:3726–3731.

76. Ingram RM, Arnold PE, Dally S, et al. Emmetropisation, squint, and reduced visual acuity after treatment. *Br J Ophthalmol* 1991;75:414–416.

77. Atkinson J, Braddick O, Bobier B, et al. Two infant vision screening programmes: prediction and prevention of strabismus and amblyopia from photo- and videorefractive screening. *Eye* 1996;10:189–198.

78. Baldwin WR. Refractive status of infants and children. In: Rosenbloom AA, Morgon MW, eds. *Principles and Practice of Pediatric Optometry.* Philadelphia: JB Lippincott; 1991:104–152.

79. Zadnik K, Mutti DO, Friedman NE, et al. Initial cross-sectional results from the Orinda Longitudinal Study of Myopia. *Optom Vis Sci* 1993;70:750–758.

80. Hirsch MJ. Sex differences in the incidence of various grades of myopia. *American Journal of Optometry and Archives of the American Academy of Optometry* 1953;30:135–138.

81. Sperduto RD, Seigel D, Roberts J, et al. Prevalence of myopia in the United States. *Arch Ophthalmol* 1983;101:405–407.

82. Ingram RM, Gill LE, Goldacre MJ. Emmetropisation and accommodation in hypermetropic children before they show signs of squint: a preliminary analysis. *Bull de la Societe belge d'ophthalmologie* 1994;253: 41–56.

83. Dobson V, Sebris SL, Carlson MR. Do glasses prevent emmetropization in strabismic infants? *Invest Ophthalmol* 1986; 27[Suppl]:2.

84. Ingram RM, Arnold PE, Dally S, et al. Results of a randomised trial of treating abnormal hypermetropia from the age of 6 months. *Br J Ophthalmol* 1990;74:158–159.

85. Goldschmidt E. Refraction in the newborn. *Acta Ophthalmologica* 1969;47:570–578.

86. Lissauer T, Clayden G. *Illustrated Textbook of Pediatrics.* St. Louis: CV Mosby, 1997;79.

87. Saunders KJ, McMulloch DL, Shepherd AJ, et al. Emmetropization following preterm birth. *Br J Ophthalmol* 2002;86:1035–1040.

88. Saw SM, Chew SJ. Myopia in children born premature or with low birth weight. *Acta Ophthalmol Scand* 1997;75:548–550.

89. Nissenkorn I, Yassur Y, Mashkowski D, et al. Myopia in premature babies with and without retinopathy of prematurity. *Br J Ophthalmol* 1983;67:170–173.

90. FitzGerald DE, Chung I, Krumholtz I. An analysis of high myopia in a pediatric population less than 10 years of age. *Optometry* 2005;76:102–114.

91. Laws D, Shaw DE, Robinson, et al. Retinopathy of prematurity: a prospective study. Review at six months. *Eye* 1992; 6:477–483.

92. Robinson R, O'Keefe M. Follow-up on premature infants with and without retinopathy of prematurity. *Br J Ophthalmol* 1993;77:91–94.

93. Page JM, Schneeweiss S, Whyte Hea, et al. Ocular sequelae in premature infants. *Pediatrics* 1993;92:787–790.

94. Quinn GE, Dobson V, Repka MX, et al. Development of myopia in infants with birth weights less than 1251 grams. *Ophthalmology* 1992;99:329–340.

95. Dobson V, Fulton AB, Manning K, et al. Cycloplegic refractions of premature infants. *Am J Ophthalmol* 1981;91:490–495.

96. Fletcher MC, Brandon S. Myopia of prematurity. *Am J Ophthalmol* 1955;40:474–481.

97. Graham MV, Gray OP. Refraction of premature babies' eyes. *BMJ* 1963;1:1452–1454.

98. Rodriguez A, Villarreal J, Homar Paez J. Visual acuity and retinoscopy of preterm and full-term infants during the first year of life. *Ann Ophthalmol* 1996;28:46–53.

99. Fledelius HC. Preterm delivery and growth of the eye. An oculometric study of eye size around term-time. *Acta Ophthalmol* 1992;204[Suppl]:10–15.

100. Choi MY, Park IK, Yu YS. Long term refractive outcomes in eyes of preterm infants with and without retinopathy of prematurity: comparison of keratometric value, axial length, anterior chamber, and lens thickness. *Br J Ophthalmol* 2000;84:138–143.

101. Holmstrom M, elAzazi M, Kugelberg U. Ophthalmological long term follow up of preterm infants: a population based, prospective study of the refraction and its development. *Br J Ophthalmol* 1998;82:1265–1271.

102. Shapiro A, Yanko L, Nawratzki I, et al. Refractive power of premature children at infancy and early childhood. *Am J Ophthalmol* 1980;90:234–238.

103. Gallo JE, Lennerstrand G. A population-based study of ocular abnormalities in premature children aged 5 to 10 years. *Am J Ophthalmol* 1991;111:539–547.

104. Wibaut F. Ueger die Emmetropisation und den Ursprung der Spharischen Refractionsanomalien. *Archf Ophthalmol* 1925;116:596.

105. Hirsch MJ, Weymouth FW. Prevalence of refractive anomalies. In: Grosvenor T, Flom MC, eds. *Refractive Anomalies*. Boston: Butterworth-Heinemann; 1991: 270–280.

106. Banks MS. Infant refraction and accommodation. *Int Ophthalmol Clin* 1980;20:205–232.

107. Sorsby A, Benjamin B, Sheridan M, et al. Refraction and its components during growth of the eye from age three. Medical Research Council Special Report Series No. 301. London. HMSO 1961.

108. Cook RC, Glasscock RE. Refractive and ocular findings in the newborn. *Am J Ophthalmol* 1951;34:1407–1413.

109. Mayer DL, Hansen RM, Moore BD, et al. Cycloplegic refractions in healthy children aged 1 through 48 months. *Arch Ophthalmol* 2001;119:1625–1628.

110. Mohindra I, Held R. Refraction in humans from birth to five years. *Doc Ophthalmol* 1978;28:19–27.

111. Mohindra I. A non-cycloplegic refraction technique for infants and young children. *Journal of the American Optometric Association* 1977;48:518–523.

112. Saunders K, Westall C. Comparison between near retioscopy and cycloplegic retinoscopy in the refraction of infants and children. *Optom Vis Sci* 1992;69:615–622.

113. Wesson MD, Mann KR, Bray NW. A comparison of cycloplegic refraction to the near retinoscopy technique for refractive error determination. *Journal of the American Optometric Association* 1990;61:680–684.

114. Borghi RA, Rouse MW. Comparison of refraction obtained by a near retinoscopy and retinoscopy under cycloplegia. *American Journal of Optometry and Physiological Optics* 1985;62:169–172.

115. Santonastaso A. La refrazione oculare nei primi anni di vitra. Ottal Clin Ocul (Italy) 1930;848.

116. Wood ICJ, Hodi S, Morgan L. Longitudinal change of refractive error in infants during the first year of life. *Eye* 1995;9:551–557.

117. Ehrlich DL, Braddick OJ, Atkinson J, et al. Infant emmetropization: longitudinal changes in refraction components from nine to twenty months of age. *Optom Vis Sci* 1997;10:822–843.

118. Edwards M. The refractive status of Hong Kong Chinese infants. *Ophthalmic Physiol Opt* 1991;11:297–303.

119. Ehrlich DL, Atkinson J, Braddick O, et al. Reduction of infant myopia: a longitudinal cycloplegic study. *Vision Res* 1995;35: 1313–1324.

120. Mohindra I, Held R. Refraction of humans from birth to five years. *Doc Ophthalmol* 1981;28:19–27.

121. Moore B, Lyons SA, Walline J, et al. A clinical review of hyperopia in young children. *Journal of the American Optometric Association* 1999;70:215–224.

122. Hirsch MJ. The changes in refraction between the ages of 5 and 14—theoretical and practical considerations. *American Journal of Optometry and Archives of the American Academy of Optometry* 1952;29:445–459.

123. Young FA, Beattie RJ, Newby FJ, et al. The Pullman Study—a visual survey of Pullman schoolchildren Part II. *American Journal of Optometry* 1954;31:445–454.

124. Hirsch MJ. Changes in astigmatism during the first eight years of school: an interim report from the Ojai Longitudinal Study. *American Journal of Optometry and Archives of the American Academy of Optometry* 1963;40:127–132.

125. Parssinen O. Astigmatism and school myopia. *Acta Ophthalmol (Copenhagen)* 1991; 69:786–790.

126. Lavrich JB, Nelson LB, Simon JW, et al. Medium to high myopia in infancy and early childhood: frequency, course and association with strabismus and amblyopia. *Eye Muscle Surgery Quaetrly* 1993;8:41–44.

127. Grosvenor T, Goss DA. *Clinical Management of Myopia*. Boston: Butterworth-Heinemann, 1999;10.

128. Hirsch MJ. Predictability of refraction at age 14 on the basis of testing at age 6—interim report from The Ojai Longitudinal Study of refraction. *American Journal of Optometry and Archives of the American Academy of Optometry* 1964;41:567–573.

129. Blum HL, Peters HB, Bettman JW. *Vision Screening for Elementary Schools—The Orinda Study*. Berkeley, CA: University of California Press, 1959.

130. Mäntyjärvi M. Incidence of myopia in a population of Finnish school children. *Acta Ophthalmol* 1983;61:417–423.

131. Mutti DO, Mitchell GL, Moeschberger ML, et al. Parental myopia, near work, school achievement, and children's refractive error. *Invest Ophthalmol Vis Sci* 2002;43:3633–3640.

132. Goss DA. Variables related to the rate of childhood myopia progression. *Optom Vis Sci* 1990;67:631–636.

133. Care of the patient with myopia. In: *Optometric Clinical Practice Guidelines*. St. Louis: American Optometric Association, 1997.

134. Zadnik K, Mutti DO. Prevalence of myopia. In: Rosenfield M, Gilmartin B. eds. *Myopia & Nearwork*. Boston: Butterworth-Heinemann; 1998:13–30.

135. Goss DA, Eskridge JB. Myopia. In: Amos JF, eds. Diagnosis and Management in Vision Care. Boston: Butterworths; 1987:121–127.

136. Grosvenor T. A review and a suggested classification

system of myopia on the basis of age-related prevalence and age of onset. *American Journal of Optometry and Physiological Optics* 1987;64:545–554.

137. Goss DA, Winkler RL. Progression of myopia in youth: age of cessation. *American Journal of Optometry and Physiological Optics* 1983;60:651–658.

138. Mäntyjärvi, MI. Predicting of myopia progression in school children. *J Pediatr Ophthalmol Strabismus* 1985;22:71–75.

139. Goss DA. Childhood Myopia. In: Grosvenor T, Flom MC, eds. *Refractive Anomalies.* Boston: Butterworth-Heinemann; 1991:81–103.

140. Lin LL, Shih YF, Tsai CB, et al. Epidemiologic study of ocular refraction among schoolchildren in Taiwan in 1995. *Optom Vis Sci* 1999;76:275–281.

141. Goss DA. Linearity of refractive change with age in childhood myopia progression. *American Journal of Optometry and Physiological Optics* 1987;64:775–780.

142. François J, Goes F. Oculometry of progressive myopia. *Bibl Ophthalmol* 1975;83:277–282.

143. Mäntyjärvi MI. Changes of refraction in schoolchildren. *Archives of Opthalmology* 1985b; 103:790–791.

144. Langer MA. Changes in ocular refraction from five to sixteen. MS Thesis. Indiana University. 1966.

145. Kleinstein RN, Jones LA, Hullett S, et al. Refractive error and ethnicity in children. *Arch Ophthalmol* 2003;121:1141–1147.

146. Kempf GA, Collins SD, Jarman EL. Refractive errors in the eyes of children as determined by retinoscopic examination with a cycloplegic. Public Health Bull No. 182. Washington, DC. US Government Printing Office 1928.

147. Raab EL. Hypermetropia in accommodative esotropia. *J Pediatr Ophthalmol Strabismus* 1984;21:194–198.

148. Repka MX, Wellish K, Wisnicki, et al. Changes in the refractive error of 94 children with acquired accommodative esotropia. *Binocul Vis Strabismus Q* 1989; 4:15–21.

149. Swan KC. Accommodative esotropia. *Ophthalmology* 1983;90:1141–1145.

150. Wolffe M. Refractive development in strabismic children. *British Journal of Phsysiological Optics* 1976;31:1–13.

151. Brown EVL. Net average yearly change in refraction of atropinized eyes from birth to beyond middle age. *Arch Ophthalmol* 1938;19:719–734.

152. Slataper FJ. Age norms of refraction and vision. *Arch Ophthalmol* 1950;43:466–481.

153. Augsburger AR. Hyperopia. In: Amos JF, ed. *Diagnosis and Management in Vision Care.* Boston: Butterworths; 1987:101–119.

154. Care of the patient with hyperopia. In: *Optometric Clinical Practice Guidelines.* St. Louis: American Optometric Association, 1997.

155. Abrahamsson M, Fabian G, Sjostrand. A longitudinal study of a population based sample of children II. The changeability of anisometropia. *Acta Ophthalmologica* 1990;68:435–440.

156. Abrahamsson M, Sjostrand J. Natural history of infantile anisometropia. *Br J Ophthalmol* 1996;80:860–863.

157. Flom MC, Bedell HE. Identifying amblyopia using associated conditions, acuity and nonacuity features. *American Journal of Optometry and Physiological Optics* 1985;62:153–160.

158. Hirsch MJ. Anisometropia: a preliminary report from the Ojai Longitudinal Study. *American Journal of Optometry and Archives of American Academy of Optometry* 1967;44:581–585.

159. Howland HC, Sayles N. Photorefractive measurements of astigmatism in infants and young children. *Invest Ophthalmol Vis Sci* 1984;25:93–102.

160. Gwaizada J, Scheiman M, Mohindra I, et al. Astigmatism in children: changes in axis and amount from birth to six years. *Invest Ophthalmol Vis Sci* 1984;25:88–92.

161. Mohindra I, Held R, Gwiazda J. Astigmatism in infants. *Science* 1978;202:329.

162. Atkinson J, Braddick O, French J. Infant astigmatism: its disappearance with age. *Vision Res* 1980:20:891–893.

163. Fulton AB, Dobson V, Salem BA, et al. Cycloplegic refractions in infant and young children. *Am J Ophthalmol* 1980;90:239–247.

164. Howland HC, Atkinson J, Braddick O, et al. Infant astigmatism measured by photorefraction. *Science* 1978;202:331–332.

165. Lyle WM. Astigmatism. In: Grosvenor T, Flom MC, eds. *Refractive Anomalies.* Boston: Butterworth-Heinemann; 1991: 146–173.

166. Mutti DO, Mitchell L, Jones LA, et al. Refractive astigmatism and the toricity of ocular components in human infants. *Optom Vis Sci* 2004;81:753–761.

167. Gwiazda J, Mohindra I, Brill S. et al. Infant astigmatism and meridional amblyopia. Vision Res 1985;25:1269–1276.

168. Lam CSY, Goh WSH. Astigmatism among Chinese school children. *Clin Exp Optom* 1991;74:146–150.

169. Chung I, FitzGerald DE, Hughes R. Comparison of MTI Photoscreening to visual examination of Chinese-American preschool children. *Journal of Behavioral Optometry* 2002;13:3–6,25.

170. Chan OYC, Edwards M. Refractive error in Hong Kong Chinese pre-school children. *Optom Vis Sci* 1993;70:501–505.

171. Doxanas MT, Anderson RL. Oriental eyelids: an anatomical study. *Arch Ophthalmol* 1984;102:1232–1235.

172. Mohindra I, Nagarai S. Astigmatism in Zuni and Navajo Indians. *American Journal of Optometry and Physiological Optics* 1977;54:121–124.

173. Lyle WM, Grosvenor T, Dean KC. Corneal astigmatism in Amerind children. *American Journal of Optometry and Archives of American Academy of Optometry* 1972;49:517–524.

174. Hamilton JE. Vision anomalies of Indian school children: the Lame Deer study. *Journal of the American Optometric Association* 1976;47:479–487.

175. Maples WC, Herrmann M, Hughes J. Corneal astigmatism in preschool Native Americans. *Journal of the American Optometric Association* 1997;68:87–94.

176. Montes-Mico R. Astigmatism in infancy and childhood. *J Pediatr Ophthalmol Strabismus* 2000;37:349–353.

177. Ingram RM, Gill LE, Lambert TW. Reduction of astigmatism after infancy in children who did and did not wear glasses and have strabismus. *Strabismus* 2001;9:129–135.

178. Woodruff ME. Cross sectional studies of corneal and astigmatic characteristics of children between twenty-fourth and seventy-second months of life. *American Journal of Optometry and Archives of American Academy of Optometry* 1971;48:650–659.

179. Lyle WM. Changes in corneal astigmatism with age. *American Journal of Optometry and Archives of American Academy of Optometry* 1971;48:467–478.

180. Dobson V, Fulton AB, Sebris SL. Cycloplegic refractions of infants and young children: the axis of astigmatism. *Invest Ophthalmol Vis Sci* 1984;25:83–87.

Development of Eye Movements in Infants

5

Jordan R. Pola

Over the past 40 years, many studies have investigated both the characteristics and development of oculomotor behavior in infants. These studies have used recording techniques ranging from simple observation of the direction of gaze to objective recording of eye movements in carefully controlled and executed experimental situations. A general finding coming from this work is that, at the time of birth or shortly thereafter, infants make what are typically regarded as immature eye movements, although in some important respects these eye movements are similar to adult movements. Within as little as a few weeks to several months, depending on the particular oculomotor system, the eye movements change to become virtually identical to adult movements.

Concurrent with the study of infant eye movements, the neural mechanisms underlying the generation of oculomotor behavior have been vigorously investigated in both humans and animals. This work has uncovered basic aspects of neurophysiologic activity associated with the generation of eye movements, and the functional significance of this activity as represented, in particular, by models of the oculomotor system. Especially well understood are the features of motoneuron signals and the manner in which they produce efficient eye movements in the face of the resistive mechanics of the extraocular muscles and surrounding orbital tissue (i.e., the oculomotor plant). An important general finding is that along with brainstem

motor areas, a broad range of cortical and subcortical areas discharge in association with eye movements, whether fast or slow.

A primary purpose of this chapter is to examine some of the main features of infant eye movements and their development as well as to attempt to relate these features, at least in a first-order manner, to some of the known functional properties of the oculomotor system. The review of the each type of eye movement is divided into three parts: basic features of the eye movement in adults along with a simple explanatory model of the movement; characteristics and development of the eye movement in infants; and mechanisms and processes that may underlie the infant eye movement. An outline of experimental procedures is often provided to explain how the resulting oculomotor data and conclusions were obtained.

SACCADIC EYE MOVEMENTS

Basic Features of Saccadic Movements in Adults

Saccades are high-velocity eye movements that shift the direction of gaze from one spatial location to another. These movements enable us to quickly bring the *fovea* to a new object so that the object can be seen with maximal clarity. Saccades are utilized in a wide variety of circumstances. We make voluntary saccades to look at an object (or event) that seems to be of immediate interest or importance. Saccades also occur reflexively in the direction of an event that occurs suddenly and without warning. We typically make a repeated sequence of saccades when we enter a room, are engaged in social interaction, view some panoramic scene, or simply examine a picture. This type of behavior, sometimes called a *saccadic scan-path*, allows us to rapidly acquire information about the characteristics of the physical or social circumstance. Saccades are often of relatively large magnitude, ranging from 2° to as much as 40°, in everyday circumstances. Small amplitude saccades, however, play an important role in a number of situations. Reading involves a sequence of small saccades as the eyes move along a line of text. When we look at a stationary target, we make microsaccades as part of the process of holding our direction of gaze on the target.

The latency for a saccade is traditionally given as 200 milliseconds (ms). This reflects the time it takes for the following series of events to occur: (a) the passage of visual signals to oculomotor areas of the brain; (b) the processing of oculomotor signals; and (c) the flow of oculomotor signals to the extraocular muscles. Nevertheless, substantial variation exists in the latency from one person to another, especially depending on the specifics of the stimulus situation. Consider, for example, an experiment where a subject initially views a fixation target, and then, on the appearance of a peripheral target, makes a saccade as quickly as possible to look at the target. Typically, the latency of the saccade is shorter if the fixation target disappears before the peripheral target appears (the "gap" condition), than if the fixation target disappears after the peripheral target appears (the "overlap" condition). One interpretation of this difference is that, in the gap condition, an *attention disengagement* process occurs automatically and quickly with the disappearance of the fixation target, whereas in the overlap condition, the attention disengagement process is slowed by the continued presence of the fixation target.

Saccadic eye movements are among the fastest of human motor behaviors, in some cases reaching a peak velocity of more than 800°/second (s). An important feature of these movements is that, in most situations, they have rather invariant response characteristics: Their duration increases linearly and their peak velocity increases exponentially as a function of amplitude. This stereotypic response shows that, although we often have a choice whether to make a saccade or not, once that choice is made, the mechanism for generating the movement is automatic and deterministic. For this reason, the saccadic system has traditionally been regarded as being *ballistic*, in the sense that once it is activated, it typically runs until its task—creating a saccade—is completed.

The saccadic system, for our purposes, can be represented as consisting of a cortical component and a brainstem component (Fig. 5.1). The cortical component might be viewed as being responsible for perceptual information processing (perception of and attention to a target), decision-making about where and when to execute a saccade, and initiating the sequence of events leading up to the occurrence of the saccade. In contrast, the brainstem component consists of those structures that produce and shape the actual motor signals that go to the extraocular muscles.

It is worthwhile, at this point, to consider some main features of the brainstem component, because they are relevant both to the discussion of saccades and to the other types of eye movements that are reviewed below. The brainstem component can be regarded as consisting of a *pulse generator* and a *neural integrator* (Fig. 5.1). The pulse-generator creates a *pulse* of neural activity. The pulse goes to the integrator to produce a *step* of neural activity, and also travels around the integrator to sum with the step. The resulting *pulse-step* goes to the extraocular muscles where, filtered through the mechanics of the oculomotor plant, it generates a saccadic eye movement (i.e., the pulse overcomes viscous resistance of the plant to produce the saccade, whereas the step deals with elastic resistance to hold the eye in position after the saccade).

Saccadic Movements in Infants

Saccades to a Peripheral Target

Aslin and Salapatek (1) conducted one of the first systematic studies on saccades in infants. The infants, 1 and 2 months of age, were placed on their backs in a reclining seat and looked upward to view targets reflected in a mirror. Eye

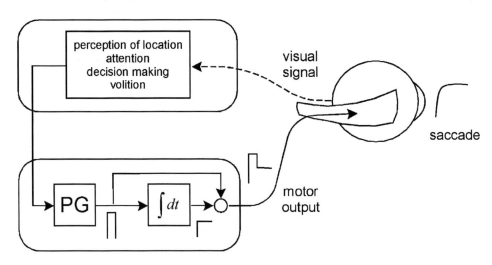

FIGURE 5.1. A model showing some of the control features of the saccadic system. The *upper box* shows cortical functions associated with the initiation of voluntary saccadic eye movements. The cortex sends its output to two brainstem motor mechanisms, a pulse generator (*PG*) and a neural integrator (*∫dt*).

movements were recorded using the electro-oculograph (EOG) technique. The study involved two types of trials, *replacement* trials and *addition* trials. In the *replacement* trials, a fixation target was turned off at the same time as a peripheral target appeared, whereas in the *addition* trials, the fixation target remained on when the peripheral target became visible. An interesting finding was that the infants often made an initial saccade in the wrong direction (i.e., the saccade occurred away from the location of the peripheral target) in both types of trials, but the probability of a saccade in the wrong direction occurred much less in the replacement trials than in the addition trials (Fig. 5.2). The likelihood of a saccade in the wrong direction increased as the distance of the peripheral target increased.

Perhaps the most striking result of this study is that when infants turned their eyes toward the location of the peripheral target, their eye movements often consisted of a succession of saccades (as opposed to a single saccade as made by an adult). The number of saccades ranged from one to five, with the likelihood of multiple saccades increasing as the eccentricity of the

peripheral target increased (Fig. 5.3). All the successive saccades tended to be of about the same amplitude, where the size of each saccade increased as the peripheral target eccentricity increased. The latency of the first saccade was much longer than the usual 200 ms. The latency for 1-month-old infants was 800, 1320, and 1480 ms when the peripheral target was located at 10°, 20°, and 30°, respectively. Furthermore, the intersaccadic latency varied from about 500 to 900 ms.

As would be expected, the percentage of successive saccades decreased over time, changing from 86% in infants 1 month of age to 75% in those 2 months of age (1), and from 55% in those 3 months of age to about 32% in infants 6 months of age (2). An important feature of these saccades is that their velocity–amplitude relation was similar to that for adults (2).

Saccades for Scanning Shapes and Patterns

Looking at a simple peripheral target is a far cry from viewing the complex stimuli that are present in the everyday visual environment. In experiments by Hainline et al. (3), infants

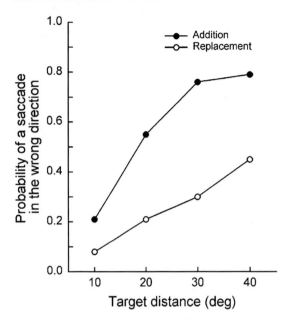

FIGURE 5.2. The probability of making a first saccade in the wrong direction to a peripheral target plotted against the distance of the target from the fovea. A saccade in the wrong direction was more likely in the *addition* condition than in the *replacement* condition. (Adapted from Aslin RN, Salapatek P. Saccadic localization of visual targets by the very young infant. *Percept Psychophys* 1975;17:293–302, with permission.)

visually scanned either geometrical shapes or simple patterns, a task that might be considered a bit closer to normal visual circumstances. The experimenter held the infants, ranging in age from 14 to 151 days, so that they could view the stimuli over the experimenter's shoul-

der. Eye movements were recorded using an infrared corneal reflection technique. In contrast to studies with a peripheral target, infants did not make a succession of saccades from one location to another when viewing either geometrical shapes or simple patterns. Instead, as with adults, they shifted their gaze from place to place using single saccades with intersaccadic intervals of 250 ms or less. Another difference was that instead of saccades of the same size, saccadic amplitude ranged from about 2° to 20°. The dynamics of the eye movements, however, were not the same with the patterns and the shapes. In particular, the saccadic peak velocity was similar for infants and adults with the patterns, but was much lower for infants with the shapes (Fig. 5.4).

Saccadic scanning in infants matures rather quickly. Bronson (4,5) showed that when infants viewed simple patterns, the range of saccadic amplitudes changed dramatically between 6 and 13 weeks of age (Fig. 5.5A). The amplitudes varied from about 1° to 5° in 6-week-old infants. They increased substantially, however, by 13 weeks of age, ranging from 1° to 15°. The fixation dwell times between the saccades also changed (Fig. 5.5B). The dwell times varied from 0.1 to 4.0 s in 6-week-old infants, but decreased to no more than about 1.0 s by 13 weeks.

Mechanisms

Infant saccadic responses to a single peripheral target have at least three notable features: the saccadic latency is exceptionally long, an initial

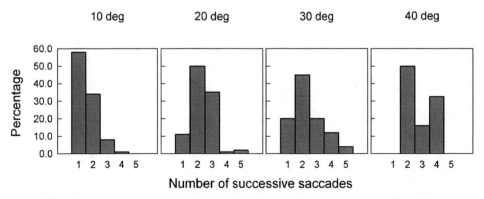

FIGURE 5.3. Percentage of successive saccades to a peripheral target at a distance of 10° to 40° from the fovea. (Adapted from Aslin RN, Salapatek P. Saccadic localization of visual targets by the very young infant. *Percept Psychophys* 1975;17:293–302, with permission.)

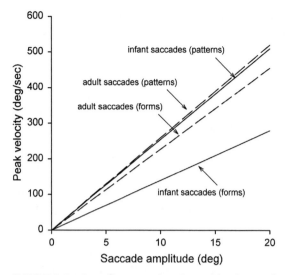

FIGURE 5.4. Best-fit curves showing peak velocity of saccadic eye movement as a function of saccade amplitude. (Adapted from Hainline L, Turkel J, Abramov I, et al. Characteristics of saccades in human infants. *Vision Res* 1984;12:1771–1780, with permission.)

saccade often occurs in the wrong direction, and a succession of saccades occurs when the eyes turn in the correct direction (1). What is responsible for these unusual behaviors? One possibility is that the long saccadic latency is a consequence of an immature attention disengagement mechanism (6). The misdirected saccades and succession of saccades may also be a product of this mechanism. Of course, in addition to, or instead of, undeveloped attention capabilities, infants may not be interested in a small peripheral target situated in an otherwise

relatively featureless background. Another possibility is that visual mechanisms for perception of spatial location are not yet developed and, as such, are not easily activated by a simple peripheral target.

Infant scanning saccades also have a number of distinctive features. Some of these may arise from the same mechanisms responsible for saccades to a peripheral target. For instance, the long dwell time between saccades when infants scan a simple pattern (4,5) could be the consequence of an immature attention disengagement process. Also, the fact that infants make lower velocity saccades when scanning shapes than when scanning patterns (3) could indicate that infants find the shapes less interesting than the patterns, or it could be a result of poor spatial localization.

The processes underlying attention, perception of location, and volition are primarily located in cortical areas of the brain (Fig. 5.1). This suggests that many of the characteristics of saccades in infants and the ways in which they differ from adult saccades are a result of immature cortical mechanisms. Direct support for a relation between cortical development and the execution of saccades comes from recordings of event-related potentials. As an example, adults show a positive cortical spike potential preceding the onset of a saccade by about 8 to 12 ms (7–9). This potential is thought to arise from the parietal cortex in association with the planning of a saccade. Infants 6 months of age do not show the potential. By 12 months, however,

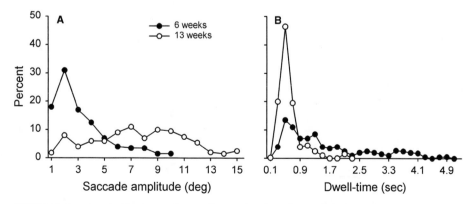

FIGURE 5.5. **A:** Distributions of saccadic amplitudes when infants visually scanned a simple pattern. **B:** Distributions of fixation dwell times. (Adapted from Bronson GW. Infants' transitions toward adult-like scanning. *Child Dev* 1994;65:1243–1261, with permission.)

a positive potential occurs that is smaller but similar in timing to the adult potential (10).

In contrast to most features of saccadic eye movements in infants, the velocity of infant saccades is similar to that of adult saccades, both for saccades made to a peripheral target (2) and for saccades made in scanning patterns (3). An implication of this is that the brainstem mechanisms responsible for generating the actual motor behavior (Fig. 5.1) are relatively mature at birth, as opposed to cortical function. That is, the pulse generator, responsible for the high velocity of the saccadic eye movement, and the neural integrator, responsible for holding the eye in its postsaccadic position, appear to be more or less fully functional at birth.

SMOOTH PURSUIT EYE MOVEMENTS

Basic Features of Smooth Pursuit Movements in Adults

We make smooth pursuit eye movements to track visually a target moving at low to moderate velocity. The primary stimulus for smooth pursuit is generally thought to be target velocity with respect to the retina (i.e., retinal-slip velocity). The pursuit system, however, seems to be able to respond to a variety of stimuli. These include, along with target velocity, target offset from the fovea, target acceleration, perceived target velocity, and possibly relative target-background motion.

Smooth pursuit movements can occur in response to unidirectional target motion, periodic target motion, or to complex quasirandom or random target motion. Smooth pursuit velocity is typically less than target velocity (i.e., smooth pursuit gain—eye velocity or target velocity is less than 1.0). Furthermore, pursuit gain decreases as target velocity increases or as the target motion becomes more complex. As pursuit gain decreases, saccades tend to occur to reduce excessive error that accumulates between the eye and target (i.e., to keep the fovea close to the target for clear viewing).

The latency of smooth pursuit is about 100 ms, notably shorter than the latency of a saccade. This latency represents the time it takes for visual signals to pass through the visual system to the smooth pursuit motor mechanisms. As in the case of the saccadic system, the smooth pursuit system can be represented as consisting of a cortical component resting atop a brainstem component (Fig. 5.6). The cortical component is involved in perception of target velocity,

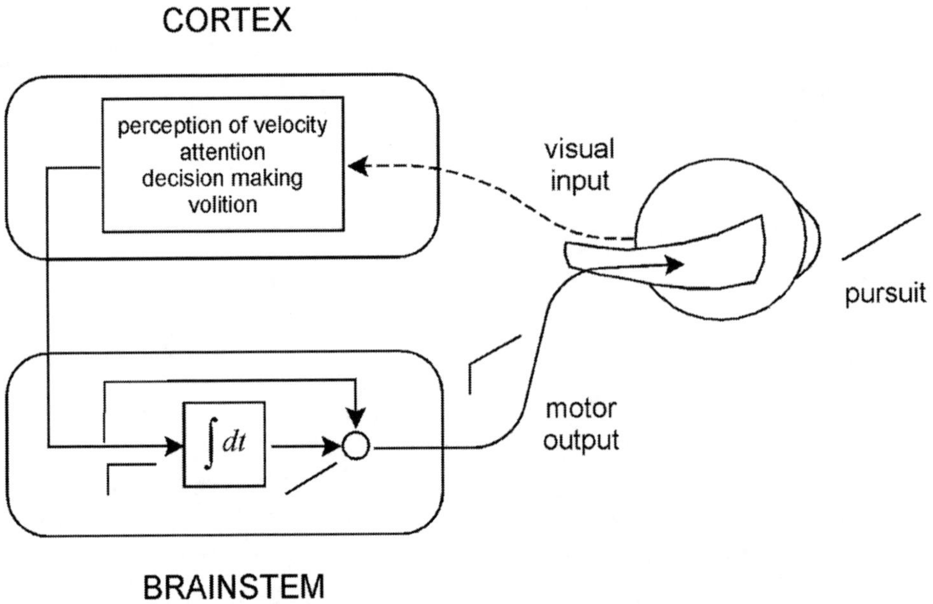

FIGURE 5.6. A model of the smooth pursuit eye movement system. The *upper box* shows cortical processes for pursuit, and the *lower box* shows a neural integrator.

attention to the target, initiation of smooth pursuit movements, and maintenance of the pursuit. According to the model, the cortex sends a velocity signal (a *step* of neural activity) to the brainstem neural integrator to produce an eye position signal (a *ramp* of neural activity). The velocity and position signals add and are delivered to the oculomotor plant to generate a smooth pursuit movement. As with the saccadic system, the velocity signal is necessary to deal with the viscous resistance of the plant, whereas the position signal is required for the elastic resistance.

Smooth Pursuit Movements in Infants

Smooth Pursuit with Binocular Viewing of a Stimulus

Kremenitzer et al. (11) conducted one of the first quantitative experiments on smooth pursuit eye movements in infants. Newborns (1 to 3 days old) observed a large (12°) black circle moving horizontally at velocities of 9° to 40°/s. Eye movements were recorded using the EOG. The newborns made occasional "smooth pursuit movement" in the direction of the target motion. The smooth movement eye velocity, however, was low overall and showed only a small

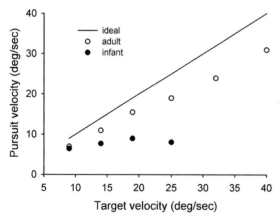

FIGURE 5.7. Smooth eye velocity in response to a black circle moving horizontally. Both infant and adult eye velocities are shown. The *line* indicates ideal eye velocity (i.e., eye velocity that perfectly follows target velocity). (Adapted from Kremenitzer JP, Vaughan HG, Kurtzberg D, et al. Smooth-pursuit eye movements in the newborn infant. *Child Dev* 1979;50:442–448, with permission.)

increase as target velocity increased (Fig. 5.7). In addition, the duration of smooth movement "epochs" was never more than several hundred milliseconds. One possible problem with this study is that the motion of the large black circle may have activated both a smooth pursuit response, dependent of the fovea, *and* a component optokinetic response, driven by the peripheral retina (see below: *Optokinetic Nystagmus*). Aslin (12) attempted to study smooth pursuit without the intrusion of optokinetic movements. He used a smaller target (2° wide, 8° high) that moved in a sinusoidal manner. The results show saccadic tracking of the target with no smooth pursuit in infants 5 to 6 weeks of age, and that smooth pursuit first appeared only after 8 weeks of age.

Both of these studies suggest that smooth pursuit movements are nonexistent or, at best weak, in infants up to several weeks of age. Recent experiments challenge this finding. Perhaps the most detailed investigation of smooth pursuit in infants was conducted by Phillips et al. (13). In this study, infants 1 to 4 months of age, observed a small (1.7°) target moving at a constant velocity. Eye movements were recorded using the EOG. An important finding was that infants as young as 1 month of age were able to make smooth pursuit movements in response to the target motion. The pursuit gain decreased as a function of target velocity (Fig. 5.8A). At higher target velocities, however, the gain increased as the infants became older. As an example, at a target velocity of 24°/s, pursuit gain was 0.48 in infants 1 month of age, but increased to 0.77 by 4 months of age. In the case of adults, the gain was approximately 1.0. The duration of smooth pursuit epochs also increased with age (Fig. 5.8B). For example, at a target velocity of 8°/s, the duration was about 200 ms in infants 1 month of age, increasing to about 450 ms in those 4 months of age. For adults, the duration was in excess of 1 second. As might be expected, the frequency of catch-up saccades was inversely related to the duration of pursuit epochs. Thus, the number of catch-up saccades rapidly decreased with age, approaching that for adults (Fig. 5.8C). Pursuit latency in infants was remarkably long, varying from 300 to 500 ms, whereas the latency for adults was about 150 ms.

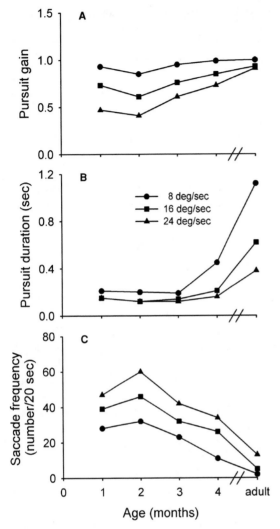

FIGURE 5.8. Pursuit gain, duration, and associated saccade frequency plotted against age. (Adapted from Phillips PO, Finocchio DV Ong L, et al. Smooth pursuit in 1- to 4-month-old human infants. *Vision Res* 1997;37:3009–3020, with permission.)

Lengyel et al. (14) conducted a similar study, except that it involved infants less than 1 month of age. The stimulus was a square (9.4°) target moving at 7.50°/s. Smooth pursuit movements occurred in infants as young as 1 week of age. Pursuit gain for these infants was about 0.75 and it remained close to this value up to 16 weeks of age. Pursuit epochs had a duration of between 2 and 3 s in the youngest as well as the oldest infants. This duration, it should be noted, is much longer than that found in the above studies.

Smooth Pursuit with Monocular Viewing

Binocular viewing (as in the above-mentioned studies) has a potential to mask some features of the oculomotor response, given neurologic yoking between the two eyes (i.e., Hering's law). For example, if right eye visual signals were stronger than left eye signals, the right eye would tend to dominate in the generation of smooth pursuit. Jacobs et al. (15) explored smooth pursuit as infants observed a moving target (a toy elephant) with one eye, the other eye patched. Consistent with the results from binocular studies (see above), smooth pursuit gain increased with age (Fig. 5.9). But instead of being the same in both directions, the gain was greater with target motion in the temporonasal direction than in the nasotemporal direction for infants between 1 and 5 months of age. This difference tended to decrease with age and was gone after 5 months of age, at which time the gain became essentially the same as found in adults.

Eye-Head Pursuit

In most oculomotor studies, the subject's head is restrained so that the only option is eye movements. Without head restraint, as in everyday circumstances, visual tracking can involve head movements as well as eye movements. Von Hofsten and Rosander (16) investigated the development of such eye-head tracking. Infants, without head restraint, observed a 10° "happy-face"

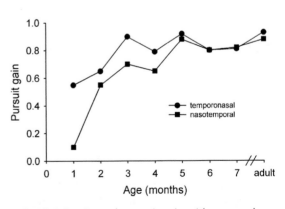

FIGURE 5.9. Smooth pursuit gain with monocular viewing of target motion (temporonasal and nasotemporal) shown as a function of age. (Adapted from Jacobs M, Harris CM, Shawkat F, et al. Smooth pursuit development in infants. *Aust N Z J Ophthalmol* 1997;25:199–206, with permission.)

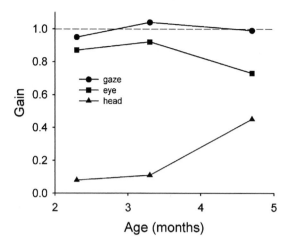

FIGURE 5.10. Smooth gaze, eye, and head tracking of target motion at ages ranging from 2 to 5 months. (Adapted from von Hofsten C, Rosander K. Development of smooth pursuit tracking in young infants. *Vision Res* 1997;37:1799–1810, with permission.)

moving according to either a sinusoidal or triangular function. The results (Fig. 5.10) show that the gain of gaze tracking (the combination of eye and head) was roughly 1.0 in infants ranging from about 2 to 5 months of age—the gaze tracking was nearly perfect. The relative contributions of the eye and head to the gaze tracking varied, however, with the infants' age. In those 2 month of age, the head tracking gain was less than 0.10, whereas the eye tracking gain was about 0.85. After 5 months, however, the head tracking gain had increased to 0.5, and as a consequence the eye tracking gain decreased.

Mechanisms

Smooth pursuit movements in infants generally have low gain and short duration epochs (13). A likely factor responsible for both of these is that visual cortical mechanisms for target velocity are not fully developed (i.e., the neural response is not commensurate with the target velocity). Another related possibility is that cortical processes concerned with paying attention are immature.

Pursuit gain is low in infants with monocular as well as binocular viewing; with the monocular viewing, however, the gain tends to be greater with target motion in the temporonasal direction than in the nasotemporal direction (15). Evidence shows that under monocular

conditions the visual cortex responds to target motion in both directions, whereas, for example, the pretectal nucleus of the optic tract (NOT) responds more strongly to motion in the temporonasal direction (see *Optokinetic Nystagmus* below). This suggests that in infants, whose cortex is immature, the pretectum is responsible to some extent for the asymmetric pursuit response. As the cortex matures, it plays a larger role in generating pursuit, so that over time, the asymmetry decreases and finally disappears.

That infants between 1 and 4 weeks of age are able to make smooth eye movements in response to target motion (13,14) means that, at an early age, cortical and pretectal velocity signals travel to the brainstem integrator where they are transformed into appropriate eye position signals. The integrator in infants seems to be intact and functioning in a mature manner. This, of course, is consistent with what appears to be the case in the saccadic system.

VERGENCE EYE MOVEMENTS

Basic Features of Vergence Movements in Adults

We make convergence eye movements to look from a far to a near object. These movements, in simplest form, are an exponential rotation of the eyes toward the nose. Similarly, we make divergence movements in looking from a near to a far object, an exponential rotation of the eyes away from the nose. Besides horizontal vergence movements, we can make vertical vergence and cyclovergence movements. Here, we are concerned with only horizontal vergence.

The stimuli for vergence include disparity between the object images on the two retinas, blur of the object images, and proximity of the object. Under most normal circumstances, all three of these stimuli are probably used to some extent. Under specialized experimental situations, however, either one or another of the stimuli alone is able to drive vergence movements. The vergence response to disparity alone occurs after a latency of about 160 ms, and consists of an exponential change in eye position with a time constant of about 200 ms (the time taken for the eye to rotate to 63% of it final position). The response to blur (no disparity) has a similar latency, but involves a somewhat slower change in eye position. It should be noted that the latency and the exponential characterization of the response are only rough generalizations and, in fact, may be highly variable from one study to another and across subjects.

The maximal velocity of vergence varies according to target location. The velocity is greater during convergence (the eyes turning toward a near target) than during divergence (the eyes turning toward a far target). When attempting to look at a target displaced from fixation both laterally and in depth, a combination of vergence and saccadic movements is required. In this circumstance, the vergence velocity is often considerably greater than when vergence occurs by itself.

Besides making vergence movements from one location to another, we can make such movements in following a smoothly moving target as it approaches or recedes. These two types of responses raise the possibility that at least two vergence systems may exist, a *fast* vergence system and a *slow* vergence system.

Single cell recordings in monkeys suggest that the vergence system is functionally organized in a manner similar to the saccadic and smooth pursuit systems. Thus, the fast vergence system might consist of a pulse generator that sends a pulse into and around a neural integrator, with the resulting pulse-step producing a vergence movement (Fig. 5.11). The pulse generator and integrator may be distinct from those in the saccadic system. Similarly, the slow vergence system might involve cortical and/or subcortical velocity signals that travel to a neural integrator.

Vergence Movements in Infants

Static and Dynamic Vergence

A number of early experiments claim that infants cannot make vergence eye movements until at least 2 months of age (17–22). All of these studies used a corneal reflection technique to record the position of the eyes, with the assumption that the center of the pupil indicates the direction of gaze (i.e., the visual axis). The center of the pupil and the direction of gaze, however, do not necessarily coincide (23). What this means, of course, is that the early studies may not have accurately appraised the infants' vergence capabilities.

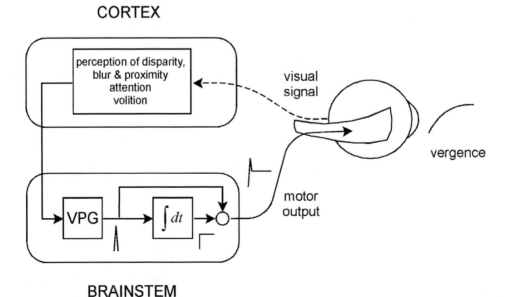

FIGURE 5.11. A model of the vergence eye movement system showing cortical processes for vergence. A vergence pulse generator (*VPG*) and a neural integrator.

Slater and Findlay (24) conducted three experiments on vergence movements in infants using corneal reflection, but included a correction factor to determine the actual direction of gaze. The primary concern in these studies was the posture of the eyes after the completion of vergence movements (i.e., static vergence). In the first experiment, infants 1 to 8 days of age viewed a far stimulus followed by a near stimulus, or vice versa. The far stimulus was a vertical row of lights at a distance of 20 inches (50.8 cm), and the near stimulus was a similar vertical row at a distance of 10 inches (25.4 cm). The results of the study show that the infants were able to make vergence movements in the direction of the far stimulus or the near stimulus. The average amount of vergence was about 2.6°, however, whereas a fully appropriate amount would have been 3.1°. Thus, the resulting mean vergence error was about 0.5°. Furthermore, the vergence posture for each stimulus was not stable, but tended to fluctuate over a range of about 2° between under- and oververgence. In the second experiment, the infants viewed a vertical row of lights at distances of 10 and 5 inches (25.4 and 12.7 cm). The vergence was about the same as above when the stimulus was at 10 inches, but was much less or nonexistent with the stimulus at 5 inches (12.7 cm). The third experiment required the infants to look at three different stimuli (a vertical strip, a combination triangle-plus-square, and an arrangement of squares) located at a distance of 10 inches (25.4 cm). Most of the infants were able to make some degree of vergence with all three stimuli, showing that the infant vergence system is capable of dealing with a variety of visual circumstances.

In a subsequent investigation, Aslin (25) used corneal photography to record the characteristics of the ongoing vergence eye movements (i.e., dynamic vergence). In one experiment, infants 1, 2, and 3 months of age observed a luminous cross as it moved closer or farther away. The stimulus moved at either a low or high velocity over a distance between 6 and 22 inches (15 and 57 cm). It was arranged so that the cross provided all of the traditional cues for vergence: disparity, blur, and proximity. In line with Slater and Findlay (24) findings, the infants could make vergence movements in the direc-

tion of the stimulus motion, converging as the stimulus moved closer and diverging as the stimulus moved farther. The younger infants showed lower amplitude vergence than the older infants, especially when the stimulus moved at the higher velocity. In a second experiment, infants 3, 4.5, and 6 months of age were tested for vergence when the only cue was disparity (an infant's attention was attracted by a stimulus, after which a wedge prism was introduced in front of the infant's eyes). The important result was that those 3 and 4.5 months of age showed little or no vergence response with disparity as the sole stimulus. By 6 months of age, however, clear and consistent vergence occurred with disparity alone.

The Development of Disparity Vergence

The research by Slater and Findlay (24) and Aslin (25) suggests that vergence eye movements can occur within the first weeks of infancy, but that a substantive vergence response to disparity does not appear until somewhat later. Thorn et al. (26) investigated the details of the development of the vergence response and its relation to cortical disparity mechanisms. They tested 34 infants biweekly over a period starting shortly after birth until about 22 weeks of age. At the beginning of a vergence trial, an examiner jiggled a toy located about 0.5 m in front of an infant's face. When the infant looked at the toy, the examiner moved the toy slowly toward the infant's nose and at the same time observed the infant's eyes. Convergence in response to the toy motion was reported according to three categories: no convergence; first sign of convergence; and full convergence. Disparity mechanisms were explored using preferential looking toward a fusible stimulus versus a nonfusible stimulus (i.e., a rivalrous stimulus).

The proportion of infants showing first sign of convergence, full convergence, and fusion preference is plotted against age in Fig. 5.12. Each set of data was fitted with a normal ogive. Convergence and fusion preference first appeared in some of the infants at about 5 weeks of age. The mean first sign of convergence occurred at 12.1 weeks, whereas the mean full convergence occurred at 13.7 weeks, a difference of 1.6 weeks. Mean fusion preference occurred

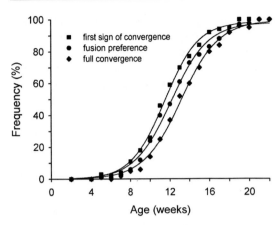

FIGURE 5.12. Cumulative functions for first sign of convergence, full convergence, and fusion preference. (Adapted from Thorn F, Gwiazda J, Cruz AAV, et al. The development of eye alignment, convergence, and sensory binocularity in young infants. *Invest Ophthalmol Vis Sci* 1994;35:544–553, with permission.)

at 12.8 weeks, halfway between the first sign of convergence and full convergence. It was not until 22 weeks had passed that all infants had achieved full convergence as well as fusion preference.

Mechanisms

Blur and proximity may be the primary stimuli driving vergence eye movements during the first few weeks of infancy, with disparity playing a lesser role (25). The mutual development of cortical disparity mechanisms and vergence (26), however, suggests that disparity becomes a major stimulus for vergence between about 2 and 6 months of age. In any case, studies (24) show that newborn infants can make vergence movements to both far and near targets, although with some inaccuracy and instability. This implies that at an early age, consistent with the findings for saccadic and smooth pursuit movements, brainstem motor mechanisms (e.g., a vergence pulse generator and neural integrator) are reasonably functional. In short, cortical mechanisms responsible for governing vergence develop over a period of months, whereas brainstem motor mechanisms for vergence are in place at birth or shortly thereafter.

THE VESTIBULO-OCULAR REFLEX

Basic Features of the Vestibulo-Ocular Reflex in Adults

All of the eye movements considered thus far are driven by visual stimuli. In contrast, the vestibulo-ocular reflex (VOR) is activated by rotation of the head. Sensory signals for the VOR arise from three semicircular canals (one for each spatial dimension, roughly speaking) located near the inner ear on each side of the head. The VOR is typically a sawtoothlike pattern of nystagmus consisting of alternating slow-phase eye movements and fast-phase (saccade-like) movements. When a person rotates, the slow movements occur opposite to the direction of the rotation, and the fast movements occur in the same direction as the rotation. The purpose of the slow movement is to keep the eyes reasonably stable with respect to the surrounding environment, so that objects can be clearly observed. The fast movements reset the position of the eyes to allow further slow movements.

The two principal modes of studying the VOR are with periodic rotation (e.g., rotation from left to right at a given frequency) and with constant velocity unidirectional rotation (e.g., rotation to the left). With periodic rotation in the dark, the gain of the VOR (slow-phase velocity/head-velocity) is between 0.6 and 0.7. If subjects are allowed to view visual stimuli such as a small stationary target or a full field of stationary contours, however, the gain increases to about 1.0. This increase is caused, in the case of the small target, by the activation of the smooth pursuit system, the fixation system, or both, and in the case of the full field, to the optokinetic system (see below). With constant velocity rotation in the dark, the slow-phase velocity decreases exponentially with a time constant of about 20 s. The VOR can be inhibited if a subject views, or even imagines, a target moving along with the head as it rotates.

Acceleration of the head is responsible for activating the semicircular canals. The effect of this acceleration is displacement of the endolymph-cupula within a canal and, as a consequence, stimulation of hair cells located within the cupula. The mechanics of the canal (the endolymph-cupula), however, are such that the head acceleration is *filtered*, resulting in a

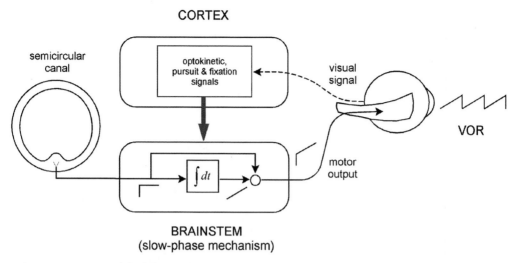

FIGURE 5.13. A model of the vestibulo-ocular system showing vestibular velocity signals going to the brainstem neural integrator. Pursuit, optokinetic, and fixation signals can also affect vestibular eye movements.

neural signal proportional to head velocity. As the model in Figure 5.13 shows, the velocity signal travels both into and around the brainstem integrator to generate slow-phase vestibular eye movements. The slow-phase movements not only compensate for rotation, but also trigger a saccadic pulse generator (not shown) to produce fast phases. The model also indicates that the pursuit, optokinetic, and fixations systems can influence vestibular eye movements.

The Vestibulo-Ocular Reflex in Infants

Periodic Rotation

Finocchio et al. (27) investigated the gain of the VOR in infants (slow-phase velocity/head-velocity) in several stimulus situations. The infants sat in a chair that was rotated horizontally from side to side through an arc of about 40°. Eye movements were recorded using the EOG, under three conditions: VOR in the dark, VOR with a stationary small target, and VOR with a stationary full field of vertical alternating white and black stripes. Gain is shown in each of the three conditions as a function of age (Fig. 5.14). The gain in the dark was approximately 1.0 in infants from 1 month of age (the youngest in the study) to 4 months of age (the oldest). What is interesting is that this is much greater than the gain for adults. When either the target or

the full-field stimulus was present, the gain was again about 1.0 for the infants. The gain was also close to 1.0 in these two conditions for adults. In addition to gain, the study looked at the frequency and amplitude of the fast phases of the VOR (Fig. 5.15). These data have several interesting features. First, the frequency of the fast phases was somewhat lower in the infants than in adults. Second, the amplitude tended to increase between 1 and 4 months of age, whereas it was relatively low in adults.

Along with gain, phase lag is an important aspect of the VOR (e.g., the phase lag should be about 180° for the eyes to remain reasonably stable in space). Cioni et al. (28) recorded the amplitude and phase lag of the VOR in infants and children. The infants were 1 to 4 weeks of age and the children were 4 to 7 years of age. They were rotated sinusoidally in the dark, and eye movements were recorded using the EOG. Amplitude and phase lag of the movements of both the infants and children appear in Fig. 5.16. For the infants, both the amplitude and phase were less than optimal at low frequencies: the amplitude was less than the maximal value of 100 and the phase lag was less than 180° when the frequency was between 0.05 and 0.25 Hz. In contrast, the children's amplitude was at or near the maximum from the lowest to the highest frequencies, and their phase lag was close to 180° except at the lowest frequency of 0.05 Hz.

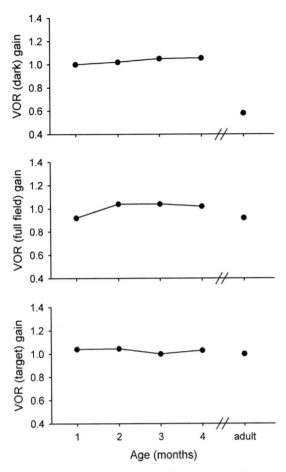

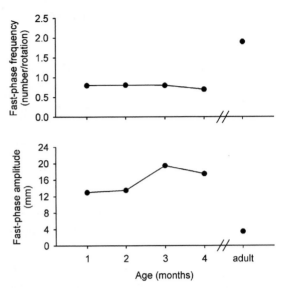

FIGURE 5.15. Fast-phase frequency and amplitude of the vestibulo-ocular reflex (VOR), plotted against age. (Adapted from Finocchio DV, Preston KL, Fuchs AF. Infant eye movements: quantification of the vestibulo-ocular reflex and visual-vestibular interactions. *Vision Res* 1991;31:1717–1730, with permission.)

FIGURE 5.14. Gain of the vestibulo-ocular reflex (VOR) as a function of age in three different background conditions: complete darkness, a field of stripes, and a small target. (Adapted from Finocchio DV, Preston KL, Fuchs AF. Infant eye movements: quantification of the vestibulo-ocular reflex and visual-vestibular interactions. *Vision Res* 1991;31:1717–1730, with permission.)

Constant Velocity Rotation

When infants are rotated at a constant velocity in the dark, the slow-phase velocity of the VOR gradually decreases in an exponential manner. In newborns, the duration of the exponential decrease is remarkably short with a time constant of about 1.0 s (29). As infants grow older, the duration of the exponential increases. Thus, in infants 5 months of age, the time constant increases to about 7.5 s and by 15-months of age, the time constant achieves a value of approximately 9.0 s (30). In adults, the time constant

can have a value of as much as 20 s (see *Basic Features of the Vestibulo-Ocular Reflex in Adults*).

Mechanisms

An interesting feature of the VOR is that its gain is at the maximal value of 1.0 in infants, but becomes notably lower (0.59) in adults (27). What is responsible for this change? Infants are immature perceptually and behaviorally, with few strategies for evaluating and effectively interacting with their surrounding world. Thus, in the first few months of life, a gain of 1.0 provides an automatic, reliable means of stabilizing the position of the eyes for good acuity (27). As the infants interact with their environment, however, optokinetic nystagmus (OKN), which is discussed below, comes into play, providing support for the stabilization. Thus, as time passes, it is no longer necessary for the VOR gain to remain at its original high value. Similarly, after about 5 months, visual tracking is often accomplished with a combination of eye and head movements (see above: *Smooth Pursuit Eye Movements*). This tracking requires suppression of the VOR and, over time, such suppression might also contribute to a decrease in the gain (27).

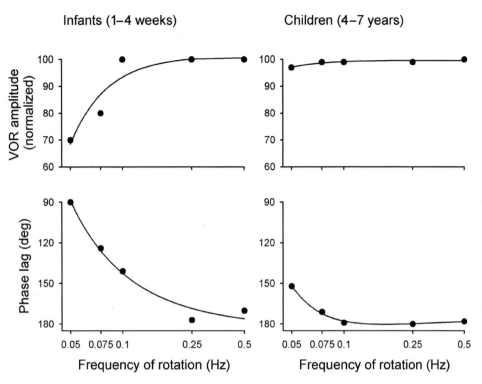

FIGURE 5.16. Vestibulo-ocular reflex (VOR) amplitude and phase-lag plotted against frequency of sinusoidal rotation. The *two graphs on the left* show the responses for infants, and the *graphs on the right* give the responses for children. (Adapted from Cioni G, Favilla M, Ghelarducci B, et al. Development of the dynamic characteristics of the horizontal vestibulo-ocular reflex in infancy. *Neuropediatrics* 1984;15:125–130, with permission.)

The high gain of the VOR in infants shows that some aspects of the vestibulo-ocular system are relatively mature at an early age. That is, the semicircular canals send velocity signals to the neural integrator where they are transformed into eye position signals. This is in accord with the above discussion on saccades and smooth pursuit. On the other hand, the phase lag of the VOR in infants raises the possibility that the integrator may not be completely formed. A fully functioning integrator should create eye position signals that reflect the time-varying features of the changing head position. But the phase lag in infants is less than 180° at low frequencies of rotation (28). That is, eye position does not completely compensate for head position at the low frequencies. A generally accepted view is that the retinal image slip arising from inappropriate phase lag activates neural machinery concerned with the adjustment of oculomotor behavior. A result of such adjustment may be

the 180° phase lag across all frequencies that appears later on in children (28).

In contrast to gain, the very short time constant of the VOR in newborns (29) indicates that the vestibulo-ocular system involves processes that are barely functional at birth. The VOR can be understood as arising from the combined effects of two velocity signal mechanisms, one residing in the mechanics of the semicircular canals, and the other in central neural circuits. The cupula, as part of the mechanics of the canals, is displaced from its resting position as the head begins to rotate at a constant velocity, but then returns to its resting position. This return occurs quickly, regardless of age, and therefore the resulting signal cannot account for the change from the short time constant (1 s) in newborns to the much longer time constant (20 s) in adults. The vestibulo-ocular system, however, also has a central *velocity storage* mechanism (31) that serves to transform the signal from the canals into a longer duration signal. Thus, it would appear that the canals, together with an immature velocity storage mechanism, are responsible for the short time constant VOR in newborns, and that development of the velocity storage mechanism over a period of months, if not years, underlies the gradual increase in the time constant (30).

OPTOKINETIC NYSTAGMUS

Basic Features of Optokinetic Nystagmus in Adults

Optokinetic nystagmus is a response to the motion of a large visual field. Similar to the VOR, it consists of a sawtoothlike pattern of alternating slow-phase eye movements and fast-phase (saccadelike) eye movements. The slow-phase movements occur in the same direction as the field motion with approximately the same velocity as the field, assuming that the velocity of the field is low to moderate. Thus, these slow movements roughly stabilize the image of the field at the retina, permitting a clear view of the field. The fast phases occur opposite to the direction of the field motion resetting eye position so that additional slow phases can occur. A typical experimental stimulus for OKN is a field of vertical alternating black and white stripes, moving horizontally at a constant velocity. OKN responds to the onset of the field motion with a latency of about 100 ms. The slow-phase velocity at first increases rapidly and then more slowly until it roughly matches the field velocity. The fast increase is thought to reflect the dynamics of the smooth pursuit system, whereas the slower subsequent rise is optokinetic. When a subject *actively* attends to the field motion, the slow-phase gain (slow-phase velocity/head velocity) tends to be higher than when a subject *passively* regards the field.

Such eye movements might seem like an oddity because, in the normal everyday world, it would be exceptional for a large portion of the visual field to move as a unit. This apparent oddity, however, vanishes when it is understood that OKN works cooperatively with the VOR to stabilize eye position against head rotation. As the head rotates, say, to the left, visual signals coming from relative head-field motion create optokinetic slow-phase responses to the right, at

the same time as vestibular signals create VOR slow phases to the right. OKN, with its slower build-up to a steady response, serves to stabilize the eyes against long duration rotation, whereas the VOR, with its fast response but slow decay, stabilizes the eyes during the onset of rotation and for short duration rotation.

Visual field motion generates velocity signals in visual cortical areas and also in a number of subcortical nuclei [e.g., the pretectal nucleus of the optic tract (NOT) and the dorsal terminal nucleus of the accessory optic system (DTN)]. As Fig. 5.17 shows, the velocity signals go to the neural integrator, resulting in the slow phases of OKN. The pulse generator for the fast phases is not shown.

Optokinetic Nystagmus in Infants

When infants view binocularly, the motion of a large field, their OKN is relatively robust whether the motion is leftward or rightward. That is, their optokinetic response is symmetric with respect to the direction of the field motion. When they view monocularly the field motion, the OKN changes dramatically, however, it is much weaker when the field motion is nasotemporal than when it is temporonasal (32–35). This asymmetry is large when the infants are a few weeks old, but gradually decreases as the infants grow older. Figure 5.18 presents the ratio of the slow-phase velocity of OKN in the two directions (slow-phase velocity in the nasotemporal direction/slow-phase velocity in the temporonasal direction) plotted against age, when the field velocity was 25° (35). For infants less than 1 month of age, the ratio was less than 0.2 (large asymmetry). As the infants became older, the ratio increased in roughly a linear manner, so that by about 6 months of age the ratio had a value of approximately 1.0 (no asymmetry). That is, the nasotemporal OKN became essentially as strong as the temporonasal OKN.

Most studies investigate OKN with a field consisting of large stripes. A problem associated with this type of stimulus is that it can elicit a limited range of the potential response features of the optokinetic system. Lewis et al. (36) conducted an experiment to determine monocular *optokinetic acuity* with both nasotemporal and temporonasal field motion.

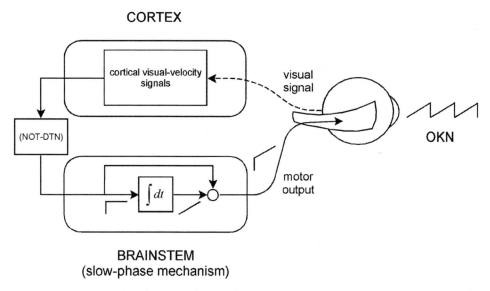

FIGURE 5.17. A model of the optokinetic system showing cortical velocity signals, subcortical nuclei, and a neural integrator. The pulse generator for fast phases of optokinetic nystagmus (OKN) is not included.

Optokinetic acuity is defined as the narrowest stripes that elicit OKN. In the study, infants 3 to 18 months of age viewed the horizontal motion of a large field of vertical stripes. The stripes varied in spatial frequency from 0.05 to 5.0 cycles/s.

Figure 5.19 shows that optokinetic acuity with temporonasal field motion was almost as high in 3-month-old infants as in those 18 months of age. This is in line with the general finding that temporonasal OKN tends to be robust

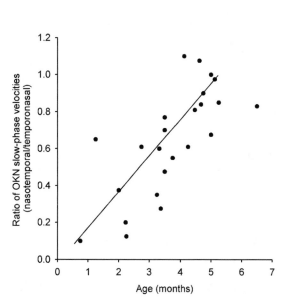

FIGURE 5.18. The ratio of optokinetic nystagmus (OKN) slow phase velocities (nasotemporal / temporonasal) as a function of age. (Adapted from Naegele JR, Held R. The postnatal development of monocular optokinetic nystagmus in infants. *Vision Res* 1982;22:341–346, with permission.)

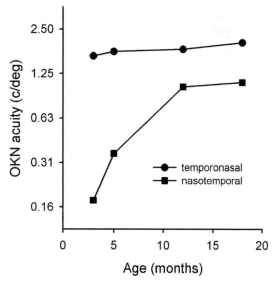

FIGURE 5.19. Optokinetic nystagmus (OKN) acuity for monocular viewing of temporonasal and nasotemporal field motion, plotted against age. (Adapted from Lewis TL, Maurer D, Chung JYY, et al. The development of symmetrical OKN in infants: quantification based on OKN acuity for nasalward versus temporalward motion. *Vision Res* 2000;40:445–453, with permission.)

(32–35). On the other hand, optokinetic acuity with nasotemporal field motion, although low in infants 3 months of age, gradually increased over the following 15 months. The low acuity is consistent with the finding that nasotemporal OKN is weak in younger infants. The fact that the acuity increased until about 18 months of age, however, shows that processes associated with nasotemporal OKN continue to develop well beyond 6 months of age, in contrast to most previous reports (32–35).

Mechanisms

The model in Fig. 5.20 shows that neurons in the pretectal nucleus of the optic tract and the dorsal terminal nucleus of the accessory optic system (NOT-DTN) receive direct input from the nasal retina of the contralateral eye. Along with the direct input, the neurons in NOT-DTN get input from both the contralateral and ipsilateral visual cortical areas [e.g., superior temporal sulcus (STS) and the primary visual cortex (V1)]. The direct input provides velocity signals for temporonasal field motion, whereas the cortical input supplies velocity signals for temporonasal and nasotemporal field motion.

One consequence of this neural arrangement is that, in infants, with an immature cortex, the direct input from the retina to NOT-DTN provides the primary signal for generating OKN (37). Thus, when infants view monocularly, the direct input causes strong OKN with temporonasal field motion but much weaker or even no OKN with nasotemporal field motion (i.e., asymmetric OKN). As the infants become older and their visual cortex matures, the cortical input gradually comes to dominate the neurons in NOT-DTN (37). As a result, the infants' monocular response by about 6 months of age shows robust OKN with nasotemporal field motion as well as with temporonasal motion (i.e., symmetric OKN).

Early visual deprivation can affect cortical function, which, in turn, could interfere with the usual course of OKN development. A disruption of visual stimulation can occur in infants who, for example, have unilateral esotropic strabismus or a unilateral congenital cataract. In the long term, these conditions can lead to poor

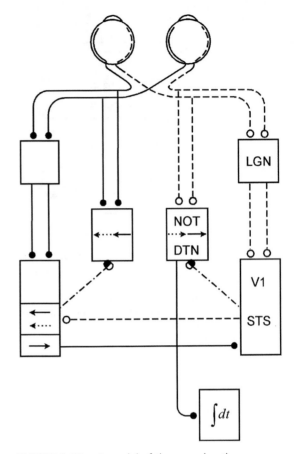

FIGURE 5.20. A model of the neural pathways involved in the generation of optokinetic eye movements. The *solid lines* show projections concerned with the right visual field and the *broken lines* show projections for the left visual field. *Arrows* indicate the direction of stimulus motion represented in each of several locations of the visual system. LGN, lateral geniculate nucleus; V1, the primary visual cortex; STS, superior temporal sulcus; NOT, nucleus of the optic tract; DTN, dorsal terminal nucleus. (Adapted from Distler C, Hoffman KP. Development of the optokinetic response in macaques: a comparison with cat and man. *Ann NY Acad Sci* 2003;1004:10–18, with permission.)

cortical binocular function and also asymmetry of monocular OKN (38). Early correction of the strabismus or cataract, however, generally results in normal development of both the binocular function and OKN.

These considerations might seem to imply that good binocular vision is a prerequisite for normal development of OKN. Cases are seen, however, where infants with reasonably intact binocular function show asymmetric OKN (38). Such observations raise the possibility that lack of binocular vision *per se* may not be the main causal factor of the asymmetry (38). What might occur is that visual deprivation has some number of injurious effects on visual function. One of these may be a lack of sufficient development of visual motion pathways from cortical areas to NOT-DTN. Instead of binocular vision, the quality of these pathways may be directly responsible for the asymmetric OKN.

SUMMARY AND DISCUSSION

A primary aim of this chapter was to present in detail some of the important characteristics of eye movements in infants. A second purpose was to point out two general features of infant eye movements and their underlying mechanisms. One of these is that, at the time of birth or shortly thereafter, the eye movements, although apparently immature, bear a resemblance to adult eye movements in a number of important respects. The other is that within a relatively short period of time, several weeks to months, the infant eye movements change to become virtually identical to adult movements. The earliest eye movements seem to be a consequence of brainstem mechanisms that are relatively mature at birth, and the manner in which these movements evolve is largely a result of a gradual maturation of cortical areas of the brain.

The cortical mechanisms considered in this review, for the most part, are concerned with visual information processing as it relates to the production of eye movements. Thus, the perception of target location is necessary for making saccades, the perception of target velocity is essential for the generation of smooth pursuit movements, and binocular vision is central in the execution of vergence movements. An important cognitive mechanism associated with eye movements is attention. This seems to play a role in making saccadic movements, especially to targets that have motivational significance, and also in generating smooth pursuit movements when it is necessary to follow target motion with little or no error. The perceptual processes develop over a period of weeks to months, whereas cognitive processes can continue to change over several years.

The brainstem mechanisms that receive the most attention here are the pulse generator for creating saccadic eye movements and the neural integrator for transforming eye velocity signals to eye position signals. It might seem that these two mechanisms represent a rather limited aspect of the brainstem, and although this may be the case functionally, it is not so anatomically. Originally, the pulse generator was thought to be largely *reticulo-centric* (39), that is, confined to reticular formation nuclei. But a number of studies now indicate that the production of saccades is not limited to one or another area of the brainstem. Horizontal saccades depend on pontine reticular nuclei (e.g., the paramedial pontine reticular formation), whereas vertical and torsional saccades involve mesencephalic nuclei. More important, however, it has recently been proposed that the pulse generator is *cerebello-centric*, where the cerebellum, as a central component, works together with the reticular nuclei and the superior colliculus (40). Thus, instead of a simple local entity, it appears that the pulse generator is functionally distributed over a variety of different neural structures. Similarly, the process of neural integration is not confined to a small, localized area of the brainstem. In the case of horizontal eye movements, the integrator involves at least two lower brainstem nuclei, the vestibular nuclei and the nucleus prepositus hypoglossi, together with aspects of the cerebellum (41). For vertical and torsional eye movements, the integrator involves upper brainstem nuclei together with the cerebellum (41). In short, the variety of structures concerned with the process of pulse generation and integration shows that a wide range of brainstem and related areas are reasonably mature in newborn infants.

The differences between the developmental features of the cortex and the brainstem are not surprising. Cortical mechanisms for perception and cognition become especially important as we separate from our parents and caretakers over a period of months and years. In contrast, the brainstem contains mechanisms concerned with, for example, arousal, breathing, blood pressure, digestion, and heart rate, all of which are essential for basic physiologic survival.

These brainstem functions suggest that the newborn's oculomotor brainstem mechanisms are not just a basis on which to establish mature behavior. Instead, they may be an integral part of the process of satisfying physiologic needs by providing interaction with caretakers. As mentioned, the high gain of the VOR in infants is important to stabilize the position of the eyes for good visual acuity. This would appear to be especially important in observing close-by objects, such as the mother. It may also be the case that infants' ability to make adultlike saccades in scanning simple patterns is a reflection of their ability to scan facial expressions in the service of social interaction, and especially to look for signs of approval. Eye movements in infants, then, may be misunderstood if they are regarded as simply immature. A more correct view may be that they are an adaptation for functioning within a very limited environment, with their development unfolding according to the requirements of an expanding world.

ACKNOWLEDGMENTS

I wish to thank Nancy Oley for providing many helpful comments on the manuscript.

REFERENCES

1. Aslin RN, Salapatek P. Saccadic localization of visual targets by the very young infant. *Percept Psychophys* 1975;17:293–302.
2. Richards JE, Hunter SK. Peripheral stimulus localization by infants with eye and head movements during visual attention. *Vision Res* 1997;37:3021–3035.
3. Hainline L, Turkel J, Abramov I, et al. Characteristics of saccades in human infants. *Vision Res* 1984;12:1771–1780.
4. Bronson GW. Changes in infants' visual scanning across the 2- to 14-week age period. *J Exp Child Psychol* 1990;49:101–125.
5. Bronson GW. Infants' transitions toward adult-like scanning. *Child Dev* 1994;65:1243–1261.
6. Matsuzama M. Development of saccade target selection in infants. *Percept Mot Skills* 2001;93:115–123.
7. Kurzberg D, Vaughan HJ. Topographic analysis of human cortical potential preceding self-initiated and visual triggered saccades. *Brain Res* 1982;243:1–9.
8. Balaban CD, Weinstein JM. The human pre-saccadic spike potential: influences of a visual target, saccade direction, electrode laterality and instructions to perform saccades. *Brain Res* 1985;347:49–57.
9. Moster LM, Goldberg G. Topography of scalp potentials preceding self-initiated saccades. *Neurology* 1990;40:644–648.
10. Cisbra G, Tucker LA, Voleins A, et al. Cortical development and saccade planning: the ontogeny of the spike potential. *Neuroreport* 2000;11:1069–1073.
11. Kremenitzer JP, Vaughan HG, Kurtzberg D, et al. Smooth-pursuit eye movements in the newborn infant. *Child Dev* 1979;50:442–448.
12. Aslin RN. Development of smooth pursuit in human infants. In: Fischer DF, Monty RA, Senders JW, eds. *Eye Movements: Cognition and Visual Perception.* Hillsdale, NJ: Lawrence Erlbaum; 1981.
13. Phillips PO, Finocchio DV Ong L, et al. Smooth pursuit in 1- 4-month-old human infants. *Vision Res* 1997;37:3009–3020.
14. Lengyel D, Weinacht S, Charlier J, et al. The development of visual pursuit during the first months of life. *Graefes Arch Clin Exp Ophthalmol* 1998;236:440–444.
15. Jacobs M, Harris CM, Shawkat F, et al. Smooth pursuit development in infants. *Aust N Z J Ophthalmol* 1997;25:199–206.
16. von Hofsten C, Rosander K. Development of smooth pursuit tracking in young infants. *Vision Res* 1997;37:1799–1810.
17. Fantz RL. The origin of form perception. *Sci Am* 1961;71:871–875.
18. Salapatek P, Kessen W. Visual scanning of triangles by the human newborn. *J Exp Child Psychol* 1966;3:155–167.
19. Hershenson M. Visual discrimination in the human newborn. *Journal of Comparative and Physiological Psychology* 1964;58: 270–276.
20. Wickelgren LW. Convergence in the human newborn. *Journal of Experimental Child Psychology* 1967;5:74–85.
21. Wickelgren LW. The ocular response of human newborns to intermittent visual movement. *J Exp Child Psychol* 1969;8: 469–482.
22. Greenberg DJ, Weitzmann F. The measurement of visual attention in infants: a comparison of two methodologies. *J Exp Child Psychol* 1971;11:234–243.
23. Slater AM, Findlay JM. The measurement of fixation position in the newborn baby. *J Exp Child Psychol* 1972;14:249–364.
24. Slater AM, Findlay JM. The corneal-reflection technique and the visual preference method: sources of error. *J Exp Child Psychol* 1975;20:240–247.
25. Aslin RN. Development of binocular fixation in human infants. *J Exp Child Psychol* 1977;23:133–150.
26. Thorn F, Gwiazda J, Cruz AAV, et al. The development of eye alignment, convergence, and sensory binocularity in young infants. *Invest Ophthalmol Vis Sci* 1994;35: 544–553.
27. Finocchio DV, Preston KL, Fuchs AF. Infant eye movements: quantification of the vestibulo-ocular reflex and visual-vestibular interactions. *Vision Res* 1991;31:1717–1730.
28. Cioni G, Favilla M, Ghelarducci B, et al. Development of the dynamic characteristics of the horizontal vestibulo-ocular reflex in infancy. *Neuropediatrics* 1984;15:125–130.
29. Weissman BM, DiScenna AO, Leigh RJ. Maturation of the vestibulo-ocular reflex in normal infants during the first 2 months of life. *Neurology* 1989;39:534–538.
30. Ornitz EM, Kaplan AR, Westlake JR. Development of the vestibulo-ocular reflex from infancy to adulthood. *Acta Otolaryngology (Stockholm)* 1985;100:180–193.
31. Raphan T, Matsuo V, Cohen B. Velocity storage in the vestibulo-ocular reflex arc (VOR). *Exp Brain Res* 1979;35:229–248.

32. Atkinson J. Development of optokinetic nystagmus in the human infant and monkey infant: an analogue to development in kittens. In: Freeman RF, ed. *Developmental Neurobiology of Vision.* New York: Plenum Press; 1979.

33. Atkinson J, Braddick O. Development of optokinetic nystagmus in infants; an indicator of cortical binocularity? In: Fisher DF, Monty RA, Sanders JW, eds. *Eye Movements: Cognition and Visual Perception.* Hillsdale, NJ: Lawrence Erlbaum; 1981.

34. Schor CM. Development of OKN in human infants. *American Journal of Optometry and Physiological Optics* 1981;58:80.

35. Naegele JR, Held R. The postnatal development of monocular optokinetic nystagmus in infants. *Vision Res* 1982;22: 341–346.

36. Lewis TL, Maurer D, Chung JYY, et al. The development of symmetrical OKN in infants: quantification based on OKN acuity for nasalward versus temporalward motion. *Vision Res* 2000;40: 445–453.

37. Distler C, Hoffman KP. Development of the optokinetic response in macaques: a comparison with cat and man. *Ann NY Acad Sci* 2003;1004:10–18.

38. Westall CA, Eizenman M, Kraft SP, et al. Cortical binocularity and monocular optokinetic asymmetry in early-onset esotropia. *Invest Ophthalmol Vis Sci* 1998;39:1352–1369.

39. Pola J. Models of the saccadic and smooth pursuit systems. In: Hung JK, Ciuffreda KJ, eds. *Models of the Visual System.* New York: Kluwer Academic/Plenum Publishers, 2002.

40. Quaia C, Lefevre P, Optican LM. Model of the control of the saccades by superior colliculus and cerebellum. *J Neurophysiol* 1999;82:999–1018.

41. Leigh RJ, Zee DS. *The Neurology of Eye Movements,* 3rd ed. New York: Oxford University Press; 1999.

6

Development of Accommodation in Human Infants

Mark Rosenfield

Ocular accommodation is the process whereby changes in the refractive power of the crystalline lens allow clear vision to be maintained across a range of viewing distances. Contraction of the ciliary muscle pulls the choroid forward and the attachment of the zonules inward, thereby relaxing the tension of the zonular fibers. This allows the crystalline lens to become more convex because of both the elastic forces in the lens capsule and the viscoelastic properties of the lens substance (1–3).

An infant needs to be able to accommodate accurately to resolve objects at a close viewing distance. With the exception of a few infants having uncorrected myopia (4–8), they will have poor near visual resolution without adequate accommodation. This is critical for normal visual development to proceed, because it depends on the brain receiving clear and focused images from each of the two eyes (9).

The earliest evidence for active accommodation in human infants comes from studies that have observed differences in refractive error when measured both with and without the use of pharmaceutical cycloplegic agents to paralyze active accommodation. For example, analysis by Howland (8) of the data presented by Santonastaso (10) indicated that for 19 infants under 15 days of age, the mean spherical refractive error measured with and without cycloplegia was +0.98 D and −7.03 D, respectively. Earlier, Jaeger (11) used the direct ophthalmoscope to determine the refractive

error of 100 infants between 9 and 16 days of age without cycloplegia, and reported that 78% were myopic. It should be noted that the direct ophthalmoscope is generally regarded as an inaccurate instrument for assessing refractive error (12,13). Nevertheless, most studies that have measured refractive error under cycloplegia have observed a much lower prevalence of myopia. For example, Cook and Glasscock (4) using cycloplegic retinoscopy on 1000 eyes of children during "postdelivery care" found that approximately 25% were myopic. Similar levels of myopia prevalence in infants ($N = 356$) using atropine cycloplegia were reported by Goldschmidt (5). Furthermore, a significant difference was observed in the refractive error of 2-day old infants when assessed with and without cycloplegia (14). It was concluded that these differences provided evidence of active accommodation in the newborn infant.

Having demonstrated that newborns do indeed possess the ability to accommodate, subsequent studies have examined the accommodative response to a range of stimulus demands in young infants. This assessment of the accommodative stimulus-response profile is commonly carried out in adults, and a typical adult accommodative stimulus-response function is illustrated in Fig. 6.1 (1,15,16).

One of the first studies to examine this function in infants was carried out by Haynes et al. (14). Here, dynamic retinoscopy was used to measure the accommodative response of

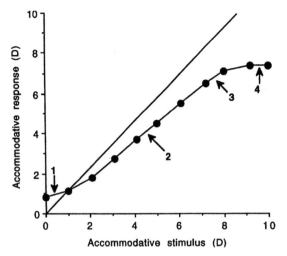

FIGURE 6.1. Static accommodative stimulus-response curve for a normal adult subject. 1, initial nonlinear region; 2, linear region; 3, transitional soft saturation region; 4, hard saturation region. The *diagonal line* represents the unit ratio (or 1:1) line. (Redrawn from Ciuffreda KJ, Kenyon RV. Accommodative vergence and accommodation in normals, amblyopes and strabismics. In: Schor CM, Ciuffreda KJ, eds. *Vergence Eye Movements: Basic and Clinical Aspects*. Boston, Butterworths, 1983;101–173.)

22 normal infants ranging from 6 days to 4 months of age. The fixation target was composed of a white card, which was mounted on the retinoscope, and contained a red annulus with an outside diameter of 3.8 cm. Black marks and dots were printed randomly within the red area.

Haynes et al. (14) reported that before 1 month of age, accommodation appeared to be locked at a single focal distance having a median value of 19 cm (5.3 D). The flexibility of the response improved with increasing age, however, so that adult-like responses were achieved by 4 months of age. Further, to demonstrate that the infants were indeed capable of accommodating, the refractive state was measured in 11 infants when they were sleeping, and compared with the findings for the same children when they were awake and alert. The authors reported that the refractive state varied by an average of 5 D under these two conditions.

In reevaluating the data presented by Haynes et al. for the nine infants who were less than 1 month of age, it is apparent that almost all of these subjects showed poor responsivity to the changing stimulus (i.e., maintained a relatively stable response). A wide range of accommodative response levels was observed, ranging from approximately 3.5 D to 8.75 D. Accordingly, the often-quoted statement based on this study that the accommodation of newborn infants is fixed at a value around 5 D is unjustified. Rather, it would be more accurate to state that a very wide range of accommodative responses was observed, but little change in accommodation resulted from alteration of the target distance.

An extensive series of investigations by Banks (17) also used dynamic retinoscopy to examine accommodative stimulus-response profiles in infants between 1 and 3 months of age. In the first experiment, accommodation was measured in 20 infants longitudinally at weekly intervals from 1 week up to at least 2 months of age. Three stimulus values were tested, namely 1.00, 2.00, and 4.00 D. Summary data are shown in Fig. 6.2, and longitudinal data for a single subject is illustrated in Fig. 6.3. Banks noted three changes with increasing age, namely (a) an increase in the gradient of the stimulus-response function, (b) a decrease in variability within each age group, and (c) a decline in the mean accommodative error (i.e., the difference between the accommodative stimulus and response). In comparing his findings with those of Haynes et al., Banks noted that the mean gradients of the stimulus-response function observed in his study for infants 1, 2, and 3 months old were 0.51, 0.75, and 0.83 D/D, respectively. In comparison, for similar aged children, Haynes et al. observed mean gradients of 0.06, 0.50, and 0.76 D/D, respectively.

To explain the discrepancy between his findings and those of Haynes et al., particularly in the children under 1 month of age, Banks suggested that the form and size of the target adopted by Haynes et al. might have represented a poor accommodative stimulus in such young children. The angular subtense of the annulus would have varied from 23° at a viewing distance of 10 cm to 2° at a viewing distance of 100 cm. Thus, the "black marks and dots," which were printed randomly on the target, probably subtended less than 15 minutes of arc at the furthest viewing distance. Although

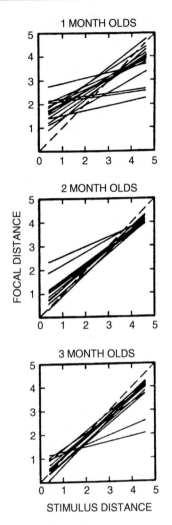

FIGURE 6.2. Accommodation stimulus-response function for 14 infants at 1, 2, and 3 months of age. Focal distance (plotted in diopters) refers to the distance at which the eye is focused, and reflects the accommodative response. Best-fitting lines were calculated from the responses of each infant. The *diagonal dashed line* represents the unit ratio (or 1:1) line. (From: Banks MS. The development of visual accommodation during early infancy. *Child Dev* 1980;51:646–666, with permission.)

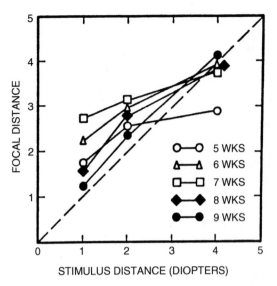

FIGURE 6.3. Accommodation stimulus-response function measured on a longitudinal basis for a single infant between 5 and 9 weeks of age. Focal distance (plotted in diopters) refers to the distance at which the eye is focused, and reflects the accommodative response. The *diagonal dashed line* represents the unit ratio (or 1:1) line. (From Banks MS. The development of visual accommodation during early infancy. *Child Dev* 1980;51:646–666, with permission.)

estimates of unaided visual acuity in newborn infants vary widely depending on the method of assessment (18), a value between 20/400 and 20/800 (19,20) would correspond to a minimum angle of resolution between 20 and 40 minutes of arc. Accordingly, much of the detail present in the target used by Haynes et al. is likely to have been too small for the subjects

to be able to resolve, thereby explaining why little change in accommodation was observed in the youngest subjects, with the accommodative response appearing to be "locked" at a single response value.

Additionally, results from the measurement of visual resolution at different viewing distances in infants may also support the proposal that these individuals have the ability to vary their accommodative response. For example, Salapatek et al. (21) used a preferential looking procedure to determine the visual acuity threshold to square wave gratings in 33 full-term infants varying from 24 to 63 days of age. Gratings were presented at distances of 30 cm and 150 cm for all subjects, and some subjects were also tested at 60 cm and 90 cm viewing distances. The authors reported that acuity thresholds were "relatively constant" regardless of the viewing distance. Similar findings were observed by Atkinson et al. (22), who compared visual acuity at distances of 30 cm and 60 cm in infants as young as 5 weeks of age, and found equivalent results at the two viewing distances. If the infants lacked the ability to alter their accommodative response, then one would have predicted a significant decline in visual acuity when the position of the target was altered, provided the change in stimulus exceeded the depth-of-field of the eye. As will be noted in a later section of this chapter, the depth-of-field [which can be defined as the range of object distances within which the visual acuity does not deteriorate (23), and is dioptrically equivalent to the depth-of-focus] tends to be large in young infants. These findings, therefore, do not conclusively demonstrate a change in accommodation.

In an alternative procedure to dynamic retinoscopy, other investigators have used objective photorefraction to assess the refractive state of an accommodating subject. Early studies (24,25) used orthogonal photorefraction to assess accommodation in infants. Here, a fiber-optic bundle delivers a point of light to the center of a 35 mm camera lens, and a photograph is obtained after refraction at the eye through an array of four 1.50 D cylindrical lenses that surround the fiber-optic bundle. The cylindrical lenses produce a star pattern, with the length of the cross arms being proportional to the refractive power of the respective meridian. Although this technique measures the magnitude of defocus, it does not indicate its sign (i.e., whether it is myopic or hyperopic). An alternative procedure, eccentric photorefraction, where the light source is not centered in the camera aperture, can be used to determine both the magnitude and sign of the refractive error.

Braddick et al. (25) used orthogonal photorefraction to examine accommodative responsivity in infants as young as 1 day old. Targets were presented at viewing distances of 1.5 m and 0.75 m. For an emmetropic observer, these correspond to accommodative stimuli of 0.67 and 1.33 D, respectively. The camera operator, serving as the visual target, attracted the infant's attention by shaking colored rattles or playing an attention-seeking game such as peek-a-boo. For the 0.75-m viewing distance, the eye was considered "in-focus" if the point conjugate with the retina lay within a range of 1.2 D in front of the camera (i.e., was focused between 1.3 and 2.5 D). At the 1.5-m viewing distance, the in-focus range was considered to fall between 0.37 and 1.27 D. The size of these in-focus zones was determined by the region within which the observed reflexes were vignetted by the fiber-optic head. For the 0.75-m target, Braddick et al. reported that approximately 50% of the infants 1 to 9 days of age were consistently in-focus at the distance, rising to a level of greater than 80% at 2 to 3 months of age. Even in the infants 1 to 9 days of age, approximately 85% were considered in-focus for this relatively distant target on at least one of the three or four occasions when accommodation was measured. For the more distant 1.5-m target, however, none of the infants 1 to 9 days of age was found to be in-focus consistently, although between 10% and 40% were "inconsistently" focused at this distance. By 2 to 3 months of age, approximately 85% and 60% of the subjects were consistently in focus at the 0.75- and 1.5-m distances, respectively, which rose to 100% for both distances at 6 to 8 months of age.

A subsequent study by Dobson et al. (26) also used photorefraction to measure the accommodative response of infants 3 month of age. Here, the target was composed of either a horizontally or vertically oriented square-wave grating [1.6 cycles per degree (cpd)] or orthogonal 19-min stripes positioned at target distances of 1.5 m and 0.55 m. This corresponds to a change in accommodative stimulus of 1.15 D. The mean change in accommodation for both astigmatic and nonastigmatic subjects was approximately 0.8 D, which indicated that the subjects exhibited a change in accommodative response that was somewhat less than the stimulus, but no significant difference was found between the three types of stimuli tested.

Recent investigations have used video photorefraction to measure the refractive state of the eye in infants and children (27). The advantage of a video-based system is that it allows the captured images to be viewed almost immediately, thereby avoiding the risk of discovering that defective images have been obtained only after the child has left the laboratory or clinic. Static digital recording devices would also have the same advantage. Video photorefraction has also been used to examine the dynamics of the accommodative response, and Howland et al. (27) used this technique to

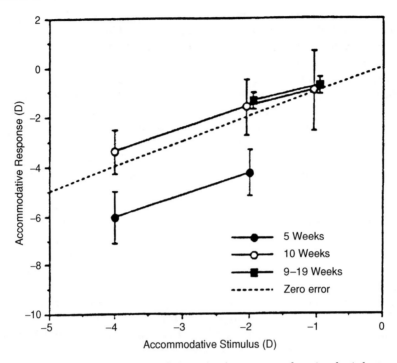

FIGURE 6.4. Mean accommodation stimulus-response function for infants 9 to19 weeks of age (*N* = 15); 10 weeks of age (*N* = 4); and 5 weeks of age (*N* = 4). Accommodation was measured using an objective, open-field, infrared optometer. *Error bars* indicate ±1 SEM. (From Aslin RN, Shea SL, Metz HS. Use of the Canon R-1 autorefractor to measure refractive errors and accommodative responses in infants. *Clin Vis Sci* 1990;5:61–70, with permission.)

demonstrate that the speed of accommodation in infants between 4- and 9-months of age was up to 4.6D per second. This is very similar to findings in adult subjects presented by Campbell and Westheimer (28) and Charman and Heron (29).

Objective infrared optometers can also be used to measure accommodation in infants. The use of such devices has a number of significant advantages over both photorefraction and dynamic retinoscopy. For example, they are extremely rapid (taking less than 1 s per reading), fully objective, and allow the refractive state to be measured over a wide range of ametropias (typically ±15.00 D spheres and 6.00 D cylinders). Accordingly, Aslin et al. (30) used the open-field Canon R-1 infrared autorefractor to measure accommodation in infants ranging from 31 to 118 days of age. This optometer has been used in a wide range of accommo-

dation studies in older children and adults (31–33). Binocular accommodative stimuli ranging between 1.00 and 4.00 D were tested. Mean results are shown in Fig. 6.4, and Aslin et al. noted that accommodative accuracy was "moderately good" for 15 subjects 9 to 19 weeks of age and "quite good" for 4 who were 10 weeks of age. The mean gradient of the accommodative stimulus response function for these two age groups was 0.61 and 0.82 D/D, respectively. Additionally, the mean accommodative error (i.e., the difference between the accommodative stimulus and response) was 0.44 and 0.35 D, respectively. Thus, by 10 weeks of age, the accommodative response, both in terms of the gradient and accommodative error, was similar to values obtained in adult subjects.

Interestingly, the findings for the four subjects 5 weeks of age showed a very high gradient of the function (0.90 D/D), but also a large accommodative error. These subjects exhibited large leads of accommodation (i.e., the accommodative response exceeded the stimulus), with a mean error of 2.16 D. Similar findings were also reported by Shea (34) using the same make of infrared optometer. She observed that infants under 3 months of age consistently over accommodated for targets at viewing distances between 34 and 67 cm, with some of the errors reaching 3.00 D.

The rationale for the excess accommodation in the youngest infants is unclear, although Aslin et al. (30) suggested that the four 5-week-old infants tested in their investigation may have been in an "exceptionally attentive state" as indicated by the high accommodative stimulus-response gradient (0.9 D/D). The inaccurate accommodative responses in the youngest infants could also be related to the large depth-of-focus of the eye, although this would still not account for the infant over- rather than under-accommodating to the target stimulus. Banks (17) and Green et al.(35) noted that the depth-of-focus of the eye is inversely proportional to the product of the pupil diameter and the visual acuity. Thus, inaccurate accommodation

could either result from larger pupil diameters in the youngest infants, when compared with older infants, children, and adults, or from reduced visual acuity. Accordingly, Banks (17) measured pupil diameter using a photographic technique in infants 1, 2, and 3 months of age ($N = 6$ for each age range) while viewing targets at 0.25, 0.50, and 1.00 m, respectively. The mean pupil diameter, averaged across the three test distances was 4.2, 4.6, and 4.6 mm for the infants 1, 2, and 3 months of age, respectively, whereas a mean pupil diameter of 5.2 mm was observed for an adult control group. The effect of age was not significant. Banks therefore concluded that increased pupil diameter does not account for any differences in depth-of-focus between the youngest and older infants.

Significant improvements in both visual acuity and contrast sensitivity have been observed, however, between 1 and 3 months of age (22,36–38). These are shown in Fig. 6.5. Banks (17) estimated the change in depth-of-focus that would occur with increasing age, and his findings are illustrated in Fig. 6.6. It should be noted that these results predict a depth-of-focus in adults

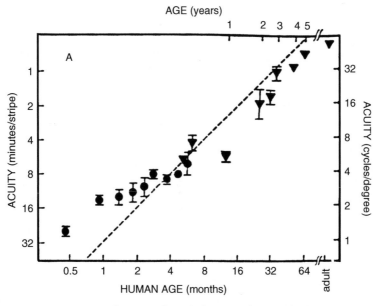

FIGURE 6.5. Mean change in forced-choice preferential looking visual acuity, plotted as a function of age, in humans. The *dotted line* represents a mnemonic that acuity in cycles per degree is roughly equivalent to the age in months. (From Teller DY. First glances: The vision of infants. *Invest Ophthalmol Vis Sci* 1997;38:2183–2203, with permission.)

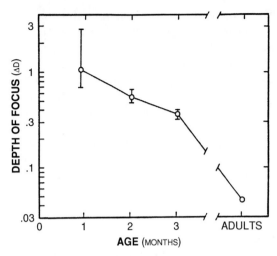

FIGURE 6.6. Estimated depth-of-focus in diopters for infants 1, 2, and 3 months of age and adults. (From Banks MS. The development of visual accommodation during early infancy. *Child Dev* 1980;51:646–666, with permission.)

of approximately ±0.05 D, which is considerably smaller than the more typical value of ±0.4 D that has generally been reported (39). Indeed, even the predicted value of ±1.0 D in infants 1 month of age would be too small to account fully for the leads of accommodation of up to 3.00 D that have been observed in this age group (30,34). Nevertheless, Banks concluded that infants accommodate as accurately as they require to maintain constant image clarity. Because their depth-of-focus is large, considerable errors in accommodation can exist without any resulting loss of visual acuity. Thus, the sensory component of the accommodation system appears to be responsible for the inaccurate accommodative responses in infants under 3 months of age, rather than any deficiencies in the motor system.

Besides examining the overall accommodative response, other studies have examined subcomponents of accommodation in infants, and these will be considered in the next sections. Using Heath's (40) classification of accommodation, which is analogous to the classification of vergence proposed by Maddox (41), four accommodative subcomponents have been identified, namely tonic, proximal, convergent, and blur-driven accommodation.

TONIC ACCOMMODATION

In the absence of an adequate visual stimulus, accommodation adopts an intermediate position of approximately 0.5 to 1.0 D in adults. Because this was believed to reflect the level of tonic innervation to the ciliary muscle, this component has been termed *tonic accommodation*. The response, however, probably represents an aggregate finding resulting from multiple stimuli (42).

The only published report to date detailing the measurement of tonic accommodation in infants appears to be that of Aslin and Dobson (43), who used photorefraction to measure the refractive state of the eye in darkness. A diffuse, infrared light source and an infrared sensitive television monitor were used to ensure that the subject's gaze was directed toward the photorefraction camera. The mean value of tonic accommodation (±1 SD) for the 3-month ($N = 4$), 6-month ($N = 3$), 12-month ($N = 5$), and adult ($N = 3$) groups was 1.59 D (0.34), 1.37 D (0.21), 1.35 D (0.16), and 1.14 D (0.04), respectively. Although these differences were not significant, it is interesting to note that a trend of decreasing tonic accommodation occurs with age. Further studies with larger sample sizes would be valuable. Nevertheless, this finding is also consistent with measurements of tonic accommodation in adults. Here, a consistent decline in response with age has also been reported (44,45).

PROXIMALLY INDUCED ACCOMMODATION

Proximally induced accommodation (PIA) can be defined as accommodation resulting from knowledge of apparent nearness of an object of regard (46). A number of investigations have demonstrated that awareness of target proximity can produce a significant increase in the open-loop accommodative response in adults (46–49). PIA in infants was examined by Currie and Manny (50). Accommodation was measured using eccentric photorefraction in eight infants who were tested at 1.5 and 3.0 months of age (±1 week). Four monocular stimulus conditions were tested, namely (a) a 0.5° checkerboard at 0.25 m (accommodative stimulus = 4.00 D), (b) a 0.5° checkerboard at 1.0 m (accommodative stimulus = 1.00 D), (c) a 0.5° checkerboard at 1 m viewed through a −3.00 spherical lens (accommodative stimulus = 4.00 D), and (d) a diffuse light at 0.25 m (nominal accommodative stimulus = 4.00 D). The first condition will stimulate both blur- and proximally induced accommodation, whereas the third condition will stimulate primarily blur-driven accommodation. Accordingly, PIA can be calculated as the difference between the responses for these two conditions.

When examining the data for the infants 1.5 months of age viewing the 0.25-m checkerboard, three of the eight subjects had responses within ±1.00 D of the target stimulus (4.00 D), whereas the remaining five subjects all exhibited overaccommodation, with the responses ranging from 5.16 D to 6.5 D. When viewing the 1-m target through the −3.00 D lens (blur-only condition), however, only one of the eight subjects had a response that fell within the 3.00 to 5.00 D range, two had responses of approximately 6.00 D, and the remaining four subjects (data was not shown for one individual) all demonstrated underaccommodation, with responses of 2.00 D or less. Five of the six subjects showed lower responses for the blur-only condition, compared with the 0.25-m target, with the difference between the two conditions ranging between 0.4 D and 5.5 D.

At 3 months of age, the accommodative responses to the 0.25-m checkerboard were much more accurate, with seven of the eight subjects showing a response that lay within the 3.00 to 5.00 D range (i.e., within ±1.00 D of the stimulus). When viewing the 1-m target through the −3.00 D lens, however, only two subjects had a response that fell within ±1.00 D of the stimulus. Three subjects showed a reduction in accommodation ranging from 1.2 to 6.5 D when viewing the blur-only stimulus, whereas two subjects had an increase in accommodation of approximately 1.00 D for the blur-only condition.

It is clear that most of subjects accommodated more accurately to the target positioned at 0.25 m, when both blur and proximal stimuli were presented, compared with the blur-only condition. This would imply that target proximity (i.e., awareness of nearness) may play a significant role in the infants' accommodative response. An alternative explanation, how-

ever, may be that the infants responded poorly to the dioptric blur stimulus created by the −3.00 D lens. Both Gwiazda et al. (32) and Chen and O'Leary (51) have observed reduced accommodative responses in older children when viewing relatively distant targets through minus lenses. Accordingly, it is perhaps not surprising that the youngest infants responded poorly to the blur-only stimulus. Currie and Manny (50) noted that because most of the targets in the infant's world are usually at a close viewing distance, their accommodation may be "preprogrammed" for near targets. Alternatively, they may simply fail to attend to the more distant targets. Another possibility is that the subjects may be inefficient at reducing their accommodative response for a low dioptric stimulus, hence the tendency to overaccommodate under many test conditions. The observation that 50% of the infants 1.5 month of age had responses under 2.00 D when viewing the 1-m target through the −3.00 D lens would not support the latter proposal.

Interestingly, several subjects exhibited high accommodative responses to condition (d) i.e., a diffuse light at 0.25 m. Although this condition would have a nominal dioptric stimulus value of 4.00 D, in reality it was likely to constitute a very poor stimulus to blur-driven accommodation, and any response is likely to be derived solely from knowledge of the target proximity. Four of the subjects 1.5 months of age and three of those 3 months of age, however, showed accommodative responses of at least 4.00 D, suggesting again that target proximity appears to be a powerful cue to accommodation in these individuals.

CONVERGENT ACCOMMODATION

In adults with normal binocular vision, the processes of accommodation and convergence [disjunctive eye movements to achieve and maintain binocular fixation (52)] combine to obtain and maintain focused images of the object of regard on the fovea (15). These functions act synkinetically so that vergence will initiate an accommodative response, termed *convergent accommodation*, and, conversely, accommodation will drive convergence, termed *accommodative convergence* (53). Fincham and Walton (54) observed that in subjects between

12 and 24 years of age, the convergent accommodation in diopters was equal to the convergence measured in meter angles. They suggested that the accommodative response in this age range could be driven entirely by vergence cues. Although other studies have observed lower values for the ratio between convergence accommodation and convergence (53,55–57), it is apparent that convergence can provide substantial input to the accommodative response.

If infants fail to converge accurately on the object of regard, this may account for the inaccurate accommodative responses observed, particularly for the relatively distant targets, such as those positioned around 1 m and beyond. Evidence for poor attention to targets located at this range may be drawn from McKenzie and Day (58), who presented findings from two experiments demonstrating that the duration of visual fixation varied as a function of viewing distance in infants, with the longest fixation occurring for the closest targets. In their first experiment, an 18-cm cube was presented at a viewing distance of 90 cm for ten, 10-s trials, with 5-s intervals being allowed between each trial. Following these ten trials, either an 18-cm or a 6-cm cube was presented at viewing distances of 30 cm and 90 cm. The length of fixation was timed manually, with fixation being determined by the position of the corneal reflections within the pupil. The experiment was carried out on two groups of subjects, either between 6 and 12 weeks of age, or between 13 and 20 weeks of age. No significant change in fixation time was observed between the 10 repeated trials when viewing the 90-cm target, thereby indicating no habituation of fixation to this target distance. Furthermore, a significant increase in fixation time was found when targets were presented at a viewing distance of 30 cm, compared with the targets positioned at 90 cm. This increase in fixation time was independent of the size of the target, and did not vary significantly with the age of the subjects. The finding that fixation time varied as a function of viewing distance was confirmed in a second experiment, which also showed that the effect was present whether the actual size of the target remained constant as it was advanced toward the subject (thereby producing increasing angular size at the eye) or al-

ternatively, when the target size was adjusted to maintain constant angular subtense at the eye.

To determine whether the failure of infants to accommodate accurately results from poor convergence on the object of regard, Hainline et al. (9) measured both accommodation and vergence simultaneously in 653 infants ranging in age from 26 to 365 days. Accommodation was assessed using paraxial photorefraction and convergence was quantified from the position of the anterior corneal reflection relative to the center of the pupil for each eye. Target distances ranged from 2 m to 0.25 m. In addition, the infants' refractive error was estimated by extrapolating the accommodative stimulus-response function for a stimulus of 0 D. Because this function is generally nonlinear within this low dioptric stimulus range in adults, with a lead of accommodation typically being found in older subjects (1,15,16) (see Fig. 6.1), such an extrapolation may overestimate the prevalence of myopia. Conversely, because a cycloplegic agent was not instilled (as this would have prevented examination of the accommodative response), latent hyperopia (i.e., that hyperopia masked by accommodation) may also have been missed.

Four types of behavior were identified, namely (a) monotonic changes in both accommodation and convergence in the appropriate direction, (b) monotonic changes in accommodation in the appropriate direction but poor convergence responses, (c) monotonic changes in convergence in the appropriate direction but poor accommodation responses, and (d) poor accommodation and convergence. Interestingly, more than 75% of the youngest infants (26–45 days) showed good convergence [groups (a) or (c) above], while approximately 36% of these subjects had responses that were categorized in the first group (i.e., good accommodation and convergence). The percentage of subjects falling in this optimum category increased to around 70% for those 74 to 87 days of age, and this prevalence remained relatively constant for the older subjects. This finding would suggest that most of even the youngest subjects tested, were in fact attending to the fixation target.

In examining the accommodative responses, the mean gradient of the accommodative

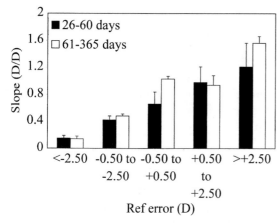

FIGURE 6.7. Mean slope of the accommodative stimulus-response function plotted as a function of the distance refractive error (plus and minus values represent hyperopia and myopia, respectively) for infants between 21 and 60 days of age (*N* = 82 eyes) and between 61 and 365 days of age (*N* = 571 eyes). *Error bars* indicate 1 SEM. (Data from Hainline L, Riddell P, Grose-Fifer J, Abramov I. Development of accommodation and convergence in infancy. *Behav Brain Res* 1992;49:33–50, with permission.)

stimulus-response function, plotted as a function of the refractive correction, is shown in Fig. 6.7. It is apparent that with the exception of the myopic subjects, relatively high values were found, particularly in the hyperopic subjects. The authors noted that for the youngest subjects overaccommodation was again typically observed for all but the 0.25-m target. This is consistent with other studies (30,34). The very low gradients recorded for the myopic subjects can be explained by the stimulus levels tested. For example, an individual who is 3.00 D myopic would not accommodate for any target further away than 0.33 m, and would only have to accommodate 1.00 D for the 0.25 cm target (the closest target distance that was tested). A significant limitation of the photorefraction technique is the limited dioptric range over which accommodative responses can be measured. Aslin et al. (30) noted that vignetting of the rays reflected from the fundus as a result of the limited diameter of the camera lens produces a plateau in the magnitude of the defocused image for larger refractive errors. This asymptote can begin for errors as small as 3.00 D, and limits the maximal myopic er-

ror that can be measured to around 4.00 to 5.00 D.

The first study to examine the interaction between accommodation and convergence in infants directly was that of Aslin and Jackson (59). They measured convergence by comparing the separation of the pupil centers when the subjects viewed either far (viewing distance = 2 m) or near (viewing distance = 15 cm) targets. Red and green filters and targets were used in some situations to create dissociated viewing conditions, so that the accommodative stimulus would be visible to only one eye, although both eyes could be seen for the assessment of convergence. Subjects ranged in age from 8 to 30 weeks. An increase in convergence was observed when the target was advanced under monocular viewing conditions, even in infants 8 weeks of age, which the authors concluded resulted from accommodative convergence. Bobier et al. (60) pointed out that the change in vergence response could have been driven by knowledge of the proximity of the near target (i.e., proximal accommodation) rather than blur-induced accommodation.

Accordingly, Bobier et al. measured both accommodation and vergence while base-out prisms were introduced to change the vergence stimulus. Accommodation was quantified using eccentric photorefraction. For eight infants between 3 and 6 months of age (mean = 4.5 months), the mean stimulus CA:C ratio (i.e., the increase in convergent accommodation produced by a unit change in the vergence stimulus) was 0.17 D/Δ. Because the interpupillary distance in infants is smaller than that found in older subjects, the vergence demand will be reduced in the younger individuals. Accordingly, to account for these anatomic differences, vergence was also quantified in meter angles (MA). A meter angle is defined as the reciprocal of the target distance in meters, and is equal to the product of the vergence demand in prism diopters and the interpupillary distance in centimeters. Using these units, the mean CA:C ratio for the eight infants was 0.73 D/MA. For an adult control group using the same procedures, Bobier et al. found a significantly lower mean ratio of 0.25 D/MA. The authors suggested that the decline in CA:C with age may reflect the loss of accommodative amplitude in adulthood [a finding replicated elsewhere (55,61)] or may be accounted for by the larger depth-of-focus present in infants (17,35).

Subsequently, Turner et al. (62) measured both accommodation and vergence to quantify the response AC:A ratio (change in accommodative convergence produced by a unit change in accommodation) in infants. They observed that for infants between 1 and 54 weeks of age, if a response AC:A ratio could be measured reliably, then it did not vary significantly with increasing age. For example, a mean ratio of 0.93 MA/D was recorded from 56.5% of the subjects between 1 and 8 weeks of age ($N = 26$), compared with ratios of 1.06 and 1.09 MA/D for children between 17 and 26 weeks, and 27 and 54 weeks of age, respectively. It should be noted that these values excluded findings from those individuals in whom flat accommodative or vergence responses were obtained when the stimulus demands were varied.

These findings demonstrate that the synkinesis between accommodation and vergence is present in infants by 2 to 3 months of age. Turner et al. (62) also noted, however, that accommodation and vergence appear to develop at different rates. In their study, they found that accommodation developed earlier than vergence. This finding differs from the earlier Hainline et al. (9) investigation, which reported that vergence developed first. Nevertheless, the establishment of a synkinetic relationship at an early stage is important. These interactions appear to vary with age, and Turner et al. also noted that the ability of both blur- and proximally induced accommodation to stimulate vergence varies during the first year of life.

BLUR-DRIVEN ACCOMMODATION

As noted previously, the improvement in the accuracy of the accommodative response over the first 3 months of life appears to result from an improvement in sensory function, which reduces the depth-of-focus of the eye. Under naturalistic viewing conditions, accommodation is stimulated by convergence of the eyes and knowledge of apparent nearness of the object of regard, as well as retinal defocus. To quantify

blur-driven accommodation in adults, Rosenfield (63) noted that measurements should be taken with a fixed target under monocular conditions, to ensure that convergent and proximally-induced accommodation remains constant. The accommodation stimulus can then be varied by the introduction of plus and minus lenses.

Such a procedure was undertaken by Currie and Manny (50), as described in the earlier section on proximally-induced accommodation. A blur-only stimulus was created by subjects monocularly viewing a target at a distance of 1 m through a −3.00 D spherical lens. Of the seven subjects 1.5 months of age examined for this condition, only one had a response that fell within ±1.00 D of the stimulus, two had responses of approximately 6.00 D, and the remaining four subjects all demonstrated significant underaccommodation, with responses of 2.00 D or less. Of the eight subjects 3 months of age who were tested under the same conditions, only two had a response within ±1.00 D of the stimulus. Two subjects had accommodative responses of approximately 6.00 D, whereas the remaining four subjects had responses of approximately 2.00 D or less. Given that infants have a tendency to overaccommodate the observation that 50% of infants both 1.5 and 3 months of age showed very low responses (<2.00 D) would suggest minimal or zero response to the blur-only stimulus.

Interestingly, in a study of emmetropic children between 2 and 5 years of age, Chen and O'Leary (51) compared accommodative accuracy when accommodation was stimulated either in free space (directly viewing a near target) or by viewing a far target through a minus lens. They observed a mean lag of accommodation for the free space and minus lens conditions of 0.24 D (SEM = ±0.03 D) and 0.69 D (SEM = ±0.08 D), respectively. No significant correlation was observed between the accommodative lag and the age of the subjects. These findings indicate that preschool children may also respond poorly to accommodative stimuli created by the introduction of minus lenses.

These results confirm the observation that infants respond poorly to blur-only stimuli, presumably because of their poor level of visual resolution, and require input from both target proximity and vergence stimulating convergent accommodation to produce a more accurate accommodative response. Even in adult subjects, blur-only stimuli can fail to produce an appropriate accommodative response without clear instructions. This is commonly found when performing the clinical minus lens amplitude of accommodation procedure (1). Subjects must be encouraged to clear the target at all times, otherwise a reduced response will be obtained. Clearly, such instructions and encouragement will be ineffective in young infants.

SUMMARY

The results of the studies described above indicate that accommodation generally reaches adult levels around 3 to 4 months of age. Before that time, accommodation does appear to be able to respond to changes in stimuli, although with significantly reduced gain compared with the normal findings in older children and adults. This attenuated responsivity appears to be related both to the increased depth-of-focus in newborn infants (which is a consequence of their poor visual acuity) and to poor attention and limited responses to retinal defocus. Other cues (e.g., awareness of target proximity), however, may provide input to the accommodative response, which may account for the leads of accommodation frequently observed in this neonatal population.

It is important to consider why an infant requires the ability to accommodate in the earliest days of life. Because most newborns are hyperopic at birth (4–6), they will have poor visual resolution for both distant and near targets without appropriate accommodation. Probably little requirement exists for clear distance vision at this early age, because most of the significant targets for very young infants are placed at close viewing distances. Thus, adequate near visual acuity is a more important function, which can only occur if accommodation results in the object of regard being focused on or close to the retina. Additionally, normal visual development depends on the brain receiving clear, focused images from each of the two eyes (9).

The measurement of accommodation in infants presents many methodological difficulties. Obviously, subjective responses are not possible, whereas objective testing must be precise, rapid, and encompass a wide range of responses. Maintaining fixation and attention on the stimulus is critical, and the effects of uncorrected refractive error must be considered when quantifying the stimulus demand. Refractive error in infants, however, cannot be measured accurately without the use of a cycloplegic pharmaceutical agent to paralyze accommodation. Obviously, the use of such therapy precludes any measurement of accommodation until the effects of the drug are no longer manifest.

Although many investigations into the development of accommodation in infants have been carried out over the last 30 years, many unanswered questions remain. For example, why do infants under 3 months of age frequently show excessive accommodative responses (leads of accommodation) to near targets? Older children and adults rarely exhibit a response to a near target that exceeds the stimulus demand (1,15,16). A possible explanation for the high response could be the effects of target proximity combined with a large depth-of-field. This would produce a high, but relatively inaccurate, accommodative response. Proximal accommodation could be measured in infants by quantifying the change in response to monocular open-loop targets [such as a low spatial frequency difference of Gaussian (DOG) grating] positioned at different viewing distances. Alternatively, relaxation of accommodation, which is facilitated by sympathetic innervation to the ciliary muscle (64), may be poorly developed in these youngest infants. To date, this autonomic function does not appear to have been investigated in this population. Other areas worthy of further investigation in infants include measurement of tonic accommodation in a large sample, and the construction of a quantifiable model showing the development of the synkinetic relationship between accommodation and vergence in infants. These and other avenues of research will enhance our knowledge of the development of accommodation in infants over the first months of life.

REFERENCES

1. Rosenfield M. Accommodation. In: Zadnik K, ed. *The Ocular Examination.* Philadelphia: WB Saunders; 1997:87–121.
2. Weale RA. Presbyopia. *Br J Ophthalmol* 1962;46:660–668.
3. Kikkawa Y, Sato T. Elastic properties of the lens. *Exp Eye Res* 1963;2:210–215.
4. Cook RC, Glasscock RE. Refractive and ocular findings in the newborn. *Am J Ophthalmol* 1951;34:1407–1413.
5. Goldschmidt E. Refraction in the newborn. *Acta Ophthalmol* 1969;47:570–578.
6. Fulton AB, Dobson V, Salem D., et al. Cycloplegic refractions in infants and young children. *Am J Ophthalmol* 1980;90:239–247.
7. Wood ICJ, Hodi S, Morgan L. Longitudinal change of refractive error in infants during the first year of life. *Eye* 1995;9:551–557.
8. Howland HC. Early refractive development. In: Simons K, ed. *Early Visual Development. Normal and Abnormal.* New York: Oxford University Press; 1993:5–13.
9. Hainline L, Riddell P, Grose-Fifer J, et al. Development of accommodation and convergence in infancy. *Behav Brain Res* 1992;49:33–50.
10. Santonastaso A. La refrazione oculare nei primi anni di vita. *Ann Ottalmol Clin Ocul* 1930;58:852–885.
11. Jaeger E. *Ueber die Einstellung des dioptrischen Apparates im menschlichen Auge.* Vienna: Verlag Weissnichtwem, 1861.
12. Borish IM. *Clinical Refraction,* 3rd ed. Chicago: Professional Press, 1970.
13. Duke-Elder S, Abrams D. *System of Ophthalmology,* Vol V. *Ophthalmic Optics and Refraction.* London, Henry Kimpton, 1970.
14. Haynes H, White BL, Held R. Visual accommodation in human infants. *Science* 1965;148:528–530.
15. Morgan MW. Accommodation and its relationship to convergence. *American Journal of Optometry and Archives of the American Academy of Optometry* 1944;21:183–195.
16. Ciuffreda KJ, Kenyon RV. Accommodative vergence and accommodation in normals, amblyopes and strabismics. In: Schor CM, Ciuffreda KJ, eds. *Vergence Eye Movements: Basic and Clinical Aspects.* Boston: Butterworths; 1983:101–173.
17. Banks MS. The development of visual accommodation during early infancy. *Child Dev* 1980;51:646–666.
18. Dobson V. Visual acuity testing in infants: from laboratory to clinic. In: Simons K, ed. *Early Visual Development. Normal and Abnormal.* New York: Oxford University Press; 1993:318–334.
19. Yamamoto M, Brown AM. Vision testing of premature infants using grating acuity cards. *Folia Ophthalmologica Japonica* 1985;36:796–799.
20. Dobson V, Schwartz TL, Sandstrom DJ, et al. Binocular visual acuity in neonates: the acuity card procedure. *Dev Med Child Neurol* 1987;29:199–206.
21. Salapatek P, Bechtold G, Bushnell EW. Infant visual acuity as a function of viewing distance. *Child Dev* 1976;47:860–863.
22. Atkinson J, Braddick O, Moar K. Development of contrast sensitivity over the first 3 months of life in the human infant. *Vision Res* 1977;17:1037–1044.
23. Bennett AG, Rabbetts RB. *Clinical Visual Optics,* 2nd ed. London: Butterworths; 1989:344–346.
24. Howland HC, Sayles N. A photorefractive characterization of focusing ability of infants and young children. *Invest Ophthalmol Vis Sci* 1987;28:1005–1015.
25. Braddick O, Atkinson J, French J, et al. A photorefractive study of infant accommodation. *Vision Res* 1979;19:1319–1330.
26. Dobson V, Howland HC, Moss C, et al. Photorefraction of normal and astigmatic infants during viewing of patterned stimuli. *Vision Res* 1983;23:1043–1052.
27. Howland HC, Dobson V, Sayles N. Accommodation in infants as measured by photorefraction. *Vision Res* 1987;27:2141–2152.
28. Campbell FW, Westheimer G. Dynamics of accommodation responses of the human eye. *J Physiol* 1960;151:285–295.
29. Charman WN, Heron G. Spatial frequency and the dynamics of the accommodation response. *Optica Acta* 1979;26:217–228.
30. Aslin RN, Shea SL, Metz HS. Use of the Canon R-1 autorefractor to measure refractive errors and accommodative responses in infants. *Clinical Vision Science* 1990;5:61–70.
31. Rosenfield M, Ciuffreda KJ. Proximal and cognitively-induced accommodation. *Ophthalmic Physiol Opt* 1990;10:252–256.
32. Gwiazda J, Thorn F, Bauer J, et al. Myopic children show insufficient accommodative response to blur. *Invest Ophthalmol Vis Sci* 1993;34:690–694.
33. Zadnik K, Satariano WA, Mutti DO, et al. The effect of parental history of myopia on children's eye size. *JAMA* 1994;271:1323–1327.
34. Shea SL. Dynamic accommodative responses of young infants. *Invest Ophthalmol Vis Sci* [Suppl] 1992;33:1100.
35. Green DG, Powers MK, Banks MS. Depth of focus, eye size and visual acuity. *Vision Res* 1980;20:827–836.
36. Banks MS, Salapatek P. Acuity and contrast sensitivity in 1-, 2-, and 3-month old human infants. *Invest Ophthalmol Vis Sci* 1978;17:361–365.
37. Teller DY. First glances: The vision of infants. *Invest Ophthalmol Vis Sci* 1997;38:2183–2203.
38. Daw NW. *Visual Development.* New York, Plenum Press; 1995:32–44.
39. Campbell FW. The depth of field of the human eye. *Optica Acta* 1957;4:157–164.
40. Heath GG. Components of accommodation. *American Journal of Optometry and Archives of the American Academy of Optometry* 1956;33:569–579.
41. Maddox EE. *The Clinical Use of Prisms and the Decentering of Lenses.* Bristol, John Wright & Sons; 1893:83–106.
42. Rosenfield M, Ciuffreda KJ, Hung GK, et al. Tonic accommodation: A review. I. Basic Aspects. *Ophthalmic Physiol Opt* 1993;13:266–284.
43. Aslin RN, Dobson V. Dark vergence and dark accommodation in human infants. *Vision Res* 1983;23:1671–1678.
44. Whitefoot H, Charman WN. Dynamic retinoscopy and accommodation. *Ophthalmic Physiol Opt* 1992;12:8–17.
45. Mordi JA, Ciuffreda KJ. Static aspects of accommodation: age and presbyopia. *Vision Res* 1998;38:1643–1653.
46. Rosenfield M, Gilmartin B. Effect of target proximity on the open-loop accommodative response. *Optom Vis Sci* 1990;67:74–79.
47. Wick B, Currie D. Dynamic demonstration of proximal vergence and proximal accommodation. *Optom Vis Sci* 1991;68:163–167.
48. Rosenfield M, Ciuffreda KJ, Hung GK. The linearity of proximally-induced accommodation and vergence. *Invest Ophthalmol Vis Sci* 1991;32:2985–2991.

49. Rosenfield M, Ciuffreda KJ. Effect of surround propinquity on the open-loop accommodative response. *Invest Ophthalmol Vis Sci* 1991;32:142–147.

50. Currie DC, Manny RE. The development of accommodation. *Vision Res* 1997;37:1525–1533.

51. Chen AH, O'Leary DJ. Free-space accommodative response and minus lens-induced accommodative response in pre-school children. *Optometry* 2000;71:454–458.

52. Von Noorden GK. *Burian-Von Noorden's Binocular Vision and Ocular Motility.* St. Louis: CV Mosby; 1985:86.

53. Rosenfield M, Gilmartin B. Assessment of the CA/C ratio in a myopic population. *Am J Optom Physiol Opt* 1988;65:168–173.

54. Fincham EF, Walton J. The reciprocal actions of accommodation and convergence. *J Physiol* 1957;137:488–508.

55. Rosenfield M, Ciuffreda KJ, Chen HW. Effect of age on the interaction between the AC/A and CA/C ratios. *Ophthalmic Physiol Opt* 1995;15:451–455.

56. Schor CM, Kotulak JC. Dynamic interactions between accommodation and convergence are velocity sensitive. *Vision Res* 1986;26:927–942.

57. Hung GK, Semmlow JL. Static behavior of accommodation and vergence: computer simulation of an interactive dual-feedback system. *IEEE Trans Biomed Eng* 1980;BME-27:439–447.

58. McKenzie BE, Day RH. Object distance as a determinant of visual fixation in early infancy. *Science* 1972;178:1108–1110.

59. Aslin RN, Jackson RW. Accommodative-convergence in young infants: development of a synergistic sensory-motor system. *Canadian Journal of Psychology* 1979;33:222–231.

60. Bobier WR, Guinta A, Kurtz S, et al. Prism induced accommodation in infants 3 to 6 months of age. *Vision Res* 2000;40:529–537.

61. Bruce AS, Atchison DA, Bhoola H. Accommodation-convergence relationships and age. *Invest Ophthalmol Vis Sci* 1995;36:406–413.

62. Turner JE, Horwood AM, Houston SM, et al. Development of the response AC/A ratio over the first year of life. *Vision Res* 2002;42:2521–2532.

63. Rosenfield M. Accommodation and Myopia. In: Rosenfield M, Gilmartin B, eds. *Myopia and Nearwork.* Oxford: Butterworth Heinemann; 1998:91–116.

64. Gilmartin B. A review of the role of sympathetic innervation of the ciliary muscle in ocular accommodation. *Ophthalmic Physiol Opt* 1986;6:23–37.

7 Development of Binocular Vision

Robert H. Duckman and Jojo W. Du

Binocular vision refers to the condition where the two eyes view a common portion of visual space. In vertebrates, the size of this overlap ranges from 0° to about 190° in humans (1). In visual space, objects occupy a three-dimensional space; the x- and y-dimensions give the object visual direction, and the z-dimension gives the object depth information. The x- and y-axes information can be obtained from the geometric retinal image. The z-axes information, however, is not available to a single retina, but requires the input from two retinae. For humans, the eyes are frontally placed and laterally separated. This separation is crucial in providing the two eyes with slightly different views of an object. These small differences in retinal images, known as *disparity*, provide the critical z-axes information giving rise to depth perception.

Traditionally, Worth (2) classified binocular function into three hierarchically related levels:

1. Bifoveal fixation
2. Fusion
3. Stereopsis

In normal adults, the presence of bifoveal fixation is a necessary prerequisite for fusion, and fusion is essential for stereopsis. It is currently known, however, that bifoveal fixation is not a sufficient condition for functional fusion or for stereoscopic abilities. This chapter considers each of these three levels of binocular func-

tion to describe the mechanisms underlying the development of bifoveal fixation and fusion, leading to the pinnacle of binocular function, stereopsis, the ability to discriminate disparate information giving a three-dimensional depth percept.

Stereopsis is an acquired ability; thus, newborn babies do not perceive binocular depth until a sudden onset at age 3 to 5 months. This sudden onset is followed by a period of rapid maturation that finalizes between 4 and 6 months of age, in which the adultlike stereoacuity is achieved. The oculomotor system is not mature at birth, but develops rapidly in parallel with the anatomic development of the eye, vision, and the visual pathway. Binocularity and stereopsis can only manifest if the eyes are accurately aligned. At this early age, infants are very sensitive to conditions that interfere with visual development. Common vision problems (e.g., uncorrected refractive errors, strabismus, and visual deprivation) present during this period of plasticity can cause a permanent reduction of stereoacuity by hampering the development of stereopsis. Early detection of these anomalies within the critical period carries high potential for recovery and normal vision development, because the potential to develop normal visual function seem to be inversely related to age.

Early research on infant binocular vision failed to separate monocular and binocular cues to depth. Owing to poor experimental design, results described in those initial studies could be affected by monocular cues of depth or technical artifacts. Based on those results, consistent conclusions regarding the binocular component of depth perception could not be delineated. Subsequent studies were designed with the focus of increasing understanding of binocular cues. Further research was made more accurate by studying binocular cues in isolation from monocular ones, thus leading to more conclusive information.

OCULAR ALIGNMENT AND CONVERGENCE

As the eyes track an object, they move in synchrony via yoked eye movements. This results in synchronous retinal images. When both foveae are directed toward the same target, a condition known as *bifoveal fixation* results. Similar retinal images and, hence, bifoveal fixation are thought to be required for binocular fusion and stereopsis. In preverbal infants, the development of bifoveal fixation has been studied indirectly by measuring ocular alignment and vergence control. Although ocular alignment and vergence control improves with age (3), several lines of evidence suggest that this is not the limiting factor on early binocular function. Early studies of ocular alignment suggested that infants often exhibit divergence (4,5), indicating a lack of bifoveal fixation and, thus, accounting for the lack of binocular function and stereopsis. This is in contrast to more recent findings that most newborn infants are orthotropic (6), thus indicating that cortical development, rather than ocular alignment, is the limiting factor on early binocular function.

Early eye alignment experiments conducted by Wickelgren (5) and Maurer and de Graaf (4) presented visual targets and recorded the relative position of the two pupil centers using corneal photography (5). Their research concluded that infant visual axes are generally diverged. This technique had a pitfall, however; it measured eye alignment with respect to the center of the pupil (optic axis), but did not take into account that the optical axis did not coincide with the visual axis (line from the target to the fovea). This optic axis-visual axis discrepancy is called the *angle alpha*. The results

from their experiments, therefore, could be affected by errors in their methodology. Later in 1975, Slater and Findlay (7) concluded that binocular fixation was present at birth with a limited response to static targets (10 and 20 inches). Although the corneal photography method was used, previous limiting factor of the angle alpha was overcome by using an average correction method (2).

Interestingly, Aslin (8) provided evidence that inaccuracies in binocular fixation during early infancy are not the result of a divergence bias. The resting position of binocular alignment in infants and adults was estimated by obtaining photographic measures of interpupillary distance in total darkness. The mean dark vergence position in the adult group corresponded to a distance of approximately 100 cm. The mean dark vergence positions were 25 and 50 cm for infants aged 1 to 4 months and 6 to 18 months, respectively. Hence, these results provide evidence that young infants' inadequate convergence to near target distances is not the result of a divergence bias. Moreover, these results suggest that the young infants' oculomotor system can most easily maintain binocular fixation at relatively near viewing distances. The correspondence between the optic-visual axis discrepancy and interocular separation during development and the validity of the estimates of dark vergence in infants is uncertain, however.

Although clinical observational reports indicate newborn infants often exhibit substantial eye turns, mostly exotropia (9), Hainline and Riddell (3) proposed that some eye turns were caused by the confusion of versions and vergences (as evaluated from a single photograph taken of an off-axis infant) as well as the large angle kappa of newborn infants. Angle kappa is the angle between the visual line, which connects the point of fixation with the nodal points and the fovea, and the pupillary axis, which is a line through the center of the pupil perpendicular to the cornea.

Thorn et al. (6) used the Hirschberg test to examine the ocular alignment in 34 healthy infants; they reported that most infants are orthotropic in the first month. This is in contrast with previous large sample ($N = 1031$–3316) studies that used the examiner's face as a fixation target as infants attend to a face better than to a light (10–12). Besides the large angle kappa of newborn infants, Thorn et al. (6) have found the task of judging the position of their own reflection from an infant's cornea to be far more difficult than the Hirschberg test. Another confounding factor, when using the examiner's face as a fixation target, is that the facial features on which the infant fixates change with age (3). In any case, all studies concur that a substantial proportion of newborns are orthotropic and that this proportion increases with age (13). Owing to the limited cooperation of infants, methods available to test ocular alignment prove to be insufficient. Hence, examiners have resorted to an indirect measure of ocular alignment.

To successfully fixate bifoveally, not only do the eyes need to be relatively well aligned in the stationary state, but they also need to be capable of changing its alignment in the appropriate direction should the object of interest move. To determine whether bifoveal fixation is a limiting factor for stereopsis, a number of researchers measured the ability of young infants to change their vergence in response to static and dynamic targets.

Using corneal photography, Aslin (14) recorded changes in binocular eye alignment in infants 1, 2, and 3 months of age in response to a luminous target that moved along the infant's midline. In his experiments, angle alpha was not affected by changes in the target distance because the light creating the corneal reflection was created by the moving target itself, and was not a fixed light source as in previous experiments (5). The results indicated that infants have the ability to converge and diverge in the appropriate direction as early as 1 month of age, but they cannot consistently converge to near targets until 2 months of age. Moreover, as age increases, the ability to respond appropriately to faster target motion also increases (14).

Because disparity is a likely cue for the visual system to indicate the necessity for a change in convergence, Aslin (14) also observed the saccadic refixation response to wedge prisms, clinically known as the *four-prism diopter base out test* commonly used to test for foveal suppression. The introduction of a prism during bifoveal fixation induces a shift in the image of the target as viewed by the affected eye, thus creating diplopia. A typical response to the four prism-diopter base out test consists of biphasic eye movements: a saccade followed by a convergent movement. If the affected eye is suppressed, the disparity created by the prism is not detected, and no eye movement occurs. If suppression is not present, the affected eye detects the disparity created by the prism and diplopia results. Eye movements will then be initiated to realign the foveae to reattain fusion. A five- or ten-prism diopter wedge prism, which displaces the image 2.5° and 5° nasally, respectively, was placed alternately in front of each eye of infants 3, 4.5, and 6 months of age. Refixational eye movements in response to disparity induced by wedge prisms were not present consistently until 6 months of age. This agreed with earlier results by Parks (15), whose clinical reports indicate that saccadic response to a prism test was not present in infants until 4 to 6 months of age.

Birch et al. (16) examined the hypothesis of whether the development of vergence accounts for the onset of stereopsis by comparing the ages of onset for stereopsis with and without vergence requirements. The presentation of stimuli near the horopter, which is a geometric surface in visual space that passes through the point of bifoveal fixation and contains all corresponding retinal points where single vision results (Fig. 7.1), did not significantly alter the age of onset of stereopsis. Hence, the development of accurate vergence is not the limiting factor in the development of stereopsis, but rather, the onset of stereopsis is dependent on the development of neural mechanisms (16).

Moreover, Hainline and Riddell (3) measured monocular and binocular eye positions of 631 infants (aged 17–120 days) from photographic images of eyes when static targets were presented (25–200 cm). Many of even the youngest infants showed good ocular alignment, both monocularly and binocularly, although the youngest infants displayed the greatest variability in vergence. This suggests that oculomotor constraints are not a significant barrier to the development of higher forms of binocularity.

When infants are tested using tasks that require dynamic changes in vergence, a different picture emerges. Ling (17) moved a target

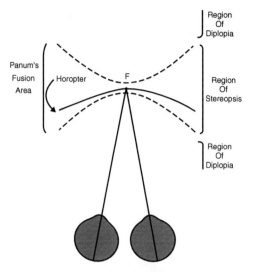

FIGURE 7.1. A schematic of an observer bifoveally fixating a point in space and the resulting specification of the horopter, Panum's fusion area, the region of stereopsis and the region of diplopia.

consisting of a black disc (2 inches in diameter) along the infant's midline from a distance of 3 to 36 in (at 2 inches/second); she concluded that systematic vergence eye movements throughout the range of target distances employed do not appear until 7 weeks postnatally. Aslin (14) also reported that infants do not consistently converge to dynamic targets until 2 months of age, and do not converge without delay until 3 months. This is in agreement with the Coakes et al. (18) study where their results showed that convergence is well established by 3 months.

This discrepancy could result from the use of static versus dynamic targets. Studies that employ static targets (3) report good eye movement control, even in early infancy. When dynamic targets are used (14,17), however, few report good eye movement control, especially in the youngest infants. This suggests that different mechanisms could mediate static versus dynamic vergence and that these may have different developmental time courses during infancy. It is important to note that, although appropriate vergences are made in response to a near target, it is by no means suggestive of bifoveal fixation, but merely that the infant is fixating with consistent retinal points, which may or may not correspond to the fovea. Nevertheless, it appears that neural mechanisms, not bifoveal fixation (although necessary, but not limiting), are the limiting factor in the development of stereopsis.

FUSION

Fusion is the combining of two retinal images into a single percept. When the two foveae are aimed toward the same object in visual space, each eye receives similar stimulation and, thus, gives rise to a fused percept of an object. Beside the foveae, many retinal loci can yield fusion. These loci comprise the horopter. Single vision, however, can also occur at areas around the horopter, known as *Panum's fusion area* (Fig. 7.1). This area for single vision is wider at the periphery. Any object located in front or behind Panum's fusion area does not stimulate corresponding retinal points, resulting in diplopia.

The development of binocular single vision is accompanied by the development of oculomotor systems that function to keep images from the two eyes aligned. Binocular single vision is composed of sensory fusion and stereopsis. Fusion is often referred to as unification—a process by which the images formed on the retinas of the two eyes are combined into a single percept. As a prerequisite to achieve fusion, the eyes must be able to align themselves in such a manner that the retinal images of the fixated object can be easily placed and maintained on the fovea of the two eyes. Any object located outside of Panum's fusion area while the subject is fixating on a target, does not stimulate corresponding retinal points, resulting in diplopia in the absence of suppression. As demonstrated by psychophysical and electrophysiologic measurements, human infants display a rapid onset of fusion at 3 to 5 months of age, which correlates with the development of stereopsis (19). To determine whether fusion is a prerequisite for stereopsis, fusion has been measured in normal healthy infants as well as in those with strabismus.

In normal healthy infants, fusion is not present at birth, but develops at approximately 3 months of age, corresponding to the development of stereopsis. To study the development of binocular function in infancy, Braddick and Atkinson (20) examined visual evoked potential

(VEP) induced by random dot patterns that alternated between correlated (fusible) and anticorrelated (rivalrous) states and found the median age at which binocular VEP first could be detected to be 11.4 weeks. Gwiazda et al. (21) determined the age of onset of fusion preference to be 12.4 weeks, and that female infants (9.9 weeks) developed fusion-rivalry discrimination earlier than male infants (13.8 weeks). In concordance with Gwiazda et al. (21), Thorn et al. (6) used forced-choice preferential looking (FPL) and found similar ages of onset of fusion (12.8 weeks) and that the shift of preference from rivalrous to fusible stimuli occurred during a brief period, often less than 2 weeks. Using both FPL and VEP protocols, which showed high concordance, Birch and Petrig (22) reported that few infants aged 2 to 3 months demonstrated fusion; most infants aged 5 months and older demonstrated fusion and reached adult levels by 6 to 7 months of age in 149 healthy, full-term infants. Together, studies on the ages of onset of fusion show close agreement. These findings suggest that sensory fusion is not present at birth but develops rapidly over the first 6 months of life.

To determine the effect of anomalous visual experience on fusion capabilities, a number of studies examined fusion in children with early-onset infantile esotropia to gain insights into the sequence of events that lead to strabismus. Eizenman et al. (23) measured VEP responses to dynamic random dot correlograms (RDC) in children with early-onset esotropia before and after surgical alignment. Before surgical alignment, 38% of children showed detectable VEP responses (significantly different to age-matched normals), compared to 85% after surgery (not significantly different to age-matched normals), suggesting that children with early-onset esotropia have the capacity for fusion and that a congenital sensory fusion defect is not the cause of esotropia (23). Although the critical period for fusion development is longer than that of stereopsis (24), early surgical alignment increases the probability of obtaining sensory fusion (23,25). This contrasts the views of Ing and Rezentes (24). Using the Worth 4-dot test, Ing and Rezentes examined the proportion of infants with congenital esotropia who achieved fusion after surgical alignment as a function of age at alignment and duration of misalignment (24). It was found that the age at alignment, as well as duration of misalignment, had no effect on fusion status. Consistent with the results of Schor (26) that fusion can exist in the absence of stereopsis, Ing and Rezentes (24) proposed that the development of fusion has a longer time window when compared with the development of stereopsis: 94% (24) established fusion compared with 74% (27) achieving stereopsis in the same children with congenital esotropia. Interestingly, Birch et al. (19) showed that, although surgical correction of infantile esotropia during the first year of life is not associated with higher prevalence of stereopsis, it is associated with better stereoacuity among those children who achieve stereopsis following surgery. Similarly, Rogers et al. (28) showed that 50% of the children with infantile esotropia who had corrective surgery before 1 year of age developed gross stereopsis 2 weeks following surgery and 50% showed some degree of binocular summation. The presence and the quality of stereopsis was significantly improved for patients whose eyes were aligned by 1 year of age or with a duration of misalignment equal or less than 12 months (29). Together, these findings support the hypothesis that early surgical alignment optimizes the development of stereopsis.

Moreover, Fawcett and Birch (30) examined the link between motion VEP asymmetry and bifoveal fusion. They found a significant relationship between the asymmetry index and bifoveal fusion, suggesting that the symmetry of motion VEP responses is highly predictive of their performance on the four prism base-out test, and that motion VEP is a marker for bifoveal fusion, thus providing an alternative measure of bifoveal fusion to the base-out prism test. Motion VEP are asymmetric in young normal human infants before the onset of binocularity, but they become symmetric as binocular function is established (31). Development of infantile esotropia interrupts this process and the motion VEP remains asymmetric (31). Tychsen et al. (32) determined how early versus delayed repair of induced strabismus in monkeys influenced the development of motion VEP. Control and early repair monkeys exhibited symmetric motion VEP, whereas delayed repair and naturally strabismic monkeys had asymmetric motion VEP responses. It seems that delayed repair causes permanent motion VEP maldevelopment and early repair restores normal development of visual motion pathways in the cerebral cortex. These results provide additional evidence that early strabismus repair is beneficial. As with bifoveal fixation, it appears that the ability to fuse retinal images may be a necessary, but not the limiting factor for depth perception. Perhaps other factors (e.g., neural mechanisms) also play a role.

STEREOPSIS

Although fusion enables the observer to view a single object from two retinal images, *stereopsis* enables the observer to utilize retinal disparity to calculate the z-axes information to appreciate depth. Stereopsis, then, capitalizes on a unique source of information about the relative positions of objects in visual space. Stereopsis, however, relies on fine coordination, accurate functioning of the eyes, and suitable cortical connections. If the eyes are misaligned (strabismus), if only one eye is fully functional (amblyopia), or if the cortical connections are damaged or incompletely developed (as in infants), then stereopsis will be impaired.

Stereopsis is the appreciation of relative depth owing to retinal disparity. If an object does not stimulate corresponding retinal points, it results in retinal disparity. Retinal disparity works because of the slightly different retinal images created by the separation of the two eyes in space. When the degree of retinal disparity exceeds Panum's fusion area, physiologic diplopia is perceived. Alternatively, when the degree of retinal disparity is less, the image falling inside the Panum's fusion area enables a three-dimensional percept (2).

Retinal disparity is the predominant binocular cue for depth perception. Other binocular cues that contribute information to depth perception include convergence and accommodation, but these provide less binocular information overall than retinal disparity. Binocular cues have been described as being innate, whereas the monocular cues to depth perception are empiric cues that must be learned (2).

On the other hand, monocular cues for depth perception include relative size and height, occlusion, geometrical perspective, and light and shadow.

Normal stereopsis is required for certain vocations. Understanding its mechanisms is crucial in developing remedial interventions should the system breakdown to optimize stereoacuity.

Onset of Stereopsis

Shea et al. (33) and Fox et al. (34) used visual pursuit combined with preferential looking techniques in the first systematic study of the development of stereopsis. The infants viewed a dynamic random dot stereogram (RDS) containing a $10° \times 5°$ vertical rectangle cyclopean pattern (i.e., the stimulus contained no monocular cues and the motion of the cyclopean pattern was not visible to either eye alone). The 45- and 134-minute of arc stereoscopic rectangle was moved left or right. Infants were deemed to have stereoscopic vision if their eyes followed the moving cyclopean pattern as judged by an observer who was unaware of the direction of movement (Fig. 7.2). By 3 to 4 months, some infants demonstrated stereoscopic vision, denoted by the infant following the movement of the rectangle. By 7 months, nearly 100% of the infants displayed stereoscopic vision.

Held et al. (35) used the preferential looking procedure to evaluate stereoscopic responses to line or contour stereograms in infants 2 to 7 months of age. The disparities were varied from 3480 to 60 seconds of arc. Their study demonstrated that few infants 2 months of age responded, whereas virtually all those 7 months of age responded to the 60-second disparity target. Furthermore, responses to crossed disparity occurred approximately 1 month before uncrossed disparity. This agreed with Atkinson and Braddicks' study (36) of stereoscopic discrimination in infants 2 months of age where they found that some infants of this age could perform stereoscopic discriminations. Using preferential looking techniques, Birch (37) found few infants younger than 4 months of age who demonstrated discrimination for any stimulus pairing; for the infants tested at 4 months of age, however, 82% preferred the stereoscopic

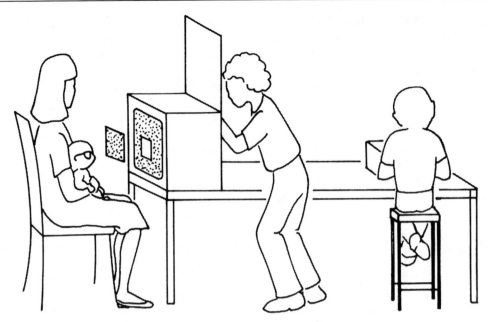

FIGURE 7.2. A schematic of the preferential looking setup employed by Shea et al. and Fox et al. to study the development of stereopsis. While wearing goggles, the infants viewed a dynamic random dot stereogram (RDS) containing a 10° × 5° vertical rectangle cyclopean pattern. This stereoscopic rectangle was moved left or right. Infants were deemed to have stereoscopic vision if their eyes followed the moving cyclopean pattern as judged by an observer who was unaware of the direction of movement. (From Shea SL, Fox R, Aslin RN, et al. Assessment of stereopsis in human infants. *Invest Ophthalmol Vis Sci* 1980;19(11):1400–1404; and Fox R, Aslin RN, Shea SL, et al. Stereopsis in human infants. *Science* 1980;207(4428): 323–324, with permission.)

stimuli to the zero-disparity stimuli, and this increased to nearly 100% in those 5 to 6 months of age.

Using RDS cards, Calloway et al. (38) found that stereopsis was not demonstrable in infants younger than 8 weeks of age. By 9 to 16 weeks of age, the mean stereoacuity level was 2.91 log seconds of arc, further increasing to 2.53 at 17 to 24 weeks, reducing slightly to 2.65 at 25 to 36 weeks of age. At 37 to 56 weeks of age, the mean stereoacuity value was recorded as 2.53 log seconds of arc.

Following the onset of stereopsis, stereoacuity continues to develop (39). Although children below 24 months of age can be expected to have stereo thresholds in the range of 300 sec arc, a transition occurs at approximately 24 months of age, after which stereoacuity approaches adult levels.

Besides preferential looking techniques, recording VEP from the surface of the scalp can also be used to investigate binocular func-

tions in preverbal infants. Amigo et al. (40) first showed that the comparison of the amplitude of VEP recorded during binocular and monocular viewing can offer an easy and satisfactory method for screening out defects of binocular coordination. They recorded VEP in response to phase-alternating gratings from normal and stereodefective subjects (adults and children) under both monocular and binocular viewing conditions. The amplitude of the binocular VEP was found to exceed the larger monocular VEP in normal, but not in stereodefective, subjects. From this, they concluded that VEP provides an objective method for screening out defects of binocular vision.

Subsequently, Braddick et al. (41) used VEP as a measure of cortical binocularity in infants. In infants 4 to 8 weeks of age, less than 50% showed significant VEP to the cyclopean RDS compared with control condition. By 3 to 5 months of age, all infants showed significant VEP. Braddick et al. (41) concluded that the human infant has a functional binocular visual cortex by 3 months of age, with some individuals showing cortical binocularity at an earlier age.

This finding is supported by a subsequent longitudinal study of VEP elicited by dynamic RDC to assess the cortical binocular function in infants starting between 35 and 50 days (42). The median age for the first evidence of binocular function was 91 days, with individual variation from 54 to 105 days. A number of newborns with ages ranging from 6 hours to 15 days, with a median age of 1.5 days, were also tested. Interestingly, the newborns showed a VEP with the contrast stimulus, but none showed a VEP with the binocular stimulus. Hence, conclusions were that even in infants who can demonstrate a VEP with the spatial and temporal parameters of the stimulus used, no evidence of functional binocularity was seen at birth (20,42).

Julesz et al. (43) developed a robust technique that permits the quick determination of stereopsis by measuring VEP to dynamic RDC that alternate between binocularly identical and uncorrelated dynamic noise. They concluded that using RDC is more advantageous over RDS for several reasons. First, RDC elicited larger VEP compared with RDS. Second, if RDC is presented as red/green anaglyphs, it is insensitive to head tilt, which could occur in infants. Third, RDC can be back projected onto large screens viewed from near distances such that the subject is surrounded by the stimulus (i.e., so they cannot look away). Hence, VEP elicited by RDC represent a quick and objective method for determining stereopsis in subjects who cannot communicate through language. Others, however, believe that VEP responses elicited by RDC reflect the fusion rather than the stereopsis status (44).

Although VEP is useful to detect the presence of cortical binocularity, Giuseppe and Andrea (45) found no clear relationship between the degree of binocularity, as measured by the Titmus stereo and TNO tests, and the amplitude of binocular VEP, thus limiting the clinical application of binocular VEP recordings in the diagnosis of binocular vision disturbances.

Shea et al. (46) recorded VEP elicited by a temporally modulated checkerboard patterns in infants 2 to 10 months of age, and in stereo-deficient and normal adults. In stereonormal adults, binocular VEP summation was less than 100% compared with 145% in infants and, in stereodeficient adults, binocular VEP summation was not significantly greater than zero. The significantly higher level of binocular VEP summation in infants was the result of much larger binocular VEP amplitudes, whose monocular amplitudes were similar to those of adults. Shea et al. (46) proposed that VEP amplitude is mediated by two independent pools of monocular cortical neurons and that binocular VEP amplitude in adults saturates at a lower level than in infants. Thus, the enhanced binocular VEP in infants may represent the summed response of two monocular pools of neurons rather than the activation of binocular cortical neurons (46).

In a longitudinal study of three infants, Penne et al. (47) recorded binocular VEP summation. In the first 2 months of life, no summation occurred, indicating that in the first 2 months of life, the eyes do not seem to cooperate as in adults. Between the second and third month, summation values rose markedly and, after the third month, its value was greater than 100%, thus reflecting increasing binocular interaction.

This large binocular VEP summation may also reflect the activity generated by the development of excitatory inputs to binocular cells during the critical period for development of stereopsis (48). Leguire et al. (48) recorded binocular VEP summation in normal infants and in those who were esotropic. Normal infants showed no significant binocular VEP summation at 1.5 months of age, developed a rapid increase between 1.5 and 3 months, peaking at 3 months, and then gradually declined from 3 to 58 months. The peak at 3 months corresponded to the general age range for the onset of binocular eye alignment, fusion, and stereopsis. Infants who were esotropic after surgical ocular alignment, however, showed a reduction in the initial increase and the peak of binocular VEP summation. Thus, Leguire et al. (48) proposed that the binocular VEP summation function reflects the human critical period for the development of binocular vision.

Using a novel system, Skarf et al. (49) recorded VEP responses to both RDC and RDS. Their system used alternating field stereoscopy

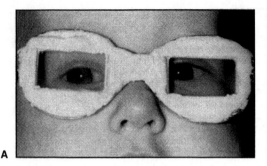 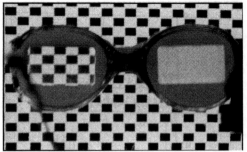

FIGURE 7.3. Alternating field stereoscopy used by Skarf et al. to record visual evoked potentials (VEP) in infants (49). **A:** An infant wearing liquid crystal glasses. Note the clarity of the shutters in the 'open' mode and the ease with which the eyes can be observed. **B:** The liquid crystal glasses in front of the stimulus screen showing one shutter open and the other electronically closed. Note the uniform translucent appearance of the liquid crystal when closed shutter blocks all pattern transmission. (From Skarf B, et al. A new VEP system for studying binocular single vision in human infants. *J Pediatr Ophthalmol Strabismus* 1993;30(4):237–242, with permission.)

that rapidly alternated between the right and left images on a screen. This is coupled with spectacles incorporating light-scattering liquid crystal lenses that also alternated between clear and opaque modes in synchrony with the video monitor (Fig. 7.3). In 40 infants, responses to correlograms, which reflect binocular fusion, have been detected as early as 5 weeks of age, and responses to stereograms, which require disparity sensitivity, have been recorded in babies as young as 12 weeks of age. This is in agreement with the Birch and Petrig study (22); both VEP and preferential looking techniques with RDS showed an abrupt onset of stereopsis between 3 to 5 months.

Subsequent to the foregoing studies, Petrig et al. (50) used dynamic RDS, with and without stereopsis, to elicit VEP. Their physiologic analysis of the emergence of stereopsis matched the psychophysical analysis of Shea et al. (33), Fox et al. (34), and Held et al. (35). In summary, the previously described studies demonstrate that stereoscopic responses begin to emerge at 3 to 4 months and are fully developed by 7 months of age. It is interesting to note that the onset of stereopsis occurs at an age when interocular visual acuity differences are rapidly declining (37,51), suggesting that the third to fifth month of life may mark a period of binocular competition, culminating in small interocular acuity differences and the onset of binocular function.

Most infants show the first evidence for stereopsis between 2 and 6 months of age, with an average onset age of 4 months (2).

Following the abrupt onset of stereopsis, the stereoacuity threshold decreases rapidly down to 1-minute of arc within a few weeks, presumably reflecting the development of cortical processing (16,52). The situation before the onset of stereopsis (prestereoptic system), however, is less clear. Held (52) proposed the superposition hypothesis where the two monocular images are simply added point-for-point for each set of corresponding loci on the retinae (Fig. 7.4A). Using FPL, Shimojo et al. (53) measured the preferences for the interocularly orthogonal (rivalrous) to the interocularly identical (fusible) stripes in infants (Fig. 7.4B). Initially, most infants preferred the rivalrous stripes to the fusible stripes. Because infants prefer grids over gratings (i.e., more complex pattern over less complex pattern; Fig. 7.4C), they suggested that prestereoscopic infants see a grid because they lack the binocular suppression mechanism responsible for binocular rivalry. Then at some age, all infants showed a sudden shift of preference to the fusible pattern. This shift occurred within 2 weeks at approximately 3.5 months of age, with a range of 2 to 6 months of age (Fig. 7.4D). This suggests that, in the prestereoptic system, most of the cortical cells are binocular; that is, it is eye nonselective, leading to a loss of eye-of-origin information at early stages of visual processing. In the poststereoptic system, however, most of the cortical cells are monocular and are eye selective (Fig. 7.4E), thus maintaining separate monocular representations of visual inputs together with eye-of-origin

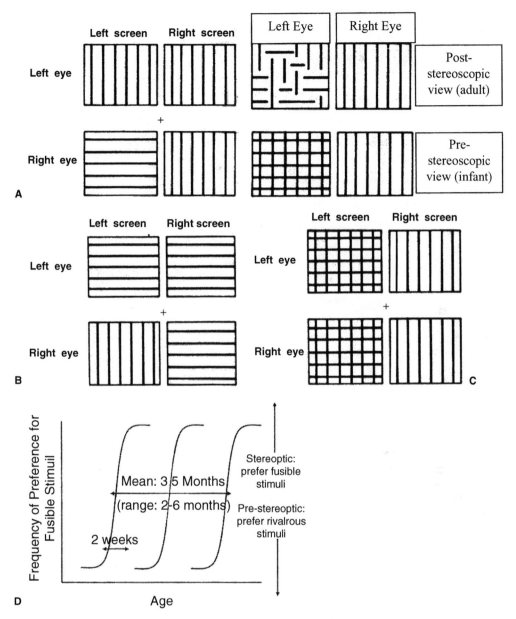

FIGURE 7.4. Superposition hypothesis. **A:** In the poststereoscopic system, binocular rivalry occurs when viewing a rivalrous stimuli created by interocularly orthogonal stripes (*left screen*). In the prestereoscopic system, the superposition hypothesis proposes that the two monocular images (created by vertical stripes viewed by the left eye and horizontal stripes viewed by the right eye) are simply added point-for-point for each set of corresponding loci on the retinae, creating a grid. **B:** Interocularly orthogonal (rivalrous) and interocularly identical (fusible) stripes were used in a preferential looking technique. **C:** Infants prefer more complex (grids) over less complex stimuli (stripes). **D:** Changes in preference of stimuli with age. *(Continued)*

Pre-steroptic binocular vision in infants

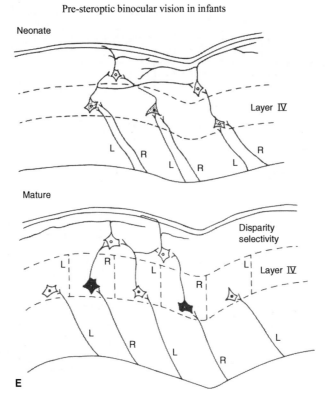

E

FIGURE 7.4. *(Continued)* **E:** Comparison of the neonate and mature visual systems. (From Shimojo S, et al. Pre-stereoptic binocular vision in infants. *Vision Res* 1986;26(3):501–510, with permission.)

information up to higher levels of processing to enable disparity discrimination.

A follow-up study (21) also demonstrated a dramatic shift of preference from interocularly orthogonal stripes to the interocularly identical stripes with an average age of onset for stereopsis of 11 weeks (range, 5–18 weeks) also occurring over a short time frame (1.5–2.5 weeks). A more recent attempt to repeat the aforementioned studies refutes the superposition hypothesis (54). With differences in protocol, Brown and Miracle (54) reported that infants never showed any systematic trend to prefer the rivalrous dichoptic plaid over the fusible stripes at any age. Instead, the preference changed smoothly from near chance performance at 5 to 6 weeks to 80% preference for the fusible stimuli at 14 to 16 weeks, contrary to previous studies (21,53). In an attempt to explain their results, Brown and Miracle (54) proposed the alternation hypothesis; in young infants, the visual

signals arriving from the two eyes are not sufficiently strong to be seen reliably and simultaneously, suggesting that in the prestereoptic system, infants see an alternation of images. As the infant matures, the signals become stronger and can be seen simultaneously, thus binocular fusion and binocular rivalry would emerge, leading to a preference for the fusible stimuli. Further studies are needed to provide support or to further refute the superposition hypothesis.

A number of studies have investigated the age of onset and rate of development of stereoacuity, but few examined the differences between crossed (target perceived to be in front of the plane of fixation) and uncrossed (target perceived to be behind the plane of fixation) mechanisms. In a large sample ($N = 128$) cross-sectional study, Birch et al. (55) assessed the development of crossed and uncrossed disparities. At 3 months of age, 64% of infants failed the crossed disparity stimuli compared with 90% for the uncrossed disparity stimuli. At 5 months of age, 74% of infants reached 1-minute of arc-crossed stereoacuity, whereas only 34% of infants perceived the 1-minute of arc uncrossed stereogram. Crossed stereoacuity was found to develop earlier but at approximately the same rate as uncrossed stereoacuity. No higher overall preference was seen, however, for crossed over uncrossed stimuli (preference for crossed over uncrossed stimuli of equal disparity was found only when crossed stereoacuity had reached that level while uncrossed stereoacuity had not). Furthermore, not only does crossed-disparity detectors develop before uncrossed-disparity detectors (55), VEP elicited by convergent and divergent stimuli also differ. The latency differences between the two response modalities indicate that convergent disparities are processed faster than the divergent disparities (56).

With the development of sensitivity of binocular disparity, the infant's spatial perception also improves. Granrud (57) investigated the relation between the development of binocular vision and infant spatial perception. Under binocular viewing conditions, infants 4 to 5 months of age reached more consistently for the nearer of the two objects than under monocular viewing conditions. Also, infants identified as disparity sensitive reached more consistently for the nearer object than infants identified as disparity insensitive. Moreover, infants who were disparity sensitive showed size constancy by recovering from habituation when viewing a novel object. Hence, the development of sensitivity to binocular disparity is accompanied by a substantial increase in the accuracy of infant spatial perception. Although the reaching response of infants is a different approach to the study of depth perception in preverbal subjects, it is not without pitfalls. Such procedures assume that the infant is capable, first of processing the disparity information, and second, then is able to convert this into motor actions. This technique, therefore, does not purely measure disparity sensitivity and spatial perception.

Optokinetic nystagmus (OKN) asymmetry has been reported to be associated with strabismus (58). OKN is a rhythmic involuntary eye movement elicited by moving patterns (59). It consists of a slow component with eye movements in the same direction as the movement of a target and a fast component with saccadic eye movement in the opposite direction .(60). OKN asymmetry usually refers to faster slow-phase eye movement (relative to stimulus velocity) elicited by temporal to nasal stimulus motion compared with nasal to temporal stimulus motion when viewed monocularly. Although OKN asymmetry is associated with deficiencies in binocular and stereovision (58), OKN asymmetry is also associated with other pathologies such as amblyopia (61) and unilateral congenital cataract (62). Hence, it is not a specific marker for stereopsis.

Anatomic and Physiologic Basis of Stereopsis

Physiologically, stereopsis is thought to take place in Brodman area 17 of the cerebral cortex. Single-cell animal recordings in this area have identified two different types of complex cells: 80% of these are binocular and 20% are monocular (63). Binocular cells respond to a stimulus of light presented to either eye, whereas monocular cells respond only to input from one eye. The distribution of binocular and monocular cells in the primary visual cortex is often referred to as *ocular dominance columns*. Ocular dominance columns are eye-specific zones of thalamic innervation in layer 4 (64) and altered sensory experience during the critical period can change the structure of the columns (65–68). Single cell recordings in animals, which could not be done on humans, and their similarities to the human oculomotor system, significantly advanced our understanding of the anatomic and physiologic basis of stereopsis. Bishop et al. (69) has identified a group of binocular cells that respond maximally to various retinal disparities. Barlow et al. (70) demonstrated that the cells identified by Bishop et al. respond maximally to a retinal disparity at a specific spatial location. These findings are important in establishing the neurophysiologic basis of stereopsis.

By using single cell recordings, Pettigrew (71) measured the development of disparity detectors in the cat. Before the fourth postnatal week, Pettigrew found that no response occurred to disparity stimuli; however, after the fifth week, responses to retinal disparity improved rapidly to almost adult levels. Disruption of binocular vision by occlusion or strabismus between 4 and 16 weeks in cats resulted in a shift in the ocular dominance histogram (i.e., most cells became monocular, with a resultant loss of specificity of binocular cells to respond to disparity). This period of neurologic plasticity is known as the critical period. After the critical period (16 weeks in the cat), disturbances in binocular vision have little permanent effect on disparity detectors. Removal of the obstacle to binocular vision during the critical period results in a variable recovery.

Livingstone (44) studied VEP in response to random-dot, two-color dynamic correlograms and stereograms at a number of luminances. Interestingly, the VEP response to stereograms was greatly reduced at equiluminance, whereas the response to correlograms was greater at equiluminance than at nonequiluminance. These results suggest that a significant fraction of cells that receive input from both eyes can respond to correlation or anticorrelation shifts, yet are not involved in stereopsis. This supports the hypothesis that VEP to correlograms reflect fusion, whereas those to stereograms reflect stereopsis.

Skrandies (72) presented electrophysiologic data obtained in healthy subjects evoked by the presentation of RDS to study 'stereo channels' in isolation because RDS do not contain contrast, luminance, or color information. Stereoscopically evoked brain activity, compared with that elicited by conventional contrast patterns, showed small, but consistent, differences. The RDS elicited smaller amplitude and longer latency (conduction time) than the contrast stimuli; suggesting that fewer neurons are activated in synchrony by disparate stimuli, and differences underlying neural assemblies process contrast and stereoscopic stimuli, respectively. The locations of the maxima and minima elicited by the two stimuli also differ (maxima: stereo stimuli more anterior; minima: stereo stimuli is more posterior to the stereo maxima location), providing further evidence that different mechanisms mediate stereoscopic and contrast stimuli.

The basic set of cortical connections is present at birth in the primate visual system. The maintenance and refinement of these innate connections are highly dependent on normal visual experience, and prolonged exposure to binocularly uncorrelated signals early in life severely disrupts the normal development of binocular functions. In monkeys, both the binocular and monocular response properties of neurons in the primary visual cortex (V1) are immature at birth, but rapidly improve to near adultlike maturity by 4 weeks of age (73,74). This rapid cortical maturation just precedes the age at which stereopsis emerges (75). Owing to the plasticity of infant brains, early abnormal visual experience can disrupt the normal development of binocular functions. Extracellular, single-unit recordings in rhesus monkeys showed that a brief period (2 weeks) of misalignment after the emergence of stereopsis is sufficient to reduce the sensitivity of V1 units to interocular spatial phase disparity (disparity sensitivity) and higher prevalence of binocular suppression (76). Longer periods of induced strabismus resulted in little additional loss of disparity sensitivity, suggesting that corrective measures should be taken before the known onset age of stereopsis to optimize outcomes.

Zhang et al. (77) investigated how brief periods of ocular misalignment at the height of the critical period alter the cortical circuits that support binocular vision in monkeys. After only 3 days of wearing goggles containing 15-D prisms oriented base-in over each eye, an increase was seen in the prevalence of V1 neurons whose binocular responses were weaker than their monocular responses (i.e., binocular suppression). This suggests that the first significant change in V1 caused by exposure to binocularly uncorrelated signals is binocular suppression, and this suppression originates at sites beyond where binocular signals are initially combined (77). This is in agreement with psychophysical data. In strabismic subjects with alternating fixation, the suppression of the deviated eye was most intense in a region corresponding to the fovea of the fixating eye, but was reduced or absent in the periphery. This is also accompanied by suppression of the peripheral visual field of the fixating eye (78). To compensate for the strabismus, it seems that the human visual system developed cooperative suppression such that in parts of the visual field, the two eyes tended to replace each other.

The critical period concept is conjectural in humans, because single-cell recordings have never been performed. The similarity of neuroanatomy, development, and psychophysical functions among cats, monkeys, and humans strongly suggests, however, that a critical period exists in humans. The critical period does not begin at birth, but seems to begin with the emergence of a function. Thus, the emergence of stereopsis is important in establishing the critical period.

CRITICAL PERIOD

Ample evidence, from animal physiology and clinical experience, indicate that the binocular organization of visual cortex remains highly modifiable for a period after it is initially established (13). Thirty years ago, Banks et al. (79) reported interocular transfer (IOT) of the tilt aftereffect in 24 patients with strabismus and provided the first evidence of a critical period for susceptibility of binocular vision in humans. IOT of the tilt aftereffect was used as a measure of binocularity because it was previously shown that IOT highly correlated with stereopsis (80), and that esotropic subjects who exhibited poor stereopsis also had low IOT of the tilt after effect (81). Normal binocular experience (NBE) is defined as the difference between the age at testing and the period of abnormal binocular experience, which is the period between esotropia onset and corrective surgery. Significant correlation exists between the period of NBE and IOT scores, indicating the relative importance of abnormal binocular experience for ages between 0 to 10 years, with the most critical period being 1 to 3 years (79). The results, however, were slightly different for congenital (onset <6 months) versus late onset (onset ≥6 months) esotropia (Fig. 7.5). Banks et al. (79) concluded that infants with congenital esotropia required early surgery, whereas immediate surgery is not required for those with late onset esotropia, perhaps because late onset esotropia had a period of NBE.

In 1983, Mohn and van Hof-van Duin (82) pointed out that a less clear-cut relationship exists between stereoacuity and IOT of the tilt aftereffect because stereoblind subjects always showed some IOT and some patients with

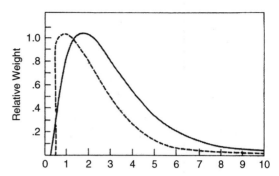

FIGURE 7.5. Developmental weighting function of congenital esotropia (*solid line*) and late-onset esotropia (*broken line*). These functions indicate the relative importance of abnormal binocular experience from birth to age 10 years. The developmental weighting functions were slightly different for congential versus late onset esotropia, thus, indicating that different treatment strategies should be employed. (From Banks MS, Aslin RN, Letson RD. Sensitive period for the development of human binocular vision. *Science* 1975;190(4215):675–677, with permission.)

normal stereoacuity may show reduced or no IOT. Henceforth, Fawcett et al. (83) set out to define the critical period for susceptibility of human stereopsis to an anomalous binocular visual experience by developing a quantitative model of the critical period using data from a large clinical population with a diversity stereoacuity outcome. They examined how the effect of an anomalous binocular visual experience on long-term stereoacuity outcomes varied as a function of onset and duration of constant eye misalignment in two groups of children: infantile and accommodative esotropia. In children with infantile strabismus, the critical period for susceptibility of stereopsis begins at 2.4 months and peaks at 4.3 months of age. In cases of accommodative esotropia, the critical period is delayed (beginning at 10.8 months and peaking at 20 months). When the data are combined, the critical period begins soon after birth and peaks at 3.5 months, and continues to at least 4.6 years. In concordance with Banks et al. (79), stereoacuity outcome correlated significantly with NBE (83), but the specific ages of the critical period differ (79). With a better understanding of critical periods, better treatment plans can be targeted to those at risk.

This plastic period of development may be mediated by motility of dendritic spines in the visual cortex. Cortical dendritic spines are highly motile postsynaptic structures onto which most excitatory synapses are formed. In normal mice, spines were motile during days 21 to 42 postnatal. Motility was reduced between days 21 and 28, and then remained stable through day 42. Binocular deprivation before eye-opening, by lid suture, up-regulated spine motility during the peak of the critical period. Deprivation at the start of the critical period had no effect on spine motility, whereas continued deprivation through the end of the critical period slightly reduced spine motility (84). It appears that neuronal plasticity is mediated by cortical dendritic spine motility and this motility is affected by visual deprivation.

Monocular deprivation during a critical period of development abolishes cortical binocularity. The requirements for recovery, however, are less well characterized. In ferrets, cortical binocularity and orientation selectivity responses can fully recover even if prolonged deprivation was initiated at the peak of plasticity. Interestingly, ferrets who had never received visual experience through the deprived eye, failed to recover binocularity although normal binocular vision was restored at halfway through the critical period (85). This indicates that a potential for recovery of cortical binocularity and orientation selectivity exist, and also illustrates the importance of early binocular visual experience even before the onset of the critical period for ocular dominance plasticity.

Generally speaking, the critical period starts sometime after the onset of development of a visual property. The critical period depends on a number of factors, including the anatomic level of the system (cells at higher levels of the system have longer critical periods) and visual function (a property processed by higher levels of the visual system has a critical period lasting longer than that at a lower level) being studied, previous visual history, and the severity of the deprivation (a severe change can have an effect over a longer period than a milder change) (86). From a clinical point of view, it should follow that the visual function with an early critical period should be treated before visual functions with a later critical period. Hence, a good rehabilitative program should treat the visual properties in a logical sequence. In the absence of definite information, however, the optimal forms of treatment have yet to be elucidated.

A recent study compared the effect of intensive and reduced occlusion therapy regimens on binocular sensory outcomes, visual acuity, and the prevalence of strabismus in children after surgery for congenital unilateral cataract (87). The intensive occlusion group was patched 80% of waking hours and the reduced occlusion group patched 25% to 50% of waking hours. A higher proportion of subjects in the reduced occlusion group had stereopsis or fusion compared with the intensive group. Interestingly, no differences were found in visual acuity between the groups, but a higher prevalence of strabismus in the intensive compared with the reduced occlusion group. These results suggest that a reduced occlusion protocol may be associated with better binocular sensory outcomes and a reduced prevalence of strabismus without compromising visual acuity in children after congenital unilateral cataract surgery.

RISK FACTORS

Identification of risk factors for esotropia could play an important role in determining which children may benefit from shorter follow-up examination intervals, and how to prevent and early treat the condition. Accommodative esotropia, if left untreated, often leads to concomitant esotropia. Thus, determining the risk factors for accommodative esotropia among hyperopic children is of great importance. Extensive twin and family studies suggest a significant genetic component to the cause of strabismus (88). In a recent study that aimed to identify risk factors for accommodative esotropia, 23% of children with accommodative esotropia had an affected first-degree relative and 91% had at least one affected relative (89). Furthermore, random-dot stereoacuity was abnormal in 41% of the children with accommodative esotropia and subjects with significant hyperopia and anisometropia were at increased risk for developing accommodative esotropia. A positive family history, subnormal random-dot stereopsis, and hyperopic anisometropia each pose a significant risk for the development of accommodative esotropia (Fig. 7.6). Spectacle correction of hypermetropia reduces the prevalence of

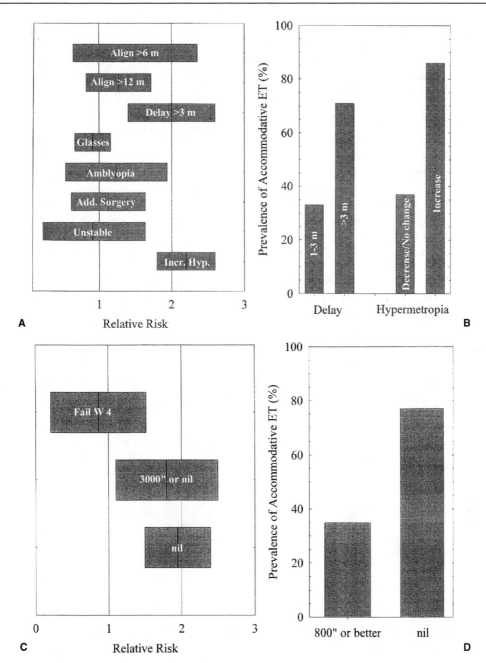

FIGURE 7.6. Risk factors for the development of accommodative esotropia. **A:** Relative risk of accommodative esotropia as a function of age at alignment (<6 months vs. >6 months and <12 months vs. >12 months), delay in alignment (<3 months vs. >3 months), presurgical glasses (yes/no), amblyopia treatment (yes/no), additional surgical procedures (yes/no), unstable alignment (yes/no), and increase in hypermetropia (yes/no). **B:** Prevalence of accommodative esotropia as a function of delay in alignment and change in refractive error. **C:** Relative risk of accommodative esotropia as a function of peripheral fusion (pass vs. fail Worth 4-dot test at near) and stereopsis (random dot stereopsis <800 vs. 3000 arc second or nil and 3000 arc second or better vs. nil). **D:** Prevalence of accommodative esotropia as a function of stereopsis. (From Birch EE, et al. Risk factors for accommodative esotropia among hypermetropic children. *Invest Ophthalmol Vis Sci* 2005;46(2):526–529, with permission.)

accommodative esotropia by 50% (90), possibly by minimizing any potential adverse effects that hypermetropia may have on binocular motor and sensory function. Assessment of the presence or absence of these risk factors, in conjunction with the overall degree of hyperopia, should help to identify those children who are most likely to benefit from preventative treatment before the onset of esotropia.

Moreover, development of stereopsis depends on contrast sensitivity and spatial tuning (26). Hence, refractive anomalies (e.g., anisometropia) that limit high-frequency spatial resolution and binocular integration present a major obstacle to the development of binocular vision.

As accommodative esotropia is common following surgical alignment of infantile esotropia, Birch et al. (91) examined whether accommodative esotropia is a preexisting condition that is unmasked at the time of strabismus surgery, or whether it is a sequela of infantile esotropia. Findings were that 60% of the children developed accommodative esotropia at 22.8 ± 14.9 weeks after corrective surgery (91). Of the twelve risk factors examined, a delay in alignment (>3 months between esotropia onset and surgery), increasing hyperopia (sustained increase of 0.50 D/year) and absent or poor stereopsis were deemed to be significant risk factors, but accommodative esotropia was not found to be a preexisting condition (91).

In nonstrabismic patients, anisometropia is associated with a significant increase in the incidence of amblyopia and decrease in binocular function (degree of stereopsis) when compared with patients who are not anisometropic (92).

Our understanding of the development of binocular vision leapt in the past decades. Previously thought as a hierarchically organized system may, in fact, be a complicated network with crosstalk and feedback loops. Advances in technology and objective techniques available provide hope for further discoveries in this field where the subjects of interest are often difficult to examine and nonverbal. Binocularity is no doubt an important topic in the study of visual development and with unanswered questions remaining, it will no doubt continue to be a focus of research.

REFERENCES

1. Howard IP. *Binocular correspondence and the Horopter.* In: Howard IP, ed. *Seeing in Depth.* Howard. Ontario: I. Porteous, 2002;1–40.
2. Aslin RN, Dumais ST. Binocular vision in infants: a review and a theoretical framework. *Adv Child Dev Behav* 1980;15:53–94.
3. Hainline L, Riddell PM. Binocular alignment and vergence in early infancy. *Vision Res* 1995;35(23–24):3229–3236.
4. Maurer HJ, de Graaf AS. [Amblyopia as a complication of cerebral angiography (author's transl)]. *Fortschr Geb Rontgenstr Nuklearmed* 1974;120(6):733–739.
5. Wickelgren LW. Convergence in the human newborn. *J Exp Child Psychol* 1967;5(1):74–85.
6. Thorn F, Gwiazda J, Cruz AA, et al. The development of eye alignment, convergence, and sensory binocularity in young infants. *Invest Ophthalmol Vis Sci* 1994;35(2):544–553.
7. Slater AM, Findlay JM. Binocular fixation in the newborn baby. *J Exp Child Psychol* 1975;20(2):248–273.
8. Aslin RN. Dark vergence in human infants: implications for the development of binocular vision. *Acta Psychol (Amst)* 1986;63(1–3):309–322.
9. Archer S. Detection and treatment of congenital esotropia. In: Simons K, ed. *Early Visual Development: Normal and Abnormal.* Oxford: Oxford University Press, 1993.
10. Archer S, Sondhi N, Helveston EM. Strabismus in infancy. *Ophthalmology* 1989;96:133–137.
11. Nixon R, Helveston EM, Miller K, et al. Incidence of strabismus in neonates. *Am J Ophthalmol* 1985;100:798–801.
12. Sondhi N, Archer SM, Helveston EM. Development of normal ocular alignment. *J Pediatr Ophthalmol Strabismus* 1988;25:210–211.
13. Braddick O. Binocularity in infancy. *Eye* 1996;10(Pt 2):182–188.
14. Aslin RN. Development of binocular fixation in human infants. *J Exp Child Psychol* 1977;23(1):133–150.
15. Parks MM. Growth of the eye and development of vision. In: Gellis SLAS, ed. *The Pediatrician's Ophthalmology.* St Louis: CV Mosby, 1966;15–5.
16. Birch EE, Gwiazda J, Held R. The development of vergence does not account for the onset of stereopsis. *Perception* 1983;12(3):331–336.
17. Ling B. A genetic study of sustained fixation and associated behavior in the human infant from birth to six months. *J Genetic Psychol* 1942;61:227–277.
18. Coakes RL, Clothier C, Wilson A. Binocular reflexes in the first 6 months of life: preliminary results of a study of normal infants. *Child Care Health Dev* 1979;5(6):405–408.
19. Birch EE, Stager DR, Everett ME. Random dot stereoacuity following surgical correction of infantile esotropia. *J Pediatr Ophthalmol Strabismus* 1995;32(4):231–235.
20. Braddick O, Atkinson J. The development of binocular function in infancy. *Acta Ophthalmol Suppl* 1983;157:27–35.
21. Gwiazda J, Bauer J, Held R. Binocular function in human infants: correlation of stereoptic and fusion-rivalry discriminations. *J Pediatr Ophthalmol Strabismus* 1989;26(3):128–132.
22. Birch E, Petrig B. FPL and VEP measures of fusion, stereopsis and stereoacuity in normal infants. *Vision Res* 1996;36(9):1321–1327.

23. Eizenman M, Westall CA, Geer I, et al. Electrophysiological evidence of cortical fusion in children with early-onset esotropia. *Invest Ophthalmol Vis Sci* 1999;40(2):354–362.

24. Ing MR, Rezentes K. Outcome study of the development of fusion in patients aligned for congenital esotropia in relation to duration of misalignment. *J AAPOS* 2004;8(1):35–37.

25. Ing MR. Early surgical alignment for congenital esotropia. *Trans Am Ophthalmol Soc* 1981;79:625–663.

26. Schor CM. Development of stereopsis depends upon contrast sensitivity and spatial tuning. *Journal of the American Optometric Association* 1985;56(8):628–635.

27. Ing M. Outcome study of stereopsis in relation to duration of misalignment in congenital esotropia. *J AAPOS* 2002;6:3–8.

28. Rogers GL, Bremer DL, Leguire LE, et al. Clinical assessment of visual function in the young child: a prospective study of binocular vision. *J Pediatr Ophthalmol Strabismus* 1986;23(5):233–235.

29. Ing MR, Okino LM. Outcome study of stereopsis in relation to duration of misalignment in congenital esotropia. *J AAPOS* 2002;6(1):3–8.

30. Fawcett SL, Birch EE. Motion VEPs, stereopsis, and bifoveal fusion in children with strabismus. *Invest Ophthalmol Vis Sci* 2000;41(2):411–416.

31. Birch EE, Fawcett S, Stager DR. Why does early surgical alignment improve stereoacuity outcomes in infantile esotropia? *J AAPOS* 2000;4(1):10–14.

32. Tychsen L, Wong AM, Foeller P, et al. Early versus delayed repair of infantile strabismus in macaque monkeys: II. Effects on motion visually evoked responses. *Invest Ophthalmol Vis Sci* 2004;45(3):821–827.

33. Shea SL, Fox R, Aslin RN, et al. Assessment of stereopsis in human infants. *Invest Ophthalmol Vis Sci* 1980;19(11):1400–1404.

34. Fox R, Aslin RN, Shea SL, et al. Stereopsis in human infants. *Science* 1980;207(4428):323–324.

35. Held R, Birch E, Gwiazda J. Stereoacuity of human infants. *Proc Natl Acad Sci U S A* 1980;77(9):5572–5574.

36. Atkinson J, Braddick O. Steroscopic discrimination in infants. *Perception* 1976;5(1):29–38.

37. Birch EE. Infant interocular acuity differences and binocular vision. Vision Res 1985;25(4):571–576.

38. Calloway SL, Lloyd IC, Henson DB. A clinical evaluation of random dot stereoacuity cards in infants. *Eye* 2001;15(Pt 5):629–634.

39. Ciner EB, Schanel-Klitsch E, Herzberg C. Stereoacuity development: 6 months to 5 years. A new tool for testing and screening. *Optom Vis Sci* 1996;73(1):43–48.

40. Amigo G, Fiorentini A, Pirchio M, et al. Binocular vision tested with visual evoked potentials in children and infants. *Invest Ophthalmol Vis Sci* 1978;17(9):910–915.

41. Braddick O, Atkinson J, Julesz B, et al. Cortical binocularity in infants. *Nature* 1980;288(5789):363–365.

42. Braddick O, Wattam-Bell J, Day J, et al. The onset of binocular function in human infants. *Hum Neurobiol* 1983;2(2):65–69.

43. Julesz B, Kropfl W, Petrig B. Large evoked potentials to dynamic random-dot correlograms and stereograms permit quick determination of stereopsis. *Proc Natl Acad Sci U S A* 1980;77(4):2348–2351.

44. Livingstone MS. Differences between stereopsis, interocular correlation and binocularity. *Vision Res* 1996; 36(8):1127–1140.

45. Giuseppe N, Andrea F. Binocular interaction in visual-evoked responses: summation, facilitation and inhibition in a clinical study of binocular vision. *Ophthalmic Res* 1983;15(5):261–264.

46. Shea SL, Aslin RN, McCulloch D. Binocular VEP summation in infants and adults with abnormal binocular histories. *Invest Ophthalmol Vis Sci* 1987;28(2):356–365.

47. Penne A, Baraldi P, Fonda S, et al. Incremental binocular amplitude of the pattern visual evoked potential during the first five months of life: electrophysiological evidence of the development of binocularity. *Doc Ophthalmol* 1987;65(1):15–23.

48. Leguire LE, Rogers GL, Bremer DL. Visual-evoked response binocular summation in normal and strabismic infants. Defining the critical period. *Invest Ophthalmol Vis Sci* 1991;32(1):126–133.

49. Skarf B, Eizenman M, Katz LM, et al. A new VEP system for studying binocular single vision in human infants. *J Pediatr Ophthalmol Strabismus* 1993;30(4):237–242.

50. Petrig B, Julesz B, Kropfl W, et al. Development of stereopsis and cortical binocularity in human infants: electrophysiological evidence. *Science* 1981;213(4514):1402–1405.

51. Birch EE, Shimojo S, Held R. Preferential-looking assessment of fusion and stereopsis in infants aged 1–6 months. *Invest Ophthalmol Vis Sci* 1985;26(3):366–370.

52. Held R. Binocular vision—behavioral and neural development. In: Mehler V, Fox R, eds. *Neonate Cognition: Beyond the Blooming, Buzzing confusion.* Hillsdole, NJ: L. Erlboum. 1985:37–44.

53. Shimojo S, Bauer J Jr., O'Connell KM, et al. Prestereoptic binocular vision in infants. *Vision Res* 1986;26(3):501–510.

54. Brown AM, Miracle JA. Early binocular vision in human infants: limitations on the generality of the superposition hypothesis. *Vision Res* 2003;43(14):1563–1574.

55. Birch EE, Gwiazda J, Held R. Stereoacuity development for crossed and uncrossed disparities in human infants. *Vision Res* 1982;22(5):507–513.

56. Sahinoglu B. Depth-related visually evoked potentials by dynamic random-dot stereograms in humans: negative correlation between the peaks elicited by convergent and divergent disparities. *Eur J Appl Physiol* 2004;91(5–6):689–697.

57. Granrud CE. Binocular vision and spatial perception in 4- and 5-month-old infants. *J Exp Psychol Hum Percept Perform* 1986;12(1):36–49.

58. Valmaggia C, Proudlock F, Gottlob I. Optokinetic nystagmus in strabismus: are asymmetries related to binocularity? *Invest Ophthalmol Vis Sci* 2003;44(12):5142–5150.

59. Westheimer G, McKee SP. Visual acuity in the presence of retinal-image motion. *J Opt Soc Am* 1975;65(7):847–850.

60. Yee R, Honrubia BR, V. Pathophysiology of optokinetic nystagmus. In: Honrubia BM. *Nystagmus and Vertigo: Clinical Approaches to the Patient.* London: Academic Press; 1982:251–275.

61. Westall CA, Schor CM. Asymmetries of optokinetic nystagmus in amblyopia: the effect of selected retinal stimulation. *Vision Res* 1985;25(10):1431–1438.

62. Lewis TL, Maurer D, Brent HP. Optokinetic nystagmus in normal and visually deprived children: implications for cortical development. *Canadian Journal of Psychology* 1989;43(2):121–140.

63. Hubel DH, Wiesel TN. Receptive fields, binocular interaction and functional architecture in the cat's visual cortex. *J Physiol* 1962;160:106–154.

64. Feller MB, Scanziani M. A precritical period for plasticity in visual cortex. *Curr Opin Neurobiol* 2005;15(1):94–100.

65. Hubel DH, Wiesel TN, LeVay S. Plasticity of ocular dominance columns in monkey striate cortex. *Philos Trans R Soc Lond B Biol Sci* 1977;278(961):377–409.

66. LeVay S, Wiesel TN, Hubel DH. The development of ocular dominance columns in normal and visually deprived monkeys. *J Comp Neurol* 1980;191(1):1–51.

67. Shatz CJ, Stryker MP. Ocular dominance in layer IV of the cat's visual cortex and the effects of monocular deprivation. *J Physiol* 1978;281:267–283.

68. Hensch TK. Critical period regulation. *Annu Rev Neurosci* 2004;27:549–579.

69. Bishop PO, Coombs JS, Henry GH. Receptive fields of simple cells in the cat striate cortex. *J Physiol* 1973;231(1):31–60.

70. Barlow HB, Blakemore C, Pettigrew JD. The neural mechanism of binocular depth discrimination. *J Physiol* 1967;193(2):327–342.

71. Pettigrew JD. The effect of visual experience on the development of stimulus specificity by kitten cortical neurones. *J Physiol* 1974;237(1):49–74.

72. Skrandies W. The processing of stereoscopic information in human visual cortex: psychophysical and electrophysiological evidence. *Clin Electroencephalogr* 2001;32(3):152–159.

73. Chino YM, Smith EL 3rd, Hatta S, et al. Postnatal development of binocular disparity sensitivity in neurons of the primate visual cortex. *J Neurosci* 1997;17(1):296–307.

74. Hatta S, Kumagami T, Oian J, et al. Nasotemporal directional bias of V1 neurons in young infant monkeys. *Invest Ophthalmol Vis Sci* 1998;39(12):2259–2267.

75. O'Dell C, Boothe RG. The development of stereoacuity in infant rhesus monkeys. *Vision Res* 1997;37(19):2675–2684.

76. Mori T, Matsuura K, Zhang B, et al. Effects of the duration of early strabismus on the binocular responses of neurons in the monkey visual cortex (V1). *Invest Ophthalmol Vis Sci* 2002;43(4):1262–1269.

77. Zhang B, Bi H, Sakai E, et al. Rapid plasticity of binocular connections in developing monkey visual cortex (V1). *Proc Natl Acad Sci U S A* 2005;102(25):9026–9031.

78. Sireteanu R. Binocular vision in strabismic humans with alternating fixation. *Vision Res* 1982;22(8):889–896.

79. Banks MS, Aslin RN, Letson RD. Sensitive period for the development of human binocular vision. *Science* 1975;190(4215):675–677.

80. Mitchell D, Ware C. *J Physiol (Lond)* 1974;236:707.

81. Movshon J, Chambers BEI, Blakemore C. *Perception* 1972;1:483.

82. Mohn G, van Hof-van Duin J. On the relation of stereoacuity to interocular transfer of the motion and the tilt aftereffects. *Vision Res* 1983;23(10):1087–1096.

83. Fawcett S, Wang YZ, Birch EE. The critical period for susceptibility of human stereopsis. *Invest Ophthalmol Vis Sci* 2005;46(2):521–525.

84. Majewska A, Sur M. Motility of dendritic spines in visual cortex in vivo: changes during the critical period and effects of visual deprivation. *Proc Natl Acad Sci U S A* 2003;100(26):16024–16029.

85. Liao DS, Krahe TE, Prusky GT, et al. Recovery of cortical binocularity and orientation selectivity after the critical period for ocular dominance plasticity. *J Neurophysiol* 2004;92(4):2113–2121.

86. Daw N. Critical periods and amblyopia. *Arch Ophthalmol* 1998;116:502–505.

87. Jeffrey BG, Birch EE, Stager DR, et al. Early binocular visual experience may improve binocular sensory outcomes in children after surgery for congenital unilateral cataract. *J AAPOS* 2001;5(4):209–216.

88. Michaelides M, Moore AT. The genetics of strabismus. *J Med Genet* 2004;41(9):641–646.

89. Birch EE, Fawcett SL, Morale SE, et al. Risk factors for accommodative esotropia among hypermetropic children. *Invest Ophthalmol Vis Sci* 2005;46(2):526–529.

90. Atkinson J. Infant vision screening: prediction and prevention of strabismus and amblyopia from refractive screening in the Cambridge Photorefraction Program. In: Sminos K, ed. *Early Visual Development, Normal and Abnormal.* New York: Oxford University Press; 1993:335–348.

91. Birch EE, Fawcett SL, Stager, Sr. DR. Risk factors for the development of accommodative esotropia following treatment for infantile esotropia. *J AAPOS* 2002;6(3):174–181.

92. Weakley, Jr. DR. The association between non-strabismic anisometropia, amblyopia, and subnormal binocularity. *Ophthalmology* 2001;108(1):163–171.

Development of Color Vision in Infants

8

Israel Abramov and James Gordon

Color vision is often ignored in clinical practice because it is assumed that even if a deficit is found, nothing can be done about it. No magical glasses can be prescribed.

It is important, however, to understand the topic and to test infants for color vision: Specific color deficits are often early markers for other diseases. For example, S-cone deficits are associated with diabetes, retinopathies, and dementias (1,2). Also, teaching aids for preschoolers are often color-coded and scholastic tests in the pre-K range include correct use of color names. A toddler who has problems with color vision may fail to use color names correctly, which can be wrongly ascribed to cognitive problems.

To understand infants' color vision, we must first understand the mechanisms of normal adult color vision. Only then can we examine whether color vision exists in infants, whether it is innate, and how it compares with adult color vision.

BASIC REQUIREMENTS FOR COLOR VISION

Color vision is the ability to discriminate lights of different spectra, regardless of their relative intensities. For example, consider a bi-partite field illuminated on the left with one wavelength and on the right with another wavelength (Fig. 8.1A). If the observer can adjust the intensity of the right side so that it appears the same as the left (cannot be distinguished from it), then that observer does not have complete color vision as do most of the general human population.

An observer with any form of color vision must have at least two types of receptors whose spectral sensitivities are different. This derives from the *univariance* of visual receptors. Each receptor contains a photopigment whose molecules absorb incident photons; each photon that is absorbed initiates a small electrical signal; this receptor signal is the same for any photon that is absorbed. The magnitude of the electrical signal is simply related to the total number of photons that the receptor's pigment absorbs. Wavelength determines only the probability that a photon will be absorbed; once the photon is absorbed, response is independent of wavelength.

Figure 8.1A shows the spectral sensitivity curve of a single type of receptor; in this case, a human adult's L-cone; the curve shows the percentage of incident photons that will be absorbed (for simplicity, the curve is set at 100% at its "best" wavelength, although in a real receptor that amount would be considerably less than 100%). The field is illuminated on the left with light of wavelength 590 nm and on the right with 630 nm. Initially, if the same number of photons is delivered at each wavelength, the two sides will appear different, simply because the receptors illuminated by the light on the left will absorb a greater percentage of 590-nm photons than will the receptors illuminated by 630-nm photons. An example is given in the inset table (with the

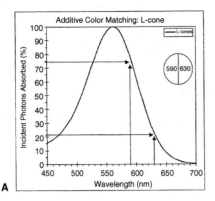

Stimulus		Photons Absorbed by Cones	
Wavelength (nm)	Photons	L-cone	M-cone
590	1,000	775	
630	1,000	230	
590	1,000	775	
630	3,370	775	

A

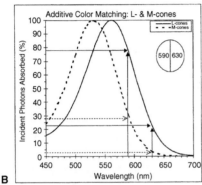

Stimulus		Photons Absorbed by Cones	
Wavelength (nm)	Photons	L-cone	M-cone
590	1,000	775	300
630	3,370	775	35
590	2,580	2,000	775
630	26,800	6,160	775

B

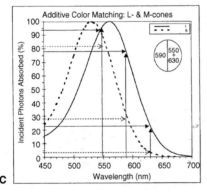

Stimulus		Photons Absorbed by Cones	
Wavelength (nm)	Photons	L-cone	M-cone
590	1,000	775	300
550	290	280	240
plus	plus	plus	plus
630	2,150	495	60
		775	300

C

FIGURE 8.1. Photopigments and additive color matching. Bi-partite stimulus field illuminated on the left with a light of 590 nm; participant adjusts *intensity* of light on the right (matching field) to make the two half-fields appear identical. Tables show the numbers of photons incident on the cones, and the numbers absorbed. **A:** Assuming all the cones contain the same photopigment, as shown, the intensity of the matching field can be adjusted to produce the same number of absorptions from both half-fields. **B:** Assuming the participant has the two cone types shown and that they are equally distributed across the entire field, the intensity of the matching field can be adjusted to equate the two sides for either one or the other cone type, but not simultaneously for both. **C:** Same as **(B)**, except that the matching field is an additive mix of two wavelengths; these can be adjusted separately so that the *total* numbers absorbed by each cone type are the same across the entire field. (Based on Gordon J, Abramov I. Color vision. In: Goldstein EB, ed. *The Blackwell Handbook of Perception, Ch. 4*. Oxford, UK: Blackwell; 2001:92–127.)

caution that the numbers are only for illustrative purposes; it is physically impossible to guarantee delivery of an exact number of photons). If the number of photons is readjusted to take into account the differences in percentages absorbed, however, the numbers absorbed by the receptors on each side will be the same, the electrical signals from receptors on each side will be the same, and the two sides will appear identical.

Only if the two sides of the field illuminate two different types of receptor will it be impossible to make the two sides appear the same simply by readjusting intensity. This is illustrated in Figure 8.1B, which shows spectral sensitivities of two adult cone types: M- and L-cones. From the table with the figure, it can be seen that the numbers of photons delivered on each side can be adjusted either to equate them for absorptions by the M-cones or by the L-cones. It is impossible, however, to adjust intensities so that each cone type on each side of the field simultaneously absorbs the same number of photons, which is what is needed for the two sides to appear identical. If a second wavelength is introduced on one side, however, a match is possible. Figure 8.1C shows the addition of photons of 550 nm to the photons of 630 nm on the right side. Now, the intensities of these two wavelengths can be separately adjusted so that the receptors on the right absorb some photons at one wavelength and some at the other wavelength such that the total number of photons absorbed by each receptor type is the same as the numbers absorbed by the receptors from the single wavelength presented on the left. The two sides match!

What do we mean by "match?" To most adults, light of 590 nm "looks" yellow, 550 nm looks green, and 630 nm looks red. Once the match is made, both sides appear identical and both appear yellow, although physically the stimuli are very different. The appearance of a light is a sensory response and is the result of processing by a particular nervous system. Chromatically different stimuli that elicit identical sensory responses are referred to as *metamers.*

Additive color mixing of the sort described above tells how many *independent dimensions* are needed to describe a particular form of color vision. The light(s) that are combined to make a match are referred to as *primaries*, and the number of primaries corresponds to the number of dimensions. If all receptors have the same photopigment, only one primary is needed to match all other lights (Fig. 8.1A) and such an observer is described as a *monochromat.* (Note that most humans are monochromats when they are fully dark-adapted and vision is governed only by the rods, all of which contain the same photopigment.). If two primaries are needed (Fig. 8.1C), the observer is a *dichromat*, and if three are needed the observer is a *trichromat.*

ADULT COLOR VISION

Trichromacy

The normal human retina has four distinct populations of receptors: rods and three types of cone whose spectral sensitivities are shown in Fig. 8.2A. The curves are for a situation in which the same numbers of photons at each wavelength is delivered to the retinal receptors; the cones are labeled S, M, L for the simple reason that one is more sensitive to longer wavelengths, one to middle wavelengths, and one to shorter wavelengths. The wavelengths of maximal sensitivity of the different cone types are approximately 430, 530, and 560 nm. Figure 8.2B shows the same receptor functions, but now in terms of equal numbers of photons at each wavelength delivered to the cornea. Sensitivity to the shorter wavelengths seems greatly depressed. This is an artifact caused by the usual procedure in psychophysical studies of color vision in which the light stimulus is measured at the cornea: the ocular media, especially the lens, absorb many of the shorter wavelength photons before they reach the retina and so these lights seem less effective for vision; of course, one can allow for this by readjusting the number of photons delivered to the cornea (more on this later).

Because receptors are sensitive to some degree to the entire spectrum, it is misleading to refer to cones as red, green, or blue receptors; all receptors are simply light receptors. For wavelengths longer than about 520 nm, how-

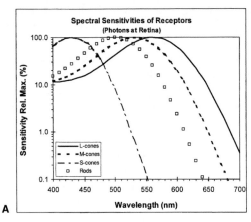

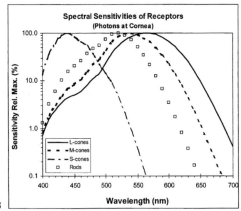

FIGURE 8.2. Spectral sensitivities of the four types of receptors in the human retina: rods and three types of cones (L-, M-, and S-cones). **A:** Sensitivities when the same numbers of photons at each wavelength are delivered directly to the receptors. **B:** Sensitivities of the same receptors when equal numbers of photons are delivered to the cornea. The differences at the shorter wavelengths are caused by losses in light transmission through the ocular media.

ever, the S-cones are so insensitive compared with L- and M-cones that these longer wavelengths effectively stimulate only the latter two types of cones; thus, anyone with normal color vision is a dichromat when the spectrum is limited to middle and long wavelengths. And, that is why a color-normal observer can make the match shown in Figure 8.1C: 590 nm ≡ 550 nm + 630 nm, which is known as the Rayleigh match, enshrined in the Nagel anomaloscope. The necessary ratio of intensities of the 550 and 630nm lights is determined by the exact form of the L- and M-cone spectra (see Fig. 8.1C),

which makes the anomaloscope a useful diagnostic tool; any significant deviation from the settings of the general population means that the observer has cones with unusual spectra. A genetic dichromat who lacks either M- or L-cones only has one photopigment in the spectral range of the anomaloscope; that person is effectively a monochromat over this range and so can match 590 nm with any ratio of 530 + 560 nm lights.

The Rayleigh match is deliberately limited to part of the spectrum because most color defects, especially of the genetic variety, involve only M- and L-cones. A person lacking L-cones is termed a *protanope*, one lacking M-cones is a *deuteranope*, and one lacking S-cones (a very rare person) is a *tritanope*. A normal adult has three classes of cones and is a *trichromat*; to match all possible lights, that individual needs to mix three primaries in the additive mixing field. Thus, merely making a normal Rayleigh match does not guarantee trichromacy; a *tritanope* is a dichromat, but has the usual M- and L-cones and so would make normal Rayleigh matches.

Although we will continue to refer to three types of cone, it should be noted that this is not strictly correct. In fact, multiple forms of the genes exist that code for the L- and M-cone photopigments and many individuals express multiple forms (3,4). All individuals with normal color vision, however, still require only three primaries to match all other lights; regardless of how many different L- and M-cones we have, we are still rigorously trichromats, meaning that somehow the nervous system must combine signals from the variants of each cone type into signals that behave as if they came from single cone types (5).

Neuronal Color Channels

Possession of different cones does not, by itself, guarantee color vision. There must also be a nervous system that compares the responses of the various cones to assess which responded more strongly and, thereby, gain information about the portion of the spectrum that stimulated the retina.

We start with retinal ganglion cells because they represent the output after all the processing at the level of the retina. Responses of ganglion cells in the primate retina can be divided into two broad classes: *spectrally opponent* and *spectrally nonopponent* types. As with all ganglion cells in the higher mammals, they have circular receptive fields with concentric zones of

excitation and inhibition; they are all *spatially* opponent, but what matters for color vision is which receptors drive these antagonistic responses. Two examples of the different organizations are shown in Fig. 8.3.

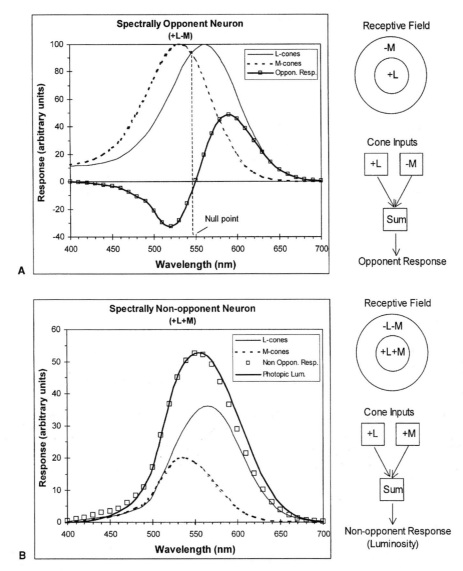

FIGURE 8.3. Spectral responses of two types of primate ganglion cells to lights of equal intensities covering their entire receptive fields. **A:** Spectrally opponent neuron that combines equally weighted responses of L- and M-cones, where one excites the neuron (+L) and the other inhibits it (−M). Spatial organization of the receptive field is on *upper right*; *lower right* shows a schematic combination of the responses of the two cone types. **B:** Spectrally nonopponent neuron that combines, with the same signs, the responses of the L- and M-cones. Spectral responses of the neuron to the cone inputs weighted as shown, closely matches the Commission Internationale de l'Eclairage (CIE) photopic luminosity function, V_λ. (Redrawn from Gordon J, Abramov I. Color vision. In: Goldstein EB, ed. *The Blackwell Handbook of Perception, Ch. 4.* Oxford, UK: Blackwell; 2001:92–127.)

Both examples deal only with responses driven by L- and M-cones. Although these cones are more or less uniformly interspersed across each region of the retina, the responses from each of the receptive field's concentric zones can be strongly biased toward one or the other cone type. Thus, for the spectrally opponent neuron in Fig. 8.3A, the center's excitatory responses are driven by L-cones, whereas M-cones drive the inhibitory inputs that predominate in the surround. This neuron is reporting the net sum of its cone inputs (by convention, excitatory inputs are positive and inhibitory ones are negative). The result is that the neuron's responses are spectrally opponent; a monochromatic light that covers the receptive field elicits one type of response for wavelengths to which the L-cone is the more sensitive, and the opposite sort of response when the M-cone is the more sensitive. Note, that a point in the spectrum exists to which this neuron does not respond, the point at which the L-and M-cones are equally sensitive so that their opposed inputs cancel. The location of this null point depends on the relative strengths of the L- and M-cone inputs to the particular cell.

By contrast, the neuron in Fig. 8.3B is spectrally nonopponent: both L- and M-cones contribute to responses of the excitatory center and the inhibitory surround so that any wavelength elicits the same type of response. In this example, it is assumed that L-cones are weighted more strongly and that the excitatory center is stronger than the surround, leading to the spectral responses shown.

The axons of the ganglion cells form the optic nerves that terminate in the lateral geniculate nucleus (LGN) of the thalamus. In primates (e.g., humans and macaque monkeys, species with very similar color vision), the LGN is a distinctively layered structure. The upper layers are termed *parvocellular* and the cell bodies of their neurons are small generically; they are called *P-cells*. The lower layers are *magnocellular*, cells that have larger bodies, called *M-cells* (beware of the distinction between M-cell and M-cone). A new category of very small cells, lying between some of the layers, has recently been described: these are termed *koniocellular* (K-cells) (6).

In macaques, all P-cells and some K-cells are spectrally opponent, whereas M-cells are spectrally nonopponent. All these cells have a spontaneous rate of firing action potentials in the absence of any light stimulus; excitation is signaled by an increase in firing rate from spontaneous, whereas inhibition is signaled by a decrease. The spectrally opponent cells can be divided into four subtypes, based on their spectral responses to monochromatic lights (7,8). Differences in the signs and relative weights of cone-derived inputs determine the particular responses: two (P-cells) are driven only by L- and M-cones, but with reversed signs (+L-M and +M-L), and the other two (K-cells) are driven by all three cone types (S vs. L+M). M-cells fall into two basic classes: some are excited to some degree by all wavelengths, whereas others are inhibited by all wavelengths; however, both types are driven only by L- and M-cones under light-adapted (photopic) conditions and by rods under dark-adapted (scotopic) conditions (9).

Psychophysiologic Linking Hypotheses

Normal human color vision is trichromatic, which means that it is defined by three independent dimensions, such as the intensities of the three primaries needed to match additively any other light. But this simply reduces color to this set of intensity axes, or some linear transformation of them as in a standard CIE chromaticity diagram (10). The matches specify when two lights appear the same, not what they appear like—red, pink, turquoise, and so on. Many possible trios of independent dimensions could be used. Sensations of color *appearance* are usually described using the three dimensions of *hue* (red, orange, yellow, and so on), *saturation* (quantity of hue: is it washed out and desaturated, or pure and saturated?), and *brightness* (in its everyday meaning of dim vs. bright).

How do we get from responses of neurons to such sensations? We must specify the linkages, the ways in which neuronal responses must be combined, presumably at higher levels of the central nervous system, to arrive at the sensations in which we are interested (11). Several things can be stated immediately: First, only the spectrally opponent cells can signal hue; when wavelength is changed, they are the only ones whose responses change qualitatively, rather than just quantitatively. Second, the spectrally nonopponent cells respond in the same qualitative fashion to the entire spectrum, and so can only signal some intensive aspect of the stimulus (e.g., luminosity). Indeed, the nonopponent cells are probably the entire basis for the spectral sensitivity function; when the eye is light-adapted, the sensitivity of these cells matches the psychophysical photopic luminosity function (the particular function in Fig. 8.3B is the photopic luminosity function), and when dark-adapted, their sensitivity matches the scotopic luminosity function (9).

As far as hue is concerned, the four types of spectrally opponent LGN neurons were originally thought to underlie the four basic hue sensations of red (R), yellow (Y), green (G), and blue (B) (7). That early hypothesis, however, was incomplete. It is now clear that the responses of the LGN cells do not exactly match color appearance functions, such as those obtained from direct hue-scaling psychophysics. The LGN opponent cells, however, are the necessary inputs to higher cortical levels at which they are compared with each other and recombined to produce mechanisms that directly specify hue sensations (5,8,12, 13).

The cortical recombination of spectrally opponent LGN responses produces two generic hue mechanisms: +R-G and +Y-B (the signs are arbitrary and serve only to distinguish qualitatively opposed responses). In this model, when the +R-G hue mechanism is excited, the sensation includes red; the exact sensation depends on the simultaneous activity in the other hue mechanism, +Y-B. If both are excited, the sensation will include some red and some yellow, the precise ratio depending on the degree to which each mechanism is excited. Note that the hue mechanisms have spectral null points, at which their opposed inputs cancel each other; for example, the +R-G mechanism has such a point at approximately 575 nm. At that point, the sensation includes neither red nor green, but the other mechanism, +Y-B, is strongly excited, leading to a sensation of unique yellow. Similar comparisons apply to all the other points in the spectrum; across the spectrum, hue shades continuously from R through RY, to Y, GY, G, BG, B, and finally BR.

The final sensory dimension of saturation probably involves a comparison of responses of spectrally opponent and nonopponent neurons. For example, if only the luminosity-signaling nonopponent cells respond to some stimulus, then a sensation of light would occur, but with no hue—the stimulus would have elicited a sensation that was completely desaturated. As soon as one or more of the opponent neurons also responds, a sensation of some hue must occur, whose saturation would be determined by the total hue-signaling responses relative to all the responses elicited by the stimulus.

A genetic dichromat cannot have the same range and variation of hue sensations for the simple reason that the opponent neuronal channels can only compare responses of two cone types. One consequence is that there will be some narrow portion of the spectrum in which the responses of these two cones are equal to each other; at that point, the responses of the opponent channels will cancel each other, eliminating any sensation of hue. The only sensation at that point will be caused by nonopponent channels that will produce a sensation that is completely desaturated. Each dichromat has a spectral neutral point. The spectral region of this neutral point varies with the type of dichromacy; protanopes and deuteranopes have neutral points in the vicinity of 490 to 510 nm, with those of deuteranopes being slightly longer; tritanopes have their neutral point in the vicinity of 465 to 475 nm.

TESTING INFANTS' COLOR VISION

Infants cannot respond to verbal instructions, and their motoric and cognitive abilities are limited; their vision cannot be evaluated in the same way as that of an adult. Additionally, several *a priori* reasons exist why infant color vision may not be simply a miniaturized version of adult color vision. We describe first the major testing techniques and then consider some of the general problems in evaluating infants' color vision in particular. Only then can will we be equipped to face the often contradictory findings on their color vision. The goal is to develop psychophysical and physiologic methods that relate behavior and physiology to physical stimuli.

Many of the methods were initially developed to examine infants' capacities beyond the purely visual. We concentrate on the variants that have been used to assay color vision.

Behavioral Methods

Habituation

An infant presented with a novel stimulus will "take notice" of it, usually with some sort of orienting response. Basically, a stimulus is presented over and over until it is no longer "novel" and the infant stops responding to its presentation—"habituation" has occurred. At that point, another stimulus that is physically different from the first is presented. If the infant detects the change, dishabituation occurs and the infant reorients to the changed stimulus. Discrimination thresholds can be measured by refining the change in the stimulus that is needed to elicit dishabituation.

Orienting responses, especially in very young infants, are based mostly on eye movements. In most studies, an eye-tracking apparatus is not used and infant's gaze is assessed by experienced testers looking carefully at the infant's face when a stimulus is presented and, typically, there is acceptable agreement among testers. Usually, one measures the amount of time spent looking at the stimulus before looking away. Habituation is indicated by a short latency to looking away and dishabituation by a subsequent increase in looking time.

For testing color vision, one method used a series of large, neutral stimuli (whites, grays) of markedly different intensities, presented in random order until the infant's looking time dropped to some low, criterion level; because the only difference among the stimuli was intensity, it was assumed that this dimension became less "interesting." At that point, a test stimulus was presented: either another neutral stimulus, but of an intensity not included in the habituation series, or a chromatic stimulus; dishabituation should occur if the infant perceives a change that is not simply in intensity (14,15).

Forced-choice Preferential Looking

Infants generally prefer to look at "something" rather than "nothing." The method of forced-choice preferential looking (FPL)(16) is widely used in many forms of vision testing: the infant looks at a large, uniform field on which an optically projected test stimulus is embedded either on the left or right side. If the infant orients toward the side with the stimulus, the stimulus is assumed to be visibly different from the surrounding field for the infant.

To avoid biases caused by the tester's knowledge of where the stimulus was presented, the tester can only see the infant's face (directly, or on a TV monitor) and must vote, based only on the infant's responses, where the stimulus was located (Fig. 8.4A). If the infant cannot detect the difference between the stimulus and the surround, the tester's voting accuracy must fall to 50%; the tester's percent correct increases as the stimulus becomes more discriminable and elicits more obvious orienting responses.

The resulting psychometric function can be used to derive a threshold (Fig. 8.4B). For example, if a test stimulus differs from the surround only in intensity (I), the function can be used to define the increment in intensity (ΔI) that produces a just noticeable difference at that value of I: some level of percent correct is chosen to represent threshold (in this two-alternative case, usually 75%) and the associated I is found by interpolation. Sensitivity is simply the reciprocal of that threshold.

To extend this approach to measuring color vision, the test stimulus can be chromatically different from the surround. Any indication of discrimination by the infant, however, may not result from a perception of a difference in hue; the chromatic stimulus may appear achromatic, but of a different intensity from the surround. The common way of ruling this out is to present the test stimulus at different intensities across trials, so that on any one trial it is above, below, or equal to the intensity of the surrounding field. The assumption is that at least one of the test intensities will match surround intensity for the individual infant being tested. Thus, if the infant is color-blind, at some stimulus the test stimulus matches the surround, and the tester's performance will drop to chance; however, if the infant has color vision and can discriminate the test from the surround regardless of intensity, the tester should detect mostly the orienting responses (Fig. 8.4C). Choice of the set of

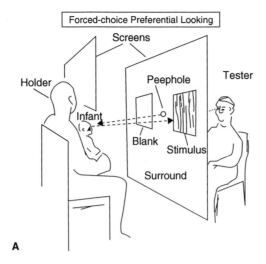

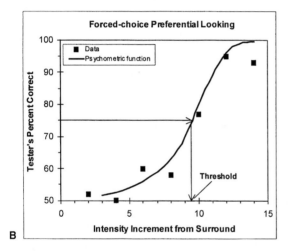

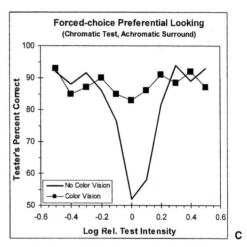

FIGURE 8.4. Forced-choice preferential looking psychophysical procedure. **A:** Typical arrangement for testing infants. Tester must choose which side of a large field contained the test stimulus based only on observation of infant's orienting responses. To avoid biasing the infant's behavior, the holder cannot see the stimulus array. **B:** Typical data showing tester's performance when infant is presented with achromatic test stimuli of different increments above the intensity of the surround. Data are fitted with a psychometric function and threshold found by interpolation. **C:** Typical data for a chromatic test and an achromatic surround. One infant shows no evidence of chromatic discrimination and performance dips to chance when test and surround intensities are the same. The other discriminates test from surround at all intensities of test relative to surround and is presumed to have some form of color vision.

intensities to use is not simple; we deal with some of the issues below.

A simpler variant that does not require an optical system to produce stimuli is derived from the Teller Acuity Cards (TAC) widely used to measure acuity (17). The version for testing color vision uses large gray cards with a central peephole for the tester to view the infant (18).

A chromatic sample from the Munsell series of colored papers is attached on one side or other of the peephole to test whether it attracts the infant's attention; because the tester is unaware of the side on which the test stimulus appears, the procedure still has the benefits of forced-choice psychophysics. The background cards have different gray levels to ensure that discrimination is based only on chromatic differences between sample and the gray background (see *Controlling Intensity,* below).

Finally, failure to demonstrate discrimination may not be true failure to discriminate by the infant. An infant may detect a stimulus change but not *prefer* to look at it (19). Ideally, stimuli should be equated initially for an infant's spontaneous preference, not an easy thing to do.

Eye Movements

Visible, moving stimuli can capture attention and elicit pursuit eye movements. This is especially so when a large part of the visual field consists of a repeating pattern drifting in one direction, as, for example, a grating moving continuously within a large aperture. Such large patterns reflexively entrain optokinetic nystagmus (OKN) with alternating phases of smooth pursuit of the pattern and return saccades (20). Such stimulus-evoked eye movements can be measured by eye-tracking optical and electronic systems, and even married to FPL: a grating of alternating black and white stripes can drift horizontally either leftward or rightward; a tester viewing only the output of the tracker must choose on each trial the direction of stimulus motion. On successive trials, the pattern can be degraded to find the threshold at which the tester no longer reliably detects the motion (21).

The above procedure can be referred to as *directionally appropriate movement* (DAM), and can be used to study color vision using a grating whose stripes alternated only in wavelength. A variant is the *motion nulling* (MN) technique, in which two gratings drift in opposite directions. Each, by itself, would elicit DAM in its direction; when both are present and equally visible, their elicited motion tendencies cancel—motion is nulled. For example, one grating might be of yellow and black bars drifting across a screen in one direction; superimposed on this, is another grating, one with blue and black bars, drifting in the opposite direction. Each direction will tend to elicit OKN in its direction. Intensity of one of the chromatic bars is varied until a motion null is found (i.e., no longer is any overt OKN present because the two gratings have been made equally visible and the opposed OKN tendencies have canceled each other). The relative intensities of the chromatic bars define the infant's sensitivity to those wavelengths; repeating the process with other wavelengths can yield a complete spectral function (22).

Typically, the MN is found by having a tester observe the infant's eyes and specify whether clear following eye movements occurred. Note, this method assumes that the neuronal center controlling OKN receives the same spectral information as do the other areas subserving color vision. Evidence suggests that the rules are not the same for infants and adults (23). In adults, the luminance contrast needed to detect a drifting grating is the same as the contrast needed to identify the direction of the motion; however, for isoluminant chromatic gratings, more than detection contrast is needed to identify direction. With infants, however, both the detection and direction-discrimination contrast thresholds are similar.

Metamers

When the spectral sensitivities of the receptors are known, it is possible to create, by additive combination, stimuli of different spectral content but which will elicit the same responses from the receptors (i.e., metamers can be fashioned; see *Basic Requirements for Color Vision*).

Infants are known to have cones at birth, but their spectral sensitivities are not necessarily known. If, however, we *assume* their spectral sensitivities are the same as those of adults, we can ask which, in fact, are present and functioning. If adult metamers are equivalent for the infant, then the hypothesized photopigments exist and contribute to the infant's vision. Because four receptor types can contribute to infants' discriminations (L-, M-, and S-cones and rods), four primary lights must be added to create complete metamers. This cumbersome arrangement can be simplified by confining the spectrum to middle and long wavelengths, as in the examples in Fig. 8.1. Now, only three primaries suffice, which can be combined to create a set of metamers for any pair of L- and M-cones, and rods; when one metamer is replaced by another spectrally different one, any response to the change must be caused by a functioning version of the third receptor type (24). Furthermore, the magnitudes of any changes can be used to measure the spectral sensitivity of that third unmatched receptor (25).

More generally, the spectra of the cones can be used to define a color space (26), within which it is possible to modulate a stimulus such that only specific combinations of cones respond to the changes. For example, stimuli can be modulated only along an L/M axis: the stimuli can vary in appearance from R, through Y, to G without changing the stimulation of S-cones, which would not contribute to any discrimination.

Any of the behavioral methods described, as well as the physiologic methods discussed below, could be used to test whether adult metamers are also infant metamers at any given age.

Physiologic Methods

Many physiologic methods are available for studying sensory systems. Only two, however, have been productively applied to infant vision: the electroretinogram (ERG) and the visually evoked potential (VEP).

ELECTRORETINOGRAM

Recording an ERG can be invasive in that often a contact lens with an electrode is applied directly to the cornea. This records the gross potential developed across the retina in response to a light flash. Typically, to increase signal-to-noise ratio, responses are averaged across several stimulus presentations. Both response and noise amplitudes, however, are lower in infants than adults so that fewer repetitions are required.

The advantage of the ERG is that its component waveforms are well-known and can be related to specific neuronal layers. Because all the retinal neurons, except for the ganglion cells, contribute to the response, the ERGs is a good indicator of distal processing in the visual system. But this means that ERGs are rod-dominated, because most receptors are rods; obtaining cone-driven (photopic) ERGs, calls for special methods (e.g., intense backgrounds and fast flicker rates) (27).

VISUALLY EVOKED POTENTIALS

The VEP is a much less-invasive technique; it is recorded from electrodes placed on the scalp over the visual areas of the cerebral hemispheres, usually the occipital lobe. The VEP is a special case of the electroencephalogram, which is a very noisy response and rarely shows a clear response to a single presentation of a simple visual stimulus. As with the ERG, the responses must be averaged across many trials. Because of the distance of the electrodes from the responding tissue and the complexity of cerebral architecture, it is not always obvious which areas contribute to the recorded responses and to what degree. It is widely accepted, however, that in adults VEPs, unlike ERGs, are dominated by photopic mechanisms (27).

It must also be emphasized that these methods describe particular neuronal mechanisms, and not necessarily those that underlie awareness and many of the behavioral methods. For example, when stimuli are presented on a computer monitor, flicker occurs at the frame-rate of the display; while participants are completely unaware of this flicker, their occipital VEPs will show large responses associated with the frame rate (28).

General Problems with Tests of Infants

None of the above methods is "fool-proof." Ultimately the *caveats* found in virtually every paper can only be resolved by convergent lines of evidence from different studies, using different methods, and making different assumptions.

Group Functions

It is difficult to get complete data sets from every infant, mostly because of limited attention spans. Infants, therefore, are often lumped together by age to compute group average functions. Because each infant contributes only some of the data, it is difficult to estimate error variances associated with each point on a function. And even when each infant contributes an entire set of data, each infant may have been tested across several sessions on separate days. Furthermore, choosing which infants to include in an average depends on arbitrary age boundaries for each group. For example, a group designated as 2-month-old infants could span a range of 7 to 9 weeks, variations that represent appreciable fractions of an infant's entire existence.

More generally, it is not always clear why many data from infants display so much variability, even within one laboratory and with one procedure. Such variance must logically be apportioned between measurement error and true between-infant differences. To sort these apart requires very large numbers of trials per infant and very expert testers; if this is done, however, the variability in any set of data may be greatly reduced, implying that infants of a given age may be more homogenous than the usual group functions suggest (29).

Area of Retina

Even in adults, the retina is not a homogenous structure. Most obviously, central fovea is largely free of rods. Considerable differences also are seen in distributions of the different cone types; the fovea contains very few S-cones (30); also, the ratio of L- to M-cones changes drastically across the retina, with the periphery being dominated by L-cones. Additionally, the sizes of neuronal receptive fields increase greatly as one moves away from the fovea, suggesting marked changes in combinations of the different cones. Surprisingly, all these changes have relatively modest impact on adult color vision across much of the retina, provided extrafoveal stimuli are enlarged to account for increasing receptive field sizes (31).

The problem is compounded in infants; at birth, the fovea is anatomically so immature that it is unlikely to be functional (32). Cones continue to mature at least throughout the first 5 years of life, by which time extrafoveal regions appear adultlike (33). At age four, however, foveal cones' outer segments, which contain the photopigment, are still only half those of an adult and are packed only half as densely (34). These studies deal only with morphology of cones in general; it is still possible that the different cone types mature at different rates.

In short, it matters which part of the retina is used in any test. With infants, however, it is difficult to instruct them to look at some small fixation spot that would enable the experimenter to control retinal position of a test stimulus.

Testing Method

The often unspoken assumption is that any of the testing methods can be used to demonstrate that infants have color vision and to examine its attributes. Each method, however, taps information from different populations of neurons. For example, eye movements are at the root of many of the methods. These are complex responses driven by responses of neurons in many brain areas, some of which may not be privy to all the information from the retina about the stimulus and its attributes. Similarly, motion perception is weighted toward responses of M-cells in the LGN, which are spectrally nonopponent and do not contribute to sensations of hue.

With adults, it is possible to take some color function obtained with standard psychophysics and compare it with a similar function obtained by testing an adult in as close a way as possible to the procedure used with infants; if the two agree, the particular method has access to the appropriate information. For example, using one of the eye movement based methods, adults have been tested to show that the direction of their OKN responses correlated well with perceived motion (22). The absolute sensitivities, however, may not be the same; thresholds for detection of luminance contrast are usually higher when derived from a tester's votes about direction of OKN than when the participant votes directly, and these are higher than those from a traditional psychophysical technique (35). Thus, the indirect methods used with infants may underestimate their capabilities.

Stimulus Size and Wavelength

To test color vision, one must use spectrally different stimuli. Optimally, these stimuli are narrow-band, generated either from interference filters or monochromators. In much of the infant work, however, these were often not done, mostly because of limitations of the available instruments. Stimuli were either colored papers (e.g., the Munsell papers) or were from broad-band filters. With adults, this is a relatively minor problem; based on standard functions for additive trichromatic matches, each stimulus is equivalent to a dominant wavelength mixed with some standard "white"; the degree of white in the match determines its purity, or closeness to a monochromatic light. In many studies of infants, broad-band stimuli are referred to by the wavelength equivalents for adults, which may not be appropriate.

Adult color vision is typically measured in the fovea and stimuli rarely exceed 1° in diameter. Stimuli in studies of infants are often very large [e.g., 12° × 14° (36); 4° to as much as 32°] (15). Large size, in itself, can be a problem; cats, who have notoriously poor color vision, will often show wavelength discrimination independent of intensity when stimuli are large (37), as will human adult dichromats (38).

Controlling Intensity

Color vision is the ability to discriminate among spectrally different stimuli regardless of any perceived differences in intensity. The problem is simplified when testing adults; they can be instructed to ignore any differences in brightness. This is obviously harder to achieve with nonverbal observers (e.g., infants or animals). It is straight-forward, with such observers, to test whether stimuli appear different, but it is more difficult to show the basis for any difference. To test for color vision, the stimuli must first be equated for brightness or luminosity.

Ideally, the first step is to measure the spectral sensitivity function, and then use it to equate the intensities of all the test stimuli. But which is the correct function to use? In principle, adults have two spectral sensitivity functions: one defines sensitivity under light-adapted, photopic, conditions and is based on responses of cones; the other is for dark-adapted, scotopic, conditions based on responses of rods. A purely rod-based system cannot have color vision, because all rods contain the same photopigment; the scotopic sensitivity function is inappropriate for testing color vision.

The problem with testing infants is that we may not be able to use an adult photopic function; we cannot assume that infant and adult functions are the same, nor do we know which area of retina is being used. For the same reason, we cannot use a photometer to equate the different stimuli for luminance because such lu-

minance measurements are based on the standard adult function.

Even if we begin by measuring spectral sensitivity to obtain a *standard* infant luminosity function, the problem is that a range of thresholds exists within any group of infants. Measuring each participant's spectral sensitivity is prohibitively time consuming. If a group function is used to control intensity, additional steps are needed to account for variations among individuals (39). One approach is to vary intensity systematically to generate psychometric functions, as shown in Fig. 8.4, to ask whether behavior changes with intensity or is independent of it. Another tactic that is commonly applied is to "jitter" the intensities of the chromatic stimuli. Initially, all are equated according to a chosen luminosity function; on subsequent trials, their intensities are randomly varied over some small range. Such jittering from trial to trial may make intensity a less salient discriminative cue in the hope that the infant will ignore that cue.

Intensity jittering has been used with infants (39) and with other nonverbal observers such as cats (40) and nonhuman primates (41). The problem is to choose a range of intensities that encompasses the range of possible variations. With adults, the range has to cover individual variations about a common mean function. With infants, the luminosity function changes with age (see below), so that the range of jitter must be sufficient to cover different versions of that function. In practice, this means a large range must be used, with attendant increase in testing time, to rule out all possible interpretations, including the possibility that rods underlie many discriminations (42). Because of instrument limitations, many infant studies use average luminances that would be in the mesopic range for adults, a range in which the spectral sensitivity function is at some intermediate point between scotopic and photopic.

SPECTRAL SENSITIVITY

Scotopic Spectral Sensitivity

Although color is usually thought to be a photopic phenomenon, scotopic vision cannot be ignored. Across most of the retina the vast majority of receptors is rods and, in an immature system, these rods may combine with one or more cone types to provide the ability to discriminate among wavelengths. In principle, it should be simpler to measure infants' scotopic sensitivity; it is not necessary to disentangle responses driven by receptors with different photopigments because all rods contain the same photopigment, rhodopsin. We will use this *simpler*

situation to illustrate many of the problems discussed in general above.

Infants' Spectral Sensitivity

Figure 8.5A shows mean spectral sensitivities of fully dark-adapted 1-month-old ($N = 13$) and 3-month-old ($N = 14$) infants (43). The method

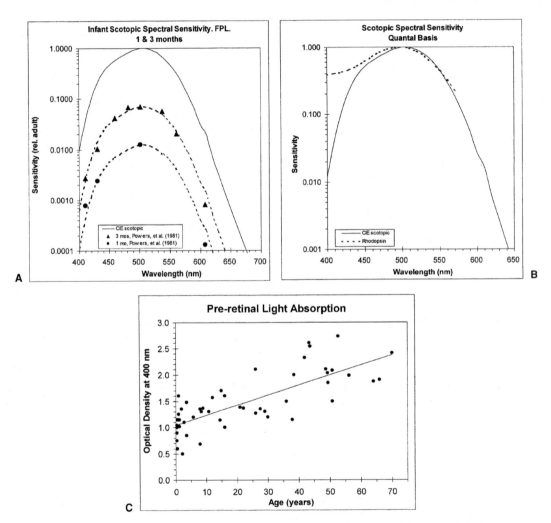

FIGURE 8.5. Scotopic spectral sensitivity. **A:** Infants' sensitivities relative to adults. Forced-choice preferential looking (FPL) with two groups of fully dark-adapted infants (1- and 3-months of age). (Data points from Powers MK, Schneck M, Teller DY. Spectral sensitivity of human infants at absolute visual threshold. *Vision Res* 1981;21:1005–1016.) Curves are the CIE scotopic function, V′$_\lambda$, slid vertically for best-fit to the infant data. **B:** Spectral sensitivity, on a quantal basis, of rhodopsin compared with the standard function, V′$_\lambda$. The deviations at shorter wavelengths are caused by absorption of light by preretinal structures. **C:** Optical density, across age, of the ocular media at 400 nm, derived from the difference between behavioral spectral sensitivity curves and the rhodopsin curve. (Redrawn from Werner JS. Development of scotopic sensitivity and the absorption spectrum of the human ocular media. *J Opt Soc Am A* 1982;72:247–258.)

was FPL (see above, *Methods*), using 17° test fields and monochromatic lights (interference filters); intensity ranges were chosen to yield psychometric functions from which thresholds were derived by interpolation. The solid curve is the standard adult curve from young adults (CIE, V'_λ) (10); infant sensitivities are plotted relative to the maximum of the adult curve. The adult curve has been slid down for best fit to the infant curves. Clearly, infant and adult spectra are the same. Compared with adults, however, 1-month-old infants are approximately 80 times, and 3-month-olds about 15 times less sensitive.

The shift in sensitivities toward adult values (Fig. 8.5A) raises additional questions, especially regarding area of retina being tested. From dark-adapted ERG, it has been shown that rod responses from peripheral retina reach 50% of adult values by the age of about 3 months; however, close to the fovea, rod responses only reach these levels by about 5 months (44). This retinal variation accords with post-natal retinal changes: maturation of parafoveal rods is delayed compared with maturation of peripheral rods (33).

Preretinal Light Absorption

The good agreement with the standard adult curve, however, is a possible problem. Light transmission by the ocular media changes with age, which changes the amount of light delivered to the cones. The lens, in particular, becomes denser and more yellow, meaning that it absorbs and filters out shorter wavelengths more than longer wavelengths. These changes and their values in any given individual can be assessed by measuring scotopic spectral sensitivity, which is determined solely by the well-known spectrum of rhodopsin, the photopigment in the rods. In Fig. 8.5B, we plot the standard scotopic function together with rhodopsin. (Note: in this case, for comparison with a photopigment function, sensitivity has been converted to a quantal basis; that is, number of quanta at each wavelength to reach threshold, rather than energy at threshold, which is the more usual measure for visual functions.) The deviations at shorter wavelengths must be caused by losses in ocular transmission.

The deviations from rhodopsin have been used to estimate optical density of the ocular media at very short wavelengths. The results from VEP, across the life-span, are shown in Fig. 8.5C (45). Although density of the ocular media increases continuously with age, also large individual differences are seen at any one age. Nonetheless, because infants' media, on average, have a density of 1.0, they are about 0.5 log units (factor of 3) less dense than young adults. Thus, we might expect their scotopic sensitivities at very short wavelengths to be higher by the same factor. The discrepancy is not caused by comparing VEP and FPL findings; using a similar approach, but with FPL, it has been found that 10-week-old infants media have a median density of 0.75 log units (46). A possible explanation is, that at any age are seen, large individual differences in sensitivities and media densities.

Purkinje Shift

The transition from photopic to scotopic vision, the Purkinje shift, is not abrupt. A considerable range is seen of adaptation states, corresponding to different levels of average light intensity, over which the function is termed *mesopic* and shifts gradually from one limit to the other. In the mesopic range, both rods and cones contribute to any function that is measured with stimuli extending into the retinal periphery. Stimuli that are clearly in the photopic range have luminances that begin at approximately 10 cd/m²; stimuli that are clearly scotopic have luminance less than 0.001 cd/m²; everything in between is mesopic (10).

The Purkinje shift in 3-month-old infants has been examined using eye movements elicited by drifting gratings, specifically using the MN paradigm (see *Methods*): stimuli were superimposed blue-black and yellow-black gratings moving in opposite directions; relative intensities were varied to find the values at which motion was nulled; absolute intensities ranged from adult scotopic thresholds to photopic levels (47). At the lowest absolute intensities, the relative spectral intensities for motion nulls approximated those for the standard adult scotopic function, V'_λ; at the highest levels, they approximated values expected from the standard adult photopic function, V_λ (see below). In both adults and infants, the transition was gradual from approximately 0.01 to 10 cd/m^2.

Photopic Spectral Sensitivity

Adults' Photopic Sensitivities

No one true photopic function exists, even for adults (48). Figure 8.6A shows different versions of this function; all have been equated at their peaks to emphasize differences in the shapes of the functions. The figure includes the standard human photopic function for the fovea, the CIE's V_λ; this is an amalgam of data from older adult observers and is derived from a procedure known as) at fast flicker rates that cannot be followed by rods. In HFP, each test wavelength is alternated with a fixed standard; the intensity of the test light is varied until flicker is no longer seen; at which point, the test light elicits the same magnitude of response as does the standard.

Other methods yield curves of different shapes. For example, a very different function is obtained when one uses an intense achromatic field to suppress the rods and then measures sensitivity to incremental flashes of different wavelengths; the result is a broader, trilobed curve; the peaks of this curve do not correspond to the peaks of the three cone types, but probably are related to peaks of the spectrally opponent neuronal responses (49) (Fig. 8.6A).

Additionally, we show a photopic function obtained with HFP, but for the peripheral retina at 45° from the fovea; this function may include marked rod contributions even under photopic conditions (50).

Finally, because infants' ocular media are clearer than those of adults, we include a version of the standard V_λ that we have readjusted to remove the effects of transmission losses through the eye; this correction is based on estimates in adults of densities of lens and macular pigment (10); it is the same function we used to show the differences in sensitivities of cones when stimulus lights are measured at the cornea rather than at the retina (Fig. 8.2).

Infants' Photopic Sensitivities

Figure 8.6B shows photopic sensitivities of light-adapted 2-month-old infants obtained from VEP in two different laboratories using similar procedures; complete functions were obtained from each infant [$N = 5$, (51); $N = 7$ (51)]. In both cases, the maximal stimulus intensities near the peaks of the curve were well into the adult photopic range [40 cd/m^2 (51); 25 cd/m^2 (52)]. The combination of adaptation state, stimulus intensities, and use of VEP make it highly likely that the functions are dominated by cone responses. The degree of agreement between the data sets illustrates the variations typically found across studies. For comparison,

---

FIGURE 8.6. Photopic spectral sensitivity. **A:** Adults' functions including the CIE standard photopic function, V_λ, obtained by flicker-photometry; V_λ corrected to remove the effects of preretinal absorption, mostly by lens and macular pigment; photopic sensitivity of peripheral retina, using flicker-photometry (data from Abramov I, Gordon J. Color vision in the peripheral retina. I. Spectral sensitivity. *J Opt Soc Am A Opt Image Sci Vis* 1977;67:203–207; trilobed sensitivity function obtained from increment thresholds on an intense achromatic field (data from Harwerth RS, Sperling HG. Effects of intense visible radiation on the increment-threshold spectral sensitivity of the rhesus monkey eye. *Vision Res* 1975;15:1193–1204.). **B:** Photopic sensitivities, from VEP, of 2-month-old infants, compared with the corrected V_λ in **(A)**. (Data from Dobson V. Spectral sensitivity of the 2-month infant as measured by the visually evoked cortical potential. *Vision Res* 1976;16:367–374 and Moskowitz-Cook A. The development of photopic spectral sensitivity in human infants. *Vision Res* 1979;19:1133–1142.). **C:** Same as **(B)**, except for 4-month-old infants. (Data from Moskowitz-Cook A. The development of photopic spectral sensitivity in human infants. *Vision Res* 1979;19:1133–1142 and Bieber ML, Volbrecht VJ, Werner JS. Spectral efficiency measured by heterochromatic flicker photometry is similar in human infants and adults. *Vision Res* 1995;35:1385–1392). **D:** Photopic sensitivities, from FPL, of 2-month-old infants, compared with adult peripheral photopic sensitivity in **(A)**, and CIE scotopic function, V'_λ. (Data from Clavadetscher JE, Brown AM, Ankrum C, et al. Spectral sensitivity and chromatic discriminations in 3- and 7-week-old infants. *J Opt Soc Am A Opt Image Sci Vis* 1988;5:2093–2105.) **E:** FPL photopic sensitivities of 3-month infants from increments on an intense achromatic field, compared with the corrected V_λ in **(A)**. (Data from Peeples DR, Teller DY. White-adapted spectral sensitivity in human infants. *Vision Res* 1978;18:49–53.)

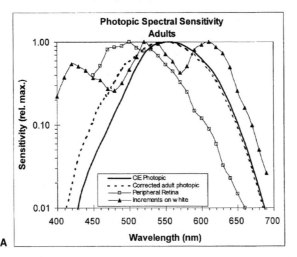

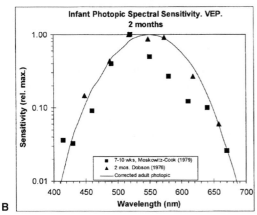

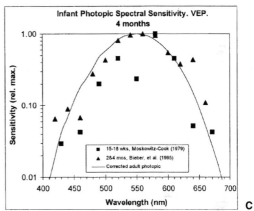

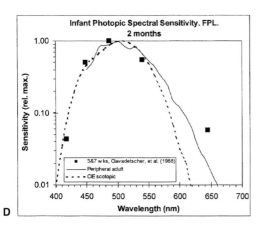

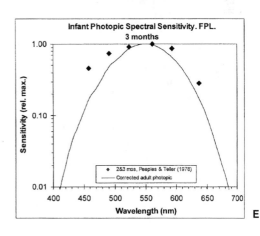

we include the standard adult V_λ function with all preretinal light losses removed (Fig. 8.6A).

Figure 8.6C shows VEP-derived functions for 4-month-old infants. One study used the same procedures as with the 2-month-old infants [$N = 5$, (51)]. Although the other used HFP with a mesopic intensity for the standard (0.6 cd/m^2), the combination of a fast flicker rate and VEP was probably sufficient to elicit photopic responses; 2- and 4-month-old infants were tested and, because no differences were seen between these groups, the data were pooled [$N = 42$, (53)].

Photopic functions have also been derived from FPL chromatic discrimination tests; intensities of chromatic test stimuli are varied above and below the intensity of the surround; if no color vision exists, performance should drop to chance when these intensities elicit equal responses from the infant; but even if some color vision is present, performance can show a dip toward chance at the matching intensities. The relative intensities of these dips can be used to derive a spectral sensitivity function.

Using such a procedure, functions were obtained for groups of 3- and 7-week-old infants; because no age-related differences were seen, the data were pooled and are shown in Fig. 8.6D (53), which is discussed further below under *Chromatic Discriminations*. Clearly, this 2-month function differs from the VEP curve in Fig. 8.6B. For comparison, we show the standard adult *scotopic* curve, V'_λ, as well as an adult photopic curve from the peripheral retina (50). One conclusion, from the agreement of these curves at their peaks, is that young infants' spectral sensitivities are heavily influenced by rods; however, the deviation at long wavelengths indicates cone contributions, presumably from L-cones. A note of caution: some of the rod dominance may result from the surround's intensity, to which test lights were being matched, which was only about 2 cd/m^2, which is in the mesopic range, at least for adults.

Forced choice preferential looking has also been used together with eye movements (DAM) to find the threshold intensities at which an infant will follow a chromatic test stimulus projected onto an intense (100 cd/m^2) white field (55). The results for a single infant at each of 2- and 3-months of age did not

differ and were pooled; we have ascribed them to 3-month-old infants and they are shown in Fig. 8.6E, together with a standard adult function corrected for ocular transmission losses. In this case, the peaks are at the wavelengths of adult *photopic* curves. The broadness of the infants' curve probably results from measuring increment thresholds on a white field (Fig. 8.6A).

We can probably conclude from these data that young infants and adults have similar photopic spectral sensitivities. This is bolstered by a variety of other studies that compared sensitivities at only two or three spectral points, which permitted testing of larger groups; for example, eye-movement MN techniques have shown that, by 3-months of age, the adult function is a good approximation of the infant function, especially if allowance is made for the clearer ocular media of infants (22,29,35,56).

The problem, however, is which adult function to use for equating stimuli to be presented to infants? Clearly, the choice must be dictated by the specific viewing conditions, which greatly affect even adults' functions. Even then, intensities must still be jittered or otherwise varied to encompass the possible range of sensitivities for each infant; the advantage of starting with an adult function that fits the particular stimulus conditions is that the range of jitter may be limited. Finally, we note that tolerable agreement with an adult photopic function does not mean that infants must possess functional L- and M-cones. The standard adult function, V_λ, is dominated by L-cones (Fig. 8.3B).

CHROMATIC DISCRIMINATION

Emergence of Color Vision

Because it is difficult to bring complex optical systems into neonatal nurseries, studies of color discriminations by newborns are based on colored papers with broad-band reflectance spectra, which complicates precise stimulus specification (as a compromise, we will refer to these stimuli by their appearance to adults). Also, each infant usually participates in only one condition and conclusions are based on group behaviors. Nonetheless, newborns do seem to show some color discriminations.

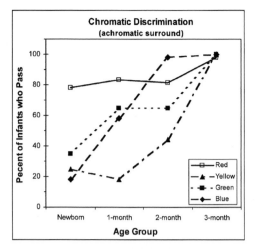

FIGURE 8.7. Infants' chromatic discriminations from habituation procedures. Percentages of infants in each of four age cohorts who successfully discriminate large, broad-band chromatic stimuli (colored papers) from achromatic surrounds (gray cards) of varying intensities. Newborns appear to discriminate only red from achromatic independent of intensity. By 3 months of age, all the hues can be discriminated from achromatic. (Redrawn from Adams RJ, Courage ML, Mercer ME. Systematic measurement of human neonatal color vision. *Vision Res* 1994;34:1691–1701.).

When tested with habituation procedures, they could discriminate 8° red squares from white; with increasing sizes of stimuli, they could also discriminate green and yellow from white, but failed to discriminate even a 32° blue square from white (15). More recently, using a color version of an acuity-card procedure, it was shown that newborns, as a group, could reliably discriminate only red from an achromatic surround (57). By 1 month of age, performance improved somewhat, especially for blue and green versus gray; and, when data were pooled with those from older infants tested in the same way, performance improved to the point that by 3 months of age all infants could discriminate red, yellow, green, and blue from gray (Fig. 8.7).

Similar conclusions were reached about younger infants in a very careful FPL study that used monochromatic lights, thus avoiding many of the problems associated with broad-band stimuli, and rigorously controlled the range of

intensities of the chromatic stimuli by first measuring each infant's isoluminant point (54).

The surround in this study was not achromatic, but set at 547 nm ("yellowish-green" to adults). A test stimulus of similar wavelength was used to measure discriminations based only on intensity differences; psychometric curves dipped close to 50% correct responses from the tester when intensities were equal, and rose gradually with test intensities below and above that point. Group averages of these intensity discrimination functions for 3- and 7-week-old infants are shown as the solid lines in Fig. 8.8. These curves can be used to decide whether discrimination of other test wavelengths from the surround was indeed based on perception of chromatic differences, as would be indicated only if performance at all the jittered test intensities remained well above chance (Fig. 8.4C). But even in those cases, curves of many infants showed dips toward chance; these dips represent isoluminant values for the infant and were used to derive the spectral sensitivity functions in Fig. 8.6D.

Test wavelengths were 417, 448, 486, and 645 nm (these values, seen against a 547-nm surround, were chosen to maximize differences of responses from the various adult cone types and to optimally stimulate adult spectrally opponent and nonopponent neuronal mechanisms). Because each infant has a slightly different spectral sensitivity curve, individual psychometric curves showed dips at slightly different values. Therefore, simply pooling infant data to get group averages might obscure failures to discriminate. To avoid this, group averages were derived from individual chromatic discrimination curves that had been shifted along the intensity axis for best coincidence with each other. The results are shown as the data points in Fig. 8.8. For the 3-week-old infants, only the curve for the 645-nm test and 547-nm surround indicates discrimination that is not entirely driven by intensity differences. By 7 weeks, however, clear evidence shows that all the test wavelengths could be discriminated from the surround largely independent of relative intensities.

In short, based on the above behavioral tests, infants between 2 and 3 months of age show that they have some ability to discriminate among chromatic stimuli across most of the visible

Chromatic Discrimination

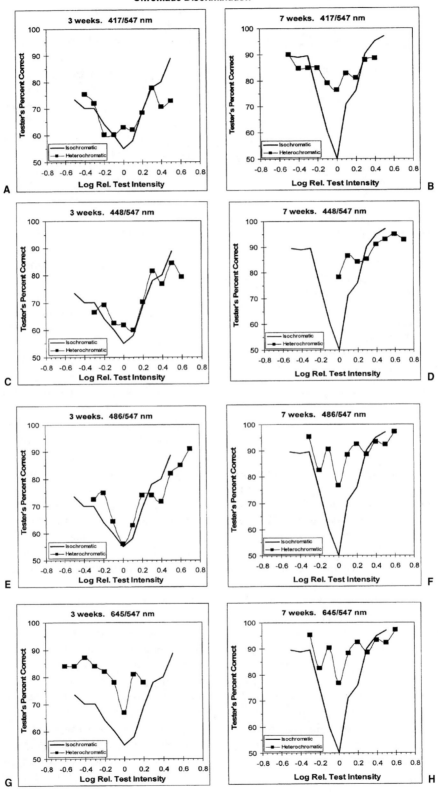

spectrum. This agrees with data from many other papers, some of which are included below, that show only limited discriminations by 1-month-old infants.

Cone Types and Neuronal Mechanisms

The early emergence of ability to discriminate long wavelengths (adult "reds") from achromatic surrounds (Fig. 8.7) must be based on comparison of responses of two spectrally different receptors, but which ones? It is difficult, however, to rule out rods as one of the types, especially given the form of the young infant's behavioral photopic spectral sensitivity (Fig. 8.6D).

Given the tight genetic specification of the cone photopigments, it is unlikely that infants will start with radically different cone types, except for relatively minor variations because of densities of the photopigments in the cones, and so on. It is possible, however, that functional versions of the different cone types mature at different rates. Thus, the well-studied spectra of adult cones can be used as a starting point to ask which are present and when.

L- and M-Cones: Behavioral Methods

One can investigate the presence of L- and M-cones by suppressing rods (e.g., by using photopic intensities, foveal stimuli, and so on) and limiting stimuli to wavelengths longer than 540 nm; this spectral range is the *Rayleigh range* to which S-cones are by and large insensitive (Fig. 8.2). The classic approach is the Rayleigh match (Fig. 8.1) in which a wavelength at the short end of this range is additively mixed with a long wavelength to match an intermediate wavelength (Fig. 8.1). If a precise ratio similar to that of color-normal adults is needed for the match, then infants have functional versions of both these cones.

Making a Rayleigh *match*, however, is too daunting to do with infants. Instead, investigators have used Rayleigh *discrimination* in FPL, using a field that is "yellow" and the test is either "red" or "green." Assuming rod suppression, such discrimination must be caused by the presence of functional L- and M-cones. An early study with a group of 1-month-old infants found that less than half could discriminate either a broad-band long wavelength ("red") test $(3° \times 3°)$ or a 550 nm ("green") test from a 589-nm surround but by 3-month old infants and all could do so (58). The luminance of the 589-nm surround was only 1.2 cd/m^2, however, which is mesopic for adults.

One possible reason for Rayleigh discrimination failures by younger infants may be caused by using test fields that are too small for the infant. In a similar study using a 589-nm surround $(10$ cd/m$^2)$ and a 650 nm test, 1-month-old infants could make the discrimination with 8° and 4°, but not 2°, stimuli, whereas 3-month-old infants could make the discriminations even with 2° stimuli (11,59). This dependence of color vision on stimulus size is reminiscent of the finding that, for adults, small stimuli that are sufficient in the fovea elicit degraded color vision in the periphery; peripheral stimulus size must be increased to match the sizes of local *perceptive fields* (31).

From these behavioral investigations, we can probably accept that, by 3 months of age, both L- and M-cones are functioning. Furthermore, it has been shown that at least some of the neuronal mechanisms driven by these cones are present at this age. When spectral sensitivity is measured by increment thresholds on an intense background, the curve has several

---

FIGURE 8.8. Infants' chromatic discriminations from forced-choice preferential looking (FPL). Group means for 3- and 7-week-old infants tested with 417-, 448-, 486-, and 645-nm stimuli against a 547-nm surround. *Solid curves* are the group means for isochromatic intensity discriminations using a test stimulus of similar wavelength to the 547-nm surround. Data points show performance for the various chromatic combinations. For 3-week-old infants, the only heterochromatic behavior that clearly differs from isochromatic discrimination is for the combination of the 645 nm test and 547 nm surround, as shown in **(G)**. By 7 weeks, all test stimuli are discriminated from the surround independent of intensity. (Re-drawn from Clavadetscher JE, Brown AM, Ankrum C, et al. Spectral sensitivity and chromatic discriminations in 3- and 7-week-old infants. *J Opt Soc Am A Opt Image Sci Vis* 1988;5: 2093–2105.)

minima, or notches, which are usually interpreted as resulting from spectrally opponent neuronal processing (48) (Fig. 8.6A). One such notch has been shown, using FPL, in 3-month-old infants tested with stimuli in the Rayleigh range and superimposed on an intense (approximately 200 cd/m^2) 580-nm field (60).

L- and M-Cones: Physiologic Methods

We treat the findings from physiologic methods, primarily VEP, separately because their developmental sequences do not always agree with psychophysical findings. Physiologic methods often show that a mechanism exists at a younger age. We reiterate, however, that physiology cannot show that responses of such a mechanism are available to the infant or guide the infant's overt behavior.

A powerful approach is to assume that if infants have L- and M-cones they will be the same as in adults. Metamers (see *Behavioral Methods, metamers*) can be created from additive combinations of monochromatic lights. Only three wavelengths are needed, if they are confined to the Rayleigh region of the spectrum, to create equivalences for any pairing of rods, and L- and M-cones; only the remaining receptor type can respond to the changes when these stimuli replace each other. Using such stimuli and recording VEP from 4- and 8-week-old infants, it has been shown that both groups had functioning L- and M-cones, although the evoked responses were smaller at 4-weeks (24). The spectral sensitivities of the isolated L- and M-cones closely matched data from adults tested in the same fashion (25). They also agreed closely with well-known adult functions similar to those in Fig. 8.2B. Similar conclusions were reached in a longitudinal study of infants showing that responses driven by both L- and M-cones emerged clearly by about 4 weeks (61).

S-Cones: Behavioral Methods

Although it is convenient to test infant color vision mostly in the Rayleigh region, a complete description must include S-cones.

Forced choice preferential looking has been used to test whether infants can discriminate between a pair of chromatic stimuli that an adult tritanope, who lacks S-cones, would confuse (61). In the heterochromatic test for S-cones,

the surround was 547 nm at approximately 3 cd/m^2 and the test was 416 nm, at jittered intensities above and below the surround's intensity; the isochromatic control for measuring sensitivity to changes only in intensity used a test of 543 nm. Figure 8.9 shows the performance of groups of 4- ($N = 12$) and 8-week-old ($N = 17$) infants displayed in the same way as in Fig. 8.8. Although some of the 4-week-old infants showed some discrimination of the 416-nm stimulus from the surround, as a group their performance fell close to chance at the matching intensity. By 8 weeks of age, however, all showed clear discrimination independent of intensity. This is very similar to the data in Fig. 8.8 for comparable stimuli. Thus, S-cones appear to contribute to chromatic discriminations by about the same time as both L- and M-cones: 2 months.

Forced choice preferential looking has also been used with a classic method for isolating responses driven by a single cone type: chromatic adaptation. Test wavelengths, from 400 to 560 nm, were superimposed on a yellow background chosen to adapt L- and M-cones strongly, but have minimal impact on S-cones. Tested in this fashion, adults' spectral sensitivities peaked at 440 nm, clearly showing the presence of S-cones. This was not the case with most 2- and 3-month infants, however, whose yellow-adapted spectra did not differ greatly from a rod curve (63). But note that the adapting field was only approximately 50 cd/m^2.

Similarly, eye-movement methods, using drifting chromatic gratings whose spectra were chosen to be equivalent for a tritanope, failed to elicit appropriate eye movements in both 2- and 4-month-old infants (64).

It is not easy to reconcile these findings. One possibility is that centers controlling eye movements do not receive the same color information as do other perceptual centers (see *General Problems*, above). Another possibility is that, at the low intensities in the FPL studies, rods contributed to the discriminations.

S-Cones: Physiologic Methods

Chromatic adaptation has also been used in VEP studies (65). Adults' spectral sensitivities measured from increment thresholds on a relatively intense (160 cd/m^2) yellow background peaked

Chromatic Discrimination: Tritan Confusion

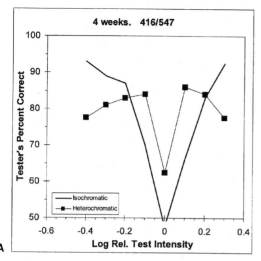
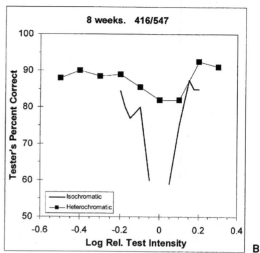

FIGURE 8.9. Discriminations that require functioning S-cones. Adults tritanopes, who lack S-cones, confuse specific pairs of monochromatic stimuli, such as 416 and 547 nm. Figures are group means for 4- and 8-week-old infants tested, using forced-choice preferential looking (FPL), with 416-nm stimuli and a 547-nm surround. *Solid curves* are for isochromatic intensity discriminations using a test stimulus of similar wavelength to the 547-nm surround. Data points are for heterochromatic discriminations. Only at 8 weeks is clear evidence seen that infants can discriminate these tritan-confusion stimuli independent of intensity. (Redrawn from Varner D, Cook JE, Schneck ME, et al. Tritan discriminations by 1- and 2-month-old human infants. *Vision Res* 1985;25:821–831.)

at about 440 nm and had a main lobe that agreed with the spectrum of S-cones. Infants from 4 to 6 weeks of age ($N = 9$) showed very similar results, demonstrating the existence of cortical responses driven by functioning S-cones.

Color Appearance and Color Categories

The major characteristic of adult color vision is that the appearance of the visible spectrum can be divided into four hue categories: R, Y, G, and B. But these sensations are not like traditional categories in which exemplars can only belong to one category. The hue elicited by some light could belong to two adjacent categories (e.g., GY). Hues shade continuously from one category to the other, which is discussed in detail by others (5,13.)

Obviously, it is important to know whether and when infants perceive the same categories. The problem is that most of the techniques that can be used in this context are either very cumbersome or require verbal responses. One early attempt with 4-month-old infants used a habituation procedure (66). Stimulus lights were cho-

sen to exemplify each of the four adult categories. After habituation to one of them, infants showed dishabituation only to stimuli from a different category; stimuli differing by the same amount in wavelength, but falling within the same category, did not elicit marked dishabituation.

Although that study was strongly criticized, mostly for choices of category boundaries and for improper control of intensity, its basic findings have been replicated recently with methods that deal with many of the criticisms (67). Again, the basic procedure was habituation-dishabituation. Stimuli were colored reflectance samples (Munsell) chosen to be equally spaced in hue, rather than wavelength, and with the same chroma (saturation) and value (brightness).

Given the findings that by 4 months of age infants have the same photopic spectral sensitivity as adults (see above), using stimuli of equal value is an acceptable answer to the intensity problem. Also, using stimuli of equal chroma avoids the confound that monochromatic (spectrally pure) lights do not appear equally saturated. The study essentially replicated the findings that within-category stimuli elicited little disabituation, even when hue separations were greater than the separations across category boundaries.

Why is Infant Color Vision Poor?

One possibility why infant color vision is poor is that the poor quality of infant color vision is more apparent than real. As we have pointed out, it is difficult to get clear-cut results from infants, especially young infants. Many of the preliminary and screening tests used with adult psychophysical observers are simply too time-consuming or impossible to use with infants. Also, infants cannot be verbally instructed to ignore some dimension (e.g., brightness) and to focus just on chromatic differences. Nonetheless, there may be real bases for why infants may have poorer color vision than adults.

Noise

A major factor is that infants have noisier, less precise visual systems. Studies that derive entire psychometric curves from individual infants and adults in the same situation typically report that infants have much shallower functions—greater variability is seen in an individual infant (29,35).

The role of noise was specifically addressed in a study that used eye movements to measure individuals' psychometric functions for luminance contrast *detection* and luminance contrast *discrimination* (68). Contrast of drifting gratings (13 cd/m^2 mean luminance) was increased to find detection threshold for DAM (see, *Behavioral Methods*); contrast discrimination was measured by pitting test gratings of various contrasts against a standard grating of fixed contrast (9.5% or 28%) to find the MN. Young infants (7-weeks of age) had much higher thresholds for detecting the gratings, but had discrimination thresholds similar to those of adults. The accepted models of where and how noise affects performance predict this outcome if infants' performance is mostly limited by intrinsic contrast noise (noise that is present whether or not the stimulus is present); fits of the model to the data suggest that infants have about 100 times more intrinsic contrast noise. Moreover, the way noise combines with the visual signal at

different contrast levels is different; in infants, the combination can be modeled as a linear process, whereas in adults it is highly nonlinear.

Finally, an often-ignored noise is contributed by the tester in FPL. Thresholds are lower when adult participants vote on their own perceptions of the stimuli compared with thresholds derived from testers' voting on their percepts of participants' orienting or eye-movement responses (35).

Poor Contrast Sensitivity

Sensitivity of infants to contrast is worse than that of adults. For example, spatial contrast sensitivity functions measured with luminance-modulated gratings show that at 4 months of age, infants' peak sensitivity is about 30 times less than the adults' peak (69). Added to this, if sensitivity to chromatic variations matures more slowly than sensitivity to intensity (luminance) variations, then infants' color vision would appear even worse.

Behaviorally, eye movements have been used with drifting gratings to measure both these contrast thresholds in the same 3-month-old infants, as well as adults (35). Chromatic gratings were composites of out-of-phase R and G gratings, each set to the same luminance based on careful preliminary measures on infants and adults. Luminance gratings were simply the in-phase additive combination of the R and G gratings and, thus, appeared Y and black; luminances were constant at about 40 cd/m^2. Threshold contrasts that elicited OKN were derived from complete psychometric curves. Infants' luminance and chromatic thresholds were considerably higher than those of adults, the exact degree depending on the technique used for the adults. The *ratios* of chromatic-to-luminance thresholds, however, were essentially the same for infants and adults (approximately 3), showing that infants' sensitivities to chromatic variations are not markedly worse than their sensitivity to luminance variations.

Visual evoked potential studies have yielded similar conclusions about the absolute sensitivities of infants and adults and about the ratios of chromatic-to-luminance thresholds (70,71). Additionally, these studies extended the range of infant ages to include 1 through 8 months.

Maturation of the Nervous System

We have already discussed the considerable maturational changes in the anatomy of the receptors and the retina in general (see *General Problems,* "Area of Retina.") We must, however, include changes in the central nervous system (72,73). Massive and prolonged changes occur, especially in the anatomy of the primary visual cortex (also know as V1, area 17, or striate cortex). Total volume increases to adult size by about 4 months. Initially, occurs a period of rapid production of synapses, which peaks between 2 and 4 months and ends at about 8 months; the changes are roughly equally distributed through all cortical layers. Synaptic proliferation is followed by an extended period, up to age 3, when synapses are eliminated. Presumably, this elimination is designed to weed out unwanted or ineffective synapses. This confers a considerable degree of plasticity on the developing cortex and allows for a *tuning* of responsivity to match visual conditions experienced by the growing child. Some 40% of the synapses are eliminated between 8 months and 11 years. Many of these unwanted synapses seem to be excitatory (74).

In the face of all these changes, it is not surprising that very young infants do not have full-blown adult color vision. The timing of the major anatomic changes also agree with the findings that infants' color vision is probably close to that of adults before the end of the first year. Note, however, that the anatomic changes continue at least until puberty, which suggests that color vision continues to change, albeit in small measure, throughout childhood.

Beyond Infancy

A detailed review of color vision across the life-span is not feasible here. Some comments, however, may help evaluate the significance of some of the issues we have discussed.

We start with VEP because this methodology is the basis for many of our conclusions about infants' vision. In a lengthy longitudinal and cross-sectional study, starting at 1 week of age, responses were recorded to the onsets of chromatic and luminance-varying gratings (61). The chromatic gratings were chosen to

stimulate preferentially, either the spectrally opponent channels associated only with L- and M-cones (Fig. 8.3A), or those that also included inputs from S-cones. Luminances were all photopic, at about 50 cd/m². Clear responses appeared between 1 and 2 months, but changed continuously throughout the first year; latencies to the first major peak in the response waveform reached adult levels between 2 and 3 months. From infancy to puberty, however, the waveforms were inverted when compared with adult responses; completely adultlike responses appeared only at about 12 to 14 years. As with the anatomic changes discussed, this long maturational sequence in the VEP suggests that color vision becomes adultlike only in the early teens.

Behavioral studies also show lengthy development. For example, a group of normal 6-year-olds, tested in an apparatus disguised as a video game, showed higher thresholds than adults for responses of both S- and L-cones isolated by chromatic adaptation, as well as for luminance-varying spatial contrast (75). Similarly, color discrimination, as measured by error rates in the Farnsworth-Munsell 100-Hue Test, improves over the ages of 5 to about 20 years (76).

A more comprehensive study, using an FPL apparatus, measured the ability to discriminate chromatic test stimuli from chromatic backgrounds across the life-span (77). Infants were tested with FPL, whereas adults responded verbally. The chromatic differences were chosen to lie along three different dichromatic axes in color space. One set would be confused by a tritanope (lacking S-cones), one by a deuteranope (lacking M-cones), and one by a protanope (lacking L-cones). A person with normal color vision, however, would discriminate along all three axes. Along all three axes, the developmental changes were the same: chromatic discrimination thresholds declined from 3 months until the minimum at about age 20 years; thresholds decreased by a factor of 2 for each doubling of age. Beyond 20 years of age, a slow increase in thresholds occurred. The similarity of the changes across the three color axes implies that chromatic mechanisms do not change with respect to each other across the life-span.

CONCLUSIONS

A variety of behavioral and physiologic methods has been developed to study infants' vision. Some behavioral methods (e.g., FPL) measure the ability of the entire organism to make a discrimination. Other behavioral methods (e.g., those based on eye movements) may tap different neuronal mechanisms, ones that do not have the same color properties as those that underlie perception. Similar problems exist with the assorted physiologic methods. Moreover, the existence of any given physiologic response does not mean that the information is available to perceptual mechanisms.

The nature of color vision in very young infants is open to a variety of interpretations. The infant is a nonverbal participant and cannot be instructed to look in a particular place nor to ignore irrelevant differences among stimuli. This raises the general problem of controlling intensity so that discriminations are based only on chromatic differences, independent of intensity. It is not easy to measure infants' photopic spectral sensitivity to obtain a starting point for equating the intensities of chromatically different stimuli.

Despite all these *caveats*, we can assert the following: Newborns can make discriminations among some chromatic stimuli, showing that they have a rudimentary form of color vision. Full-blown color vision similar to that of adults, however, is in place only by 3 to 4 months of age. By these ages, functional versions of all three cone types exist and have spectra similar to those of adults. But even then, infants' thresholds are still well above those of adults. It takes several more years to arrive finally at adult levels of color vision.

REFERENCES

1. Adams AJ. Non-invasive "dissection" of early stages of eye disease using color. In: Baldwin WR, ed. *Vision Science Symposium/A Tribute to Gordon G. Heath.* Bloomington, Indiana: Indiana University; 1988:47–67.
2. Cronin-Golomb A. Vision in Alzheimer's disease. *The Gerontologist* 1995;35:370–376.
3. Nathans J, Thomas D, Hogness DS. Molecular genetics of human color vision: the genes encoding blue, green and red pigments. *Science* 1986;232:193–202.
4. Neitz M, Neitz J. Molecular genetics and the biological basis of color vision. In: Backhaus WGK, Kliegl R,

Werner JS, eds. *Color Vision: Perspectives from Different Disciplines.* Berlin: de Gruyter; 1998:101–119.
5. Gordon J, Abramov I. Color vision. In: Goldstein EB, ed. *The Blackwell Handbook of Perception, Ch. 4.* Oxford, UK: Blackwell; 2001:92–127.
6. Hendry SHC, Reid RC. The koniocellular pathway in primate vision. *Annual Review of Neuroscience* 2000;23:127–153.
7. De Valois RL, Abramov I, Jacobs GH. Analysis of response patterns of LGN cells. *Journal of the Optical Society of America.* 1966;56:966–977.
8. Derrington AM, Krauskopf J, Lennie P. Chromatic mechanisms in lateral geniculate nucleus of macaque. *J Physiol* 1984;357:241–265.
9. Lee BB, Pokorny J, Smith VC, et al. Luminance and chromatic modulation sensitivity of macaque ganglion cells and human observers. *Journal of the Optical Society of America A* 1990;7:2223–2236.
10. Wyszecki G, Stiles W.S. *Color Science: Concepts and Methods, Quantitative Data and Formulae.* New York: Wiley; 1982.
11. Teller DY. Linking propositions. *Vision Res* 1984;24:1233–1246.
12. De Valois RL, De Valois KK. A multi-stage color model. *Vision Res* 1993;33:1053–1065.
13. Abramov I, Gordon J. Seeing unique hues. *J Opt Soc Am A*, 2005;22:2143–2153.
14. Adams RJ, Maurer D, Davis M. Newborns' discrimination of chromatic from achromatic stimuli. *J Exp Child Psychol* 1986;41:267–281.
15. Adams RJ, Maurer D, Cashin HA. The influence of stimulus size on newborns' discrimination of chromatic from achromatic stimuli. *Vision Res* 1990;30:2023–2030.
16. Teller DY. The forced-choice preferential looking procedure: a psychophysical technique for use with human infants. *Infant Behavior and Development.* 1979;2:135–153.
17. McDonald MA, Dobson V, Sebris SL, et al. The acuity card procedure: a rapid test of infant acuity. *Invest Ophthalmol Vis Sci* 1985;26:1158–1162.
18. Mercer ME, Courage ML, Adams RJ. Contrast/color card procedure: a new test of young infants' color vision. *Optom Vis Sci* 1991;68:522–532.
19. Civan AL, Teller DY, Palmer J. Infant color vision: spontaneous preferences versus novelty preferences as indicators of chromatic discrimination among suprathreshold stimuli [Abstract]. *Journal of Vision* 2003;712a. http://journal of vision.org/3/9/712/, doi:10.1167/3/9/712</misc1>.
20. Hainline L, De Bie J, Abramov I, et al. Eye movement voting: a new technique for deriving spatial contrast sensitivity. *Clinical Vision Science* 1987;2:33–44.
21. Hainline L, Abramov I. Eye movement-based measures of development of spatial contrast sensitivity in infants. *Optom Vis Sci* 1997;74:790–799.
22. Teller DY, Lindsey DT. Motion nulls for white versus isochromatic gratings in infants and adults. *J Opt Soc Am A* 1989;6:1945–1954.
23. Dobkins KR, Teller DY. Infant motion:detection (M:D) ratios for chromatically defined and luminance-defined moving stimuli. *Vision Res* 1996;36:3293–3310.
24. Knoblauch K, Bieber ML, Werner JS. M- and L-cones in early infancy: I. VEP responses to receptor-isolating stimuli at 4- and 8-weeks of age. *Vision Res* 1998;38:1753–1764.
25. Bieber ML, Knoblauch K, Werner JS. M- and L-cones in early infancy: II. Action spectra at 8 weeks of age. *Vision Res* 1998;38:1765–1773.

26. MacLeod DIA, Boynton RM. Chromaticity diagram showing cone excitation by stimuli of equal luminance. *J Opt Soc Am A Opt Image Vis Sci* 1979;69:1183–1186.
27. Riggs LA, Wooten BR. Electrical measures and psychophysical data on human vision. In: Jameson D, Hurvich LM, eds. *Handbook of Sensory Physiology.* Vol. VII/4. Berlin: Springer-Verlag; 1972:690–731.
28. Williams PE, Mechler F, Gordon J, et al. Entrainment to video displays in primary visual cortex of macaques and humans. *J Neurosci* 2004;24:8278–8288.
29. Pereverzeva M, Chien SH, Palmer J, et al. Infant photometry: are mean adult isoluminance values a sufficient approximation to individual infant values? *Vision Res* 2002;42:1639–1649.
30. Curcio CA, Allen KA, Sloan KR, et al. Distribution and morphology of human cone photoreceptors stained with anti-blue opsin. *J Comp Neurol* 1991;312:610–624.
31. Gordon J, Abramov I. Color vision in the peripheral retina. II. Hue and saturation. *J Opt Soc Am A* 1977;67:202–207.
32. Abramov I, Gordon J, Hendrickson A, et al. The retina of the newborn human infant. *Science* 1982;217:265–267.
33. Hendrickson AE, Drucker D. The development of parafoveal and midperipheral retina. *Behav Brain Res* 1992;19:21–32.
34. Yuodelis C, Hendrickson A. A qualitative and quantitative analysis of the human fovea during development. *Vision Res* 1986;26:847–855.
35. Brown AM, Lindsey DT, McSweeney EM, et al. Infant luminance and chromatic contrast sensitivity: optokinetic nystagmus data on 3-month-olds. *Vision Res* 1995;35:3145–3160.
36. Peeples DR, Teller DY. Color vision and brightness discrimination in two-month-old human infants. *Science* 1975;189:1102–1103.
37. Loop MS, Bruce LL, Petuchowski S. Cat color vision: the effect of stimulus size, shape and viewing distance. *Vision Res* 1979;19:507–513.
38. Nagy AL, Boynton RM. Large-field color naming of dichromats with rods bleached. *J Opt Soc Am A* 1979;69:1259–1265.
39. Teller DY, Bornstein M. Infant color vision and color perception. In: Salapatek P, Cohen LB, eds. *Handbook of Infant Perception.* Vol 1. New York: Academic Press; 1987;185–232.
40. Mello NK, Peterson NJ. Behavioral evidence for color discrimination in cat. *J Neurophysiol* 1964;27:324–333.
41. De Valois RL, Morgan HC, Polson MC, et al. Psychophysical studies of monkey vision. I. Macaque luminosity and color vision tests. *Vision Res* 1974;14:53–67.
42. Brown AM. Development of visual sensitivity to light and color vision in human infants: a critical review. *Vision Res* 1990;30:1159–1188.
43. Powers MK, Schneck M, Teller DY. Spectral sensitivity of human infants at absolute visual threshold. *Vision Res* 1981;21:1005–1016.
44. Fulton AB, Hansen RM. The development of scotopic sensitivity. *Invest Opthalmol Vision Sci* 2000;41:1588–1596.
45. Werner JS. Development of scotopic sensitivity and the absorption spectrum of the human ocular media. *J Opt Soc Am A* 1982;72:247–258.
46. Hansen RM, Fulton AB. Psychophysical estimates of ocular media density of human infants. *Vision Res* 1989;29:687–690.
47. Chien SH, Teller DY, Palmer J. The transition from scotopic to photopic vision in 3-month-old infants and adults: an evaluation of the rod dominance hypothesis. *Vision Res* 2000;40:3853–3871.
48. Wagner G, Boynton RM. Comparison of four methods of heterochromatic photometry. *J Opt Soc Am A* 1972;62:1508–1515.
49. Harwerth RS, Sperling HG. Effects of intense visible radiation on the increment-threshold spectral sensitivity of the rhesus monkey eye. *Vision Res* 1975;15:1193–1204.
50. Abramov I, Gordon J. Color vision in the peripheral retina. I. Spectral sensitivity. *J Opt Soc Am A* 1977;67:203–207.
51. Dobson V. Spectral sensitivity of the 2-month infant as measured by the visually evoked cortical potential. *Vision Res* 1976;16:367–374.
52. Moskowitz-Cook A. The development of photopic spectral sensitivity in human infants. *Vision Res* 1979;19:1133–1142.
53. Bieber ML, Volbrecht VJ, Werner JS. Spectral efficiency measured by heterochromatic flicker photometry is similar in human infants and adults. *Vision Res* 1995;35:1385–1392.
54. Clavadetscher JE, Brown AM, Ankrum C, et al. Spectral sensitivity and chromatic discriminations in 3- and 7-week-old infants. *J Opt Soc Am A* 1988;5:2093–2105.
55. Peeples DR, Teller DY. White-adapted spectral sensitivity in human infants. *Vision Res* 1978;18:49–53.
56. Maurer D, Lewis TL, Cavanagh P, et al. A new test of luminous efficiency for babies. *Invest Ophthalmol Vis Sci* 1989;30:297–303.
57. Adams RJ, Courage ML, Mercer ME. Systematic measurement of human neonatal color vision. *Vision Res* 1994;34:1691–1701.
58. Hamer RD, Alexander KR, Teller DY. Rayleigh discrimination in young human infants. *Vision Res* 1982;22:575–587.
59. Packer O, Hartmann EE, Teller DY. Infant color vision: the effect of test field size on Rayleigh discriminations. *Vision Res* 1984;24:1247–1260.
60. Brown AM, Teller DY. Chromatic opponency in 3-month-old human infants. *Vision Res* 1989;29:37–45.
61. Crognale MA. Development, maturation, and aging of chromatic visual pathways: VEP results. *Journal of Vision.* 2002;2:438–450.
62. Varner D, Cook JE, Schneck ME, et al. Tritan discriminations by 1- and 2-month-old human infants. *Vision Res* 1985;25:821–831.
63. Pulos E, Teller DY, Buck SL. Infant color vision: A search for short-wavelength-sensitive mechanisms by means of chromatic adaptation. *Vision Res* 1980;20:1639–1649.
64. Teller DY, Brooks TEW, Palmer J. Infant color vision: Moving tritan stimuli do not elicit directionally appropriate eye movements in 2- and 4-month-olds. *Vision Res* 1997;37:899-911.
65. Volbrecht VJ, Werner JS. Isolation of short-wavelength-sensitive cone photoreceptors in 4–6-week-old human infants. *Vision Res* 1987;27:469–478.
66. Bornstein MH, Kessen W, Weiskopf S. Color vision and hue categorization in young infants. *J Exp Psychol Hum Percept Perform* 1976;1:115–129.
67. Franklin A, Davies IRL. New evidence for infant colour categories. *Br J Exp Psychol* 2004;22:349–377.
68. Brown AM. Intrinsic contrast noise and infant visual contrast discrimination. *Vision Res* 1994;34:1947–1964.
69. Teller DY. Spatial and temporal aspects of infant color vision. *Vision Res* 1998;38:3275–3282.

70. Allen D, Banks MS, Norcia AM. Does chromatic sensitivity develop more slowly than luminance sensitivity? *Vision Res* 1993;33:2553–2562.

71. Morrone MC, Burr DC, Fiorentini A. Development of infant contrast sensitivity to chromatic stimuli. *Vision Res* 1993;33:2535–2552.

72. Huttenlocher PR, de Courten C, Garey LJ, et al. Synaptogenesis in human visual cortex-evidence for synapse elimination during normal development. *Neurosci Lett* 1982;33:247–252.

73. Huttenlocher PR, de Courten C. The development of synapses in striate cortex of man. *Human Neurobiology* 1987;61:1–9.

74. Zemon V, Eisner W, Gordon J, et al. Contrast-dependent responses in the human visual system: Childhood through adulthood. *Int J Neurosci* 1995;80:181–201.

75. Abramov I, Hainline L, Turkel J, et al. Rocket-ship psychophysics: assessing visual functioning in young children. *Invest Ophthalmol Vis Sci* 1984;25:1307–1315.

76. Roy MS, Podgor MJ, Collier B, et al. Color vision and age in a normal North American population. *Graefes Arch Clin Exp Ophthalmol* 1991;229:139–144.

77. Knoblauch K, Vital-Durand F, Barbur JL. Variation of chromatic sensitivity across the life span. *Vision Res* 2001;41:23–36.

PART 2

Evaluation of Visual Function

The Pediatric Case History

9

Robert H. Duckman and Jessica Yang

The case history is an essential collection of data for *any* health care provider. The information collected will help direct the examination. This is especially true for the visual evaluation of the pediatric patient. Depending on the information gathered during the case history, the clinician starts to formulate a list of tests that need to be done, an order in which they should be done, and even diagnosis possibilities. Of course, this presupposes that the information is accurate. In general, I find that parents tend to be very good observers, but not necessarily accurate in their observations. For example, it is commonplace to have a parent report that "Johnny's eyes cross." But when asked which one crosses, they are unsure. When parents report that an eye crosses, they should be trusted until you can prove them wrong. The clinician who is working without a "good" case history (e.g., adopted children, children in foster placements, or a child who is visiting a relative and the relative is not sure about the historical information) is at a decided disadvantage and needs to do more to rule out various diagnoses. The case history becomes the *road map* for the examination.

As with *any* other patient coming in to have their eyes examined, the single most important question in the pediatric case history, and the first one to ask, is what is the *chief complaint?* What is (are) the problem(s) that you have no-ticed and what are your (the parents[s]) concerns? That is, "what is the reason(s) you are here?" Students will usually "jump the gun" in their questioning and start asking about the pregnancy, birthweight, and so on, which are urgently important, but *not yet!* Make sure you know and understand the real or perceived problem. This single piece of information provides a starting point and a direction in which to go. And, remember, whatever happens during the examination, you must *always* come back and address the parents' primary concerns (i.e., the chief complaint). Once you have a clear picture of why the patient is in the office, you can continue with other aspects of the case history.

With children, it is best to mail the parent a patient information questionnaire, to be filled out at home by both parents and then returned *before* the examination. The reason this is a good idea is that it is difficult and time consuming to have one parent in the waiting room trying to fill out a questionnaire with the child crying or running around. At home, the parents can sit down *after* the children are asleep and respond to the questions jointly. Invariably, historical information with the joint input of both parents is more reliable, especially when more than one child is in the family and the facts can be confused so easily. Then, the history is returned to the doctor and reviewed by the doctor *before* the examination visit. By doing this, the eye care professional can see what the chief complaint is, can review the child's birth and medical history, try to come up with a group of *possible* diagnoses, and set up a strategy—a series of tests to be done and a prioritization of the order in which the tests should be done. This will maximize the very limited window of opportunity you will have when examining the child. Children, especially young ones, will attend to the testing and cooperate for a finite period of time. Once you exceed that period of time, not too much good information can be collected. If you use the beginning of the examination time with what could be a lengthy case history, you may limit how much useful time you will get with the child. Mailing a history form at the time the child is appointed and letting the parents know it is needed back *before* the examination time generally works well.

The history form mailed to the parent is best done in a checklist format whenever possible. The less you *ask* the parent to do, the more information you will get. Because many questions cannot be answered in a check-off configuration, allow space at the end of each section for the parent to annotate or explain. I used to utilize a seven-page case history where almost all the answers needed to be written and invariably, the first page was complete and each subsequent page had fewer and fewer questions answered. By the time I got to the last page, nothing was written. Changing to a check-off format history questionnaire has provided much more comprehensive information from parents on each patient.

At times when the history is mailed out, sent back to the office, and reviewed before the examination, unresolved issues remain. It may be necessary to further explore some of the information on the history at the examination visit, but it will take significantly less time than if the mail-in questionnaire had not been used. So, although fine-tuning of the history taken from the mailed questionnaire is necessary at times, it should not significantly jeopardize the examination, especially if there are appropriate stimuli in the examination room for the child. I can foresee in the very near future, putting the history form on the World Wide Web, and having parents send back an electronic history form. In this format, even the

fine tuning can be done *before* the examination date.

My personal experience in working with children is that most present for vision evaluations for a specific problem. Although the number of parents bringing in children, especially infants and toddlers, for routine visual evaluations to *make sure* everything is okay, is growing, it is still the least frequent reason that they are brought in for examination.

The most frequent reasons that parents bring infants or toddlers in for eye examination include:

1. Strabismus, real or imagined (e.g., wide epicanthal folds or pseudoesotropia)
2. Nasolacrimal duct occlusion
3. Conjunctivitis
4. Gets very close to things when looking at them
5. Consistent rubbing the eyes
6. Significant family eye history of vision problems
7. Second opinion
8. Failure on a preschool or school vision screening
9. Doing poorly in school; reading problems
10. Referred by an occupational therapist

Once you have probed the chief complaint, next direct your attention to the medical history.

THE MEDICAL HISTORY

The medical history, for the child, should be structured into three periods of time:

1. **Prenatal**—addresses the exposures during pregnancy
2. **Perinatal**—addresses the birthing of the child and associated complications
3. **Postnatal**—addresses the development of the child after birth.

All three periods are important because each provides information about risk factors or events to which the fetus or child was exposed, and the outcomes of these exposures.

Prenatal Period

The prenatal period starts with conception. Women, however, do not usually know that they are pregnant until several weeks, sometimes months, later. During this time period of *ignorance*, mothers often expose their babies to many things that are toxic and which, had they known they were pregnant, would have been eliminated from their lifestyle (e.g., smoking, drinking). It is unclear how much these toxins affect the fetus in the beginning weeks, but they can have a significant impact later on in the pregnancy.

Several types of exposure can have an effect on the pregnancy and the fetus. These include:

1. Toxic substances such as tobacco, alcohol, or drugs
2. Infectious agents such as toxoplasmosis, cytomegalovirus (CMV), syphilis, chickenpox
3. Genetic or congenital malformations such as Down syndrome, Fragile X syndrome, spina bifida, and so on
4. Metabolic disorders such as diabetes mellitus, thyroid disease, and poor maternal nutrition

Toxic Substances

The most common substances a pregnant woman exposes her unborn child to are tobacco and alcohol. These two substances, used very frequently in the United States and more frequently in other countries, are part of our lifestyle. We know that tobacco usage and alcohol endanger the viability of the fetus and most women will stop using both as soon as they learn they are pregnant. A significant time period can pass, however, before a woman is aware that she is pregnant—weeks or even months. During this time, some or a significant amount of exposure can occur to firsthand or secondhand smoke. Nicotine is a strong vasoconstrictor and decreases circulation to the fetus. Also, carbon monoxide bonds with hemoglobin to form carboxyhemoglobin, which reduces oxygen available to the fetus. What we do know about cigarette smoking and fetal development indicates that the child's physical status and developmental integrity can be significantly compromised by exposure to these toxic substances.

SMOKING AND PREGNANCY

Cigarette smoking has been shown to be harmful to the viability of pregnancy. It can lead to increased spontaneous abortion in the first trimester. In addition, the mother and fetus are at increased risk for premature placenta abruption, preterm delivery, decreased birthweight, and sudden infant death syndrome (1). Infants who are born to women who smoke during pregnancy weigh, on average, are 150 to 300 g less than those children born to nonsmokers. In addition, smoking mothers are twice as likely to have small for gestational age (SGA) babies as mothers who do not smoke (2). The effects that smoking has on fetal growth and preterm delivery increase with increasing age of the mother (3). The older the mother is, the greater the risk to the fetus is her smoking.

Cigarette smoke is known to contain carbon monoxide and nicotine (see above). These components of cigarettes seem to affect birthweight and shorten the term of the pregnancy. The chemical bonding of carbon monoxide to hemoglobin produces carboxyhemoglobin and this creates fetal hypoxia. Fetal hypoxia is associated with sudden infant death syndrome (SIDS) (4). In addition, nicotine and carbon monoxide are strong vasoconstrictors and, therefore, will cause decreased blood flow to the fetus and increase maternal blood pressure and heart rate. Cigarette smoking decreases the appetite and, therefore, can decrease the amount of nutrients consumed by the pregnant woman. Cigarette smokers are less likely to consume micronutrient supplementation and more likely to consume alcohol and other substances that negatively interact with metabolism. Many other components of cigarette smoke (e.g., lead and cadmium) could cause damage to the fetus, but the effects of these are not known.

ALCOHOL AND PREGNANCY

The worst case scenario of fetal exposure to alcohol is *fetal death*. If the fetus does survive the alcohol consumption by the mother, especially if it occurs early in the pregnancy, the child is, however, at high risk for fetal alcohol syndrome (FAS). FAS is a very significant developmental problem. The changes produced by fetal exposure to alcohol are permanent and irreversible. FAS babies are always retarded and display a myriad of physical and neurologic anomalies. Of all the causes of mental retardation, this is the most preventable form. No direct relationship exists between how much alcohol the pregnant woman consumes and the expression of FAS, but all FAS babies are born to mothers who have consumed significant amounts of alcohol during the pregnancy. It is estimated that approximately 50% of U.S. women drink socially and about half of all U.S. pregnancies are unplanned and, therefore, about 25% of all newborns have been exposed to some alcohol in early gestation (5). FAS in its *full-blown* form includes physical abnormalities of structure and size and mental retardation. The characteristics manifest in the FAS child depend on during which trimesters of pregnancy the alcohol abuse takes place. If the drinking is during all three trimesters, the expression affects the physical appearance, the physical size, and mental function. If the drinking starts in the second trimester, it usually affects only physical size and mental function with no abnormal physical features. And if the drinking is only during the third trimester, neither physical appearance nor size is affected but the mental function is. The physical findings most characteristic of babies with FAS include growth retardation for height and weight, which persists after birth by at least two standard deviations; central nervous system (CNS) dysfunction, including mental retardation, microcephaly, and hyperactivity (6). The Mayo Clinic's web page (7) reports that drinking alcohol during any part of the pregnancy will expose the fetus to risk, but the most critical period and one in which the fetus is most susceptible is the first trimester. It is known that if the mother drinks, the alcohol crosses the placenta to the fetus. Therefore, if the mother drinks, the fetus drinks. The Centers for Disease Control (8) defines FAS as the severe end of a spectrum of effects that can occur when the fetus is exposed to alcohol *in utero*. As mentioned, fetal death is the most extreme expression of this developmental anomaly. FAS is characterized by abnormal facial features, and growth and CNS problems. Stromland (9) describes FAS to include possible vision impairment and ocular anomalies affecting all parts of the eye, including optic nerve hypoplasia, coloboma of the iris, and choroid, microcornea, cataract, and others. The expression on the physical features of the face characteristic of the child with FAS include telecanthus with shortened palpebral fissures, flat philtrum, short upturned nose, epicanthal folds, and ptosis (6). These children have very significant visual anomalies. FAS, however, is now considered a spectrum disorder and great variability is seen among the signs in different children. Two other terminologies used to describe children with problems relating to prenatal alcohol exposure and are *alcohol-related neurodevelopmental disorder* (ARND) and *alcohol-related birth defects* (ARBD), which can include problems involving kidneys, heart, bones and hearing. Children with FAS and ARND can exhibit the following: poor coordination, hyperactivity, learning disabilities, developmental disabilities (e.g., speech and language delays), mental retardation or low IQ, and poor reasoning and judgment skills.

Infectious Agents

Many infectious agents can affect the fetus during pregnancy. Some of these effects are very significant, whereas others are not. All infectious agents cannot possibly be covered in this chapter. We therefore, will consider the ones that are more common and most important.

RUBELLA

Rubella, more commonly known as *German measles,* is a mild childhood viral illness that can be devastating to the fetus if the mother is infected within the first trimester. Rubella was a much more serious threat in the past because no immunization was available. Since 1969, children started receiving immunization for rubella and, since that time, no major outbreak of rubella has occurred in the United States. Cases of congenital rubella syndrome (CRS) still present clinically, however. The designation of CRS indicates significant impairment in the child, usually described as a triad including, but not limited to, congenital cataracts, deafness, and mental retardation. If the mother is infected later in the pregnancy the risk significantly decreases.

CHICKENPOX (VARICELLA) AND FIFTH DISEASE (PARVOVIRUS B19)

Relatively mild childhood viral illnesses that can harm the fetus in a pregnant woman who becomes infected include chickenpox (varicella) and fifth disease (parovirus B19). If the fetus becomes infected, it can be born with congenital varicella syndrome, which can include blindness, seizures, mental retardation, paralyzed limbs, and so on. The March of Dimes website (10) states that "a susceptible pregnant woman who is exposed to an infected household member is at about 90% risk of contracting chickenpox." They also state, however, that only about 2% of infected mothers have babies with defects caused by the virus. As with other infectious conditions, the timing of the infection is important. Women who contract the varicella virus in the first half (20 weeks) of the pregnancy face a meaningful risk of having a child with a birth defect.

Fifth disease has a similar pattern of infection and defect. Fifth disease is the fifth in a series of rash-associated childhood illness including measles, scarlet fever, rubella, and fourth disease (origin of infection is unknown). Fifth disease is caused by parvovirus B19, which can cause serious anomalies to the fetus. The most serious of these is anemia, which can be sufficiently severe to abort the pregnancy. Again, the risks are much greater if infection is in the first 20 weeks of the pregnancy and then almost no risk thereafter.

CYTOMEGALOVIRUS

Cytomegalovirus is a very common viral infection in the United States. Most people do not know they have it because no or very mild symptoms are present. It is estimated that by age 30 years, about 50% of all adults in the United States have been infected. If a pregnant woman becomes infected, she will almost always pass it on to the fetus. In some cases, this can result in very serious, possibly even life-threatening repercussions in the fetus (11,12). The range of manifestation of the cytomegaloviral infection *in utero* to the fetus can range from no involvement to death. The infected fetus may demonstrate low birthweight and deliver prematurely; neurologic involvement (seizures, microcephaly, hydrocephaly, mental retardation, developmental delay, learning disabilities) is frequently seen. Ocular findings are characteristically chorioretinal lesions, which obviously would affect visual function, dependent on the location of the lesions. The rate of intrauterine transmission of the CMV is directly related to gestational age of the fetus, with the rate of transmission increasing with increasing gestational age. Infected neonates can be born symptom-free and then develop some of the anomalies during the first 2 years.

HUMAN IMMUNODEFICIENCY VIRUS

No apparent defects are caused to the fetus of a mother who is human immunodeficiency virus positive (HIV+). A high transmission rate is seen of the virus to the infant perinatally (during delivery). Drug therapy regimens may be used to decrease rates of perinatal transmission, which can cause problems to the fetus. In the middle 1990s, zidovudine was used in cases of pregnant HIV+ mothers and the transmission rate fell from 30% to 8%. The drug is, however, known to cause significant birth defects (13).

TOXOPLASMOSIS

Toxoplasma gondii is a one-celled parasite that can sometimes cause devastating effects on the fetus if the mother becomes infected for the first time during the pregnancy. Toxoplasmosis, the disease caused by the parasite, can infect the developing fetus. It is one of a group of infections, contracted *in utero* that comprises the Torch Syndrome. TORCH is an acronym for toxoplasmosis, other agents, rubella, cytomegalovirus, and herpes simplex.

The severity of the involvement to the fetus is related to the timing of the maternal infection occurs. The earlier in the pregnancy the infection occurs, the more severe the expression of the infection (14). Toxoplasmosis can cause widespread damage to body organs such as the brain, liver, and spleen. Ocular findings include chorioretinal lesions, optic atrophy, cataract, and strabismus. The infecting agent forms cysts inside its host. These cysts remain in the host for a lifetime. Whenever the cysts rupture, a *flare-up* occurs.

Genetic and Congenital Anomalies

An almost unlimited number of genetic and congenital anomalies exist. We cannot address all, so we discuss the most common and frequently encountered in the general population. These include Down syndrome, fragile X syndrome, cerebral palsy, hydrocephalus, and spina bifida. These all have their individual ocular manifestations: refractive errors, binocular dysfunctions, and ocular disease. A thorough case history enables us to manage the visual issues facing these special children. (See Chapter 25)

Down Syndrome

Chromosomal abnormalities happen in two ways. When an error occurs during the process of cell division, it can leave either the sperm or the egg cell with more or less than the normal 23 unpaired chromosomes. Another possibility is that the cells have a normal number of chromosomes but have a section of one chromosome that is deleted, duplicated, inverted, or transposed with a part of another chromosome. Very often, the embryonic product of these unions will not survive. In fact, up to 70% of first trimester miscarriages result from chromosomal abnormalities. Of surviving fetuses, the most common chromosomal abnormality is Down syndrome, which affects about 1 of 800 to 1000 live births (15). The possibility of having a baby with Down syndrome increases with maternal age; by age 40, mothers can expect a risk of 1 in 100. Down syndrome, also called *trisomy 21*, occurs when an individual has three copies of chromosome 21.

Current medical advances have increased survival rates of children with Down syndrome, despite many physical weaknesses, such as congenital heart defects, susceptibility to pneumonia, and acute leukemia resulting from an abnormal thymus gland. It is also associated with mental retardation; however, with early intervention and special education classes, children with Down syndrome may be able to function well in society.

Children with Down syndrome are easy to recognize. They have very distinguishing features such as: short stature, thick trunk, flat nasal bridge, protruding tongue, prominent epicanthal folds, and stubby fingers.

Ocular findings include oblique palpebral fissures (16,17), prominent epicanthal folds (17), Brushfield's spots (17), iris hypoplasia (17), nasolacrimal drainage blockage (17,18), spoked vessel pattern at the optic nerve head (19), nystagmus (17,20), keratoconus (21), and cataracts (17,21,22). They often have blepharitis because of their dry skin (17). Most are hyperopic, but those with myopia have high degrees of it (9,16,17,20,23,24). Esotropia is also a common condition that affects those with Down syndrome (21,22,23).

Fragile X Syndrome

Fragile X syndrome is different from Down syndrome in that it is caused by an abnormality in a single gene and not an extra chromosome. Another difference is that it is inherited. In fact, it is the most common inherited form of mental retardation. It occurs more frequently in males than in females because it is an X-linked condition. It affects about 1 of 4000 males and 1 of 8000 females, equally in all racial and ethnic groups (25).

Children with fragile X syndrome have varying degrees of mental retardation. They often have developmental delays in all areas. Although they sometimes present with a long narrow face and large ears, they are often difficult to distinguish physically from other children.

Ocular characteristics include nystagmus, strabismus (with an equal incidence of exotropia and esotropia), accommodative insufficiency, convergence insufficiency, and no pattern of ocular health anomalies. Similar to Down syndrome, hyperopia is more common; however, those with myopia tend to manifest high refractive errors (26,27,28).

Cerebral Palsy

Cerebral palsy is caused by damage to or developmental failure of the motor areas in the brain. It can be congenital or acquired. The United Cerebral Palsy Association estimates that it affects approximately 2 of every 1000 live births. Risk factors of congenital cerebral palsy include breech birth, low Apgar scores, prematurity, nervous system malformations, infections, and maternal hyperthyroidism (29).

The four categories of cerebral palsy range from mild to severe in presentation. The ataxic type demonstrates intention tremor, decreased balance, and decreased depth perception. The athetoid or dyskinetic type shows uncontrolled, slow, writhing movements of the arms and legs. The spastic type is the most common, making up 70% to 80% of all cerebral palsy cases. This is the most severe presentation. Muscles are permanently contracted and hemiparetic tremors are present. The fourth category is the mixed type; this is usually a combination of the spastic and athetoid types. All types of cerebral palsy require physical, occupational, and speech therapy to aid in the development of motor and communication skills.

Individuals with cerebral palsy are more likely to have a hyperopic refractive error, but those who are myopic have higher refractive errors. Common ocular findings include strabismus, nystagmus, optic nerve atrophy, optic nerve colobomas, and ocular motor dysfunction. On occasion, a visual impairment may be caused by cortical defects. The more serious ocular manifestations tend to be seen in the spastic type of cerebral palsy (30).

Hydrocephalus

Cerebrospinal fluid (CSF) is a nutrient-filled fluid that surrounds the brain and spinal cord. It is produced in the ventricles, flows through the CNS, and is then absorbed into the bloodstream. Hydrocephalus occurs when CSF drainage is blocked. It can be a congenital or acquired condition and occurs in about 1 of every 500 children (31). The causes are not well defined. It can be a consequence of genetic inheritance or related to neural tube defects and prematurity. Treatment consists of the surgical placement of a shunt, which diverts the CSF to another part of the body, typically the abdominal cavity.

The most striking feature of hydrocephalus is the abnormally large head circumference. Generally, the child has a deficiency in cognitive and physical development. Many of these children benefit from rehabilitative therapies and educational assistance.

Individuals with hydrocephalus often exhibit strabismus and refractive errors. It has been found that 70% of shunt dysfunctions manifest ocular abnormalities related to increased intracranial pressure. Sudden onset of nystagmus, papilloedema, optic atrophy, or strabismus can indicate uncontrolled hydrocephalus (32,33).

Spina Bifida

Spina bifida is the result of an incomplete closure of the neural tube during pregnancy. Although it is not inherited, a child has an increased chance of acquiring the condition if it is present in a sibling. It is one of the most common serious birth defects; it occurs in about 1 of 1000 live births (34). Causes of spina bifida are not well understood; however, maternal diabetes mellitus and prenatal exposure to anticonvulsant drugs have been shown to be risk factors. Recently, it has been shown that an intake of 0.4 mg of folic acid a day can prevent 70% of these cases (35).

Three main types of spina bifida are seen, and each has a different presentation. *Spina bifida occulta* is the least disruptive of the three, and is not usually associated with any complications. The second type, *meningocele*, occurs when a cyst forms in the meninges that surround the spinal cord. This is amenable to surgical removal. The third type, *myelomeningocele*, is associated with severe neurologic problems and is oftentimes fatal. The severity of the condition depends on the location of the spinal cord defect; the higher the defect, the more severe the paralysis. Paralysis that occurs below the level of the defect is also associated with bowel and bladder problems. With current medical advances, more than 80% of these infants survive (36).

Individuals with spina bifida, as with those with hydrocephalus, often exhibit strabismus and refractive errors. Ocular findings occasionally include nystagmus, papilloedema, and optic atrophy. It has been found that 70% of shunt dysfunctions manifest ocular abnormalities related to increased intracranial pressure (32,33,37). It is important, therefore, to monitor these patients regularly with a dilated fundus examination.

Maternal Metabolic Disorders

Just as maternal infection can be passed to the fetus, the development of the fetus is affected by the maternal metabolic state. Two common conditions that affect both the pregnant woman and the fetus are hyperthyroidism and diabetes mellitus. The fetus receives all its nutrients from its mother, and so maternal nutritional intake is an important consideration of fetal health.

Thyroid Disease

Thyroid disease occurs in about 1 to 2 of every 1000 pregnancies; the most common of these is hyperthyroidism (38). Over recent years, substantial research has demonstrated the importance of maintaining normal thyroid function before and during pregnancy. Poor control has been shown to lead to decreased birthweight, mild cognitive impairment, congenital malformations, and most seriously, intrauterine death (38,39,40,41). Because thyroid disease tends to be an autoimmune condition, it is possible for maternal antibodies to cross the placental barrier and affect the fetus; however, risk of neonatal hyperthyroidism is rare. It is more likely to occur if maternal thyroid disease is poorly controlled during the pregnancy (42).

Thyroxine (T4), which is identical to the thyroxine made naturally by the maternal thyroid, is used to treat hypothyroidism; thus, it is a safe drug to take during pregnancy and breastfeeding. Hyperthyroidism is controlled by either propylthiouracil (PTU) or methimazole. Although definite contraindications for methimazole have not been specified, PTU is currently the preferred drug for pregnant women. PTU is also preferred for breastfeeding women because it has been shown that it is less likely to be excreted into breast milk (43). The infant's thyroid function should be evaluated regularly if the breastfeeding mother is on either medication.

Diabetes Mellitus

Diabetes mellitus is a disease that affects millions of Americans. During the period 1993 through 1995, the Centers for Disease control found the maternal diabetes rate to be approx-imately 25 of every 1000 women (44). It is important to understand its complications because this rate continues to increase and affect more women annually (45). Both gestational and pregestational diabetes are related to a higher frequency of congenital anomalies, cesarian sections, and future metabolic abnormalities (46). Ocular anomalies include iris vascular changes that resolve spontaneously 2 weeks after birth, and sectional optic nerve hypoplasia, also referred to as a *topless disk*, which results in long-term visual field defects with normal central vision (47–49). Encouragingly, it has been found that strict blood glucose control during pregnancy results in a significantly decreased incidence of congenital defects (50,51). Early initiation of prenatal care is essential in expectant mothers with diabetes.

Nutrition

Many changes occur in a woman's nutritional requirements when she becomes pregnant. Not only does the body undergo a multitude of physiologic modifications, it must also provide enough nutrients to nourish the fetus. Poor nutrition can lead to neonatal low birthweight (i.e., < 2500 g). To prevent this, the American College of Obstetricians and Gynecologists recommends a daily intake of

1. Four or more servings of fruits and vegetables
2. Four or more servings of whole-grain or enriched bread and cereal
3. Four or more servings of milk and milk products
4. Three or more servings of meat, poultry, fish, eggs, nuts, and dried beans and peas for protein

Most doctors advocate a daily increase in caloric consumption of about 200 to 300 kcal (52). Although some doctors suggest a multivitamin, conflicting evidence exists about whether it is more beneficial than a simple iron supplement with good eating habits (53,54). Iron is needed to form new blood cells. The fetus draws iron from the maternal supply and if insufficient amounts are in the maternal circulation, the mother can become anemic and the infant can be born prematurely with a low birth-weight (55). Two additional nutrients that have proved effective on fetal health are folic acid and vitamin D. Inadequate folic acid levels are related to premature births as well as to neural tube defects (56,57). Decreased vitamin D levels lead to reduced bone mineralization, slower growth, alterations in bone shape and increased risk of fracture, also known as *Rickett's disease* (58). For consistent and accurate findings regarding the effectiveness of other micronutrients during pregnancy, more randomized controlled clinical studies are needed.

PERINATAL PERIOD

The perinatal period, as defined by the World Health Organization, is the beginning of fetal viability at approximately 22 weeks gestational age until 7 days after birth (59). Complications during this period can cause a dramatic shock to a normally developing fetus. Conditions before the delivery that can lead to a harmful environment include pre-eclampsia or toxemia of pregnancy. At the time of the delivery, the use of forceps or suction, although helpful, can have detrimental effects. It is also important to note the incidence of a breech birth or umbilical cord complication. During pregnancy and labor, the mother is exposed to neonatal blood, which can lead to an Rh incompatibility crisis. Rh incompatibility often presents as jaundice; however, jaundice alone is commonly seen in normal infants immediately postpartum and does not always indicate a problem. If labor is extended, it might be necessary to induce the delivery or perform a cesarian section. Immediately postpartum, the child is assigned an Apgar score, which is a simple number that reveals much information about the health of the child. The score tends to be lower in low-birthweight and premature infants. Any of the previously described circumstances that are present should be elicited for a comprehensive look at a child's history.

Toxemia and Preeclampsia

Preeclampsia is a condition occurring during pregnancy, usually after 20 weeks' gestation, that includes asymptomatic hypertension, pro-teinuria, and diffuse edema. Neurologic findings (e.g., hyperreflexia and papilledema) must be watched carefully because they can be *red herrings* of eclampsia, which are seizures associated with preeclampsia. Preeclampsia occurs in approximately 6% to 8% of all pregnancies in the United States (60). Although the pathophysiology is uncertain, many risk factors have been delineated; a relative who has experienced toxemia, young maternal age, twin pregnancies, unmarried women, black women, and the presence of diabetes, hypertension, or renal disease (61). It is the second leading cause of pregnancy-related maternal deaths. If it occurs early during the pregnancy, it is related to a high perinatal mortality rate secondary to prematurity (62). Preeclampsia can lead to various fundus changes in the neonate, including: retinopathy of prematurity, vascular changes, cotton wool spots, dot and blot hemorrhages, and, rarely, optic nerve head pallor (63,64). A careful fundus evaluation of the infant will aid in the differentiation of those infants requiring more intensive care.

Forceps and Suction Delivery

Forceps are instruments used to grip a fetal head to aid in a prolonged delivery or when the fetus is malpositioned. Studies on the effectiveness and safety of their use have mixed results. For awhile, studies were showing increased morbidity. But more recent studies have shown little difference in the health of babies delivered naturally versus forceps delivery (65). The likelihood of damage caused to the neonate probably is more related to the skill of the practitioner. Forceps use is slowly becoming extinct because of medicolegal liabilities. Complications from forceps use include forceps marks, bruises and lacerations, skull fractures, facial nerve injuries, and intracranial hemorrhages. Ocular findings can range from benign to severe and can include conjunctival hemorrhage or chemosis, lid edema, hyphema, corneal abrasion, and, rarely, Purtscher's retinopathy, traumatic optic nerve injury, and choroidal rupture (66–69).

Vacuum extraction delivery with a soft cup is a gentler, more controlled alternative to forceps delivery. A carefully determined amount of pressure is applied to the fetal head to aid in the delivery. Although fewer injuries have been noted, they still do occur. The retinal hemorrhages seen tend to resolve within a few weeks. These do not seem to be associated with infant morbidity (70,71).

Breech Birth

A fetus is typically in a vertical head-down position. Occasionally, it will assume a vertical buttocks-first, or *breech*, position. This occurs approximately in 3.5% of pregnancies (72). If the fetus remains breeched beyond 36 weeks gestation, the obstetrician will attempt to shift its position. If the fetus is still breeched at the time of delivery, a cesarian section is necessary to reduce the risk of serious complications or even death (73). A planned cesarian section should be considered to avoid future visual impairments (74).

Umbilical Cord Complications

The umbilical cord contains two arteries, surrounding one vein, which connect the fetus to the placenta, thereby supplying the fetus with oxygen and nutrients and removing waste products. It is surrounded by a protective, pressure-absorbing substance called Wharton's jelly. Even with this protection, however, many types of umbilical cord complications occur relatively frequently (75). Some of these complications have no clinical significance, whereas others are severely damaging to the developing fetus. Severe defects (e.g., cardiovascular abnormalities, central nervous system defects, spina bifida, diaphragmatic hernia, hydronephrosis, dysplastic kidneys, polydactyly, and spontaneous abortion) exist in single umbilical cord arteries, velamentous insertion (incorrect insertion of the umbilical cord into the chorion), true cord knots, nuchal cord (when the cord coils around various parts of the fetal body), and cord stricture (constriction of the cord). Any of the above-mentioned anomalies can result in altered growth of neural processes, which increases the vulnerability of the fetal brain and retina during the remainder of the gestational period (76). Specific ocular anomalies noted with cord complications include exophthalmus and anophthalmus (77). As ultrasound technology improves, doctors will be able to detect these defects earlier in the pregnancy.

Rh Incompatibility and Jaundice

Rh incompatibility is the condition in which a pregnant woman with an Rh-negative blood type is exposed to Rh-positive blood cells from the fetus. This can occur during pregnancy or delivery. Once the mother is exposed, her body synthesizes anti-Rh antibodies, which can enter the fetal circulation and cause destruction of fetal blood cells. This does not usually occur in firstborns because the first maternal exposure tends to be during delivery and autosensitivity takes time to develop. The results of Rh incompatibility can range from mild to severe. The breakdown of blood cells converts hemoglobin into bilirubin, which causes the infant to become yellow, or jaundiced. In severe cases, anemia, heart failure, respiratory distress, seizures, decreased mental ability, and even death, can occur. This condition is easily prevented by Rh_0 immune globulin prophylaxis. In infants who have a history of Rh incompatibility, a higher incidence of amblyopia and strabismus has been noted (78).

Jaundice, although related to Rh incompatibility, is often seen in normal infants. At birth, liver function has not matured, leading to the accumulation of bilirubin. At times, infants with this condition are treated with phototherapy. The neonatal retina is extremely sensitive; however, with adequate shielding of the eyes during the procedure, no measurable difference is seen in retinal function of infants treated with phototherapy versus those who did not receive treatment (79,80). Without treatment, jaundice resolves within 1 to 2 weeks. Rarely, jaundice can be related to serious medical conditions other than Rh incompatibility. Some of these are galactosemia, neonatal sepsis, polycythemia, congenital hypothyroidism, cystic fibrosis, thalassemia, congenital hemolytic anemia, and congenital infections such as toxoplasmosis, syphilis, herpes, or rubella.

Induced Births

Labor induction is usually performed when the pregnancy has gone more than 2 weeks past the due date, when preeclampsia persists, in cases of a premature rupture of the membranes, or in the presence of significant maternal medical problems. Since 1989, the induced birth rate in the United States has doubled (81). Currently, about 13% of all births are induced (82). Many are concerned about these rising numbers because this process involves risks. The greatest risk in labor induction exists in the use of drugs such as cytotec (Misoprostol), prostaglandin E$_2$, (Prepidil, Cervidil, Dinoprostone), and oxytocin (Pitocin). Complications from these induction agents include (83,84).

1. Uterine hyperstimulation, which can lead to fetal distress
2. Increased likelihood of the need for a cesarian section
3. Umbilical cord prolapse, a life-threatening emergency
4. Severe maternal hypotension
5. Uteroplacental insufficiency leading to fetal hypoxia

The Apgar Score

The Apgar score is a rating ascertained at 1 minute and 5 minutes after birth. It is based on activity (muscle tone), pulse, grimace (reflex irritability), appearance (skin color), and respiration. A score above 7 generally indicates good health, whereas a score of 6 or under suggests the need for immediate care. The score does not help determine the future health or intellectual outcome of the child. A child with a low score does not necessarily develop health issues, whereas a child with serious medical conditions will always have a low score. Consequently, a low Apgar score is not invariably associated with any specific ocular condition.

Low Birthweight and Prematurity

Low birthweight refers to infants born weighing 1500 to 2499 g. Very low birthweight is a weight of 1000 to 1499 g. Extremely low birth weight is a weight of less than 1000 g. The causes can be divided into two main categories: full-term (also known as small for gestational age) or preterm. In full-term infants, low birthweight can be a result of multiple pregnancies, maternal medical problems, smoking, drug or alcohol use, low

folic acid levels, or infections during pregnancy. Preterm refers to infants born before 37 weeks' gestation.

Many systemic complications result from low birthweight. Babies born before 34 weeks' gestation are more likely to have breathing problems because of the incomplete lung development. The introduction of surfactant has greatly reduced the number of infant deaths from respiratory distress syndrome. Peri- or intraventricular hemorrhages are bleeds that occur in the brain. They usually self-resolve; however, serious cases can lead to brain damage. Some infants may present with patent ductus arteriosus, a serious heart problem, or necrotizing enterocolitis, a dangerous intestinal problem. Both of these require surgical correction.

Ocular abnormalities include optic disc atrophy, retinal hemorrhages, high refractive errors, strabismus, and oculomotor deficits (85–87). The most common of these is retinopathy of prematurity (ROP). This condition is more likely to occur at less than 32 weeks' gestation. It can either spontaneously resolve or lead to a serious condition requiring laser or cryotherapy. ROP is related to the development of myopia and strabismus (88). (For more information on ROP see Chapter 13)

POSTNATAL DEVELOPMENT

Motor Development

At birth, infants demonstrate poor motor control. The actions that they do perform are termed *generalized random movements and reflexes*. *Generalized random movements* are unorganized and involve the entire body. *Reflexes* are rapid reactive movements that are not controlled consciously. Both of these should disappear before the infant's first birthday. Controlled motor movements develop rapidly within the first year of life; these are discussed in Table 9-1. In general, an infant should be able to sit without support at 6 months, crawl at 9 months, creep at 11 months, and walk independently at 12 to 14 months (89). These are approximations, and slight delays do not always indicate that the infant is developmentally delayed. To assess whether an infant is developmentally delayed, a pediatrician performs

TABLE 9.1   Motor Development within the First Year of Life

Age (in months)	More Skill
1	Lifts head, looks and follows object moving in front of them in range of 45°; strong grasp reflex present
3	Holds chest up, grasp reflex absent, recognize faces, voices, and objects; holds objects, but does not reach for them
4	Able to roll over, tries to reach for objects but overshoots; grasps objects with both hands
5	Can support some weight; eye-hand coordination begins
6	Able to sit without support; grasps and controls small objects; holds bottle; prefers more complex visual stimuli
7	Able to crawl and stand without support, reaches for and holds objects, fixates on small objects, transfers objects from one hand to another; awareness of depth and space begin
8	Able to pull up to a standing position; picks up objects using index, fourth, and fifth fingers against thumb; begins combining syllables like "mama" and "dada," but does not attach a meaning
9	Able to sit for prolonged time; may develop a preference for use of one hand; uses thumb and index finger to pick up objects
10–11	Able to walk with assistance; says one other word besides "mama" and "dada" (hi, bye, no, go); able to manipulate objects out of tight-fitting spaces
12–13	Able to walk a few steps without assistance; attempts to build two-block tower but may fail; follows rapidly moving objects; turns pages of a book

the Denver Developmental Test, Series II. This is a screening test that evaluates several areas of development, such as personal-social, fine motor, gross motor, and language.

If a child's gross or fine motor skills are found to be delayed, that child should be referred for either occupational or physical therapy. Occupational therapy trains fine motor skills, eye-hand coordination, cognitive skills, sensory-processing deficits, and, at times, even visual perceptual skills. On the other hand, physical therapy is beneficial for gross motor skills, joint mobility, building muscle strength, and endurance. A summary of the various reasons for treatment in occupational and physical therapy are found in Table 9.2.

Speech Therapy

Speech begins with simple cooing sounds and slowly develops into complex sentences over the years. Table 9.3 provides a list of speech development norms. Some of the children coming in to see you will be having speech therapy, the reasons for it include:

1. Language problems, like difficulties with expressive vocabulary or expressive phonology (90)
2. Speech problems, for instance, pronunciation difficulties (91)
3. Cognitive problems
4. Difficulty swallowing
5. Cleft palate (92)
6. Hearing impairments
7. Generalized developmental delays (e.g., cerebral palsy, autism, and Down syndrome)

REVIEW OF SYSTEMS

Following the discussion of the medical pre-, peri-, and postnatal development of your patient, it is necessary to delve into their current health status. This is the section of the case history known as the *review of systems*. To gain an awareness of the overall health status of your patient, here we provide a checklist of items, as well as common pediatric conditions, that we consider essential in a system review.

TABLE 9.2 Reasons a Child Could be Undergoing Occupational Therapy or Physical Therapy

Occupational Therapy	Physical Therapy
Developmental delays and learning problems	Developmental delays
Sensory processing or integrative disorders	Cardiopulmonary conditions
Pervasive developmental disorders	Limb deficiencies
Mental health or behavioral problems	Orthopedic disabilities
Broken bones or other injuries	Muscle diseases
Juvenile rheumatoid arthritis	Genetic disorders
Traumatic injuries	Traumatic injuries, including head injuries
Birth injuries or birth defects	Birth injuries or birth defects
Postsurgical conditions	Postsurgical conditions
Multiple sclerosis, cerebral palsy, and other chronic illnesses	Multiple sclerosis, cerebral palsy, and other chronic illnesses

1. Allergies, including allergies to medications: Record allergens and names of medications as well as the type of reaction. Knowing medication allergies can affect the eye drops prescribed. In particular, many children have allergies to antibiotic medications such as penicillin and sulfas. Knowledge of any perennial or seasonal allergies the child has will help determine the need for any antiallergy eye medications.

2. Surgery and hospitalizations: Record dates and reasons.

3. Immunizations: Record age and type of immunizations, as well as any boosters or reactions.

4. Cardiovascular problems: Record the presence of heart murmurs or congenital heart defects. Congenital heart defects are often related to syndromic diseases, most commonly, Down syndrome and velocardiofacial syndrome. Ocular manifestations, in order of descending incidence, include retinal vascular tortuosity, optic disc hypoplasia, trichomegaly, congenital ptosis, strabismus, retinal hemorrhages, prominent eyes, and congenital cataract (93).

5. Breathing problems: A 2002 survey by the National Center for Health Statistics showed that 83 of every 1000 American children have asthma (94). Most of these children are taking inhaled steroids or beta-blockers. It is important to note that these medications in the correct dosages have been recognized as safe in terms of ocular effects (95).

6. Gastrointestinal problems: Note the presence of any diarrhea or vomiting.

TABLE 9.3 Speech Development Norms

Age	Words in Vocabulary	Number of Words in a Sentence
0–6 months	Coo-ing	None
7–12 months	First few words	None
18 months	3–5	2
24 months	10–20	2–3
30 months	300	3
3 yr	450	3–4
4 yr	1000	4–5
5 yr	–	5–6
6 yr	–	Creative sentences

7. Endocrine problems: Note the presence of insulin-dependent diabetes mellitus (IDDM), thyroid disease, or growth hormone abnormalities.

   a. Childhood IDDM is associated with a higher risk for retinopathy. It has been found that almost all individuals with childhood IDDM develop some sort of retinopathy in 20 years and almost a third have proliferative changes requiring laser treatment an average of 16 years subsequent to the diagnosis (96). Nevertheless, under the age of 12, vision screenings are not needed because of the lack of retinopathy (97).

   b. Thyroid disease is less severe in children than in adults. It manifests with lid retraction, which tends to resolve once the condition is controlled. Corneal, eye muscle, and soft tissue involvement is rare (98).

   c. It is important to perform a dilated fundus examination on children receiving growth hormone therapy, particularly if they are complaining of headaches or visual disturbances, because growth hormone therapy has been found to be linked to benign intracranial hypertension (99,100).

8. Urinary problems: Ask about pain and discomfort on urination, as well as frequency.

9. Skin problems: Inquire about rashes, excess dryness, or the presence of eczema. These conditions may be linked to blepharitis.

10. Musculoskeletal problems: Juvenile idiopathic arthritis (JIA) is associated with many cases of blindness each year because of delayed diagnoses (101). A little under one fifth of children with JIA develop anterior uveitis; of these, about one third manifests other complications (e.g., cataract, band keratopathy, glaucoma, and macular edema) (102,103). Another common affliction is keratoconjunctivitis (104).

11. Neurologic problems: Inquire about susceptibility to seizures and the presence of epilepsy. It has been shown that the translid binocular interactor (TBI) can induce seizures in those susceptible to them; use it with caution during vision therapy sessions (105).

12. Psychiatric and social problems: Ask about any behavioral problems. Attention-deficit hyperactivity disorder (ADHD) occurs in about 3% to 5% of all school-aged children (106). Oculomotor dysfunction and prolonged visual fixation are often noted with this condition (107, 108).

13. Chronic fever and unexplained weight loss or weight gain: The presence of these conditions can indicate a serious disease entity and should be referred to a primary care provider immediately.

14. Ear, nose, and throat problems: Note the presence of hearing problems, sore throats, sinus problems, or frequent colds.

15. Blood diseases: Record the presence of sickle cell or clotting disorders.

   a. The incidence of proliferative retinopathy in sickle cell anemia patients ranges from 5% to 10%, depending on the type (109). Despite this relatively low frequency of retinal pathology, it is important for these patients to receive regular eye care because other ocular anomalies are found in more than two thirds of children with sickle cell. These include conjunctival signs, retinal vascular tortuosity and dilatation, and artery/vein (AV) crossing changes (110).

16. Cancer: Note the type, treatment, and date of diagnosis. For children, the most common location for metastasis is the orbit; in such cases, a dilated fundus examination is of extreme importance (111).

17. HIV and acquired immunodeficiency syndrome (AIDS): Record treatment and current status (i.e. viral load and CD4 count). These conditions leave the patient more susceptible to ocular bacterial infections, CMV retinitis, molluscum contagiosum, macular edema, retinal hemorrhages, and sheathing of the retinal vessels (112–115).

18. Current medications: Include prior medications, when the current medications were started, and the reason they are being taken.

FAMILY OCULAR HISTORY

Because of the recent boom of gene mapping and the availability of genetic counseling, a case history would be incomplete without delving into the ocular conditions that appear in your patient's family. More than 60% of blindness in infants is caused by inherited eye diseases such as congenital cataracts, congenital glaucoma, retinal degenerations, and optic atrophy (116). Innumerable heritable eye conditions are seen, including corneal dystrophies, retinal dystrophies, ocular tumors, albinism, night vision disorders, macular diseases, choroidal dystrophies, vitreous degenerations, retinitis pigmentosa, and the phakomatoses. We will briefly discuss some of the more common inherited eye conditions, including strabismus, refractive error, color vision defects, congenital cataracts, and congenital glaucoma. Parents are sometimes unaware of the presence of some of these diseases in the family tree and so, once again, it is helpful if they are given the questionnaire before the examination date to allow them time to do a little investigating.

Strabismus

It is widely accepted that strabismus is hereditary. Recently agreed is that it is affected by multiple genes; however, no definite pattern of inheritance is found (117–121). If your patient has a first-degree relative with a strabismus, it is necessary to monitor that patient more vigorously. A higher incidence is found of similar types of strabismus but such is not always the case. For example, if a relative has esotropia, it is more likely your patient will develop esotropia versus exotropia, but not with any certainty. It is possible to develop an exotropia or no strabismus at all.

Reactive Error

The basis for the development of myopia has been at the center of many debates. It is largely agreed that it is caused by a combination of multiple genes and environmental factors such as prolonged near work and high cognitive demand (122–127). On the other hand, some believe that school-aged myopia is caused by environmental factors, whereas the early-onset high myopias are hereditary (128). It is believed that both hyperopia and astigmatism are hereditary as well, but these areas are not as intensely researched as myopia.

Color Vision

Red-green defects are the main type of inherited color vision anomalies. Such defects are found in approximately 8% of males and 0.4% of females (129). It is an X-linked condition that affects two gene loci. A female carrier has a 50/50 chance of having a male offspring who is colorblind.

It is important to determine if a child is colorblind early on because many activities in the classroom are based on colors. Some careers will have to be reconsidered (e.g., pilot, firefighter, and engineer, to name a few).

Congenital Cataracts

In contrast to age-related cataracts, which are not familial, the presence of congenital cataracts in the family must be noted. Congenital cataracts are rare and occur in about 30 of every 100,000 births in developed countries (130). Similar to refractive errors and strabismus, congenital cataracts are a consequence of multiple genes. Approximately one third of congenital cataracts are inherited, others are idiopathic or related to systemic conditions or infections (131,132). The most common form of inheritance is autosomal dominant; autosomal recessive and X-linked varieties do exist but are rare.

Congenital Glaucoma

Often confusion arises regarding the difference between infantile glaucoma and juvenile glaucoma. For our purposes, we will define *infantile glaucoma* as being present at birth or before the first birthday, whereas *juvenile glaucoma* occurs after the age of 1 year. One of the main differences is that infantile glaucoma presents with buphthalmos; it is not present in the juvenile type. Infantile glaucoma is rare and occurs in about 1 of every 12,500 newborns (133). It is inherited in the autosomal recessive fashion and only about 10% of these cases are inherited

(134,135). Juvenile glaucoma occurs even less frequently and is inherited in the autosomal-dominant fashion (135). It is imperative that both types of glaucoma be diagnosed as early as possible and referred for surgical management because they can lead to devastating visual impairments.

CONCLUSIONS

We have explored many of the things that can occur in the developing fetus, the newborn infant, and the developing child. We have traversed the pregnancy, delivered the newborn, and watched the developing human. To preserve the vision and health of the person, it is necessary to probe many different areas so that we can identify risk factors—for survival, for visual function, and for abnormal development. The sooner identification can be made, the sooner intervention can take place and the better the prognosis becomes. Destructive entities not identified can be destructive. Our job is to make sure we identify and intervene as early as possible for a visual problem or refer out as early as possible for a more global problem. A complete and thorough case history will lead the clinician in the correct direction.

REFERENCES

1. Lambers DS, Clarke KE. The maternal and fetal physiologic effects of nicotine. *Semin Perinatol* 1996;20:115–126.
2. Kramer M. Determinants of low birth weight: methodological assessment and meta-analysis. *Bull World Health Organ* 1987;65:663–737.
3. Wen SW, Goldenberg RL, Cutter GR, et al. Smoking, maternal age, fetal growth and gestational age at deliver. *Am J Obstet Gynecol* 1990;162:53–58.
4. Haustein KO. Cigarette smoking, nicotine and pregnancy. *Int J Clin Pharmacol Ther* 1999;37:417–427.
5. Marin JA, Park MM, Sutton PD. Births: preliminary data for 2001. *Natl Vital Stat Rep* 2002;50:1–20.
6. Maino DM, Maino JH, Cibis GW, et al. Ocular health anomalies in patients with developmental disabilities. In: Maino DM, ed. *Diagnosis and Management of Special Populations.* St. Louis: Mosby, 1995:193–194.
7. Mayo Clinic Staff. Fetal alcohol syndrome. The Mayo Clinic. Available at http://www.mayoclinic.com/invoke.cfm? id=DS00184. Accessed January 6, 2005.
8. National Center for Birth Defects and Developmental Disabilities. Fetal alcohol information. Center for Disease Control. Available at http://www.cdc.gov/ncbddd/fas/fasask.htm#character. Accessed January 6, 2005.
9. Stromland K. Visual impairment and ocular abnormal-

ities in children with fetal alcohol syndrome. *Addict Biol* 2004;9:153–157.
10. March of Dimes. Childhood illnesses in pregnancy: chicken pox and fifth disease. Available at http://www.marchofdimes. com/professionals/681_1185.asp. Accessed January 6, 2005.
11. Bodeus M, Hubinont C, Goubau. Increased risk of cytomegalovirus transmission in utero during gestation. *Obstet Gynecol* 1999;93:658–660.
12. Hanshaw JB. Congenital cytomegalovirus infection: a fifteen year perspective. *J Infect Dis* 1971;123:555–561.
13. Connor EM, Sperling RS, Gelber R, et al. Reduction of maternal-infant transmission of human immunodeficiency virus type I with Zidovudine treatment. *N Engl J Med* 1994;331:1173–1180.
14. Meenken C, Assies J, Van Nieuwenhuizen O, et al. Long term ocular and neurological in severe congenital toxoplasmosis. *Br J Ophthalmol* 1995;79:581–584.
15. March of Dimes. Chromosomal abnormalities. Available at http://www. marchofdimes.com/printablearticles/681_1209.asp?printable=true. Accessed January 10, 2005.
16. Haugen OH, Hovding G, Lundstrom I. Refractive development in children with Down's syndrome: a population based, longitudinal study. *Br J Ophthalmol* 2001;85:714–719.
17. da Cunha RP, Moreira JB. Ocular findings in Down's syndrome. *Am J Ophthalmol* 1996;122:236–244.
18. Coats DK, McCreery KM, Plager DA, et al. Nasolacrimal outflow drainage anomalies in Down's syndrome. *Ophthalmology* 2003;110:1437–1441.
19. Sherk MC, Williams TD. Disc vascularity in Down's syndrome. *Am J Optom Physiol Opt* 1979;56:509–511.
20. Bromham NR, Woodhouse JM, Cregg M, et al. Heart defects and ocular anomalies in children with Down's syndrome. *Br J Ophthalmol* 2002;86:1367–1368.
21. Haugen HO, Hovding G, Riise R. Ocular changes in Down syndrome. *Tidsskr Nor Laegeforen* 2004;124:186–188.
22. van Splunder J, Stilma JS, Bernsen RM, et al. Prevalence of ocular diagnoses found on screening 1539 adults with intellectual disabilities. *Ophthalmology* 2004;111:1457–1463.
23. Cregg M, Woodhouse JM, Steward RE, et al. Development of refractive error and strabismus in children with Down syndrome. *Invest Ophthalmol Vis Sci* 2003;44:1023–1030.
24. Marr JE, Halliwell-Ewen J, Fisher B, et al. Associations of high myopia in childhood. *Eye* 2001;5:70–74.
25. March of Dimes. Fragile X syndrome. Available at http://www.marchofdimes.com/printablearticles/681_9266.asp?printable=true. Accessed January 10, 2005.
26. Maino DM, Wesson M, Schlange D, et al. Optometric findings in the fragile X syndrome. *Optom Vis Sci* 1991;68:634–640.
27. Hatton DD, Buckley E, Lachiewicz A, et al. Ocular status of boys with fragile X syndrome: a prospective study. *J AAPOS* 1998;2:298–302.
28. Amin VR, Maino DM. The fragile X female: a case report of the visual, visual perceptual, and ocular health findings. *Journal of the American Optometric Association* 1995;66:290–295.
29. National Institute of Neurological Disorders and Stroke. NINDS cerebral palsy information page. Available at http://www.ninds.nih.gov/ health_and_medical/disorders/cerebral_palsy.htm. Accessed January 13, 2005.

30. McDonald E. *Treating Cerebral Palsy: For Clinicians by Clinicians.* Austin: Pro-ed, 1987.
31. National Institute of Neurological Disorders and Stroke. NINDS hydrocephalus information page. Available at http://www.ninds.nih.gov/disorders/hydrocephalus/hydrocephalus.htm. Accessed January 15, 2005.
32. Gaston H. Does the spina bifida clinic need an ophthalmologist? *Z Kinderchir* 1985;40:46–50.
33. Gaston H. Ophthalmic complications of spina bifida and hydrocephalus. *Eye* 1991;5:279–290.
34. Emedicine Consumer Health. Spina bifida. Available at http://www.emedicinehealth.com/articles/34669–1.asp. Accessed January 13, 2005.
35. National Institute of Neurological Disorders and Stroke. NINDS spina bifida information page. Available at http://www.ninds.nih.gov/disorders/spina_bifida/spina_bifida.htm. Accessed January 10, 2005.
36. Health A to Z. Spina bifida. Available at http://www.healthatoz.com/healthatoz/Atoz/ency/spina_bifida.jsp. Accessed January 10, 2005.
37. Pinello L, Bortolin C, Drigo P. Visual motor and visual defects in spina bifida. *Pediatr Med Chir* 2003;25:437–441.
38. Phoojaroenchanachai M, Sriussadaporn S, Peerapatdit T, et al. Effect of maternal hyperthyroidism during late pregnancy on the risk of neonatal low birth weight. *Clin Endocrinol (Oxf)* 2001;54:365–370.
39. Smit BJ, Kok JH, Vulsma T, et al. Neurologic development of the newborn and young child in relation to maternal thyroid function. *Acta Paediatr* 2000;89:291–295.
40. Mirabella G, Feig D, Astzalos E, et al. The effect of abnormal intrauterine thyroid hormone economies on infant cognitive abilities. *J Pediatr Endocrinol Metab* 2000;13:191–194.
41. Momotani N, Ito K, Hamada N, et al. Maternal hyperthyroidism and congenital malformations in the offspring. *Clin Endocrinol* 1984;20:695–700.
42. Brown MD. Autoimmune thyroid disease in pregnant women and their offspring. *Endocr Pract* 1996;2:53–61.
43. Bournaud C, Orgiazzi J. Antithyroid agents and embryopathies. *Ann Endocrinol (Paris)* 2003;64:366–369.
44. Center for Disease Control. Diabetes during pregnancy—United States, 1993–1995. Available at http://www.cdc.gov/reproductivehealth/mh_diabetpreg.htm. Accessed January 15, 2005.
45. Harris MI, Flegal KM, Cowie CC, et al. Prevalence of diabetes, impaired fasting glucose and impaired glucose tolerance in US adults. *Diabetes Care* 1998;21:518–524.
46. Silverman BL, Purdy LP, Metzger BE. The intrauterine environment: implications for the offspring of diabetic mothers. *Diabetes Reviews* 1996;4:21–35.
47. Ricci B, Scullica MG, Ricci F, et al. Iris vascular changes in newborns of diabetic mothers. *Ophthalmologica* 1998;212:175–177.
48. Landau K, Bajka JD, Kirchschlager BM. Topless optic disks in children of mothers with type I diabetes mellitus. *Am J Ophthalmol* 1998;125:605–611.
49. Nelson M, Lessell S, Sadun AA. Optic nerve hypoplasia and maternal diabetes mellitus. *Arch Neurol* 1986;43:20–25.
50. Kitzmiller JL, Buchana TA, Kjos S, et al. Preconception care of diabetes, congenital malformations, and spontaneous abortions. *Diabetes Care* 1996;19:514–541.
51. Sheffield JS, Butler-Koster EL, Casey BM, et al. Maternal diabetes mellitus and infant malformations. *Obstet Gynecol* 2002;100:925–930.
52. The Cleveland Clinic. Pregnancy: weight gain during pregnancy. Available at http://my.webmd.com/content/article/51/40795.htm. Accessed January 16, 2005.
53. Ramakrishnan U, Gonzales-Cossio T, Neufeld LM, et al. Multiple micronutrient supplementation during pregnancy does not lead to greater infant birth size than does iron-only supplementation: a randomized controlled trial in a semirural community in Mexico. *Am J Clin Nutr* 2003;71:720–725.
54. Vahratian A, Siega-Riz AM, Savitz DA, et al. Multivitamin use and the risk of preterm birth. *Am J Epidemiol* 2004; 160:886–892.
55. Suvacarev S. Effects of nutrition in pregnancy on hematological parameters. *Med Pregl* 2004;57:279–283.
56. Siega-Riz AM, Savitz DA, Zeisel SH, et al. Second trimester folate status and preterm birth. *Am J Obstet Gynecol* 2004;191:1851–1857.
57. Centers for Disease Control and Prevention (CDC). Spina bifida and anencephaly before and after folic acid mandate–United States, 1995–1996 and 1999–2000. *MMWR Morb Mortal Wkly Rep* 2004;53:362–365.
58. Pawley N, Bishop NJ. Prenatal and infant predictors of bone health: the influence of vitamin D. *Am J Clin Nutr* 2004;80:1748S–1751S.
59. World Health Organization, Regional Office for Europe. Promotion of effective perinatal care. Available at http://www.euro.who.int/childhealtdev/PEPC/ 20020319_1. Accessed January 16, 2005.
60. Warden M, Euerle B. Preeclampsia (toxemia of pregnancy). Emedicine. Available at http://www.emedicine.com/med/topic1905.htm. Accessed January 16, 2005.
61. Witlin AG. Counseling for women with preeclampsia or eclampsia. *Semin Perinatol* 2000;23:91–98.
62. Myatt L, Miodovnik M. Prediction of preeclampsia. *Semin Perinatol* 1999;23:45–57.
63. Sihota R, Bose S, Paul AH. The neonatal fundus in maternal toxemia. *J Pediatr Ophthalmol Strabismus* 1989;26:281–284.
64. Sihota R, Bose S, Paul AH. The neonatal fundus in maternal toxemia. *J Ophthalmic Nurs Technol* 1990;9:61–65.
65. Carmody F, Grant A, Mutch L, et al. Follow up of babies delivered in a randomized controlled comparison of vacuum extraction and forceps delivery. *Acta Obstet Gynecol Scand* 1986;65:763–766.
66. Jain IS, Singh YP, Grupta SL, et al. Ocular hazards during birth. *J Pediatr Ophthalmol Strabismus* 1980;17:14–16.
67. Khalil SK, Urso RG, Mintz-Hittner HA. Traumatic optic nerve injury occurring after forceps delivery of a term newborn. *J AAPOS* 2003;7:146–147.
68. Estafanous MF, Seeley M, Traboulsi EI. Choroidal rupture associated with forceps delivery. *Am J Ophthalmol* 2000;129: 819–820.
69. Holden R, Morsman DG, Davidek GM, et al. External ocular trauma in instrumental and normal deliveries. *Br J Obstet Gynaecol* 1992;99:132–134.
70. Lucas MJ. The role of vacuum extraction in modern obstetrics. *Clin Obstet Gynecol* 1994;37:794–805.
71. Williams MC. Vacuum-assisted delivery. *Clin Perinatol* 1995;22:933–952.

72. Baby Center. Breech birth. Available at http://www.babycenter.com/refcap/158.html. Accessed January 15, 2005.

73. Ben Aissia N, Youssef A, Said MC, et al. Breech presentation: vaginal delivery or planned caesarean section? *Tunis Med* 2004;82:425–430.

74. Tornqvist K, Kallen B. Risk factors in term children for visual impairment without a known prenatal or postnatal cause. *Paediatr Perinat Epidemiol* 2004;18:425–430.

75. Kleinschmidt R, Renziehausen K, Mattheus R. Practical significance of umbilical cord complications for the management of delivery. *Zentralbl Gynakol* 1975;97:722–728.

76. Duncan JR, Camm E, Loeliger M, et al. Effects of umbilical cord occlusion in late gestation on the ovine fetal brain and retina. *J Soc Gynecol Investig* 2004;11:369–376.

77. Morgan BLG. Umbilical cord complications. Emedicine. Available at http://www.emedicine.com/med/topic3276.htm. Accessed January 16, 2005.

78. Woodruff ME. Differential effects of various causes of deafness on the eyes, refractive errors, and vision of children. *Am J Optom Physiol Opt* 1986;63:668–675.

79. Ostrowski G, Pye SD, Laing IA. Do phototherapy hoods really protect the neonate? *Acta Paediatr* 2000;89:874–877.

80. Bhupathy K, Sethupathy R, Pildes RS, et al. Electroretinography in neonates treated with phototherapy. *Pediatrics* 1978;61:189–192.

81. Martin JA. Births: final data for 2001. *Natl Vital Stat Rep* 2002;52.

82. Harman J, Kim A. Current trends in cervical ripening and labor induction. American Family Physician. Available at http://www.aafp.org/afp/990800ap/477.html. Accessed January 16, 2005.

83. Goer H. *The Thinking Woman's Guide to a Better Birth.* New York: Perigee Books, 1999.

84. Levy H. Umbilical cord prolapse. *Obstet Gynecol* 1984;64:499–502.

85. Asproudis IC, Andronikou SK, Hotoura EA, et al. Retinopathy of prematurity and other ocular problems in premature infants weighing less than 1500 g at birth. *Eur J Ophthalmol* 2002;12:506–511.

86. Page JM, Schneeweiss S, Whyte HE, et al. Ocular sequelae in premature infants. *Pediatrics* 1993;92:787–90.

87. Newsham D, Knox PC. Oculomotor control in a group of very low birth weight (VLBW) children. *Prog Brain Res* 2002;140:483–498.

88. O'Connor AR, Stephenson T, Johnson A, et al. Long-term ophthalmic outcome of low birth weight children with and without retinopathy of prematurity. *Pediatrics* 2002;109:12–18.

89. Breckenridge ME, Murphy MN. *Growth and Development of the Young Child.* Toronto: WB Saunders Company, 1969.

90. Law J, Garrett Z, Nye C. Speech and language therapy interventions for children with primary speech and language delay or disorder. *Cochrane Database Syst Rev* 2003;3:CD004110.

91. Goorhuis-Brouwer SM, Knijff WA. Language disorders in young children: when is speech therapy recommended? *Int J Pediatr Otorhinolaryngol* 2003;67:525–529.

92. Kuehn DP, Henne LJ. Speech evaluation and treatment for patients with cleft palate. *Am J Speech Lang Pathol* 2003;12:103–109.

93. Mansour AM, Bitar FF, Traboulsi EI, et al. Ocular pathology in congenital heart disease. *Eye* 2005;19:29–34.

94. Center for Disease Control. Asthma prevalence, health care use and mortality, 2002. Available at http://www.cdc.gov/nchs/products/pubs/pubd/hestats/asthma/asthma.htm. Accessed January 15, 2005.

95. Eid NS. Update on National Asthma Education and Prevention Program: pediatric asthma treatment recommendations. *Clin Pediatr (Phila)* 2004;43:793–802.

96. Kokkonen J, Laatikainen L, van Dickhoff K, et al. Ocular complications in young adults with insulin-dependent diabetes mellitus since childhood. *Acta Paediatr* 1994;83:273–278.

97. Kristinsson JK. Diabetic retinopathy. Screening and prevention of blindness. A doctoral thesis. *Acta Ophthalmol Scand Suppl* 1997;223:1–76.

98. Gruters A. Ocular manifestations in children and adolescents with thyrotoxicosis. *Exp Clin Endocrinol Diabetes* 1999;107:S172–S174.

99. Clayton PE, Cowell CT. Safety issues in children and adolescents during growth hormone therapy—a review. *Growth Horm IGF Res* 2000;10:306–317.

100. Rogers AH, Rogers GL, Bremer DL, et al. Pseudotumor cerebri in children receiving recombinant human growth hormone. *Ophthalmology* 1999;106:1186–1190.

101. Foster CS. Diagnosis and treatment of juvenile idiopathic arthritis-associated uveitis. *Curr Opin Ophthalmol* 2003;14:395–398.

102. Vela JI, Galan A, Fernandez E, et al. Anterior uveitis and juvenile idiopathic arthritis. *Arch Soc Esp Oftalmol* 2003;78:561–565.

103. Zak M, Fledelius H, Pedersen FK. Ocular complications and visual outcome in juvenile chronic arthritis: a 25-year follow-up study. *Acta Ophthalmol Scand* 2003;81:211–215.

104. Jain V, Singh S, Sharma A. Keratonconjunctivitis sicca is not uncommon in children with juvenile rheumatoid arthritis. *Rheumatol Int* 2001;20:159–162.

105. Helveston EM, Manthey R, Ellis FD. Photo-induced convulsion after using the translid binocular interactor. *Am J Ophthalmol* 1981;92:279–281.

106. Mental Health: A Report of the Surgeon General. Children and mental health. Available at http://www.surgeongeneral.gov/library/mentalhealth/chapter3/sec4.html. Accessed January 17, 2005.

107. Munoz DP, Armstrong IT, Hampton KA, et al. Altered control of visual fixation and saccadic eye movements in attention-deficit hyperactivity disorder. *J Neurophysiol* 2003;90:503–514.

108. Mostofsky SH, Lasker AG, Cutting LE, et al. Oculomotor abnormalities in attention deficit hyperactivity disorder: a preliminary study. *Neurology* 2001;57:423–430.

109. Babalola OE, Wambebe CO. When should children and young adults with sickle cell disease be referred for eye assessment? *Afr J Med Sci* 2001;30:261–263.

110. Kaimbo Wa Kaimbo D, Ngiyulu Makuala R, Dralands L, et al. Ocular findings in children with homozygous sickle cell disease in the Democratic Republic of Congo. *Bull Soc Belge Ophtalmol* 2000;275:27–30.

111. Castillo BV Jr, Kaufman L. Pediatric tumors of the eye and orbit. *Pediatr Clin North Am* 2003;50:149–172.

112. Molyneux E. Bacterial infections in children with HIV/AIDS. *Trop Doct* 2004;34:195–198.

113. Dimantas MA, Finamor LP, Ewert V, et al. Cytomegalovirus retinitis in pediatric patients with AIDS receiving highly active antiretrovirus therapy. *Rev Assoc Med Bras* 2004;50:320–323.

114. Ikoona E, Kalyesubula I, Kawuma M. Ocular manifestations in paediatric HIV/AIDS patients in Mulago Hospital, Uganda. *Afr Health Sci* 2003;3:83–86.

115. Padhani DH, Manji KP, Mtanda AT. Ocular manifestations in children with HIV infection in Dar es Salaam, Tanzania. *Journal of Tropical Pediatrics* 2000; 46:145–148.

116. Cole Eye Institute. Inherited eye disease. Available at http://www.clevelandclinic.org/eye/patient_info/ inherited.asp. Accessed January 17, 2005.

117. Taira Y, Matsuo T, Yamane T, et al. Clinical features of comitant strabismus related to family history of strabismus or abnormalities in pregnancy and delivery. *Jpn J Ophthalmol* 2003;47:208–213.

118. Abrahamsson M, Magnusson G, Sjostrand J. Inheritance of strabismus and the gain of using heredity to determine populations at risk of developing strabismus. *Acta Ophthalmol Scand* 1999;77:653–657.

119. Paul TO, Hardage LK. The heritability of strabismus. *Ophthalmic Genet* 1994;15:1–18.

120. Mvogo CE, Ellong A, Bella-Hiag AL, et al. Hereditary factors in strabismus. *Sante* 2001;11:237–239.

121. Lorenz B. Genetics of isolated and syndromic strabismus: facts and perspectives. *Strabismus* 2002;10: 147–156.

122. Gilmartin B. Myopia: precedents for research in the twenty-first century. *Clin Exp Ophthalmol* 2004;32: 305–324.

123. Hammond CJ, Snieder H, Gilbert CE, et al. Genes and environment in refractive error: the twin eye study. *Invest Ophthalmol Vis Sci* 2001;42:1232–1236.

124. Zhan MZ, Saw SM, Hong RZ, et al. Refractive errors in Singapore and Xiamen, China—a comparative study in school children aged 6 to 7 years. *Optom Vis Sci* 2000;77:302–308.

125. Morgan I, Rose K. How genetic is school myopia? *Prog Retin Eye Res* 2005;24:1–38.

126. Farbrother JE, Kirov G, Owen MJ, et al. Linkage analysis of the genetic loci for high myopia on 18p, 12q, and 17q in 51 U.K. families. *Invest Ophthalmol Vis Sci* 2004;45:2879–2885.

127. Lam CS, Goldschmidt E, Edwards MH. Prevalence of myopia in local and international schools in Hong Kong. *Optom Vis Sci* 2004;81:317–322.

128. Ibay G, Doan B, Reider L, et al. Candidate high myopia loci on chromosomes 18p and 12q do not play a major role in susceptibility to common myopia. *BMC Med Genet* 2004;5:20.

129. St. Luke's Eye. Color blindness. Available at www. stlukeseye.com/conditions/colorblindness.asp. Accessed January 20, 2005.

130. Graw J. Congenital hereditary cataracts. *Int J Dev Biol* 2004;48:1031–1044.

131. Beby F, Morle L, Michon L, et al. The genetics of hereditary cataract. *J Fr Ophtalmol* 2003;26:400–408.

132. Rahi JS, Dezateux C. Congenital and infantile cataract in the United Kingdom: underlying or associated factors. British Congenital Cataract Interest Group. *Invest Ophthalmol Vis Sci* 2000;41:2108–2114.

133. Merin S, Morin D. Heredity of congenital glaucoma. *Br J Ophthalmol* 1972;56:414–417.

134. Kipp MA. Childhood glaucoma. *Pediatr Clin North Am* 2003;50:89–104.

135. Weisschuh N, Schiefer U. Progress in the genetics of glaucoma. *Dev Ophthalmol* 2003;37:83–93.

10 Infant, Toddler, and Children's Visual Acuity—Practical Aspects

Robert H. Duckman

Visual acuity is a clinical test that gives the clinician insights into the child's visual status. It is usually a reflection of the individual's visual function (i.e., if the acuity is normal or better, it can almost always be inferred that the patient is doing well visually). When the visual acuity is decreased, it alerts the clinician to the likelihood that some anomalous condition (e.g., pathology, refractive error, or binocular problems) is present. Of course, it is possible to have normal acuity and still have a serious problem with the eyes. Visual acuity, therefore, is only one clinical finding that can aid the clinician's strategy in the examination. Visual acuity helps in decision-making and therapy choices. When the visual acuity is lower than expected, the clinician spends much of the examination attempting to find the reason acuity is down and then trying to bring it up to expected levels. This is an important part of a vision examination whether examining an adult or a child. The difficulty lies in the fact that obtaining a visual acuity measure on a young child (birth to 5 or 6 years of age) is much more challenging than obtaining a visual acuity measure on older patients. In the early 1960s, few real ways existed to accurately quantify visual acuity in preverbal children. About the only clinical tool was the optokinetic drum. It provided some information about visual function, but nothing that was quantifiable or that could be used to gauge improvement in tracking acuity in an amblyopic eye. Now, we know that optokinetic nystagmus (OKN) (Chapter 2)

is mediated subcortically and provides little to no information about cortical visual function.

As we saw earlier (Chapter 2), visual acuity in the infant or toddler patient is not equal to an adult's acuity. This can be reconciled by the immature development of the macula and the visual cortex, and the incomplete myelinization of the visual pathways (Chapter 1). As the visual system matures, visual acuity improves and approaches the adult's level. The point at which the child's visual acuity responses reach adult levels depends on many things. The primary and most important factor, however, is the measurement tool used to quantify acuity. Different tools produce significantly different results in the measurement of acuity in children.

Visual acuity can be a critical clinical finding in children. The young child, with or without specific and as yet unidentified visual anomalies (e.g., anisometropia or strabismus), often develops amblyopia. If amblyopia is identified sufficiently early, treatment is usually prescribed. Without a reliable visual acuity measurement each time the child comes in, it is difficult to tell whether treatment is effecting change, if it is effective, and if it should be continued.

Until the 1970s, little could be done to measure acuity in preverbal children. Part of the reason for this is that up to that time, it was generally believed that infants, toddlers, and preschoolers did not have normal function and that adult function was not possible before age 5 years. Most practitioners told their patients with children that they should wait until the child was 5 years of age to have a visual examination. As the understanding of the development of the visual system became clearer through the efforts of psychophysicists and vision researchers in the 1970s and onward, it became clear that the visual system of the young child was *much* more sophisticated than people had been willing to admit. It also became clear that when a visual problem existed, it responded better to therapy (e.g., patching) the earlier it was applied. We know today that early rather than late intervention offers greater promise to the restoration of normal visual function of an eye with a functional problem.

It is our responsibility, therefore, to encourage parents to bring children in for eye examinations as early as possible and to identify and treat problems that could cause eventual loss of visual function (e.g., amblyopia in refractive anisometropia). In many cases of anisometropia, rarely are signs or symptoms seen of a visual problem. The parent assumes the child can see normally. When the child enters school and has a vision examination, however, a very significant difference is seen in acuity between the two eyes. By this time, the child may be 5 or 6 years of age and has 20/20 in one eye and 20/400 in the other eye. It is not too late to apply patching therapy at this point and improve acuity, but it will be more difficult and have a more guarded prognosis. One reason is age; another significant reason is that it is difficult for a school child to wear a patch in class. The child receives a lot of ridicule and become the brunt of a lot of teasing. So had the child in this example been tested at 6 months, it would have been easier to patch and to improve the visual acuity in the eye with the greater refractive error. It is not impossible to take the child described above and achieve improvement later on, but it will be more difficult and improvement will be slower. The child with anisometropia that is not corrected with lenses or not given a patching regimen can eventually sustain irreversible loss of visual function.

As mentioned in Chapter 2, the best acuity measurement is a recognition acuity. Obviously, an infant or toddler cannot sit and read letters, pictures, or numbers from an eye chart. Therefore, it is not possible to get a recognition acuity on these patients. Using electro-physiologic or behavioral techniques, however, the clinician may be able to obtain a threshold minimum separable acuity. This, therefore, is the best we can do with children who are very young or who cannot respond verbally or motorically, as in a matching task. These techniques, however, are certainly sufficiently sensitive to measure improvement in an amblyopic eye or ascertain the difference in acuity with the application of lenses in a child with refractive error. Because acuity age norms have been established for visually evoked potentials (VEP) (see Chapter 2) and forced-choice preferential looking (FPL) (see Chapter 2), it is possible, on repeated measures, to determine if the child's visual development is proceeding in a normal pattern.

What is the difference between VEP measurement and FPL? As mentioned in Chapter 2, VEP has advantages and disadvantages when compared with FPL. VEP is faster and, therefore, more reliable. The main factor in dealing with very young children is maintaining their interest in the task. Because the VEP acuity test requires less time, especially if a sweep VEP is used, it is more likely that the child will be able to attend for the duration of the test. FPL techniques take significantly longer to do and, therefore, may become less reliable as attention wanes with continued presentations. As an aside, I find that many young patients respond robustly to the FPL cards and then suddenly, as if deciding "this is enough," they no longer attend. When there is no clear decrease in responsiveness, but rather only an all or nothing type of response, I refer to these acuity values as "minimal visual acuity" and not threshold visual acuity. The VEP measures the electrophysiologic response of patterns of light into the eye and up to the level of the visual cortex. This test, therefore, can provide valuable information about the intactness of the visual system from the eye to the visual cortex, but it says nothing about visual processing beyond the cortex. It gives no information about what the individual child is *actually* seeing—just the limits of the child's *potential* to see. The biggest disadvantage of the VEP procedure is that the instrumentation is very expensive and if the practitioner does not need to do a lot of these procedures, it is unlikely to find its way into the practice.

The advantages of the FPL procedure are (a) it is the clearest indication of what the patient can actually see of any of the techniques available; (b) the spatial frequencies available cover a very wide range of minimum separable visual acuity values (20/2400 to 20/10); and (c) it is easier to administer and is portable so it can easily be moved around. Of course, disadvantages are seen as well. The most significant one is the extended period of time it takes to administer. No matter how streamlined the task is made, it is extremely difficult to get three measurements (OD, OS, OU) in a single testing session. Infants may like stripes, but not that much. My preference is to test acuity first because it probably demands the greatest attention. If no reason exists to suspect that one eye is seeing less well than the other (e.g., in constant right esotropia, concern would exist that the right eye is seeing less well than the left and a monocular right eye acuity test would be done first) and with no historical information suggesting an interocular difference in acuity, then I would first measure binocular acuity. Children having this procedure often get extremely upset when a patch is placed on their eye. If they do get upset, the child may not ever continue. If you start with a binocular visual acuity test, however, you will very likely get a visual acuity value. This will allow you to assess whether the acuity development is normal for the child's age. At this point, if you wish, you can attempt monocular acuity measurements. I prefer to let the monocular measurements "sit until needed." If, on the other hand, the child comes in with a constant right esotropia present since 3 months of age, my biggest concern is to get the monocular right eye acuity. In this case, I will put the patch on the left eye and proceed with the Teller acuity cards (TAC). This may likely upset the child, but, in this case, it is essential to find out what the acuity in the right eye is to determine how to manage the child's care. A binocular acuity value in this case tells *nothing* about the deprived right eye. So, if no reason is seen to suspect a difference in acuity between the eyes, start with a binocular condition. When there is concern about an interocular acuity difference, do the *deprived* eye first. When the binocular acuity is normal for the child's age, continue with the rest of the examination. If during the examination, you uncover an amblyogenic factor (e.g., refraction = OD −7.00 Sph OS Plano) that was not obvious before the examination, it becomes urgently important to go back and measure the visual acuity in the deprived eye (in this case, the right eye). In measuring the deprived eye acuity, the refractive correction should be applied in a trial frame. (By far the best infant, toddler, and even pediatric trial frame that I have come across is the product Solo Bambini by Occhialino di Prova seen in Fig. 10.1.

If the child objects to the patching and becomes behaviorally difficult, set up another appointment to measure the right eye acuity. It is a good idea to have the child wear a patch for 5 to 10 minutes at home each day on the nondeprived eye until the next visit. This to accustom the youngster to experiencing the patch in a "safe" environment. Testing is best done about

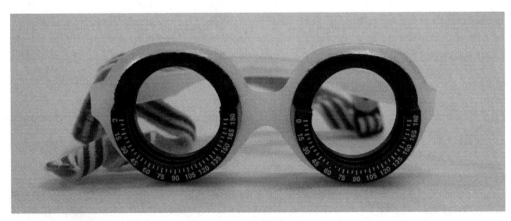

FIGURE 10.1. The Solo Bambini Baby 2 Trial Frame by Occhialino di Prova.

30 minutes after feeding or napping. The worst time to attempt to examine an infant or toddler is while they would normally be napping or when they are hungry. Appointments should be made accordingly. On the return visit, first attempt quantification of the visual acuity of the deprived eye. Once this is done in conjunction with the previous findings, a treatment plan can be formulated. For the kind of lenses to prescribe, see Chapter 20.

It is important when testing FPL to use the most expedient methodology so that it takes the least amount of time. My preference is to use a modified "staircase" presentation. In this procedure, the spatial frequencies are presented from lowest to highest cycles per degree (cpd). Rather than starting from the lowest spatial frequency, however, I start at the expected acuity card diagnostic stripe width for the child's age, then present higher and higher spatial frequency cards until reaching threshold or losing attention. Of course, if the child cannot perform at the age-appropriate diagnostic stripe width, decrease spatial frequency until a response is elicited.

Another methodology referred to as *diagnostic stripe width* (DSW) is available (see Chapter 2). As an example, if the child is 6 months of age, the DSW is equal to minimum separable acuity of 20/100 (ca. 6.5 cpd). The clinician would then show the child the card corresponding to 6.5 cpd at the utilized test distance ten or more times. If the child correctly looks to the stripes 70% of the time or greater, the child has developed to the expected acuity for that child's age. This is not necessarily a threshold acuity value and a statement cannot be made about the child's *best* possible visual acuity. What can be said, however, and in a relatively short period of time, is that this child's visual acuity development is normal (1,2). (If the child cannot demonstrate DSW, it would be in everyone's best interest to find out what the child's visual acuity threshold is and why.)

FPL using TAC or any other type of presentation takes a degree of practice to get comfortable with the technique. It is very easy to make the observations about the patient's fixations when you are well above threshold. As the clinician approaches threshold acuity, however, the observations become increasingly more difficult to make. Judgments about which side the stimulus is on in the FPL procedure should be made on the basis of

1. First fixation
2. Relative interest in the stimulus
3. How much time the child fixates one side over the other

Judgments should be practiced to take into consideration all possible subtleties. Understand, the child has a 50/50 chance of looking to the correct side. When the child does fixate to the right or left side, however, make sure the child is fixating the stimulus and not, for example, part of a hand that is holding the card or a toy off to the side of the stimulus presentation. Again, these observations are easy to make when you are well above threshold, but become increasingly more difficult as you reach the child's visual acuity threshold.

TELLER VISUAL ACUITY CARDS

Teller acuity cards (TAC) (Fig. 10.2) are recommended to test visual acuity in infants from birth to approximately 1 year of age. The cards and the procedure "top out" at about 12 months because, by this point in development, children are too fascinated with the world around them to be enamored with spatial frequency gratings. It therefore becomes necessary to look for other instruments to measure visual acuity. This is an extremely important time for the infant in terms of visual development, because it is a time when abnormal visual experience can have a very large impact on normal visual development. If, for example, the child has an amblyopic eye and therapy is being applied (e.g., patching), make sure the visual acuity is improving over time. A reliable tool is needed with which to measure visual acuity across time. If acuity is measured in

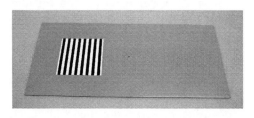

FIGURE 10.2. Teller acuity cards (Precision Vision).

an amblyopic eye when the infant is 6 months of age and is shown to be below normal while the partner eye is normal, you may want to initiate a patching regimen. Recheck the child and monitor acuity 1 to 2 months later. At the recheck visit, if visual acuity has improved, but is still below the paired opposite eye, continue with the patching regimen. Continue this for several more visits, until the child is 16 months old. Although all earlier measurements were done with TAC, the child will now no longer attend to them. The child's acuity, on whatever instrument you now use to measure acuity, cannot be equated to the acuity measurements obtained with the FPL procedure. Monocular acuities can be taken with a new visual acuity procedure and by comparing the previously normal eye with the previously amblyopic eye. One cannot say that the amblyopic eye has changed when comparing one measurement procedure with the other.

As mentioned, the TAC produce their best results when used on a population of normal infants from birth to approximately 1 year of age. It has also been used on children with developmental disabilities. Duckman and Selenow (3) found that this procedure could be used very effectively, almost without limitation on age, on neurologically impaired children. Jacobsen et al. (4) found that when the TAC were used to measure acuity of mentally retarded children, they were effective and there was good test–retest reliability.

In the ancient history of visual development research (1980), FPL was "born." Initially, the targets were very difficult to make because the presentations were made by rear-projecting spatial frequency slides against high optical transmission material such as Polacoat. The striped slide projections were matched for mean luminance with the gray slides. At the end of the procedure, therefore, a spatial visual acuity (minimum separable) would have been obtained. The last spatial frequency the infant was able to achieve, at the criterion level of 75%, becomes the visual acuity threshold for the FPL procedure. Later in the decade, Vistech Corporation, with Davida Teller, achieved a set of cards, commercially produced, which had the background gray of the card match the mean luminance of the stimulus' spatial frequency. These cards

are now considered an important clinical tool utilized throughout the country and the world. The cards have recently been plasticized, have slightly lower contrast, and need to be recalibrated. The overall utility of the cards, however, is sound and reliable. Although TAC are useful for infants from birth to about 12 months of age, age range can be extended if the child understands the instructional set "look at or point to the lines." Sometimes it is very important to get a visual acuity on a child because of expected or known amblyopia. If the child cannot respond to looking at or pointing to the stripes, it is reasonable to attempt a conditioned FPL paradigm. In this procedure, the child is conditioned, through positive reinforcement schedules, to look at or point to the stripes. It is difficult to do, but if it works, a threshold visual acuity can be obtained on the amblyopic and nondeprived eye. By the time the child is about 2.5 years of age, it should be possible to capture recognition acuities on one of the available charts.

FORCED-CHOICE PREFERENTIAL LOOKING PADDLE ACUITY

Teller acuity cards are a reliable clinical tool that is used both in clinical and laboratory settings. The TAC, however, are relatively expensive (approximately $3000) and clinicians often find it difficult to justify spending that much money on the occasional infant they see in their practices. Therefore, "budget" versions of FPL acuity testing have emerged in the form of spatial frequency paddles (approximately $200).

Several companies produce these paddles (Fig. 10.3). The paddles are calibrated for a

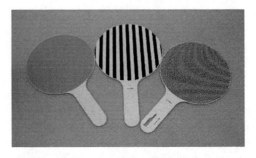

FIGURE 10.3. Spatial frequency paddles for visual acuity testing in young children.

specific distance, (usually 1 m), although with a little mathematic calculation they can be presented at any distance. The sets usually consist of four paddles and six different spatial frequencies. Each of three paddles has a different spatial frequency on each side. The fourth paddle has the luminance-matched, homogenous gray field on it. The procedure is to hold the gray over one of the spatial frequencies. Then, when the infant is attending, separate the paddles and see if the child's fixation moves with the stripes. The procedure works fairly well, but at least two problems exist with this format:

1. When introducing movement into the procedure, the child might be following the movement of the stripes without being able to resolve them.
2. Only six spatial frequencies are available, making threshold acuity impossible to achieve (i.e., without modification of the recommended procedure).

Despite these problems, this is a reasonable way to get some information on a baby's visual function in a clinical setting where purchase of a full set of TAC is not justified.

VISUALLY EVOKED POTENTIALS

Another methodology used to measure visual function in a young child is the *visually evoked potentials* (VEP) procedure. Two methods can be used for this technique: flash VEP and patterned VEP. The flash VEP is usually used with very young children or children who are incapable of fixating a target. No real attention is needed for this procedure and it can be done through closed eyes, even with the child sleeping. The stimulus is a stroboscopic light that is placed near the eye. The light from the strobe will pass through the lid and stimulate the retina. This, in turn, will create electrophysiologic responses at the level of the retinal receptor cells and then be transduced along the optic pathways to the visual cortex. This technique will confirm the integrity of the pathways, but it tells nothing about visual acuity. To get a visual acuity value from this technique—and again we have to settle for a minimum separable visual acuity—it is necessary to use a stimulus with minimum separable units (e.g., spatial frequency stripes or, more commonly, checkerboard squares). To get VEP responses, the patterns have to be phase-alternated at specific frequencies. The elements of the stimuli are presented at various angular subtenses to see what the smallest element is which gives a positive VEP response (see Chapter 2). As mentioned, the VEP equipment is very expensive. It, however, provides potential threshold minimum separable visual acuity in a relatively short period of time.

CARDIFF CARDS

The Cardiff cards represent a tool that can be used to measure visual acuity in children from 1 to 3 years of age, according to the manufacturer. The principle is similar to TAC in that it is expected that as long as the child can see the optotype (line drawings of pictures), the child will show a preference for the picture as compared with the plain gray background. The black and white lines forming the pictures become finer with each set of three cards, until the picture cannot be seen (vanishing optotype) and the preference for fixation to the picture is lost. The pictures are presented on cards with the optotype appearing either on the top or the bottom of the card. The rest of the card is a homogenous gray that matches the mean luminance of the picture. Each acuity equivalence value consists of three cards. Note, only a *minimum separable acuity* will be obtained, but the optotypes presented on each card are equated to Snellen acuity values. A total of 11 sets of cards are available, with acuity values ranging from 20/400 down to 20/20, which have been calibrated for two presentation distances—0.5 m and 1.0 m (Fig. 10.4). The patient is presented with one set of cards at a particular acuity equivalence, one card at a time. By observing the child's eye movements and fixations, the examiner must decide if the optotype is on the top or bottom of the card. If the examiner chooses correctly at least 75% of the time, then go to the next finer line drawings. This continues until the examiner correctly identifies the side of the card that the picture is on less than 75% of the time. At this point, the last *correct* (75% or better) set of responses is considered to be the child's

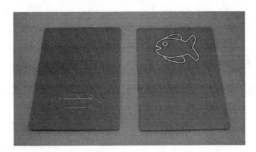

FIGURE 10.4. Cardiff cards: lower spatial frequency on the right and higher spatial frequency on the left.

visual acuity. Cardiff cards are an excellent way to determine minimum separable acuity in a child 1 to 3 years of age, *unless* that child can respond to a recognition acuity chart. It is not unusual today to find children 2 to 3 years of age who can respond in some way (either by naming or matching) to recognition optotypes, whether it be pictures, numbers, or even letters. When the child is capable of doing this, it is preferable to utilize this latter acuity type test.

As with the TAC, fixations to the pictures on the Cardiff cards are relatively easy to assess. It becomes more difficult as threshold is approached. Using the cards held horizontally instead of vertically, as intended by the manufacturer (Keeler, UK), makes the fixations easier to judge, especially as threshold is approached. If the pictures are rotated 90°, they will have the same angular subtense, but the child will be making horizontal rather than vertical eye movements. As with the TAC, attention is an important component of this methodology and must be considered when assessing acuity. If the child loses attention during the testing and becomes uncooperative, it is unlikely that a threshold will be reached, although a *minimal* visual acuity value can be obtained. The pictures seem to capture the child's attention well. If a child is not interested in "fixating" the target, ask the child to point to it. This often will get the child more *into* the task and, possibly, more responsive.

Depending on the entering chief complaint, it may be better to use the Cardiff cards binocularly before attempting monocular acuities. Adoh and Woodhouse (5) found in measuring monocular and binocular acuity with children from 12 to 36 months of age that their rate of

successfully measuring visual acuity binocularly ranged from 96% to 100%, but fell to a rate of 41% to 91% for monocular testing. They further presented age norms on the test so it could be used as a clinical tool to measure acuity in toddlers between 12 and 36 months of age.

BROKEN WHEEL CARDS

Broken wheel cards is another means of obtaining a subjective visual acuity on toddlers and preschoolers who are not yet capable of giving subjective responses or performing a matching task. They are also extremely useful in vision testing children with special needs.

The broken wheel cards are a set of seven matched pairs of cards (acuity values ranging from 20/20 to 20/100 when held at 10 feet) (Fig. 10.5) presented in a forced-choice paradigm without the need for verbal responses. Each pair of cards consists of line drawings of a matched-sized car on each, but on one car the wheels are closed circles and on the other car the wheels are broken circles (essentially embedded Landolt Cs). cards are presented at and calibrated for 10 feet. The visual acuity tester holds up one pair of cards at a time and asks the child to "point to the car with the broken wheels." The examiner notes if the response is correct, "mixes" them up and makes another presentation. It is better if the tester does not know where the car with broken wheels is until after the child responds. The child must achieve a success rate of four of four responses to say that an acuity level has been achieved. If the child correctly gets four of four, the next smaller set of cards is utilized. This continues, using smaller and smaller cars, until the child can no longer consistently identify the car with the broken wheels. Richman et al. (6) contend that the broken wheel acuity test is an easily administered test of visual acuity for preschool and exceptional children. Their data indicated that the broken wheel and Snellen tests are highly correlated and that acuities measured with broken wheel cards is equivalent to the Snellen chart with letters if using the four-of-four criterion to achieve a certainty of at least 94%.

The instructions for the use of the broken wheel cards suggests a practice run with the child with the 20/100 card presented at 50 cm

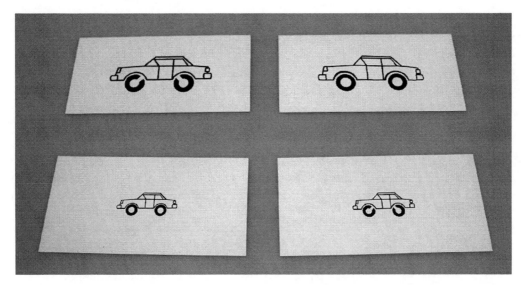

FIGURE 10.5. Broken wheel cards: Note the breaks in the wheels are embedded in the chassis of the car for contour interaction.

to teach or check that the child can do the task. To maximize time they also suggest that the test is started with the smallest optotypes first and worked back, testing binocularly first and then monocularly. Richman et al. showed that testability was greater than 90% and practice, binocular, and monocular acuities were obtained in 5 to 7 minutes. McDonald and Chaudry (7) compared four methods of assessing visual acuity in young children. These included (a) TAC (minimum separable); (b) Dot Visual Acuity Tester (detection acuity); (c) broken wheel cards (minimum separable acuity); and (d) American Optical Pictures (a recognition acuity). Their data showed the acuity cards were most useful for 2 year olds, while the broken wheel cards were best for testing 3 year olds.

LEA SYMBOLS TESTS

Lea Hyvarinen, a Finnish pediatric ophthalmologist, developed a vast array of testing devices that have been standardized using four pictures—circle, square, house, and apple—to evaluate visual function in young children. These are four symbols that have been carefully calibrated at first against the Snellen Illiterate E chart and later against the Landolt C chart as required by the International Commission for Optics (ICO) Standard. These optotypes can be presented as single characters, as a wall chart at a distance of 10 feet to 20 feet. They can be presented on a video display terminal (VDT) screen or as single optotypes in a flip book. The earliest set of symbols was created by Hyvarinen et al. (8) in 1976 and calibrated against the Snellen E chart, the reference optotype of the time. The size of the 1.0 symbols (6/6, 20/20) were found to be 7.5 minutes of arc. When the Landolt C became the reference optotype in 1988, the symbols were tested against it and a reduction of the size of the symbol optotypes was found to be necessary. The size of the 1.0 (20/20, 6/6) optotypes was reduced from 7.5 to 6.84 minutes of arc. When the generation of symbols was taken over by the computer in late 1993, edge quality improved and the optotypes had to be recalibrated again. During this particular recalibration, improvement in edge quality was found to be greater for the square than for the other figures, so each symbol had to be calibrated independently against the Landolt C.

The Lea symbols (Fig. 10.6) now have the two important basic features of good optotypes; they blur equally and are calibrated against the Landolt C (the reference optotype). Hyvarinen went on to develop Lea numbers in 1993 and had them calibrated by 1994. She felt numbers were a good way of testing individuals who did not use the Western alphabet.

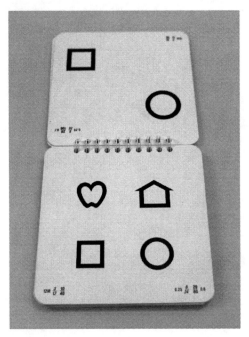

FIGURE 10.6. Lea symbols book of calibrated acuity cards. Although not shown, it comes with a template for isolation of symbols.

Today, Lea symbols are available in many different formats so that children can be tested at distance and near, logarithm of the **m**inimum **a**ngle of **r**esolution (LogMAR) or non-LogMAR presentations, verbal or matching (nonverbal) testing response formats, isolated, whole line, whole chart (folding or nonfolding), surrounded (crowding effect) optotypes, and so on. These various formats allow the clinician many different ways to obtain clinical data on children.

Depending on chronologic or developmental age, different tests or testing strategies should be used. Recommendations are

1. 18–36 months: Use the three-dimensional symbols, key cards, or flash cards to get the child familiarized with the forms and then use the "single figure book" to test distance acuity.

2. 36–48 months: Use the three-dimensional symbols, the key card, or flashcards for familiarization. At this age, the nine-line distance chart should be used to test distance acuity and the near card should be used for near acuity.

3. 60–72 months: Use the 14-line distance chart for distance acuity and the near card for near acuity.

4. 72–84 months: Use letter charts for most children in this age category. If they do not know their letters, use the 14-line symbol chart for distance and the near card at close working distance.

Although not discussed here, other charts are available that utilize Lea symbols to evaluate contrast sensitivity function.

Shallo-Hoffmann et al. (9) examined whether differences existed between the results of the HOTV test and the Lea symbols test of distance visual acuities in children 3 to 5 years of age. They found that sensitivity, specificity, and accuracy were high at 100%, 79%, and 80%, respectively. They found that children 3 years of age were more likely to finish testing when Lea symbols were utilized than when HOTV letter optotypes were used. They also found that testability varies with age rather than on which test is utilized so long as socioeconomic factors are held constant. The Vision in Preschoolers Study Group (10) also compared the HOTV (this time with crowded optotypes) with Lea symbols acuity tests. The percentage of children between 3 and 3.5 years of age whose monocular acuity could be assessed was high and equivalent for the two charts. Crowded HOTV acuities were better than the values achieved with the Lea symbols. This, however, was attributed to the difference in the format of the two tests.

Repka (11), in an editorial, discussed the importance of finding an accurate means of measuring acuity in young children. It is necessary to know what the acuity is with the *same* method of measurement over time to know clinically what is happening with an amblyopic youngster, for example. You cannot compare the acuity obtained with Allen pictures on one visit with Lea symbols on the next with HOTV on the next visit. It is important in children to use consistency of measurement and to get monocular acuity values. Repka says, "Letter optotypes have generally been too difficult for pre-school children, while traditional picture optotypes, like the Allen pictures, though much more testable, substantially reduce the sensitivity of the test for the detection of amblyopia." He felt the Lea symbols were a "reasonable alternative."

Becker et al. (12), in a population of 385 children ranging in age from 21 to 93 months, found that Lea symbols were "useful" in the testing of visual acuity in these children. Ninety subjects of their study were followed up in a hospital setting and, in these 90 children, they compared Lea symbol acuity with Landoldt C acuity. In this setting, they could measure monocular acuity on both eyes in 77% of the children using Lea symbols and 48% of the children using the Landoldt C test. They also found the older children more testable than the younger ones. Becker et al. (12) concluded that the Lea symbols were useful for visual acuity measurement in early childhood.

PATTI PICS

Patti Pics is another large repertoire of visual acuity tests intended to be used with preschool children who can either name or match the four picture optotypes. This series of tests manufactured by Precision Vision are logarithmic visual acuity tests that have been calibrated against Sloan letters, *mostly* in booklet format with crowding effects produced by pictures, bars, or surround (see Fig. 10.7).

The mean difference between Sloan letter and Patti Pics acuities was +0.01 LogMAR, which is equivalent to one half letter and the maximal difference +0.06 logMar. "In seven subjects, the Sloan letter acuities were better than Patti Pics acuities; in six subjects the Patti Pics acuities were better; and in one subject the acuities were identical. Thus, tendency exists for one optotype acuity to be better than the other. Moreover, the differences between acuities were within test–retest variability for EDTRS letter charts in adults. This means that the acuity differences were random and not caused by optotype differences (13). In addition to the Patti Pics, Precision Vision makes a series of HOTV tests (see below) for both distance and near in booklet format. Included in each test is a template for the child to use to give matching responses when verbal responses are not available.

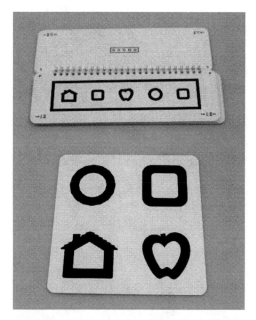

FIGURE 10.7. Patti Pics by Precision Vision.

HOTV CHART

The HOTV chart, a visual acuity test, is one of the best ways to get a recognition acuity using letters calibrated to the Snellen parameters. The four letters—H, O, T, and V—were chosen because they are symmetric around the body midline (vertical axis) and cannot be confused because of directional inversions. The letters can be shown and identified by the child, either by labeling or by matching to a HOTV display card. The HOTV chart is considered one of the best ways to measure visual acuity in children aged 3 to 5 years. It was adopted as the acuity measurement technique of choice by the Amblyopia Treatment Study (ATS). PEDIG (Pediatric Eye Disease Investigative Group), the clinical group for the amblyopia studies, developed a new procedure for quantifing visual acuity using isolated HOTV characters with crowding bars, first on the Baylor-Video Acuity Test (BVAT) instrument and later on its own program developed for the different amblyopia studies. In a study done to evaluate the reliability of their new protocol, they found in the age group 3 to 7 years a high level of testability and excellent test–retest reliability (14,15). The child does not need to know the letters or call them by name. The child just has to be able

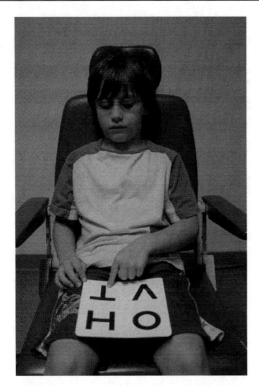

FIGURE 10.8. Baylor-Video Acuity Test (BVAT) HOTV presentation (out of view) with matching on HOTV matching card.

to match the isolated, surrounded letter on the VDT to one of the four characters on a card in front of him or her. The ATS protocol is described in the cited paper (15). It allows the clinician to get a Snellen type acuity (recognition acuity) long before the child might otherwise be able to respond to the alphabet optotypes (Fig. 10.8).

When comparing the administration of the HOTV versus the Lea symbols visual acuity tests

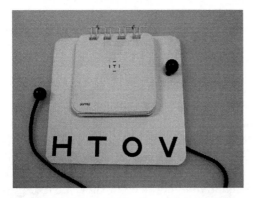

FIGURE 10.9. HOTV format near point chart with distance testing control (Precision Vision).

in a large population of children 3 to 5 years of age ($N = 777$), Hered et al. (16) found that vision screening was more rapid and more frequently achieved with children aged 4 to 5 years than with children aged 3 to 4 years. For the population as a whole, each chart gave similar results. Among children 3 years of age, testability was better for the Lea symbols and they may be more efficacious than the HOTV chart for testing children that age.

The ATS, for many years, have used crowded HOTV acuity measurements for all their studies involving measurement of monocular acuity in children between 3 and 7 years of age in a prescribed protocol, which has been described in the literature (14).

The Vision in Preschoolers Study Group (17) determined that overall sensitivity and group I sensitivity (group I conditions = amblyopia, strabismus, anisometropia, and all conditions where early detection and treatment are urgently important) were slightly higher using Lea symbols than HOTV optotypes to evaluate visual acuity in children 3 to 5 years of age. The associated P values between the two, however, were not significant.

In 1986, Fern and Manny (18) described some 46 visual acuity tests designed to assess acuity in preschool children. They objectively cited the attributes of each one and described what each test measured. Of the 46 tests, many are not easily available today, but most of the tests mentioned thus far were mentioned in the article. Fern and Manny recommended that optotypes on visual acuity charts being used to test preschoolers be

1. Isolated single optotypes
2. High-contrast optotypes
3. Without directional components
4. For younger children, a matching response rather than a verbal response
5. Presented at 3 m instead of 6 m for distance acuity testing

Many of the tests Fern and Manny discussed in 1986 are still available, but not necessarily tests of preference. Many other visual acuity tests are available today for the preschool population. A brief description of some of these follow (some have already been discussed) with the understanding and the expectation that by the time this book goes to press, there may be other newer and better ones.

ALLEN CARDS AND AMERICAN OPTICAL PICTURES

Picture acuity charts have been popular among clinicians who work with children. The two most popular are the *Allen cards* and the American Optical pictures. Both of these tests use pictures drawn to Snellen specifications and standardized against adults with known visual acuities. The Allen cards (seven optotypes) are presented to the child for recognition at a test distance of 15 feet (20/40) at 3 years of age and 20 feet (20/30) at 4 years of age. The American Optical pictures are either projected to a distance of 20 feet or the clinician can use a distance chart calibrated for 20 feet.

The best acuity that these optotypes can identify is usually 20/30 at 20 feet. Both of these picture charts are recognition acuity tasks. Schmidt (19) compared acuities obtained using Allen figures (American Optical picture chart) and broken wheel cards. She found no correlation between the two tests under binocular conditions. A greater range of visual acuity values was seen for the broken wheel cards versus the picture acuity test and a consistency was found in the acuity value measured. This makes it a "valuable clinical tool to measure acuity in young children." Schmidt further says that the broken wheel test would be greatly enhanced if the range of stimulus pairs were extended, scaling between acuity values was made consistent, and the accuracy of the elements was made more consistent.

LANDOLT C

The Landolt C test attempts to measure a minimum separable acuity in youngsters who can understand the concept of "the break in the circle." Landolt Cs are presented with the "opening" of the optotype at 3, 6, 9, or 12 o'clock. The child has to tell where the opening is. The separation at the break in the C represents 1 minute of arc and the entire C subtends 5 minutes of arc at the eye for 20/20. Norms for the Landolt C test were derived by Kozaki et al. (20).

TUMBLING E CHART

Another popular test for young children is the Tumbling E chart. For many years, people were afraid to use this test on youngsters, feeling that children did not have sufficiently developed directional concepts to be able to identify which direction the "E" is pointing. The test, however, is only asking children to make a direct match between their hand and the "E," independent of direction. Sometimes, children have difficulty moving their hand into the four possible directions and this can limit their ability to respond. The test is based on Snellen principals and is a minimum separable (not a recognition) visual acuity measure. "E" charts typically have values that go to 20/20 or even better.

KAY PICTURES

Kay pictures is another picture optotype developed to assess visual acuity in young children at distance and at near (21). The figures are "child friendly," with matching cards for children who cannot or will not speak. The figures are constructed, according to the manufacturer, exactly the same way as Snellen letters. Although the individual elements subtend a visual angle of 1 minute of arc, the total figure subtends 10′ of arc at the eye. Available are 6-m and 3-m visual acuity test booklets; the 3-m test booklet is used for younger children who will not attend at 6 m. Near point cards are also available to assess near visual acuity. The test was designed to quantify visual acuity of children from 2 to 3 years of age and claims to be more accurate than alternative tests for this age group.

Jones et al. (22) compared acuity values in preschool children utilizing the Kay pictures and LogMAR crowded-letter tests. They tested children from 2.5 to 16 years of age, but looked particularly at the children from 2.5 to 5 years of age ($N = 50$) to compare testability. The older children ($N = 53$; mean = 8.9 years ±2.3) participated to minimize confounding factors relating to the cognitive abilities of the younger children. The authors concluded that the Kay crowded-picture test is comparable to the LogMAR crowded-letter test. They also found on the target population (<5 years of age) that the Kay pictures were easier to perform than the LogMAR crowded letters and that the acuity values obtained with the two different methods are comparable.

BUST

Another picture test designed to test visual acuity of young children as well as children with vision impairment and developmental handicaps, is the BUST Vision test (23). BUST is an acronym for the Swedish words for "Visual Acuity and Picture Perception Test." The BUST was standardized against other visual acuity tests with empirical comparison. The range of visual acuity for distance acuity measurement values goes from 0.02 to 1.6 (20/1000 to 20/10). In addition, a set of BUST playing cards can be used to quantify near visual acuity on these same patients.

SNELLEN

Snellen acuities are the goal of most clinicians. In Snellen testing, one has a recognition acuity based on angular subtense of the component parts of the optotypes as well as the entire optotype itself. Snellen acuity is the standard against which others make comparisons. Snellen is a letter optotype either projected or on a wall chart. Current, with the enormous emphasis parents put on academic achievement and performance, more and more children 2, 3, and 4 years of age are coming in able to read letters of the alphabet. Do not forget to enquire about the child's abilities because it could save time and give a more accurate clinical finding because letters are used to measure visual acuity. Snellen acuity measurement has long been considered the gold standard for taking visual acuity measurements. In the past two decades or so, however, LogMAR acuity charts have been slowly gaining in popularity as the *new* gold standard of visual acuity measurement.

LOGMAR

LogMAR charts were designed by Bailey and Lovie and were used as a basis for acuity in the ETDRS (Early Treatment of Diabetes Retinopathy Study). Unlike Snellen charts, the LogMAR charts maintain a consistent ratio between optotypes and spacings, no matter what the angular subtense of the optotype is. Each acuity value has the same number of optotypes and the interaction of adjacent contours is consistent. The charts, therefore, appear as an inverted triangle of letters or other symbols (Fig. 10.10).

These charts are slowly becoming the gold standard for measuring visual acuity. Therefore, they are seen more frequently and are being manufactured as visual acuity charts for both adults and children. LogMAR chart configurations are now available with Lea symbols, HOTV symbols, letters, numbers, illiterate Es, Landolt Cs, and so on, and in chart and illuminated-panel formats, as well as flip books. In addition, computer program visual acuity charts can be displayed on VDT or in self-contained, high-contrast light boxes in either the Snellen configuration or the LogMAR configuration. HOTV charts and Lea symbol wall and stand charts, as well as numbers, letters, pictures, illiterate Es, and other formats have all been commercially produced in LogMAR configurations. HOTV, Lea symbol, Es, Landolt Cs, letters, numbers, and Allen picture configurations are available for near point charts in Snellen or LogMAR formats.

In recent years, computer-generated visual acuity charts have been emerging into the market place from companies such as Medtronic Solan (BVAT PC Visual Acuity System, with nine different optotypes), Reichert Inc. (Clear Chart Digital Acuity System), and M & S Technologies Smart System 20/20. Each of these has some very useful features to assist in the acquisition of visual acuity information in younger patients and older patients. Medtronic Solan is a computer program that displays letters, numbers, Landolt Cs, pictures, and HOTV, in single presentations with or without crowding, whole line, or whole chart. The whole chart can be displayed Snellen or LogMAR (Bailey-Lovie) format. In addition, it has other features helpful in testing pediatric patients. The Reichert Clear Chart Digital Acuity System and the M & S Technologies Smart System 20/20 are digital PC-based systems having a wide variety of optotypes that can be presented in different formats. The Reichert Clear Chart has eleven optotypes, including Allen pictures, children shapes, Retsyn pictures, HOTV letters, Es, Landolt Cs, letters, and so on. The optotypes can be presented as

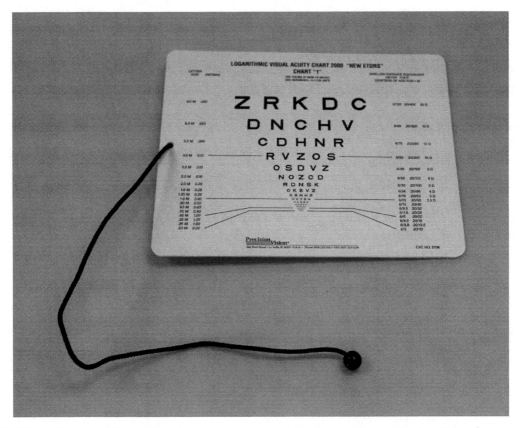

FIGURE 10.10. Logarithm of the **m**inimum **a**ngle of **r**esolution (LogMAR) near visual acuity configuration.

single letters, whole line or whole chart. Crowding bars are available. Chart acuity can be done as Snellen or Bailey-Lovie formats. The high contrast display allows acuity testing with the room lights on, which is a big advantage in working with younger children. The M & S Technologies Smart System 20/20 has similar features with high-contrast screen and an extend cartoon, which aids in maintaining distance fixation during retinoscopy and ophthalmoscopy. The M & S instrument is ATS (Amblyopia Treatment Study) and E-ETDRS (Electronic-Early Treatment of Diabetic Retinopathy Study) certified. Other systems include Thomson Software, which can display letters, Landolt Cs, tumbling Es, and Kay pictures; whole chart, single symbol, or single optotype with crowding bars.

With increased awareness of the importance of early visual examination and early intervention, new instruments of acuity measurement are introduced periodically. Currently, the visual acuity measurement tools described in this chapter are the best and most frequently used charts and optotypes today. Some of these, such as the Tumbling E and Landoldt C have been around for a long time, whereas others (e.g., Lea symbols, Patti Pics, and Kay pictures) are relatively new. It is certain that the future will bring new and hopefully better charts with which to evaluate visual function in young children.

REFERENCES

1. Dobson V, Teller DY, Lee CP, et al. A behavioral method for efficient screening of visual acuity in young infants. I. Preliminary laboratory development. *Invest Ophthalmol Vis Sci* 1978:17(12);1142–1150.
2. Dobson V. Behavioral tests of visual acuity in infants. *Int Ophthalmol Clin* 1980;20(1):233–250.
3. Duckman RH, Selenow A. Use of forced preferential looking for measurement of visual acuity in a population of neurologically impaired children. *Am J Optom Physiol Opt* 1983;60(10):817–821.
4. Jacobsen K, Grottland H, Flaten MA. Assessment of visual acuity in relation to central nervous system activation in children with mental retardation. *Am J Ment Retard* 2001;106(2):145–150.
5. Adoh TO, Woodhouse JM. The Cardiff acuity test used for measuring visual acuity development in toddlers. *Vision Res* 1994;Feb 34(4):555–560.

6. Richman JE, Petito GT, Cron MT. Broken Wheel Acuity Test: a new and valid test for preschool and exceptional children. *J Am Optom Assoc* 1984;55(8):561–565.
7. McDonald M, Chaudry NM. Comparison of four methods of assessing visual acuity in young children. *Optom Vis Sci* 1989;66(6):363–369.
8. Hyvarinen L, Nasanen R, Laurinen P. New visual acuity test for pre-school children. *Acta Ophthalmol (Copenh)* 1980;58:507–511.
9. Shallo-Hoffmann J, Coulter R, Oliver P, et al. A study of preschool vision screening tests, testability, validity and duration: do group differences matter? *Strabismus* 2004; 12(2):65–73.
10. Vision in Preschoolers (VIP) Study Group. Threshold visual acuity testing of preschool children using the crowded HOTV and Lea Symbols acuity tests. *J Am Assoc Pediatr Ophthalmol* 2003;7(6):396–399.
11. Repka, MX. Ed. Use of Lea symbols in young children. *Br J Ophthalmol* 2002;86:489–490.
12. Becker R, Hubsch S, Graf MH, et al. Examination of young children with Lea Symbols. *Br J Ophthalmol* 2002;86(5):513–516.
13. Personal correspondence from D. Luisa Mayer, Harvard Medical School to Precision Vision, April 19, 2004.
14. Moke PS, Turpin AH, Beck RW, et al. Computerized method of visual acuity testing: adaptation of the amblyopia treatment study visual acuity testing protocol. *Am J Ophthalmol* 2001;132(6):903–909.
15. Holmes JM, Beck RW, Repka MX, et al. Pediatric Eye Disease Investigator Group. The amblyopia treatment study visual acuity testing protocol. *Arch Ophthalmol* 2001;119(9):1345–1353.
16. Hered RW, Murphy S, Clancy M. Comparison of the HOTV and Lea Symbols charts for preschool vision screening. *J Pediatr Ophthalmol Strabismus* 1997; 34(1):24–28.
17. The Vision in Preschoolers Study Group. Comparison of preschool vision screening tests as administered by licensed eye care professionals in the vision in preschoolers study. *Ophthalmology* 2003;111(4):637–650.
18. Fern KD, Manny RE. Visual acuity of the pre-school child: a review. *American Journal of Optometry and Physiological Optics* 1986;63(5):319–345.
19. Schmidt PP. Allen figure and broken wheel visual acuity measurement in preschool children. *J Am Optom Assoc* 1992;63(2):124–130.
20. Kozaki M, Iwai H, Mikami C. Vision screening of three year old children. *Jpn J Ophthalmol* 1973;17:60–68.
21. Kay H. New method of assessing visual acuity with pictures. *Br J Ophthalmol* 1983;67(2):131–133.
22. Jones D, Westall C, Averbeck K, et al. Visual acuity assessment: a comparison of two tests for measuring children's vision. *Ophthalmic Physiol Opt* 2003;23:541–546.
23. http://home.swipenet.se/~ w-94583?Elisyn/bust_intro_2002.html. Accessed May 2005.

Assessment of Ocular Health

11

Shoshana Bell-Craig and Robert H. Duckman

A high incidence of ocular disease is found in the pediatric population and, therefore, a thorough assessment of ocular health is imperative (1). To prevent vision conditions that have the potential to cause permanent vision loss, it is important to diagnose and treat them early. An evaluation of ocular health should include careful inspection of the anterior segment, pupil reflexes and intraocular pressure, and assessment of the posterior segment with dilation (2).

It is always easier to examine a patient who can respond to questions clearly and who can follow instructions during an examination. Most children will cooperate and testing used to assess the ocular health of adults can be used in the pediatric population. Standard procedures, however, may not be applicable to those who are very young or unable to communicate. We can put this population at some ease by making a number of modifications (2).

EVALUATING THE EXTERNAL EYE

The standard fixed biomicroscope can be used to evaluate the anterior segment by having the infant or child propped up by the parent (Fig. 11.1). Children 2 years of age and older can usually stand on the footrest of the chair or kneel on the chair. For infants and children younger than 2 years, a portable slit lamp can be utilized. The most useful position for infants when using a portable slit lamp is to have them face up on the parent's lap with their head on the parent's knees and their legs under the parent's armpits (3).

Portable slit lamps are available from the following manufacturers.

Clement Clarke Portable Slit Lamp 904

The Clement Clarke portable slit lamp with its head and chinrest assembly, can be used for traditional style examinations or as a handheld slit lamp (Fig. 11.2). The portable slit lamp's power source is a rechargeable battery pack, enabling the examiner to be more mobile. It provides three slit widths (0.12 mm, 0.25 mm, and 0.5 mm), four slit heights (3 mm, 5 mm, 8 mm, and 14 mm), and two color filters (blue and yellow). Its standard magnification is 10× with the availability of optional 16× lenses.

Kowa SL–15 Portable Slit Lamp

The Kowa SL-15 (Fig. 11.3) is a cordless, rechargeable unit that has a halogen illumination source with a spot and three slit widths as well as a built-in cobalt blue filter. Magnification settings are the same as for the Clement Clarke, with a range from 10 to 16. The stand doubles as a battery charger and permits long-term continuous lighting for approximately 40 minutes. An optional headrest is also available to improve stability. The illumination can be reduced to one sixteenth of the maximum and may be beneficial for use with children to reduce

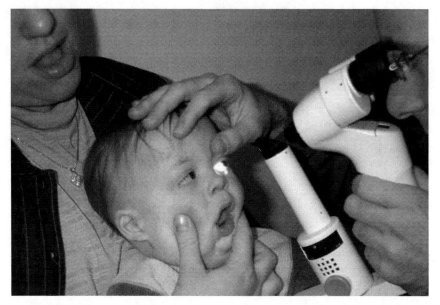

FIGURE 11.1.   Infant being examined with a handheld biomicroscope.

discomfort. (The original SL-14 model has been discontinued.)

Heine HSL 150 Pocket Slit Lamp

The Heine HSL 150 pocket slit lamp (Fig. 11.4) does not provide as many slit sizes as the Clement Clarke and Kowa, but it does have an adjustable slit image with slit size available from 0.2 mm × 10 mm to 4 mm × 14 mm. Unlike the Clement Clarke and Kowa, the blue filter is available as an option for corneal eval-

uation and does not provide as much magnification. A 6 magnification with 20-D loupe is available and, when combined with the 10-D loupe, can provide 10 magnification. It is beneficial because it increases the working distance from the patient and offers a large field of view.

Zeiss HSO 10 Hand Slit Lamp

The Zeiss HSO 10 hand slit lamp (Fig. 11.5) can be converted into an indirect ophthalmoscope.

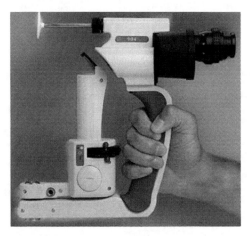

FIGURE 11.2.   Clement Clarke 904 portable slit lamp.

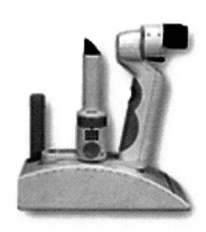

FIGURE 11.3.   Kowa SL-15 portable slit lamp.

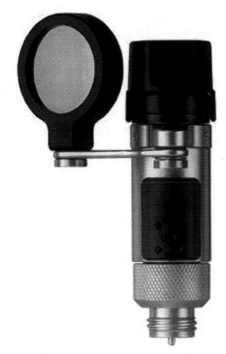

FIGURE 11.4.   Heine HSL 150 pocket slit lamp.

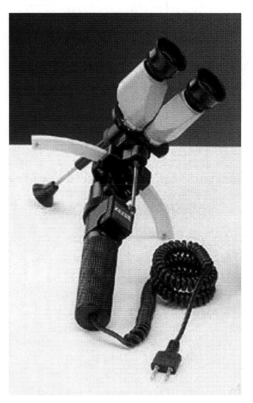

FIGURE 11.5.   Zeiss HSO handheld slit lamp.

The illumination unit can be moved with one hand and set in any position on the clamping lever so that one hand is available to hold open eyelids or improve fixation with finger puppets. The equipment includes either a power supply unit or a rechargeable battery unit so the examiner can move around freely.

In addition to using a slit lamp to evaluate the integrity of the cornea, companies have developed handheld keratometers, which are extremely patient friendly.

Portable keratometers are available from the following manufacturers.

Marco Handheld Automatic Keratometer KM-500

The KM-500 allows the examiner to observe the targeted eye from any distance. It will fire automatically when focused properly. Two rechargeable batteries provide 60 minutes of continuous use. The measurable range of corneal curvature is 33 to 67.50 D.

Nidek Handheld Auto Refractor/Keratometer ARK-30

The Nidek ARK-30 is lightweight and portable and is capable of taking measurements with an infant or child lying on a parent's lap because of its 90° correction function. It is wireless and comes with a built-in forehead rest. Nidek has also developed an autorefractor or keratometer and noncontact tonometer in one unit called the *TONOREF RKT-7700*. It allows the examiner to evaluate the external eye and obtain intraocular pressure readings without changing instruments. This unit, however, does require that the patient keep his or her chin in a chinrest.

PUPIL REFLEXES

A penlight or transilluminator is typically used to assess pupils in both the pediatric and adult population. Testing should be done with normal room illumination so as not to increase anxiety. Keep in mind, very young patients have more miotic pupils, which do not reach normal size until about the age of 6 months (Jennings 1996). Have the infant or child sit on a parent's lap and direct their fixation onto a distant target, if possible. It may be necessary to hold the eyelids open while testing for direct and consensual pupillary responses. It is increasingly difficult to determine the presence of a relative afferent defect without accurate fixation so toys set up across the room that make noise and light up are excellent targets.

INTRAOCULAR PRESSURE

Tonometry indirectly measures intraocular pressure (IOP) by determining the resistance of the cornea to indentation. The most commonly used devices are indentation (Schiotz) tonometers, applanation (Goldmann) tonometers, noncontact tonometers (pneumotonometry), and electronic indentation tonometers (3). Assessment of IOP is important, but can be difficult to obtain in a very young patient. A baseline measurement is valuable and IOP should be assessed, particularly when ocular signs and symptoms of or risk factors for glaucoma exist. Testing under sedation or anesthesia may be appropriate if IOP cannot be assessed under ordinary conditions.

Contact Tonometers

Currently, two methods are used to measure IOP in which the instrument touches the cornea—indentation and applanation. The indentation method indents and distorts the cornea using varied weights and a 3-mm plunger to indent the cornea. The device is known as the *Schiotz tonometer* and, although outdated, is still used in some clinical settings. This device has many drawbacks including the rigidity of the cornea and resistance to indentation, rigidity of the globe, and the possibility of injury and abrasion to the cornea. The more accepted method is applanating or flattening the cornea (1).

Tonometry is usually performed with the standard Goldmann applanation tonometer mounted on a slit lamp biomicroscope. It is the standard against which all tonometers are compared, and it is the preferred method to diagnose and treat glaucoma (4). Children who are able to cooperate by sitting still and fixating on a target can be evaluated using the standard Goldmann applanation tonometer. A drawback in using it with the pediatric population is that the patient must be in a horizontal plane with the tonometer. It helps to have the child kneel on the chair or stand while taking IOP measurements (1). Further drawbacks include the necessity of instilling fluorescein and an anesthetic eye drop.

Several companies (e.g., Haag-Streit, Clement Clarke, Nikon, and R. H. Burton) manufacture Goldmann-type tonometers for the slit lamp. The measurement of IOP in school-aged children is generally successful with applanation (2). Evaluation, however, has become much easier with the advent of portable instrumentation, such as handheld applanation and noncontact tonometers. The Perkins tonometer is very useful for this population.

Handheld Applanation Tonometers

Given that the standard Goldmann tonometer is mounted on a slit lamp, it is relatively nonportable. Handheld tonometers can be easily transported and do not require the patient to be positioned in an instrument. They may be less alarming to children and allow them to sit on their parent's lap or lie down. Although less frightening, most of them require both fluorescein and anesthetic ocular drops. Many companies manufacture handheld tonometers and multiple studies have been performed to assess their reliability when compared with a Goldmann tonometer. Some of these are discussed below.

CLEMENT CLARKE-PERKINS MK2 APPLANATION TONOMETER

The Clement Clarke-Perkins MK 2 applanation tonometer (Fig. 11.6) utilizes Goldmann applanation and a counterbalance system, and can, therefore, take measurements with the patient in any position, which is very beneficial in the pediatric population. As a standard, spares and

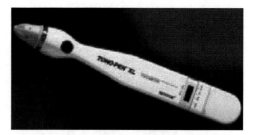

FIGURE 11.7. Medtronic Solan Tono-Pen XL.

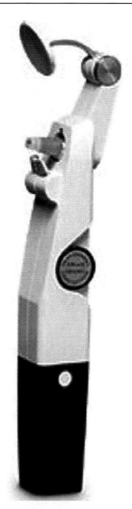

FIGURE 11.6. Clement Clarke-Perkins MK2 applanation tonometer.

accessories are supplied and the battery handle detaches for the installation and removal of batteries. Four AA batteries can be used. A rechargeable battery handle is interchangeable with the standard handle and can be left overnight to charge in the unit. The Perkins examination telescope (PET) allows magnified viewing of the fluorescein "semicircles" at arm's length. A sterile disposable prism can be used for each patient to reduce risk of contamination.

MEDTRONIC SOLAN'S TONO-PEN XL

The Medtronic Solan Tono-Pen XL is an electronic applanation tonometer. Small and handheld, it is less intimidating. A lightweight and portable instrument that fits into the hand like a pen, it allows the free hand to hold open the eyelid, if needed. The Tono-Pen is easy to use and can be positioned in a variety of ways as long as the tip is perpendicular to the patient's globe (Fig. 11.7). A protective disposable latex cover is used to reduce the possible spread of infection. A disadvantage, as with all contact tonometers, is that anesthetic must be used. However, because it does not use Goldmann doubling prisms, fluorescein is not needed. The operator repeats gentle pecking movements against the anesthetized cornea until four to ten readings are accepted and averaged. The instrument provides the final reading along with the percent variability between the highest and lowest readings (5). Because results of multiple studies have found a statistically significant difference between the Tono-Pen and Goldmann instruments, it should not be depended on to obtain reliable diurnal curves (5). The manufacturer's literature, however, claims the readings are highly correlated with Goldmann applanation tonometry.

KOWA APPLANATION TONOMETER HA-2

The Kowa HA-2 applanation tonometer (Fig. 11.8) is a Perkins-style handheld applanation tonometer that gives direct readings in mm Hg with the use of standard Goldmann doubling prisms. It uses a one-spring mechanism to produce applanation and, therefore, assures correct readings regardless of the patient's position. It can be used with one hand, which allows the other to hold the eyelid open, if necessary. The Kowa HA 2 is compact and lightweight (6). Accessories include an adjustable head rest and interchangeable 3× long relief eyepiece. Scale range of readings is from 0 to 60 mm Hg (in 1-mm Hg intervals).

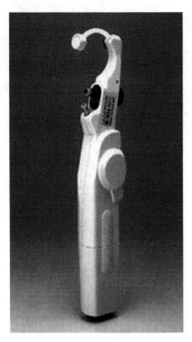

FIGURE 11.8. Kowa HA-2 portable applanation tonometer.

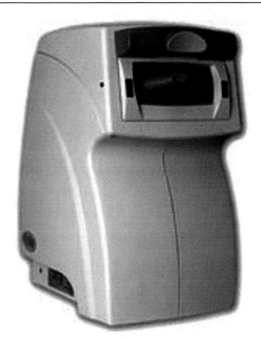

FIGURE 11.9. Reichart AT555 non-contact tonometer.

Noncontact Tonometers

Noncontact tonometers (NCTs) have several favorable characteristics such as rapidity, reliability, ease of use, and limited discomfort for the patient. The instrument does not touch the eye when taking a measurement and, therefore, does not require topical anesthesia. A puff of air indents the cornea and the instrument reads the pressure. Today's NCTs all report having a very gentle, soft puff of air and they are also much quieter than earlier models. Noncontact tonometery is very beneficial for screening, but not for following patients who have glaucoma. These instruments have been shown to be safe and to produce valid measurements (7). Some of these instruments are discussed below.

REICHERT OPHTHALMIC INSTRUMENTS AT 555 AUTO NONCONTACT TONOMETER

The Reichert AT555 (Fig. 11.9) offers no chin rest, no joystick, and no elevation controls. The patient leans against the instrument's forehead rest and views a fixation target. It has a patented hands-free automated alignment system and the operator simply presses a button to activate the

IOP measurement process. The Reichert AT555 achieves alignment of the patient's eye automatically and the puff of air is only released when the instrument is in proper alignment. Its measurement range is from 0 to 60 mm Hg.

KOWA AUTOMATED TONOMETER KT-500

Special features of the Kowa KT-500 automated tonometer include an auto-alignment function, improved softness of the air flow, and an electronically operated chin rest. Higher IOP measurements are possible without the range switching operation. The range of eye pressure measurements is 0 to 60 mm Hg in 1-mm Hg steps and measurement distance is 11 mm.

CANON TX-10

The Canon TX-10 has a fully automatic alignment system and automatically moves the measuring head to the other eye. Manual alignment is also available, if preferred. Two fixation targets are present, one internal and one external. It has a measuring range of 0 to 30 mm Hg and automatically increases to an upper limit of 60 mm Hg, if necessary. The working distance is approximately 11 mm and it can take up to a maximum of ten measurements for each eye.

The Topcon CT-80 is a fixed device with a safety mechanism to prevent patient contact. The interval time between measurements has been reduced by 30%. The CT-80 uses infrared lighting for its main illumination. This reportedly increases patient comfort by eliminating the need for harsh, bright alignment lighting. By overriding the automatic measurement setting, it can be operated manually. The working distance from the patient's eye is 11 mm, similar to that of other NCTs. The measurement range is 0 to 60 mm Hg, but, unlike the Canon TX-10, measuring IOP above 30 mm Hg is not automatic and must be selected from the screen.

MARCO NT-2000

The Marco NT-2000 features a video display of the cornea and uses a system that fires automatically when properly aligned. It is also equipped with a manual system that, when activated, will override the automatic system. It can adjust each pulse of air to maximize the patient's comfort. The working distance is 11 mm and the range of measurement is 0 to 30 mm Hg. If needed, a measurement can be taken between 30 and 60 mm Hg, but that option must be selected.

Also available from Marco Ophthalmics is the NT-4000, which is equipped with the automatic puff control function to reduce the amount of air pressure, an expanded autofocusing detection range, eyelid-checking function to reduce errors, and three selectable modes of operation—full automatic, semiautomatic, and manual.

Handheld Noncontact Tonometers

Most of the handheld NCTs are portable and cordless and are more convenient than the fixed NCT models. The handheld models are smaller and less likely to frighten an infant or young child. They may allow the examiner more ease in obtaining an IOP reading. Some of these are discussed below.

REICHERT PT100

Reichert PT100 is a portable, cordless handheld NCT. Once alignment is achieved, it automatically takes an IOP measurement. Recharging unit, infrared (IR) printer, and custom carrying case are included. According to the manufacturer, readings correlate closely to Goldmann tonometer readings. It can display up to three IOP measurements and an average for each eye. Measurement range is from 0 to 60 mm Hg.

KEELER PULSAIR EASYEYE

Keeler Pulsair EasyEye retains the handheld capabilities of earlier models, but has several additional features. The manufacturer states that it is more accurate, has an improved alignment and triggering system, and a lower-pressure air puff. It can detect if the lid or a lash has interfered with an IOP measurement and will operate only when the optimal eye instrument alignment is achieved, allowing for more reliable results. It becomes portable with the addition of an optional battery pack. The hand piece is held approximately 2 cm from the patient's cornea (5). It is beneficial for children because it can be used with the patient in any position (e.g., reclining). It can be used without anesthetic, corneal contact, or probe disinfection. Its calibrated range of IOP is 7 to 50 mm Hg in 1.0 mm Hg steps (9).

Multiple readings of IOP are suggested by the manufacturer (Keeler) and supported by Buscemi et al. (8). It can be difficult to obtain four separate readings especially when working with children or uncooperative patients. Buscemi et al. found that the variability of IOP readings on the same eye using the Pulsair instrument was up to 5 mm Hg. It is not advisable, therefore, to rely on a single value, especially when that value is borderline (8,10). Findings greater than 21 mm Hg should be further investigated with Goldmann tonometry.

As mentioned in the previous section, along with instruments used to evaluate the external eye, Nidek has developed the TONOREF RKT 7700 (Fig. 11.10), an autorefractor-keratometer and NCT in one unit.

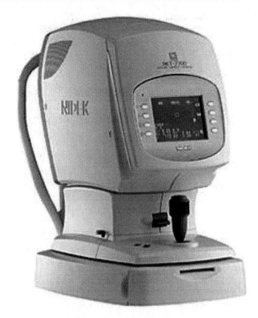

FIGURE 11.10. Nidek RKT 7700 for autorefraction, autokeratometry, and noncontact tonometry.

DILATION AND DILATORY AGENTS

The ocular pharmacologic agents used most commonly by eye care practitioners include diagnostic drugs that are used for dilation, cycloplegia, and tonometry. When dilating a child's eye, keep in mind that some significant differences exist between children and adults when using diagnostic pharmacologic agents. An increased risk of adverse reactions exists, because of children's small size and their immature mechanisms for drug excretion and biotransformation 11,14).

Anesthetics

The most common indication for the use of anesthetic agents in children is for applanation tonometry. A drop of a combination anesthetic and fluorescein agent is instilled in the eye before applanation. Another indication for the use of an ocular anesthetic is to ease discomfort before instillation of mydriatics and cycloplegics. The discomfort from the initial drop of the anesthetic itself remains a problem for many children and it also increases the likelihood that it will be more difficult to get the additional mydriatic and cycloplegic agents themselves into the already distressed child (13). The anesthetic is routinely used before instillation of other diagnostic agents to reduce discomfort and prevent the corneal surface from increasing absorption of any subsequent drops. In general, use of anesthetics is not recommended with children because it increases the potential for adverse effects (13).

Dilating Agents

Examining the anterior and posterior segments of the eye requires the use of dilating agents. Because young children will not sit still as long as adults will for ophthalmoscopic or slit lamp examination, it is important to get as good a view as possible. Two commonly used dilating agents include *phenylephrine hydrochloride* (a direct-acting adrenergic agonist) and *tropicamide* (a cholinergic antagonist). Phenylephrine provides rapid dilation with a short period of action. A potential exists for cardiovascular side effects and this drug should not be used in children under 3 years of age or in those with any history of cardiovascular problems. Pediatric use should be restricted to no more than two drops of 2.5% concentration spaced 5 minutes apart. It has been shown that phenylephrine produces greater pupil dilation when added to a cycloplegic (14). Tropicamide also provides a rapid dilation with a short duration. It is the safest dilating agent available and the recommended dosage is one drop of 0.5% or 1.0% solution with a second drop after 5 minutes (13).

Dilation of the pupils to examine the ocular media and posterior segment is essential in providing an adequate ocular examination, but children often resist instillation of mydriatic drops. As an alternative, studies have found that a spray application of diagnostic agents can be both effective and beneficial (12,15,16). Research has shown that a combination mydriatic-cycloplegic solution is an effective means of instilling eye drops in children. Some studies have reportedly seen equal effectiveness with an atomized spray of cycloplegic or mydriatic agents applied to the area around closed eyelids (12,13,15).

Wesson et al. (15) found a statistically significant difference in pupil response based on eye color, with blue irises dilating faster. They found no difference, however, after waiting 55 minutes for darker irises to dilate. The combination mydriatic solution minimizes ocular irritation and provides a less stressful encounter with a child when the eyes are closed.

OPHTHALMOSCOPES

Examination of very young children can be difficult, especially when a detailed view of the macula and optic nerve is required. Direct ophthalmoscopes can be intimidating to young children and require some degree of fixation on the part of the patient. It is likely that the observer will view only the macular area because the infant or young child will stare directly into the light. Having an assistant hold up a finger puppet or other interesting target will allow a view to be obtained of areas of the retina besides the macula. Binocular indirect ophthalmoscopes that are wireless or have portable power sources allow the examiner to move around with ease. The increased working distance is less frightening for the child; however, the light is still extremely bright. Many manufacturers have a diffused light setting to increase comfort. Using a yellow condensing lens also helps reduce the light.

To further reduce the uneasiness of children, it is important to orient them to what is going to be done. This works well if the child is more than 4 years of age. If they have some understanding of what the examiner is going to do, they may be more cooperative. If unable to perform an adequate fundus evaluation, it may be necessary to make an appropriate referral so that it can be performed while the child is sedated.

Binocular Indirect Ophthalmoscopes

The Keeler Vantage binocular indirect ophthalmoscope (BIO) has an illumination rheostat located on the headband so it is easily accessible. The illumination can be turned down to as low as 2% of the maximum to increase patient comfort. It also provides 1.6× more magnification with the standard Hi-Mag Lens. The interpupillary distance range is from 52 to 76 mm. It has a variable mirror height control, which provides the ability to view small pupils. It is the only indirect ophthalmoscope that is capable of being converted into a fundus imaging system.

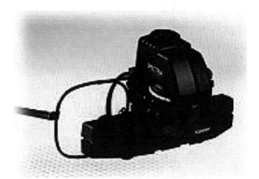

FIGURE 11.11. Keeler Spectra spectacle-mounted binocular indirect ophthalmoscope.

The Keeler All Pupil II also has the illumination controls on the headband and is lightweight. The manufacturer's literature states that it provides up to 2000 lux illumination and can be turned down to as low as 2% of the maximum.

The Keeler Spectra (Fig. 11.11) is a spectacle-mounted BIO, making it compact and portable. It is the only spectacle indirect ophthalmoscope with built-in filters. Two different aperture sizes are available, which allow examination of pupils that have not fully dilated.

The Welch Allyn 125 BIO (Fig. 11.12) has observation paths that can be adjusted from 49 mm to 74 mm. A small-pupil mode enables examination of patients with pupils as small as 2 mm. Optional is a diffuser filter, which expands the illumination beam and allows enhanced viewing

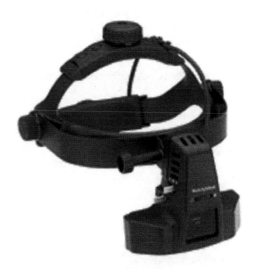

FIGURE 11.12. Welch Allyn 125 binocular indirect ophthalmoscope.

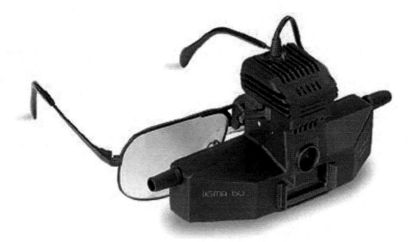

FIGURE 11.13. Heine Sigma 150 binocular indirect ophthalmoscope, which can be spectacle mounted.

of peripheral areas of the retina. It is beneficial for younger patients because it automatically decreases the illumination intensity. Using the portable power source is advantageous to moving around the room and moving the patient more easily.

Heine OMEGA 180 provides built-in red-free, cobalt blue, and yellow filters and small, medium, and large spot apertures. It has a diffused light aperture to increase comfort. The company's patented *One-Step Small* and *Variable Pupil Control* reportedly maximizes stereopsis in all pupil sizes down to 1.2 mm. The Heine Sigma 150 (Fig. 11.13) can be spectacle-mounted or worn on the head. It allows the examiner to obtain binocular views in pupils as small as 2 mm.

Monocular Indirect Ophthalmoscopes

A monocular indirect ophthalmoscope (MIO) provides a wide, panoramic view of the fundus without the need for a condensing lens. A disadvantage of the MIO, as with direct ophthalmoscopes, is the lack of stereoscopic views.

The Keeler Wide Angle Twin Mag ophthalmoscope (Fig. 11.14) is lightweight and comfortable and offers multiple aperture selections. It has a one-handed grip and fingertip controls to allow the examiner to change focus without moving position and without losing the view. It has a 40-D range of focusing adjustment and a

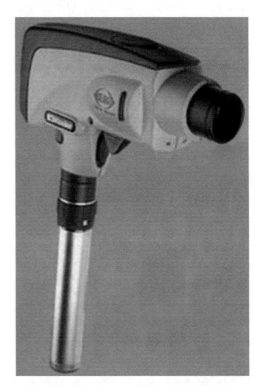

FIGURE 11.14. Keeler Wide Angle Twin Mag ophthalmoscope.

magnification of 1.0 and 2.0. It also has a corneal lens available for a corneal examination.

Welch Allyn Panoptic Ophthalmoscope (Fig. 11.15) is a handheld direct illuminating ophthalmoscope. It allows a greater working distance from the child and provides a larger view of the fundus. The manufacturer reports that

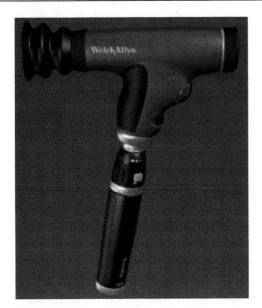

FIGURE 11.15.   Welch Allyn panoptic ophthalmoscope.

it is easier to enter small pupils and provides a wider, more panoramic view of the fundus that is 5 larger than that achieved with a standard ophthalmoscope in an undilated eye.

Keep in mind that if a view of the fundus cannot be obtained, the examination may need to be performed under sedation or attempted on another day (13).

ULTRASONOGRAPHY

Ultrasonography is important for the assessment of certain ocular and orbital diseases when direct visualization of intraocular structures is difficult or impossible. Situations that would necessitate the use of ultrasound include lid problems, corneal opacities, hyphema, miosis, hypopyon, dense cataracts, or vitreous opacities (17). Ultrasound can also be used to differentiate iris or ciliary body lesions, rule out ciliary body detachments, and differentiate between intraocular tumors and retinal detachments.

Ophthalmic ultrasonography uses high-frequency sound waves that are transmitted into the eye from a probe. This high frequency can only be transmitted through a gel-like contact substance. When the B-scan is performed through the closed eye, the eyelid compromises the image of the posterior segment. Therefore,

B-scan should be performed on the open eye. With an infant or child, however, it can be performed through the closed eyelid. Ultrasonography typically produces minimal discomfort and does not take long to obtain findings. Infants and children are best examined in their parent's arms (17).

SUMMARY

Evaluating the ocular health of an infant or child is essential in preventing vision conditions that have the potential to cause permanent vision loss. The examination has been made easier with the advent of handheld instruments. By making a few modifications, a thorough ocular health assessment can be completed. With the spectrum of instruments available, it is important to find the ones that are applicable for each practitioner.

REFERENCES

1. Catania D. The special patient. Part IV. Prepare to care for the physically challenged. *Review of Optometry* 2002;139 (04).
2. American Optometric Association. *Pediatric Eye and Vision Examination,* 2nd ed. St. Louis: American Optometric Association, 2002.
3. Kirschen D. The special patient. Get started with patients just getting started . . . in life. *Review of Optometry* 2002;139(01).
4. Luthe R. NCTs ain't what they used to be. *Optometric Management,* January 2005.
5. Armstrong T, Minckler DS, Kao S, et al. Evaluation of the Tono-pen and the Pulsair tonometers. *Am J Opthalmol* 1990;109:716–720.
6. http://www.keeler.co.uk/tonometer/kowa-ha2-tonometer.htm.
7. Cho P, Lui T. Comparison of the performance of the Nidek NT-2000 noncontact tonometer with the Keeler Pulsair 2000 and the Goldmann Applanation Tonometer. *Optom Vis Sci* 1997;74(1).
8. Buscemi M, Capoferri C, Garavaglia A, et al. Noncontact tonometry in children. *Optom Vis Sci* 1991;68(6):461–464.
9. Lawson-Kopp W, DeJong A, Yudcovitch L, et al. Clinical evaluation of the Keeler Pulsair 3000 non-contact tonometer. *Optometry* 2002;73(2):81–90.
10. Frenkel RE, Hong VYJ, Shin DH: Comparison of the Tono-Pen to the Goldmann applanation tonometer. *Arch Ophthalmol* 1988;106:750.
11. Moore B. *Eye Care for Infants and Young Children.* Boston: Butterworth-Heinemann; 1997.
12. Benavides JO, Satchell ER, Frantz KA. Efficacy of a mydriatic spray in the pediatric population. *Optom Vis Sci* 1997;74(3):160–163.
13. Press L, Moore B. *Clinical Pediatric Optometry.* USA, Butterworth-Heinemann; 1993.

14. Palmer E. How Safe are ocular drugs in pediatrics? *Ophthalmology*, 1986;93(8):1038–1040.

15. Wesson M, Bartlett J, Swiatocha J, et al. Mydriatic efficacy of a cycloplegic spray in the pediatric population. *Journal of the American Optometric Association* 1993;64(9):637–640.

16. Bartlett J, Wesson M, Swiatocha J, et al. Efficacy of a pediatric cycloplegic administered as a spray. *Journal of the American Optometric Association* 1993;64(9): 617–620.

17. Guthoff R. *Ultrasound in Ophthalmologic Diagnosis: A Practical Guide.* New York: Medical Publishers, Inc., 1991.

Abnormalities of the Anterior Segment

12

Pamela Hooker

In this chapter the most prevalent pathologies of the anterior segment encountered in the infant and pediatric population are discussed. Sight- or life-threatening disease processes are rare in this age group, but many less serious entities are commonly encountered. Etiology, prevalence, diagnosis, and treatment are all addressed.

ADNEXA AND LIDS

Capillary Hemangioma

Capillary hemangiomas are the most common benign orbital tumor in children. They can occur anywhere within the orbit or more superficially, and present with red, flat lesions that grow quickly, proptosis, or both (1). Children with capillary hemangiomas require referral to an oculoplastic surgeon if removal is to be attempted, and they should be closely monitored for the development of amblyopia if the lesion obstructs the visual axis. Occasionally, biopsy is indicated if malignancy is suspected. These lesions can spontaneously resolve, but corticosteroids are often used to speed resolution, either by local injection or systemic administration.

Dermoid

Dermoids are formed by ectodermal tissue being trapped in bony sutures during development (1). They can occur superficially, or more deeply, on the conjunctiva or cornea, and can

result in proptosis or optic neuropathy (1,2) (Fig. 12.1). The most common site for a dermoid cyst to appear is at the lateral eyebrow and the superionasal notch, and excision is usually recommended after 6 months of age. Although dermoid cysts are not themselves malignant, the potential exists for rupture of the cyst, which can lead to orbital cellulitis.

Congenital Arteriovenous Malformation

Congenital arteriovenous (AV) malformations appear in children as relatively low-flow, slow-growing lesions. Unlike capillary hemangiomas, growth of AV malformations tends to continue past the age of 1 year. If retinal involvement can be ruled out, the lesions can often be left untreated. Patients should be monitored for amblyopia development, however, if the visual axis is blocked.

Occasionally, AV malformations are found associated with Osler-Weber-Rendu or Wyburn-Mason syndromes, and patients should be referred for examination to rule out these entities.

Cellulitis

Although not as common as conjunctivitis, cellulitis is occasionally seen in the pediatric population, and can be quite serious (Fig. 12.2). Orbital cellulitis, the most common cause of proptosis in children (1), typically originates from infections in the paranasal sinuses. The most common bacterial causes include staphylococcus and streptococcus, as well as *Haemophilus*

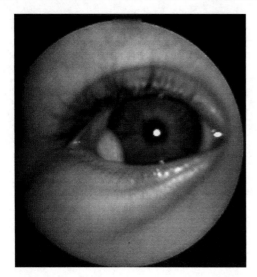

FIGURE 12.1. Dermoid cyst at corneal limbus. (Photo courtesy of Dr. Scott Richter). (See color well.)

influenzae if the child is not well immunized. Visual acuity is affected, and there is usually considerable swelling with closure of the lids and deficient extraocular motilities. Ultrasonography is a helpful diagnostic tool when the lids are too swollen to allow sufficient examination.

Treatment for cellulitis ranges from oral antibiotics on an outpatient basis (for preseptal cases) to hospitalization for intravenous administration. Occasionally, surgical draining of the sinuses is required.

Eyelid Laceration

A direct result of trauma, eyelid lacerations (Fig. 12.3) must be treated promptly to avoid intraoc-

ular infection. All patients with eyelid lacerations, regardless of age, need to have a comprehensive evaluation with dilation prior to treatment or surgical repair of the laceration to rule out any penetrating trauma to the globe. Orbital computed tomography (CT) scanning is useful for severe trauma, suspected orbital foreign body, or globe rupture.

In addition to in-office cleaning of the wound, surgical repair is often necessary, particularly if the laceration is large. Tetanus prophylaxis may also be indicated. If the laceration occurred at the lid margin, sutures are often left in place for 10 to 14 days. In other locations, sutures may be needed for only 4 to 6 days (3).

Blepharitis

Many children present with blepharitis of varying degrees. It can present with or without an accompanying conjunctivitis or meibomian gland dysfunction. A common cause of childhood blepharitis is staphylococcus infection, which usually manifests as chronic irritation of the lid, typically bilateral (4). Generally, also seen are ocular burning, conjunctival injection regardless of the presence or absence of frank conjunctivitis, and scales and collarettes around the lashes (3). Severe cases may also show neovascularization of the lid margin and possible madarosis.

Lid hygiene is the most important treatment that must be initiated in cases of active blepharitis. This typically involves lid scrubs two to three times per day with mild baby shampoo and water, as well as warm compresses to loosen

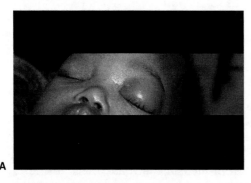
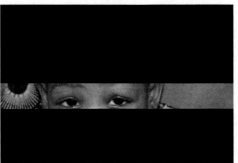

A   B

FIGURE 12.2. Preseptal cellulites. **A:** Active inflammation accompanied by high fever. **B:** Resolved condition. (Photos courtesy of Dr. Jeffrey Roth). (See color well.)

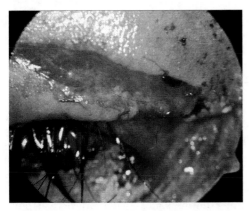

FIGURE 12.3. Eyelid laceration. (Photo courtesy of Dr. Jeffrey Roth). (See color well.)

debris and help express capped meibomian glands. Proper lid hygiene is instrumental in preventing recurrence of the condition. If necessary, topical antibiotics can also be prescribed. Ointments work well, as the medication will stay in direct contact with the affected area for extended periods. Topical steroids can be added if the case is particularly severe.

Dacryoadenitis

Dacryoadenitis is an orbital inflammation involving the lacrimal gland. The most common form of nonspecific orbital inflammation (1), it presents with pain and swelling along the upper lid in the region of the gland. Patients typically have a characteristic S-shape to the upper lid, and ptosis can be present if the swelling is significant. Diagnosis is aided with an orbital CT scan; treatment is usually with oral corticosteroids, with rapid resolution of inflammation.

Congenital Ptosis

Although ptosis can be caused by a number of entities, including birth trauma and myasthenia gravis, some children present with ptosis that is truly congenital. When faced with congenital ptosis as a possible diagnosis, it is important to rule out other conditions with careful history, paying special attention to parents' reports and earlier photographs. Intermittent conditions (e.g., nocturnal lagophthalmos) must also be considered and investigated (5).

Amblyopia is a concern in patients in whom there is visual axis obstruction. Careful visual

acuity and cycloplegic refraction should be performed to maximize the child's vision. If the visual axis is obscured, or if cosmesis is a significant issue, surgical correction of the eyelid is indicated. In general, the more severe the ptosis, the earlier the condition should be corrected to reduce the risk of severe deprivational amblyopia.

Congenital Nasolacrimal Duct Obstruction

Two to four percent of full-term newborns will show a congenital blockage of their nasolacrimal duct, a condition referred to as "nasolacrimal duct obstruction" (NLDO). One study reported an incidence of 20%, which may be more inclusive of those instances in which the condition spontaneously resolves (6). The condition, which typically manifests when the infant is between 1 and 2 weeks of age, includes a history of excessive tearing when the child is not crying. NLDO occurs when the valve of Hasner does not fully open, and most obstructions spontaneously open within 4 to 6 weeks after birth. Approximately 80% of all patients with NLDO have spontaneous resolution by the age of 1 year (5–7).

Epiphora in infants can be a sign of congenital glaucoma, a condition which must be ruled out by careful slit lamp evaluation, intraocular pressure measurement, and dilated fundus examination, as well as measurement of the corneal diameters, which are typically enlarged in congenital glaucoma. Ocular infections of various types can also cause tearing or watery discharge, and should also be ruled out before making a diagnosis of NLDO.

Duct obstruction is fairly easy to treat due to its tendency to spontaneously resolve. Parents should be instructed to perform massage over the nasolacrimal duct, rubbing downward and using petroleum jelly or other lubricant safe for the eyes to protect the sensitive skin in that area. Follow-up care should be scheduled frequently to monitor for progress and possible acute dacryocystitis, which can occur within a blocked duct. If this occurs, systemic antibiotics are indicated, with surgical drainage as needed. If the NLDO does not resolve by the time the child reaches approximately 1 year of age, probing and irrigation of the duct are indicated. Success rates above 95% have been reported if the probing is performed before 13 months of age, but the procedure is also helpful in patients older than 1 year. Occasionally, dacryocystorhinostomy is necessary for surgical bypass of the blockage in recalcitrant cases (5,8–9).

CONJUNCTIVA

Foreign Body

Children can acquire foreign bodies in as many ways as can be imagined. For most, treatment is the same as for adult patients. Symptoms can include irritation, pain, foreign body sensation, tearing, redness, a subjective history of getting something in the eye, or any combination of these. Clinical signs include injection, vertical corneal abrasions, which may stain with sodium fluorescein, and conjunctival or subconjunctival hemorrhage.

Foreign bodies should be differentiated from a number of other entities, including dry eye, blepharitis, conjunctivitis, trichiasis, recurrent corneal erosion, superficial punctate keratitis, contact lens-related problems, episcleritis, pterygium, or pinguecula. Most of these are easily discernable by outward appearance and subjective symptoms.

Clinical workup for foreign bodies includes a thorough history, slit lamp examination with measurement of intraocular pressure unless there is a known globe rupture, double lid eversion, and dilated fundus examination. Handheld slit lamps and non-contact tonometers (NCT) instruments are helpful for younger patients. In addition, B-scan ultrasonography and orbital CT scanning may be necessary.

The foreign body should be removed completely, using saline, cotton swab, spud, or forceps, as needed. The fornices should be swept for small particles as well. Antibiotic ointment with a pressure patch should be applied for the first 24 hours if the foreign body has left a central abrasion, and the child should be seen on the following day. Antibiotic drops can be used if an open abrasion remains, or the patch can be reapplied. Artificial tears and/or Celluvisc should be given for use every 1 to 2 hours once the patch is removed for residual abrasions or irritation caused by a foreign body. A follow-up visit should be scheduled for 1 week for known residual material (3).

Laceration

In addition to the eyelids, the conjunctiva can also be lacerated in cases of trauma. Symptoms with a conjunctival laceration can include pain, redness, foreign body sensation, or a history of trauma. Clinical signs that can be seen upon examination include sodium fluorescein stain of the conjunctiva, rolled conjunctival edges around the laceration, conjunctival or subconjunctival hemorrhage, and a possible direct view to the sclera if the laceration is sufficiently deep.

Work-up for conjunctival lacerations begins with a careful history to determine the nature of the injury, what type of object caused the laceration, and when the injury occurred. It is important to determine the risk of any possible penetrating injury as early as possible in the examination. Slit lamp examination with intraocular pressure (IOP) measurement (if no known globe rupture or penetrating injury) and dilation are indicated. B-scan, orbital CT, and exploratory surgery may all be necessary as well, particularly if a globe rupture is suspected.

The patient should be given antibiotic ointment three times a day (tid) for 7 days, with pressure patching as needed for 24-hour periods, depending on injury severity. Sutures are used as needed to close more significant lacerations. Follow-up visits will range from 24 hours to 1 week, depending on the extent of the injury and compliance with pressure patching and medication instillation (3).

Conjunctivitis

Neonatal

Neonatal conjunctivitis occurs in infants less than 1 month of age, and is most commonly caused by silver nitrate exposure from gonorrhea prophylaxis. Infectious varieties occur in only 1% to 12% of infants (4). Causes of neonatal infectious conjunctivitis include *Chlamydia trachomatis*, *Streptococcus* and *Staphylococcus* species, *Escherichia coli*, *Neisseria gonorrhea*, *Haemophilus* species, and herpes simplex virus. Of these, gonorrhea causes the most severe form of ophthalmia neonatorum (ON), is extremely damaging and progresses rapidly, and is thought to be responsible for up to 5% of blindness in poor countries (10). Chlamydia is thought to be the cause of up to 13% of neonatal conjunctivitis in industrialized countries (11). The high prevalence of sexually transmitted diseases in this list of etiologies is due to the likelihood from exposure to the infant's eyes during vaginal birth. For any newborn with conjunctivitis, immediate treatment should be started with antibiotics such as penicillin, erythromycin, or one or more of the cephalosporins.

Pediatric

Many different causes exist for conjunctivitis in older infants and children, which tend to be much less destructive than gonorrhea infection. Pediatric conjunctivitis can be bacterial, viral, allergic, or associated with systemic disease. The correct diagnosis is vital for proper treatment and follow-up care. Of the classifications, bacterial conjunctivitis is the most common at approximately 50% of acute cases, viral conjunctivitis accounts for 20%, and the remaining 30% are culture negative (4).

The most common bacteria that cause conjunctivitis in children are *Staphylococcus*, *Streptococcus*, *Haemophilus*, and *pneumococcus* species. Patients with bacterial conjunctivitis typically show copious mucopurulent discharge, with significant redness and swelling of the conjunctiva. Most patients are treated with broad-spectrum antibiotics without culture and followed closely for improvement. Culture must be performed if no improvement is noted over the expected time frame, and treatment adjusted accordingly (4).

Viral conjunctivitis in children is most often associated with either recent upper respiratory infection or contact with someone with a red eye. Commonly, viral conjunctivitis spreads rapidly through an entire school class, because it is easily transmitted by children sharing objects and playing with each other. Symptoms include watery mucous discharge, redness and possible swelling, possible subconjunctival hemorrhages, and palpable preauricular nodes.

The most contagious type of viral conjunctivitis is epidemic keratoconjunctivitis (EKC). Caused by adenovirus 8 or 19, it spreads extremely rapidly and can show acute symptoms for up to 3 weeks. As with all viral conjunctivitides, artificial tears and cold compresses should be used liberally, and precautions need to be taken not to share towels, pillowcases, or other household items that can come into contact with the affected eyes. Children should be kept home from school while the infection is active to reduce transmission. Antibiotics should NOT be prescribed (11).

Allergic conjunctivitis occurs in children as a result of a type I hypersensitivity reaction, with symptoms of redness, watery discharge, and itching. It is treated with mast cell stabilizers such as cromolyn sodium (Crolom or Opticrom) or lodoxamide (Alomide), or combination mast cell stabilizer and antihistamines such as olopatadine (Patanol). Allergic conjunctivitis can take the form of seasonal allergic or vernal conjunctivitis. The seasonal variety tends to show milder symptoms, and ocular signs are usually not commensurate with patient complaints. Typically, these patients have flare-ups in the spring with the re-emergence of pollens, and can be treated on an as-needed basis. Vernal conjunctivitis, on the other hand, is much more severe. In addition to the type I reaction, it also includes a type IV reaction (delayed hypersensitivity), and results in severe, giant cobblestone papillae under the upper lid. Copious ropy mucous discharge and severe itching are present. If left untreated, corneal scarring and permanent vision loss can occur. Although the disease tends to fluctuate with the seasons, being worse in spring, signs and symptoms can be present year round. Treatment includes chronic use of mast cell stabilizers or combination drops, with possible intermittent use of topical steroids (4,11).

CORNEA

Corneal Abrasion

Corneal abrasions, like foreign bodies, can occur in many ways in young children. They may have an injury from a toy, a branch, their own fingernail, or often even a sibling. Symptoms of corneal abrasions include photophobia,

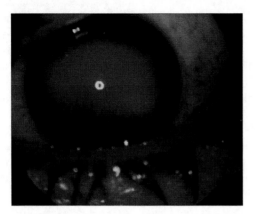

FIGURE 12.4. Corneal abrasion with sodium fluorescein stain. (Photo courtesy of Dr. Jeffrey Roth). (See color well.)

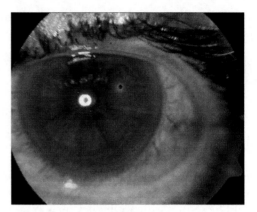

FIGURE 12.5. Corneal foreign body. (Photo courtesy of Dr. Jeffrey Roth). (See color well.)

foreign body sensation, tearing, and injection, and nearly always significant pain, particularly if the abrasion is central. Clinical signs include epithelial sodium fluorescein staining, injection, swelling, and, possibly, a mild anterior chamber reaction (Fig. 12.4). Corneal abrasions should be differentiated from foreign bodies, dry eye, blepharitis, conjunctivitis, trichiasis, recurrent corneal erosion, superficial punctate keratitis (SPK), contact lens-related problems, episcleritis, pterygium, or pinguecula. Careful slit lamp examination will usually indicate the correct diagnosis. Lid eversion is helpful to rule out a foreign body trapped in the fornix.

Treatment for corneal abrasions includes antibiotic ointment and pressure patching similar to that for foreign bodies and lacerations, but can also include the administration of a cycloplegic agent to control pain. Bandage contact lenses (BCLs) may be used in place of a pressure patch wherever one is indicated in cases where compliance with the patch may be poor and the lens can be successfully inserted. Antibiotic drops and artificial tears can then be administered directly onto the contact lens, and a BCL is more difficult to remove for young children. Follow-up care should be from 24 to 48 hours, depending on the size and centrality of the abrasion (3).

Foreign Body

Foreign bodies on the cornea are diagnosed and treated just as those on the conjunctiva,

but can show greater corneal damage in the form of abrasion or tracking. Symptoms, as with conjunctival foreign bodies, can include foreign body sensation, tearing, redness, blur, and photophobia. Signs encountered on examination can be a visible foreign body (Fig. 12.5) with or without a rust ring if the object is metallic, injection, lid edema, a mild anterior chamber reaction, SPK, and possible small infiltrates, which are usually sterile.

A careful history is needed in all cases of foreign body, whether or not corneal involvement is suspected. Important information includes the type of foreign body (if known), how and when the injury occurred, and whether any glasses or other protective eyewear was worn. Visual acuity should be taken first, as with all cases of trauma, both with and without anesthesia, to determine the best level obtainable. Careful slit lamp examination and dilation are then indicated.

If the foreign body is still in place on or in the cornea, it should be removed with saline, swab, spud, or needle, as necessary under topical anesthesia. An Alger brush may be necessary to remove a rust ring. The resulting abrasion should then be measured to determine the proper follow-up schedule. Cycloplegics, antibiotic ointment or drops, and a pressure patch or bandage contact lens are then applied. Follow-up visits should be scheduled for 24 hours in cases of a central or large abrasion, and 48 hours if the abrasion is more peripheral or small (3).

Superficial Punctate Keratitis (SPK)

Children, like adults, can present with SPK of varying causes. Reported symptoms can be pain, photophobia, redness, or foreign body sensation. Seen will be diffuse pinpoint epithelial defects that stain with sodium fluorescein, conjunctival injection, and possible watery or mucoid discharge if the SPK is more severe.

History should include information pertaining to any trauma, contact lens wear, use of drops (prescription or over the counter), and any discharge or matting of the lashes. Slit lamp examination should be performed, with attention to proper lid closure and possible laxity or trichiasis. Lid eversion is useful to rule out foreign body. Differential diagnosis and etiology for SPK includes dry eye syndrome, blepharitis, exposure keratopathy, topical drug toxicity, ultraviolet (UV) burn or photokeratopathy, and trauma.

Artificial tears and ocular lubricants are indicated to aid in corneal healing, and antibiotics can be added, as necessary, if the condition is severe. Cycloplegia may help reduce pain (3).

For patients who do not wear contact lenses, follow-up care can be on an as-needed basis, although with children it may be more prudent to schedule at least one follow up visit regardless of reported improvement in symptoms. If the child wears contact lenses, follow-up should be scheduled anywhere from 24 hours to 1 week, depending on severity. The lenses themselves should be evaluated for build-up, deposits, and tears, with wear time and care changed appropriately. Any underlying pathology in addition to the SPK should also be addressed.

Dry Eye Syndrome

Many children, particularly those who live in large urban areas, experience symptoms of dry eye syndrome. These include burning, foreign body sensation, and excess tearing exacerbated by such things as smoke, wind, heat, low humidity, and prolonged eyestrain. On examination, these patients show a thin tear meniscus and decreased tear break-up time (TBUT) and may have SPK, excess mucous, or filaments.

It is important to differentiate dry eye syndrome from entities with similar symptoms, as the treatment will differ. Other diagnoses and causes include blepharitis, exposure keratitis, nocturnal lagophthalmos, collagen-vascular disease, scarring from burns or trauma, and drug side effects.

Dry eye syndrome is typically diagnosed based on slit lamp findings in the course of a comprehensive eye examination. In some cases, a Schirmer test can be useful to quantify tear insufficiency, but this test is difficult in children, and the diagnosis can be made without it. Artificial tears, Celluvisc, or ocular ointments are appropriate for use as needed and many can be obtained over the counter. Acetylcysteine (Mucomyst) is available as a prescription for more advanced cases. Existing filaments should be removed in the office, and a pressure patch can be used in cases of severe SPK. If necessary, more intensive treatments are available, including punctal occlusion, cautery, and tarsorrhaphy.

Follow-up care is scheduled from a few days to weeks, depending on the severity of the condition. A systemic workup is recommended for severe cases of dry eye syndrome because it can be a manifestation of such diseases as sarcoidosis, juvenile rheumatoid arthritis, or ocular pemphigoid (3).

Keratitis

Keratitis, as with conjunctivitis, can occur for a variety of reasons in children, including bacterial infection, viral infection, and exposure, as well as a number of other causes. Treatment needs to address the underlying cause as well as the outward signs and symptoms for complete resolution.

Bacterial keratitis can be caused by any of the bacteria that cause conjunctivitis, and children often present with both conditions simultaneously. As with the treatment of conjunctivitis, the correct organism needs to be determined with culture, although many cases are treated with topical broad-spectrum antibiotics such as tobramycin, fluoroquinolone, or cephazolin without culture. If a corneal ulcer is present, however, a culture is imperative. For extreme cases,

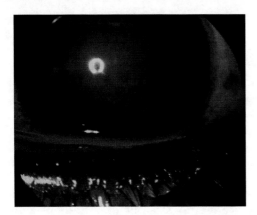

FIGURE 12.6. Corneal dendrite in herpes simplex keratitis. (Photo courtesy of Dr. Jeffrey Roth). (See color well.)

subconjunctival injection of antibiotics may be required.

Viral keratitis can be caused by either of the herpes viruses. When infection is due to herpes simplex, which can affect children of any age and is not necessarily a sign of child abuse, signs and symptoms are similar to those of an adult patient. The child will have an initial SPK, followed by classic dendritic keratitis, which stains with sodium fluorescein (Fig. 12.6). Herpes simplex keratitis may also present as a disciform keratitis, which is present underneath an intact epithelium. The stroma may become inflamed and edematous, decreasing vision and causing pain, photophobia, and tearing. If the corneal epithelium is intact, topical steroids can be used with caution. All cases should be treated with topical antivirals, as needed, and profuse artificial tears to wash away viral particles. If the viral keratitis is caused by herpes zoster, which is common in pediatric patients, the patient will have the typical vesicular skin lesions along with chills, fever, and general malaise. The virus remains dormant in the nerve ganglion, however, which can cause ocular manifestations long after the skin is clear. Dendritic lesions can appear, which look identical to those of herpes simplex, or the patient can have interstitial keratitis, chorioretinitis, optic neuritis, uveitis, or scleritis (4,11) Topical antibiotics can be used as prophylaxis in cases of open lesions on the skin, and cycloplegia is often useful to control pain. Cool compresses, lubricating ointments and artificial tears, and topical antiviral medications are all useful in reducing the time span of the active infection.

Corneal Dystrophies

Several corneal dystrophies can affect children. Although an in-depth examination of each is beyond the scope of this chapter, it is important to note these entities for proper diagnosis.

Epithelial dystrophies affecting pediatric patients include Meesmann's, Reis-Bücklers', and Cogan's dystrophy. They are all autosomal dominant in inheritance, are typically associated with recurrent corneal erosions, and usually do not affect visual acuity. Lubricating ointments can be used to treat recurrent erosions, and occasionally laser treatment to Bowman's layer is necessary to increase stability in the epithelium (11).

Stromal dystrophies include granular, lattice, gelatinous droplike, macular, and central crystalline dystrophy. Varying degrees of visual impairment are associated with these conditions, ranging from little impairment in central crystalline dystrophy to severe impairment in gelatinous droplike dystrophy. Corneal grafts can be used with varying success, with recurrence common.

Posterior polymorphous dystrophy is an endothelial dystrophy that can present in children. Patients are usually asymptomatic, and visual prognosis is good. Congenital hereditary endothelial dystrophy (CHED) is an abnormality occurring in utero, and can be visually devastating if not treated with lamellar keratoplasty within the first few months of life. It should be differentiated from congenital glaucoma; CHED shows corneal edema similar to glaucoma, but no increase is seen in either corneal diameter or IOP.

Keratoconus

In its anterior form, keratoconus is a bilateral disease process that presents with corneal thinning and protrusion, usually inferonasally. The disease onset is early, but may not be evident until the patient is between the age of 10 and 20 years. Initial findings can include distorted retinoscopy reflexes secondary to irregular astigmatism and progressive myopia, which are not correctible by spectacle prescription. A protrusion of the lower lid on downgaze (Munson's sign) and iron deposits at the base of the cone (Fleischer ring) may be seen. There may also be deep vertical striae (Vogt's) and increased visibility of corneal nerves. As the disease progresses, which tends to be slow for the first 6 to 10 years, rigid gas-permeable contact lenses may help to achieve best visual acuity. In later stages, penetrating keratoplasty may be required (11).

The entire cornea can be thinned in a rare condition known as keratoglobus. In contrast to anterior keratoconus, keratoglobus does not progress, and the cornea can perforate with only minor trauma; therefore, contact lenses are not used. Penetrating keratoplasty is difficult in these cases.

The posterior surface of the cornea can show concavity in a condition known as posterior keratoconus. This localized thinning of the cornea is associated with a normal anterior surface curvature; it is usually unilateral, nonprogressive, and occurs more often in female patients than in male patients. Its cause is unknown.

Developmental Disorders

Several developmental disorders can affect the cornea. Each can cause its own set of sequelae that must be treated as they are diagnosed. Megalocornea is a bilateral congenital condition in which the cornea has a horizontal measurement of more than 13 mm before the age of 2 years. This occurs in the absence of raised IOP, unlike in cases of juvenile glaucoma, which can also cause an increase in corneal diameter. It can be seen in conjunction with various systemic entities, or as part of Marfan, Aarskog, or Crouzon syndrome. Cornea plana is another bilateral congenital anomaly in which the cornea is flattened in association with hyperopia. It can be either autosomal dominant or recessive, the latter of which tends to be more severe. Peters' anomaly is an opacification of the cornea with underlying iridocorneal adhesions and absence of the central corneal endothelium. It is often bilateral and can be associated with glaucoma, cataract, microphthalmos, iris dysgenesis, heart defects, midline central nervous system disorders, genitourinary disease, fetal alcohol syndrome, or other systemic conditions (12).

IRIS

Uveitis

Uveitis is an entity that can easily be considered in terms of both the anterior and posterior segments of the eye. It may take the form of an iritis, a pars planitis, or a retinitis, and still be considered an inflammation of the uveal tract. Here, iritis is discussed with more posterior inflammations included with the posterior segment.

Uveitis has myriad causes, but for all of them, the first step toward proper diagnosis and treatment is a careful and thorough history. Demographics, present illness, ocular and medical history, and family history are all important, and are asked about during most standard examinations. In cases of suspected uveitis, additional questions can be helpful, including where the patient lives or has recently traveled, any pets that may be in the home, what type of foods the patient eats, and both drug and sexual history (including abuse).

Examination encompasses more than just the ocular tissues in uveitis cases, because certain systemic diseases can manifest as ocular inflammation. The joints and skin should be examined, and cranial nerve testing may be helpful. Careful slit lamp examination is indicated to check for redness, swelling, discharge, corneal involvement, precipitates, and cells and flare in the anterior chamber (Fig. 12.7). In some types of uveitis, posterior manifestations are also present in the vitreous or retina, which is discussed in the following chapter.

Uveitis can be caused by either infectious or noninfectious entities. In the anterior segment, noninfectious causes include juvenile rheumatoid arthritis (JRA), ankylosing spondylitis, Reiter's syndrome, inflammatory bowel disease, pediatric sarcoid, Fuch's heterochromic iridocyclitis, or Kawasaki disease (13,14). These causes must be carefully ruled out for proper treatment to be instituted. Infectious causes of anterior uveitis include congenital infection from such entities as syphilis, cytomegalovirus, or rubella. Also possible are viral infections such as mumps, herpes zoster, or herpes simplex.

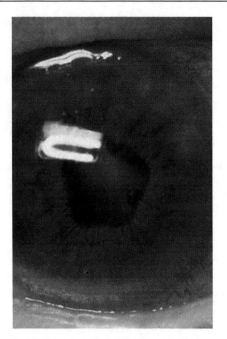

FIGURE 12.7. Posterior synechia in uveitis. (Photo courtesy of Dr. Scott Richter). (See color well.)

Finally, uveitis can also be caused by measles, influenza, Epstein-Barr virus, tuberculosis, or Lyme disease (13,14).

For most of the anterior uveitides, topical steroids will help to reduce inflammation. If the corneal epithelium is compromised, steroids must be used with caution, and antibiotics may be indicated as a preventative measure. Children with anterior uveitis may also receive comfort from mydriatics in cases of significant pain. Follow-up care is instituted on a case to case basis, depending on the cause and severity of the inflammation.

Angle Anomalies

Several congenital anomalies affect the iridocorneal angle, the most common of which is posterior embryotoxin. Seen as an anteriorly displaced Schwalbe's line, posterior embryotoxin is usually an isolated and incidental finding. Axenfeld's anomaly is a condition in which posterior embryotoxin is associated with peripheral iris adhesions to Schwalbe's line, and can be further complicated by glaucoma (12).

Rieger's Anomaly

Rieger's anomaly is a developmental anomaly that presents with varying degrees of iris hypoplasia and ectropion uveae, posterior embryotoxin, iridotrabecular bridges, and polycoria. It is accompanied by glaucoma in approximately 60% of cases, and can include such systemic features as maxillary hypoplasia, dental abnormalities, and inguinal hernias.

Aniridia

A complete absence of the iris is known as aniridia. This condition occurs in approximately 1 in 60,000 to 100,000 births (12), and usually a family history is present. Aniridia may be associated with Wilms' tumor and genitourinary abnormalities in WAGR (*W*ilms tumor, *a*niridia, *g*enitourinary abnormalities or gonadoblastoma, and mental *r*etardation) syndrome, and patients often present with nystagmus, foveal hypoplasia, lens dislocation, cataract, or corneal opacity (12).

Lens

Lenticular anomalies tend to be relatively rare in the pediatric population. When they occur, however, they are significant findings that need immediate attention. Often, lens changes appear as a leukocoria, or white pupil, which is easily apparent to the naked eye. Occasionally, leukocoria in children can be a manifestation of life-threatening illness such as retinoblastoma.

Cataract

Children can present with cataracts caused by trauma (Fig. 12.8), systemic disease, or congenital etiology. Whatever the cause, an evaluation must be made to determine the need for cataract extraction, because prolonged occlusion of one or both eyes due to cataract may result in deprivation amblyopia.

Approximately 1 in 250 newborns has some form of congenital cataract (15,16). They can occur in any layer of the lens, with varying degrees of visual impairment, from none at all to severe amblyopia, depending on location and onset. In general, the earlier a disabling cataract

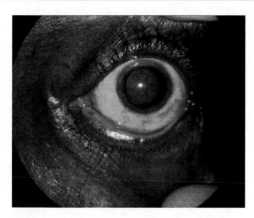

FIGURE 12.8. Rosette cataract secondary to trauma. (Photo courtesy of Dr. Jeffrey Roth). (See color well.)

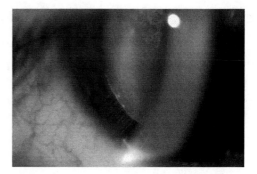

FIGURE 12.9. Subluxated intraocular lens. (Photo courtesy of Dr. Jeffrey Roth). (See color well.)

can be removed, the better the prognosis for normal visual development.

In addition to hereditary and idiopathic causes, one third of childhood cataracts are associated with systemic disease (15,16). These can include Down syndrome, Lowe syndrome, galactosemia, and various intrauterine infections. Careful slit lamp evaluation and ultrasonography can be helpful in determining both the nature of the cataract and the health of the posterior segment when the dilated view is poor.

Lens Subluxation

Subluxation of the crystalline lens, or ectopia lentis, can occur secondary to a number of clinical entities (Fig. 12.9). Among these are trauma, aniridia, congenital syphilis, and several genetic syndromes such as Marfan or Weill-Marchesani (17,18). An autosomal dominant multisystem syndrome, Marfan is the most common cause of subluxated lenses in children (19), and presents with cardiac and skeletal malformations in addition to ocular manifestations. Notable among these are excessive height, *pectus excavatum*, arachnodactyly, and hyperextendible joints. Lens dislocation occurs in 30% to 80% of these patients; other ocular sequelae can include axial elongation and megalocornea (17).

REFERENCES

1. Kazim M. Orbital diseases. In: Gallin PF, ed. *Pediatric Ophthalmology: A Clinical Guide.* New York: Thieme; 2000:295–323.
2. Hughes D. Eyelid disorders. In: Moore A, ed. *Fundamentals of Clinical Ophthalmology: Paediatric Ophthalomology.* London: BMJ Books; 2000:154–161.
3. Kunimoto DY, Kanitkar KD, Makar MS, eds. *The Wills Eye Manual: Office and Emergency Room Diagnosis and Treatment of Eye Disease,* 4th ed. Philadelphia: Lippincott Williams & Wilkins; 2004.
4. Nguyen QD, Foster CS. The red eye. In: Gallin PF, ed. *Pediatric Ophthalmology: A Clinical Guide.* New York: Thieme; 2000:204–215.
5. Leib ML. Plastic surgery. In: Gallin PF, ed. *Pediatric Ophthalmology: A Clinical Guide.* New York: Thieme; 2000:324–333.
6. MacEwen CJ, Young JD. Epiphora during the first year of life. *Eye* 1991;5:596–600.
7. Rose GE. Paediatric lacrimal and orbital disease. In: Moore A, ed. *Fundamentals of Clinical Ophthalmology: Paediatric Ophthalmology.* London: BMJ Books; 2000:162–176.
8. Stager D, Baker JD, Frey T, et al. Office probing of congenital nasolacrimal duct obstruction. *Ophthal Surg* 1992; 23(7):482–484.
9. Katowitz JA, Welsh MG. Timing of initial probing and irrigation in congenital nasolacrimal duct obstruction. *Ophthalmology* 1987;94(6):698–705.
10. Gilbert C, Foster A. Epidemiology of childhood blindness. In: Moore A, ed. *Fundamentals of Clinical Ophthalmology: Paediatric Ophthalmology.* London: BMJ Books; 2000:1–13.
11. Prydal J. Disorders of the conjunctiva and cornea. In: Moore A, ed. *Fundamentals of Clinical Ophthalmology: Paediatric Ophthalmology.* London: BMJ Books; 2000:62–81.
12. Gregory-Evans K. Developmental disorders of the globe. In: Moore A, ed. *Fundamentals of Clinical Ophthalmology: Paediatric Ophthalmology.* London: BMJ Books; 2000:53–61.
13. Weiss MJ, Hofeldt AJ. Uveitis. In: Gallin PF, ed. *Pediatric Ophthalmology: A Clinical Guide.* New York: Thieme; 2000:216–31.

14. Graham EM, Stanbury RM. Ocular inflammatory disease. In: Moore A, ed. *Fundamentals of Clinical Ophthalmology: Paediatric Ophthalmology*. London: BMJ Books; 2000:82–91.
15. Douros S, Jain SD, Garman BD, et al. Leukocoria. In: Gallin PF, ed. *Pediatric Ophthalmology: A Clinical Guide*. New York: Thieme; 2000:241–250.
16. Braunstein RE, Cotliar AM. Pediatric cataracts. In: Gallin PF, ed. *Pediatric Ophthalmology: A Clinial Guide*. New York: Thieme, 2000:251–256.
17. Butera C, Plotnik J, Bateman JB, et al. Ocular genetics. In: Gallin PF, ed. *Pediatric Ophthalmology: A Clinical Guide*. New York: Thieme; 2000:78–91.
18. Kruger E, Gorman BD, Schubert HD et al. Ocular trauma. In: Gallin PF, ed. *Pediatric Ophthalmology: A Clinical Guide*. New York: Thieme; 2000:185–203.
19. Russell-Eggitt IM. Disorders of the lens. In: Moore A, ed. *Fundamentals of Clinical Ophthalmology: Paeditric Ophthalmology*. London: BMJ Books; 2000:111–120.

Abnormalities of the Posterior Segment

13

Pamela Hooker

Ocular pathology in the posterior segment is relatively uncommon in children. When it does occur, however, it can be serious, with vision- and even life-threatening consequences. Clinicians must perform careful examinations of the posterior segment of all of their pediatric patients, including regular dilated fundus examinations. The most frequently encountered conditions will be discussed, along with current treatments and referral options.

CILIARY BODY

Posterior Uveitis

Posterior uveitis in the pediatric population has many causes. Among these are toxoplasmosis, toxocariasis, sarcoidosis, bacterial infections (e.g., tuberculosis and syphilis), viral infections (e.g., cytomegalovirus [CMV], rubella, measles, and herpes viruses), and fungal infections (1). Symptoms can include blurred vision, redness, and floaters, but usually no pain. Treatment varies according to the causative agent, but often includes systemic steroids (2).

In older children, toxoplasmosis is the most common cause of posterior uveitis (Fig. 13.1). It is caused by *Toxoplasma gondii* and is carried by cats. It can be congenital or acquired, although chorioretinitis is usually associated with the former. Lesions appear fluffy and yellow-white in active cases and are usually located adjacent to an area of chorioretinal atrophy or pigmented

scar. Often, there is an overlying vitritis. Macular involvement is usually seen, with significant visual acuity impairment (3), but toxoplasmosis cases are often self-limiting, resolving within weeks to months. In the case of an immunocompromised patient, however, more severe ocular disease can occur (4). When treatment is indicated, as in the case of lesions close to the optic nerve or macula, or in immunocompromised patients, it is usually in the form of pyrimethamine or clindamycin and steroids.

Toxocariasis is caused by infection with the intestinal parasite *Toxocara canis*, common in dogs. It can present as endophthalmitis, retinal granulomas (especially in the macula), or more widespread inflammation with the possibility of vitreoretinal abscess (1,5). The condition is generally unilateral. As with toxoplasmosis, systemic steroids are indicated to reduce inflammation. The use of antihelmintic drugs may be counterproductive because the death of the parasite can cause additional inflammation.

Posterior uveitis caused by systemic sarcoid is more common in patients between the ages of 20 and 50 years, but is occasionally seen in younger patients. Typical findings include bilateral pain and photophobia, as well as blurred vision. Severe cases may show mutton-fat keratic precipitates and iris nodules. Systemic steroids are indicated because topical steroids will be insufficient.

Bacterial infections (tuberculosis, syphilis) and viral infections (CMV, rubella, measles,

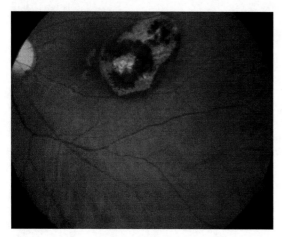

FIGURE 13.1. Toxoplasmosis (photo courtesy of Dr. Jeffrey Roth). (See color well.)

herpes zoster, herpes simplex) can also cause pediatric posterior uveitis. Approximately 6% of children with the acquired immunodeficiency syndrome (AIDS) will have CMV retinitis (1), which appears as a whitish necrotic area in the retina with associated retinal hemorrhages (5). Intravenous ganciclovir should be administered. Congenital syphilis presents as a salt-and-pepper fundus and can mimic any number of other conditions. In any case of suspected viral or bacterial infection, workup should include appropriate testing to rule out probable organisms so that the proper antibiotic or other treatment can be administered.

Panuveitis

Widespread uveitis can occur secondary to many of the above conditions if not treated promptly, as well from such entities as Behçet disease. The latter is diagnosed based on a combination of oral ulcers plus two of a number of systemic manifestations, including bilateral retinal vasculitis (6–8). Although the disease is more common in patients from 20 to 50 years of age, when a pediatric onset occurs, uveitis will more likely be one of the presenting symptoms (9). As with other cases of posterior uveitis, symptoms include blurry vision, photophobia, pain, and floaters. Complications are frequent and include hypopyon, cataract, macular edema, retinal vascular changes including branch retinal vein occlusion (BRVO) and neovascularization, and retinal detachment (1,5).

These children will need systemic steroids and referral to a specialist for possible immunosuppressive therapy.

VITREOUS

Persistent Hyperplastic Primary Vitreous

A significant developmental disorder of the vitreous is persistent hyperplastic primary vitreous (PHPV). Occasionally, the hyaloid vascular system will not be completely regressed at the time of an infant's birth. On examination it may appear as a projection of tissue from the optic disk or as a small opacity on the posterior aspect of the crystalline lens known as a *Mittendorf dot* (Fig. 13.2). More significant is the failure of proper development of the primary vitreous. When PHPV is present, it is usually associated with microphthalmia, shallow anterior chamber, lens opacities, and retrolenticular membrane, and it can present with leukocoria of the affected eye or retinal detachment (10–12). The condition may progress and cause angle-closure glaucoma. Treatment varies with the age of onset, but can include lensectomy or vitrectomy, with accompanying occlusion therapy. Contact lens fitting is indicated to manage the aphakic refractive error.

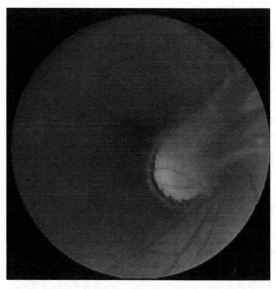

FIGURE 13.2. Persistent hyperplastic primary vitreous (PHPV) (photo courtesy of Dr. Scott Richter). (See color well.)

RETINA

Developmental Anomalies

Coloboma

Colobomas can occur in many ocular structures, including the iris, optic nerve, and retina (Fig. 13.3). Coloboma, a developmental anomaly that represents incomplete closure of the fetal fissure during gestational development, can be unilateral or bilateral. Usually, no family history of coloboma is found, but an autosomal dominant inheritance pattern has been shown in some cases.

Retinal or choroidal colobomas typically appear as a pale yellow-white area inferior to the optic disk, and may present as leukocoria if sufficiently large. They vary in size and can be associated with optic nerve coloboma. If this is the case, retinal detachment is also a concern. Visual prognosis is closely associated with the amount of macular and optic nerve involvement. An associated nonprogressive visual field defect may also be present. Associated systemic abnormalities include CHARGE association, basal encephalocele, and various chromosomal disorders (13,14).

Optic pits and morning glory syndrome have been described as mild and severe presenta-

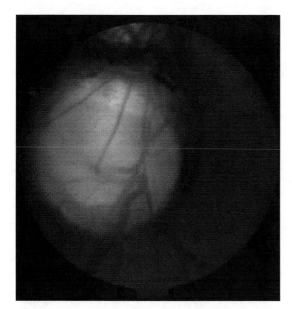

FIGURE 13.3. Optic nerve head coloboma (photo courtesy of Dr. Scott Richter). (See color well.)

tions of optic nerve coloboma, respectively (15). The latter involves a posteriorly displaced optic nerve head within a posterior staphyloma, with several layers of glial tissue covering it. The retinal vessels radiate outward like spokes on a wheel, and vision is generally poor from birth.

Vascular Anomalies

CAPILLARY HEMANGIOMA

Capillary hemangiomas in the retina typically occur as part of Von Hippel-Lindau disease (16), although they can sometimes be seen in isolation (17). They appear as elevated, red vascular lesions that vary in size and have feeder and drainage vessels. They can occur either in the retina or on the optic disk, the latter of which are more difficult to treat. By themselves, capillary hemangiomas are benign tumors, but they can cause blurred vision or vision loss from retinal exudation, epiretinal membrane formation, or vitreous hemorrhage. Treatment usually consists of either cryotherapy or argon laser, with generally good visual outcomes (18,19).

CAVERNOUS HEMANGIOMA

Cavernous hemangiomas typically appear in females in the second or third decade of life. They have a grape cluster appearance, with small aneurisms surrounded by gray-white fibrous tissue, and are usually unilateral and isolated. Most cavernous hemangiomas can be observed unless leakage is evident (14,20).

ARTERIOVENOUS (AV) MALFORMATION

Although most vascular abnormalities in children are benign when they occur in isolation, clinicians should be aware that some can be associated with systemic disease. Diabetes can cause venous beading, and leukemia can cause beading or tortuosity of retinal vessels, for example. Any vascular anomaly noted in a pediatric patient should be followed up with appropriate systemic testing.

Retinopathy of Prematurity

Retinopathy of prematurity (ROP), a vasoproliferative disorder caused by incomplete retinal vascularization, is exacerbated by oxygen exposure. Because of the increasing survival rate of premature infants, ROP is becoming more of a concern for pediatric optometrists and ophthalmologists. Peripheral vascularization reaches the nasal ora serrata at approximately 36 weeks' gestational age, but does not reach the temporal ora until 40 weeks (21). Premature infants, therefore, do not have complete retinal vascularization at the time of birth. Infants at high risk for ROP include those who are born at less than 36 weeks' gestation or weigh less than 2000 g, particularly if the child with highest risk associated with extremely low birthweight (less than 1000 g), received supplemental oxygen after birth (21). The administration of oxygen causes normal vascularization to stop, and abnormal neovascularization can occur.

According to the International Classification of Retinopathy of Prematurity (22), the disease is categorized into five stages in three retinal zones. Zone I is defined as a circle with the optic disk at the center and a diameter of twice the distance from the optic nerve to the fovea. Zone II is a circle concentric to Zone I that extends outward to the nasal ora serrata. Zone III is the remaining retina, a crescent including the superior, inferior, and temporal periphery.

Stage I disease consists of a demarcation line between vascular and avascular retina in the temporal periphery. In Stage II, this line is elevated into a ridge. Stage III disease includes neovascular vessels extending into the vitreous from this area. If retinal detachment exists, the ROP is at least Stage IV, with Stage IV-a having the macula attached and Stage IV-b having the macula detached. Total retinal detachment is seen in Stage V.

Three further classifications of ROP are *plus* disease, *rush* disease, and *threshold* disease. In *plus* disease, dilated and tortuous retinal vessels are seen in combination with dilated iris vessels (Fig. 13.4). *Rush* disease describes the involvement of Zone I with extensive disease. *Threshold* disease is reached when the child has Stage III ROP, in Zones I or II, with disease that includes either five contiguous or eight total clock hours of neovascularization.

Progression of ROP to disease is the indication for treatment, which usually consists of either cryotherapy to the avascular peripheral retina or, more recently, laser photocoagula-

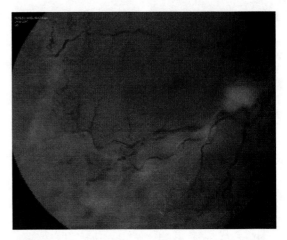

FIGURE 13.4.   Retinopathy of prematurity (ROP) with retinal detachment (photo courtesy of Dr. Jeffrey Roth). (See color well.)

tion. Cryotherapy has been shown to reduce the incidence of unfavorable outcomes in ROP by 50% (21,23). Additional surgery may be indicated for retinal detachment.

Genetic Disorders

Congenital Stationary Night Blindness

Congenital stationary night blindness (CSNB) is a genetic condition that can be inherited in an autosomal dominant, autosomal recessive, or X-linked pattern. Most patients with CSNB show either the X-linked or autosomal recessive inheritance pattern, and have nystagmus in infancy, myopia with reduction in visual acuity, and mild color vision deficiency. The autosomal dominant form does not show nystagmus and has normal visual acuity. All forms show poor night vision and reduced scotopic response on electroretinogram (ERG) (24).

Achromatopsia

Two distinct forms of achromatopsia exist: an autosomal recessive form, which is more common and also known as *rod monochromatism*; and an X-linked recessive form, also known as *blue cone monochromatism*. The autosomal recessive form, in which there is a complete lack of functional cone photoreceptors in the retina, shows absent cone responses on ERG (14), reduced vision (often with high hyperopia), rapid, fine nystagmus, and severe photophobia. In the X-linked form, presentation is milder, with

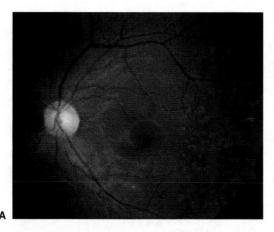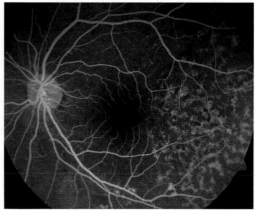

FIGURE 13.5. Stargardt's disease. **A:** Color fundus photo (see color well). **B:** Fluorescein angiography (photos courtesy of Dr. Jeffrey Roth).

typically myopic refractive error, better visual acuity, and some blue cone function (24).

Leber's Congenital Amaurosis

Also known as *infantile rod-cone dystrophy,* Leber's congenital amaurosis is an autosomal recessive inherited disorder. Children with Leber's amaurosis generally have a normal-appearing fundus, but extremely poor vision with roving eye movements, nystagmus, and high hyperopia. Pupil responses are also abnormal and ERG response is severely decreased or extinguished. The condition is typically detected within the first few months of life, and patients suspected of having Leber's amaurosis should be referred for systemic testing to rule out rare syndromes such as Joubert syndrome (24,25).

Stargardt Disease

Stargardt disease is an autosomal recessive disorder, which usually presents as a loss of central vision in school-aged children (26). In its early stages, the fundus may appear normal, although the typical presentation is a bull's-eye maculopathy that is often accompanied by flecklike yellow deposits at the level of the retinal pigment epithelium (RPE) (Fig. 13.5a). (A variant of Stargardt, *fundus flavimaculatus,* shows these flecks without maculopathy, and has a better visual prognosis.) Fluorescein angiography shows a characteristic dark choroid and central atrophy (Fig. 13.5b). Indocyanine green angiography shows large choroidal vessels in the "dark" area

and hypofluorescence of flecks (27) in contrast to the hyperfluorescence seen in fluorescein angiography. Pattern ERG is frequently reduced (28). The disease is progressive, and typically results in best visual acuity of approximately 20/200 by the patient's early twenties. These patients can also experience peripheral visual field loss and night blindness, as well as psychological difficulties such as depression (29). No treatment is known for Stargardt disease, but affected individuals may benefit from various low-vision devices and referral to a psychologist or social worker.

Best Disease (Vitelliform Dystrophy)

An autosomal dominant disease with variable penetrance, Best disease, or vitelliform macular dystrophy, is usually present from birth, although it may not be detected until later in life. The condition appears as bilateral, circular yellow lipofuscin deposits in the fovea, often compared in appearance to egg yolks (Fig. 13.6). It causes only mild visual decrease, if any, although it can result in macular choroidal neovascularization if the lesions degenerate. No current treatment is available for the underlying condition, but choroidal neovascular nets should be treated with focal laser. All affected patients and carriers of the gene for Best disease show a reduced light rise on electro-oculogram (EOG). It is important, therefore, to test all family members so that they can be followed for development of macular lesions and given proper genetic counseling (5,24).

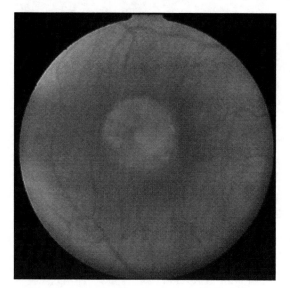

FIGURE 13.6. Macular lesion in Best disease (vitelliform dystrophy) (photo courtesy of Dr. Scott Richter). (See color well.)

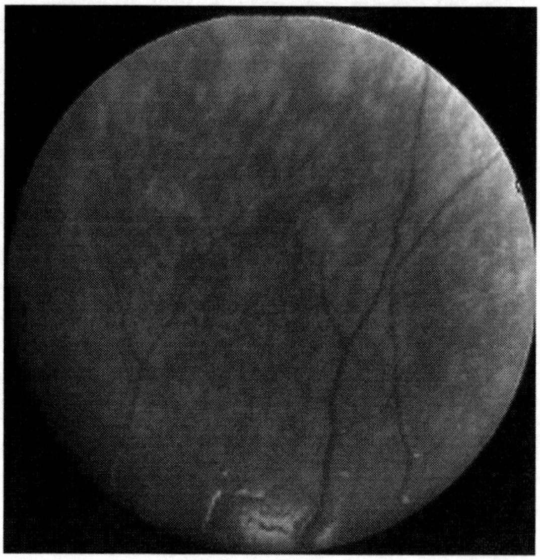

FIGURE 13.7. Retinitis pigmentosa (RP) showing typical bone spicule appearance (photo courtesy of Dr. Scott Richter). (See color well.)

Retinitis Pigmentosa

Retinitis pigmentosa (RP) describes a group of disorders involving a progressive rod-cone dystrophy. Its mode of inheritance can be X-linked recessive, autosomal recessive, or autosomal dominant, and phenotypes vary greatly even within the subgroups. In general, the X-linked recessive type has the earliest onset and worst visual prognosis (24).

Patients can present with a subjective complaint of difficulty with night vision or be asymptomatic and referred for a family history of night vision problems. Other complaints can include photopsia, headache, or fluctuating daylight vision. In addition, infants with RP can present with absent visual responses.

The progression pattern in RP is one of gradual deterioration of vision, beginning with the periphery and encroaching on central vision. An early mid-peripheral visual field loss occurs that tends to be asymptomatic, but this leads to significant constriction of the visual field and possible central vision loss if the degeneration affects the macula.

The typical appearance of RP in adults is characteristic bone spicule pigmentation in the peripheral retina (Fig. 13.7). This may not appear in children, particularly early in the disease process, because the pigmentation is a grad-

ual phenomenon. Bilateral optic nerve pallor, vascular attenuation, and cataract can also occur (14).

Because of a greater loss of rod function than cone function in RP, ERG may be useful in confirming the diagnosis and in monitoring progression. RP can be differentiated in this manner from nonprogressive disorders such as CSNB. Another possible finding is abnormal dark adaptation, although this is a difficult test to administer to children.

RP can be associated with various systemic findings. In Usher syndrome, RP is combined with deafness and possible vestibular dysfunction (the latter found in type I). This association may be found in up to 30% of patients (30). In Bardet-Beidl syndrome, there is associated obesity, mental retardation, polydactyly, and hypogonadism. Senior-Loken syndrome includes renal failure. Although a comprehensive discussion of these and other systemic conditions associated with RP is beyond the scope of this text, they can be found in detail in other sources.

No known treatment exists for the underlying disorder in RP. Affected patients may benefit from low-vision devices to maximize their remaining visual field.

X-Linked Juvenile Retinoschisis

An inherited macular disorder, X-linked juvenile retinoschisis affects mostly males, and is one of the more commonly encountered macular dystrophies in young boys. It presents as a subtle foveal schisis, cystic spaces arranged around the macula in a stellate pattern. In contrast to other types of macular edema, no staining is seen on fluorescein angiography (14). Additionally, a negative wave form shows on flash ERG that may aid in confirming the diagnosis. It is usually discovered as a result of a failed school vision screening, but can also be diagnosed in infancy, where it can appear as a large bullous schisis or vitreal hemorrhage. Peripheral schisis is seen in 50% to 70% of cases (24) and usually originates inferotemporally. Other findings associated with juvenile retinoschisis can include vascular attenuation and retinal detachment. Scleral buckle or vitrectomy is indicated, where appropriate. Prognosis tends to be poor, with visual acuity of 20/200 by the sixth or seventh decade of life.

Coats' Disease

Coats' disease is a unilateral exudative disorder that commonly affects young boys. It tends to appear within the first or second decade of the patient's life, with earlier onset usually showing a more serious presentation. The disease is characterized by diffuse retinal vascular exudation with multiple focal dilations of retinal vessels visible on fluorescein angiography. Telangiectatic retinal vessels are common. The condition can result in exudative retinal detachment, with devastating visual consequences if not discovered and treated promptly. Treatment usually involves argon laser or cryotherapy to minimize exudation and prevent extensive retinal detachment (5,24). Further surgical procedures are indicated in advanced disease (e.g., scleral buckle and vitrectomy) (31).

Familial Exudative Vitreoretinopathy

Familial exudative vitreoretinopathy (FEVR) must be differentiated from Coats' disease. In contrast to Coats' disease, FEVR is dominantly inherited, and tends to be bilateral. It presents as maldevelopment of the retinal vasculature, with the most profound changes found in the temporal retina. It can vary in expression from mild, asymptomatic disease to extensive folding and exudation in the retina. It can also result in exudative retinal detachment. Macular dragging and cataract are common late complications (32). Patients are more likely to be myopic, with anisometropia and amblyopia common. When asymmetry exists in disease presentation, patients have been found to have greater myopia in the more affected eye (33). Laser or cryotherapy is used as in Coats' disease to treat the vascular leakage (24). In general, the earlier the onset of the disease process, the poorer the visual prognosis (32).

Angioid Streaks

Although rare in children, some patients can present with breaks in Bruch's membrane radiating out from the optic nerve known as *angioid streaks*. These are usually pale areas that form an irregular or spokelike pattern, and are associated in 50% of cases with systemic disease (14) (Fig. 13.8). The most common systemic association is pseudoxanthoma elasticum; they can also be found with sickle-cell disease, Paget disease, or Ehlers-Danlos syndrome. Angioid streaks can lead to subretinal choroidal

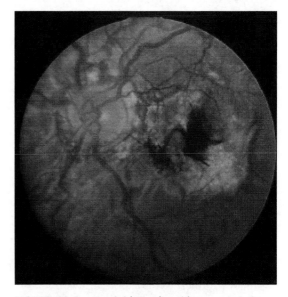

FIGURE 13.8. Angioid streaks with accompanying macular degeneration in high myopia (photo courtesy of Dr. Scott Richter). (See color well.)

neovascularization and subsequent macular degeneration, which requires focal laser and referral for management of any underlying systemic condition (34). In some cases, macular translocation can be a management option for patients with subfoveal neovascular membrane (35). Because of the increased risk of choroidal rupture and retinal hemorrhage (36) in these patients, polycarbonate lenses should be prescribed, especially for sports, and follow-up care should include dilated examinations every 6 months.

Neoplasia

Leukemia

Leukemia of various types can have ocular manifestations. The most common type of leukemia to invade the orbit is acute myeloid leukemia, which often presents as rapidly progressing proptosis, lid edema, and conjunctival chemosis. In addition to orbital signs, leukemia can have intraocular manifestations as well. Among these are optic nerve head edema and diffuse retinal vascular disease, both of which can cause visual loss (14,37). The former is considered an ocular emergency, which requires immediate radiation therapy, because it indicates central nervous system involvement (38). Optic nerve infiltration is most often seen in patients with acute lymphoblastic leukemia, which is now uncommon.

Retinopathy associated with leukemia is more common in acute forms of the disease, and usually includes hemorrhages, cotton-wool spots, vascular tortuosity, capillary attenuation, and microaneurysms. The latter three manifestations are more likely to be found in chronic forms of the disease.

The anterior segment of the eye can also be involved. The most common type to have anterior manifestations is acute lymphoblastic leukemia (20), which occasionally invades the iris and can be the first indication of relapse. Unilateral or bilateral iridocyclitis, with or without hypopyon, can be present.

Treatment for leukemia carries risks of its own. Systemic steroids can cause posterior subcapsular cataract; cytotoxic drugs can cause cranial nerve complications or corneal epithelial toxicity; and immunosuppressive drugs can open the eye to opportunistic infections (20). All cases of leukemia must be closely managed with the child's oncologist and other caregivers to detect and treat all ocular sequelae.

Retinoblastoma

One of many causes of leukocoria in infants is retinoblastoma, the most common intraocular malignancy in children (39). It occurs in approximately 1 in 15,000 to 20,000 live births (20,40), and can take one of three forms. The *endophytic* version of retinoblastoma is a white, nodular mass that can resemble cottage cheese and extends into the vitreous. The mass lesion can underlie a retinal detachment in the *exophytic* type. Retinoblastoma can also present as a diffuse inflammation resembling uveitis, the *diffuse infiltrating* form. All three forms can metastasize.

Retinoblastoma can be unilateral or bilateral and, in approximately 6% of cases, is familial (40). Typically, the tumor is diagnosed when the child is between 12 and 24 months of age, with bilateral cases usually recognized earlier. Although the most common presenting sign is leukocoria, lesions that invade the fovea can cause strabismus; therefore, all children with strabismus should have a careful dilated fundus examination.

When left untreated, retinoblastoma is almost always fatal. Current treatment, including radiotherapy and chemotherapy, gives a good prognosis, underscoring the extreme importance of early detection and treatment. A cure rate of up to 95% is achieved if treated promptly (20). In unilateral cases, because diagnosis is often made somewhat later than in bilateral cases, the tumor in the presenting eye is often large, requiring enucleation. In bilateral cases, it is common to have one eye with a larger tumor that requires enucleation, and smaller tumors in the other eye, which may respond to other forms of treatment. Visual field loss is common after such treatment, with the degree of loss dependent on tumor size, location, and type of treatment given (41). Children with retinoblastoma should have frequent and regular dilated fundus examinations, under anesthesia if necessary, to monitor for recurrence. They should also be followed closely by an oncologist to monitor for extraocular seeding or cranial involvement.

Rhabdomyosarcoma

Rhabdomyosarcoma is the most common primary orbital malignancy in children, with a rapid onset and metastatic potential (39). (This should not be confused with retinoblastoma, the most common intraocular malignancy.) It typically presents as a rapidly increasing proptosis, if the lesion is posterior to the equator of the globe, or as a rapidly enlarging mass if located superficially. It can mimic an orbital cellulitis that does not respond to treatment, which often delays proper diagnosis. The average age of detection for rhabdomyosarcoma is 7 years, although it can occur at any time from infancy into adulthood (5). A computed tomography (CT) scan is indicated to differentiate this tumor from capillary hemangioma, both of which can cause an increasing proptosis in infancy. CT will also aid in detecting bone destruction from the tumor, a common finding. Currently, chemotherapy is the first-line treatment, with radiation and surgery used as needed. Survival rates have increased greatly since the advent of combination therapy, up to approximately 90% since the 1970s (42–44).

Systemic Disease

Congenital Infection

When a mother contracts any one of a number of infections during pregnancy, serious complications can occur in the developing fetus. These infections include such entities as rubella, toxoplasmosis, syphilis, or CMV, among others.

Congenital rubella syndrome occurs when the mother is infected with rubella during the first trimester of pregnancy. Children born with this syndrome show mental and growth retardation, heart defects, deafness, thrombocytopenia, hepatosplenomegaly, and various ocular abnormalities, including cataract, glaucoma, keratitis and corneal edema, and retinal changes (24). The most common ocular manifestation is a *salt-and-pepper* retinopathy. This

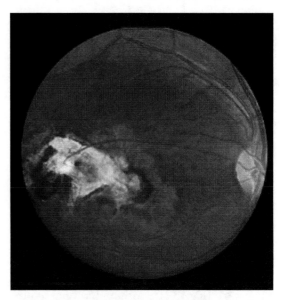

FIGURE 13.9. Toxoplasmosis (photo courtesy of Dr. Scott Richter). (See color well.)

syndrome is now rare in the United States because of widespread vaccination.

Toxoplasmosis is the most common congenital infection that affects the eye, and most cases of ocular toxoplasmosis are congenital. The most severe complications occur when the mother is infected during the first trimester, but milder sequelae are also seen with later infection. The predominant manifestation is chorioretinitis, but other manifestations can include microphthalmos, optic atrophy, and cataract (24,45) (Fig. 13.9).

Congenital CMV is relatively uncommon, occurring in approximately 0.5% of live births, and only rarely causes ocular sequelae such as optic atrophy, coloboma, cataract, or chorioretinitis (24,45).

Diabetes

Diabetes is becoming an increasing problem for pediatric patients. With the easy availability of fast food and snacks today, more children in the United States are obese than ever before. Diabetic retinopathy is therefore more of a concern to the practitioner than in the past. The presentation of diabetic retinopathy in children is the same as in adults, with cotton-wool spots, dot-blot hemorrhages, and neovascularization

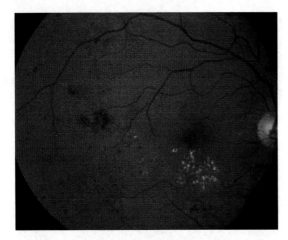

FIGURE 13.10. Diabetic retinopathy (photo courtesy of Dr. Jeffrey Roth). (See color well.)

all possible (Fig 13.10). Although retinal sequelae do not occur until the patient has typically had the condition for several years, it remains important to conduct regular dilated fundus examinations on all children either diagnosed with diabetes or at risk for it.

Retinal Detachment

Retinal detachment is uncommon in children, but can occur as a result of trauma or because of various developmental anomalies or disease processes (Fig 13.11). As in the case of adult retinal detachment, workup must include a careful history and a dilated fundus examination. Rhegmatogenous detachments not associated with trauma are found with such entities as coloboma, PHPV, aphakia, and ROP.

Exudative detachments are seen with such disorders as Coats' disease, FEVR, toxocariasis, and choroidal hemangioma. Treatment of retinal detachment in children is the same as that for adults (e.g., cryotherapy gas tamponade, or scleral buckle) (24).

Occasionally, bilateral retinal detachment is observed at birth in a condition known as *retinal dysplasia*, which is a result of failure of normal retinal and vitreous development. It is most commonly associated with Norrie's disease in boys, but can also be found in several other developmental disorders. Infants with retinal dysplasia are blind and have roving eye movements. Surgery is only indicated in instances of shallow anterior chambers, where pupillary block glaucoma becomes a concern. A lensectomy is then indicated (24).

Child Abuse

Many manifestations of child abuse, both ocular and nonocular, are seen with which the eye care practitioner must be familiar (Fig 13.12). Unusual bruising, particularly in locations not typically injured in accidents, injuries in different stages of healing, multiple hospital admissions, and inconsistent history are all red flags to possible child abuse.

Certain ocular findings are almost never accidental in nature. Bilateral periorbital ecchymosis is nearly always an indication of a direct blunt object blow to the face, and is usually inflicted, not accidental. Facial burns, especially if they are scalding burns without

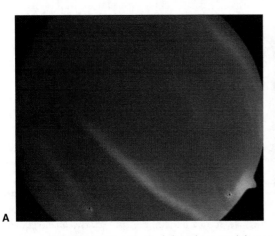

A

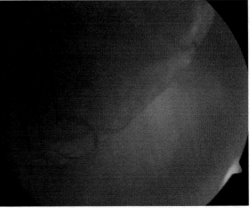

B

FIGURE 13.11. Retinal detachments (photos courtesy of Dr. Jeffrey Roth). (See color well.)

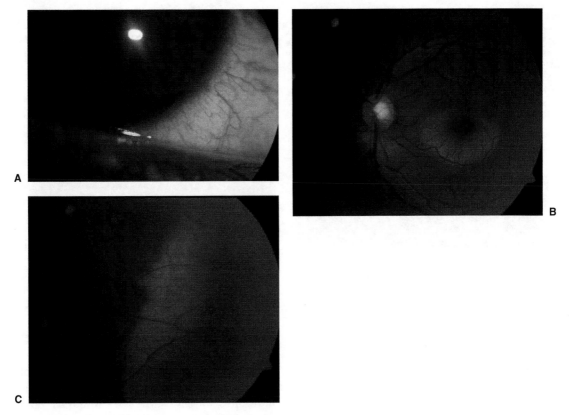

FIGURE 13.12. Possible sequelae of child abuse or other ocular trauma. **A:** Hyphema. **B:** Berlin's edema. **C:** Commotion retinae (photos courtesy of Dr. Jeffrey Roth). (See color well.)

evidence of splashing, are often an inflicted injury. Bite marks, bruises in the pattern of a particular object (e.g., electrical cord or belt), and unexplained fractures must be assessed with potential child abuse in mind (46).

Additional findings that can indicate child abuse include retinal hemorrhages, dislocated intraocular lenses, skull fractures, subdural hematomas, or small bruises under the eyes. Although these findings can be consistent with other diagnoses or history (e.g., recent car accident, Marfan's syndrome, or leukemia), when encountered without such additional history are often an indication of shaken baby syndrome. It is especially important to perform careful external evaluations and dilated fundus examinations on these patients, because small periocular bruises or retinal hemorrhages are often the only indication of further intracranial injury.

Reporting of suspected child abuse is mandatory, and practitioners should be aware of the correct reporting procedures in their state and the availability of support services.

OPTIC NERVE

Glaucoma

Glaucoma in children is a subject more appropriately discussed as a chapter or textbook of its own, because it is a complex issue with severe visual consequences. An overview is presented here, and the clinician is referred to other sources for more detail.

The most common type of pediatric glaucoma is *primary congenital glaucoma* (47,48). Patients with this type of glaucoma usually present with enlarged corneal diameters, epiphora, photophobia, and possible corneal edema that may be visible to gross observation (Fig. 13.13). Abnormal development of the drainage angle causes elevated intraocular pressure. Presentation is usually bilateral, and diagnosis is typically

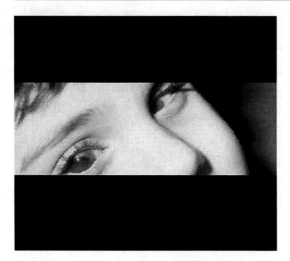

FIGURE 13.13. Buphthalmos and corneal edema in pediatric glaucoma (photo courtesy of Dr. Scott Richter). (See color well.)

made in the child between 3 and 9 months of age (48).

Children developing glaucoma after the age of 3 years fall into the category of *juvenile-onset glaucoma* (47). This is a primary open-angle form that has been shown to have autosomal dominant inheritance. Most patients with a variant are myopic and have normal gonioscopic findings. Both primary congenital and juvenile-onset glaucoma respond well to goniosurgery and filtering procedures, respectively.

Pediatric glaucoma can be associated with any of several ocular anomalies. Patients with aniridia often have glaucoma because of slowly progressing angle defects that eventually block the drainage angle. Developmental anterior segment anomalies (e.g., Axenfeld-Rieger and Peter's anomaly) can be complicated by glaucoma because they also show drainage angle maldevelopment.

Secondary glaucoma, also possible in the pediatric population, can result from trauma, neoplasm, or chronic anterior uveitis, or can occur following cataract surgery. Secondary glaucoma is more common in the pediatric population than primary glaucoma, and careful attention must be paid during evaluation of these entities to avoid missing the glaucoma.

Treatment of pediatric glaucoma is typically surgical, because medical therapy is not as effective as it is in the adult population. Medical therapy is used, however, either as a sole therapy if surgery is not an option, or as adjunct therapy. The most effective medication in children is systemic acetazolamide (48), with topical medications being used with varying success. Goniosurgery and filtration procedures are commonly used to treat patients with pediatric glaucoma, as indicated. In extreme cases, enucleation may be necessary if the eye is deformed, blind, and painful (48).

Optic Neuritis

Optic neuritis in children is typically bilateral, and is often associated with a recent viral infection or vaccination (37). It most commonly appears as prelaminar swelling and causes severe visual loss, usually over 24 to 48 hours (13), with complete recovery of vision taking up to 6 months or more. Patients may also have headache or retrobulbar pain associated with the condition.

Controversy exists over whether optic neuritis in children has the same association with multiple sclerosis that it does in adults. Some sources maintain that it is a distinct entity, whereas others more recently have suggested that 50% or more of children with optic neuritis will develop multiple sclerosis as adults (37). It is known, however, that optic neuritis can have other neurologic associations (e.g., hydrocephalus, tumors, and intracranial hypertension). It is important, therefore, for all children with the condition to have appropriate neuroimaging and lumbar puncture.

Treatment typically involves systemic steroid administration, particularly in cases of severe bilateral involvement with profound visual loss.

Optic Nerve Hypoplasia

Optic nerve hypoplasia is an uncommon developmental anomaly. It is typically bilateral, but varies greatly in the severity of its presentation and associated conditions. Mild cases can be identified on posterior pole examination but have no sequelae. Somewhat more severe cases can have associated visual field loss, decreased vision, or strabismus. The most severe presentations often include nystagmus and profound visual loss in early infancy.

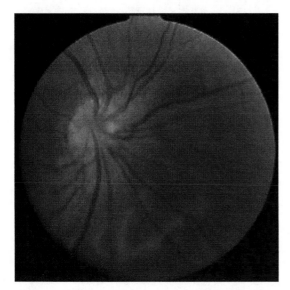

FIGURE 13.14. Optic nerve hypoplasia (photo courtesy of Dr. Scott Richter). (See color well.)

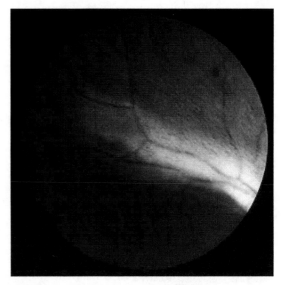

FIGURE 13.15. Myelinated nerve fiber layer (photo courtesy of Dr. Scott Richter). (See color well.)

The number of axons in a hypoplastic optic nerve is decreased, although structurally the nerve is a normal size (37). This gives a "double-ring" appearance to the nerve head, as a ring of sclera is visible (Fig. 13.14). This finding is particularly valuable in diagnosing mild cases.

Optic nerve hypoplasia has been associated with a number of central nervous system defects. Among them are absence of the septum pellucidum or corpus callosum, pituitary stalk abnormalities, and endocrine problems (e.g., growth hormone deficiency) (13,37). Close monitoring by an endocrinologist is warranted, along with neuroimaging, as necessary.

No cause for the anomaly is evident in most cases, although optic nerve hypoplasia has been associated with young maternal age, maternal ingestion of drugs (e.g., LSD or cocaine) in the first trimester, fetal alcohol syndrome, and maternal diabetes.

Myelinated Nerve Fiber Layer

In some patients, myelination of the nerve fiber layer does not stop at the cribriform plate of the optic nerve, and can be observed extending out from the disk in white, feathery opacities (Fig. 13.15). This phenomenon can be associated with high myopia or amblyopia, but generally it is a benign finding in an otherwise normal eye.

CHOROID

Congenital Hypertrophy of the RPE

Occasionally on dilated fundus examination, well-circumscribed areas of hypertrophic RPE may be seen (Fig. 13.16). This condition is known as *congenital hypertrophy of the RPE* (CHRPE) and usually presents as an isolated lesion of one to two disc diameters in the mid-peripheral retina. The presence of multiple atypical lesions may be seen associated with

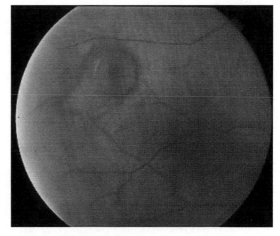

FIGURE 13.16. Congenital hypertrophy of the retinal pigment epithelium (CHRPE) (photo courtesy of Dr. Scott Richter). (See color well.)

familial adenomatous polyposis coli (FAPC), an inherited disorder of the colon in which are seen multiple polyps and an increased risk of colon cancer. These patients should be referred to their physician for evaluation and treatment of the systemic condition. A variation of CHRPE is *bear-track retinopathy*, wherein multiple small areas are seen grouped together. This finding, as with typical CHRPE, is benign and not progressive (24).

REFERENCES

1. Graham EM, Stanbury RM. Ocular inflammatory disease. In: Moore A, ed. *Fundamentals of Clinical Ophthalmology: Paediatric Ophthalmology*. London: BMJ Books; 2000:82–91.
2. Song J. Systemic management of posterior uveitis. *J Ocul Pharmacol Ther* 2003;19(4):325–343.
3. Atmaca LS, Simsek T, Batioglu F. Clinical features and prognosis in ocular toxoplasmosis. *Jpn J Ophthalmol* 2004;48(4):386–391.
4. Holland GN. Ocular toxoplasmosis: a global reassessment. Part II: Disease manifestations and management. *Am J Ophthalmol* 2004;137(1):1–17.
5. Kunimoto DY, Kanitkar KD, Makar MS, eds. *The Wills Eye Manual: Office and Emergency Room Diagnosis and Treatment of Eye Disease*, 4th ed. Philadelphia: Lippincott Williams & Wilkins; 2004.
6. Hiller N, Lieberman S, Chajek-Shaul T et al. Thoracic manifestations of Behçet disease at CT. *Radiographics* 2004;24(3):801–808.
7. Siva A, Altinas A, Saip S. Behçet's syndrome and the nervous system. *Curr Opin Neurol* 2004;17(3):347–357.
8. Tugal-Tutkun I, Onal S, Altan-Yaycioglu R et al. Uveitis in Behçet disease: an analysis of 880 patients. *Am J Ophthalmol* 2004;138(3):373–380.
9. Pivetti-Pezzi P, Accoriniti M, Abdulaziz MA, et al. Behçet's disease in children. *Jpn J Ophthalmol* 1995;39:309–314.
10. Silbert M, Gurwood AS. Persistent hyperplastic primary vitreous. *Clin Eye Vis Care.* 2000;12(3–4):131–137.
11. Sun MH, Kao LY, Kuo YH. Persistent hyperplastic primary vitreous: magnetic resonance imaging and clinical findings. *Chang Gung Med J* 2003;26(4):269–276.
12. Steele G, Peters R. Persistent hyperplastic primary vitreous with myopia: a case study. *Journal of the American Optometric Association* 1999;70(9):593–597.
13. Elston J. Visual pathway disorders. In: Moore A, ed. *Fundamentals of Clinical Ophthalmology: Paediatric Ophthalmology*. London: BMJ Books; 2000:223–235.
14. Flynn TE, Flynn JT, Chang S. Pediatric retinal examination and diseases. In: Gallin PF, ed. *Pediatric Ophthalmology: A Clinical Guide*. New York: Thieme; 2000:257–283.
15. Gregory-Evans K. Developmental disorders of the globe. In: Moore A, ed. *Fundamentals of Clinical Ophthalmology: Paediatric Ophthalmology*. London: BMJ Books; 2000:53–61.
16. Hoobyar AR, Ferrucci S, Anderson SF, et al. Juxtapapillary capillary hemangioblastoma. *Optom Vis Sci* 2002;79(6):346–352.
17. Singh AD, Ahmad NN, Shields CL, et al. Solitary retinal capillary hemangioma: lack of genetic evidence

18. Kuo MT, Kou HK, Kao ML, et al. Retinal capillary hemangiomas: clinical manifestations and visual prognosis. *Chang Gung Med J* 2002;25(10):672–682.
19. Singh AD, Nouri M, Shields CL, et al. Treatment of retinal capillary hemangioma. *Ophthalmology* 2002;109(10):1799–1806.
20. Moore AT. Intraocular tumors. In: Moore A, ed. *Fundamentals of Clinical Ophthalmology: Paediatric Ophthalmology*. London: BMJ Books; 2000:143–153.
21. Douros S, Jain SD, Gorman BD et al. Leukocoria. In: Gallin PF, ed. *Pediatric Ophthalmology: A Clinical Guide*. New York: Thieme; 2000:241–250.
22. The Committee for Classification of Retinopathy of Prematurity: an international classification of retinopathy of prematurity. *Arch Ophthalmol* 1984;102:1130–1134.
23. Multicenter Trial of Cryotherapy for Retinopathy of Prematurity: preliminary results. *Arch Ophthalmol* 1998;106:471–479.
24. Moore AT. Disorders of the vitreous and retina. In: Moore A, ed. *Fundamentals of Clinical Ophthalmology: Paediatric Ophthalmology*. London: BMJ Books; 2000: 121–142.
25. Butera C, Plotnik J, Bateman JB, et al. Ocular genetics. In: Gallin PF, ed. *Pediatric Ophthalmology: A Clinical Guide*. New York: Thieme; 2000:78–91.
26. Glazer LC, Dryja TP. Understanding the etiology of Stargardt's disease. *Ophthalmol Clin North Am* 2002;15(1):93–100, viii.
27. Hirano K, Itoh Y, Horiguchi M, et al. Indocyanine green angiography in Stargardt's disease. *Nippon Ganka Gakkai Zasshi* 1997;101(4):327–334.
28. Stavrou P, Good PA, Misson GP, et al. Electrophysiological findings in Stargardt's-fundus flavimaculatus disease. *Eye* 1998;12(pt 6):953–958.
29. Miedziak AI, Perski T, Andrews PP, et al. Stargardt's macular dystrophy—a patient's perspective. *Optometry* 2000;71(3):165–176.
30. Dufier JL. Early therapeutic trials for retinitis pigmentosa. *Bull Acad Natl Med* 2003;187(9):1685–1692; discussion 1692–1694.
31. Schmidt-Erfurth U, Lucke K. Vitreoretinal surgery in advanced Coat's disease. *German Journal of Ophthalmology* 1995;4(1):32–36.
32. Benson WE. Familial exudative vitreoretinopathy. *Trans Am Ophthalmol Soc* 1995;93:473–521.
33. Yang CI, Chen SN, Yang ML. Excessive myopia and anisometropia associated with familial exudative vitreoretinopathy. *Chang Gung Med J* 2002;25(6):388–392.
34. Gargouri HK, Cheour M, Ben Ahmed N, et al. Subretinal neovascularization in angioid streaks. *Tunis Med* 2001;79(3):161–164.
35. Roth DB, Estafanous M, Lewis H. Macular translocation for subfoveal choroidal neovascularization in angioid streaks. *Am J Ophthalmol* 2001;131(3):390–392.
36. Puig J, Garcia-Arumi J, Salvador F, et al. Subretinal neovascularization and hemorrhages in angioid streaks. *Arch Soc Esp Oftalmol* 2001;76(5):309–314.
37. Fredrick DR, Hoyt CS. Neuro-ophthalmology. In: Gallin PF, ed. *Pediatric Ophthalmology: A Clinical Guide*. New York: Thieme; 2000:100–117.
38. Rennie I. Ophthalmic manifestations of childhood leukaemia. *Br J Ophthalmol* 1992;76:641–645.
39. Castillo BV Jr, Kaufman L. Pediatric tumors of the eye and orbit. *Pediatr Clin North Am* 2003;50(1):149–172.

40. Shields JA, Shields CL. Retinoblastoma. In: Gallin PF, ed. *Pediatric Ophthalmology: A Clinical Guide.* New York: Thieme; 2000:284–294.

41. Abramson DH, Melson MR, Servodidio C. Visual fields in retinoblastoma survivors. *Arch Ophthalmol* 2004;122(9):1324–1330.

42. Orbach D, Brisse H, Helfre S, et al. Effectiveness of chemotherapy in rhabdomyosarcoma: example of orbital primary. *Expert Opin Pharmacother* 2003;4(12): 2165–2174.

43. Kazim M. Orbital diseases. In: Gallin PF, ed. *Pediatric Ophthalmology: A Clinical Guide.* New York: Thieme; 2000:295–323.

44. Rose GE. Paediatric lacrimal and orbital disease. In: Moore A, ed. *Fundamentals of Clinical Ophthalmology:*

Paediatric Ophthalmology. London: BMJ Books; 2000: 162–176.

45. Weiss MJ, Hofeldt AJ. Uveitis. In: Gallin PF, ed. *Pediatric Ophthalmology: A Clinical Guide.* New York: Thieme; 2000:216–231.

46. Figueroa J, Eis-Figueroa R. Child maltreatment. In: Gallin PF, ed. *Pediatric Ophthalmology: A Clinical Guide.* New York: Thieme; 2000:68–77.

47. Khaw PT, Narita A, Armas R, et al. The paediatric glaucomas. In: Moore A, ed. *Fundamentals of Clinical Ophthalmology: Paediatric Ophthalmology.* London: BMJ Books; 2000:92–110.

48. Walton DS. Glaucomas. In: Gallin PF, ed. *Pediatric Ophthalmology: A Clinical Guide.* New York: Thieme; 2000:232–240.

14 Quantification of Refractive Error

Amelia G. Bartolone and Daniella Rutner

Quantification of refractive error is one of the key components of a routine pediatric ophthalmic examination. The detection and treatment of uncorrected refractive error can help explain and reverse reduced visual acuity, improve alignment in accommodative esotropia, and rectify avoidance of near work, thus potentially improving academic performance. Hence, proper refraction and spectacle correction reduce the need for vision rehabilitation and increased health care costs. Because of poor visual acuity, children with uncorrected refractive error are also less likely to develop normal fine and gross motor skills necessary in writing and mathematics; reading skills may also be affected, leading to maldevelopment of language skills. Moreover, decreased visual stimulation can have an impact on social skills because the child may not see sufficiently to interact or even recognize peers. The child's refractive state can also determine if there is an accommodative cause to a strabismus.

Objective refractive techniques are used to determine the refractive status of children's eyes with no verbal response and minimal cooperation from the patient. These are the primary means to quantify refractive error in infants, preschoolers, and children with special needs. Retinoscopy is the standard method to objectively determine the refractive status of the eye. The technique locates the plane conjugate to the retina with accommodation at a minimum (the far point). Traditional techniques do not work well for preverbal or preschool children because of short attention spans and poor fixation. Therefore, several modifications to standard techniques and new technologies enhance fixation and control accommodation, producing more accurate quantification of refractive error.

This chapter reviews methods used to quantify refractive error and highlights the special needs, modifications, and techniques used in the infant, preschool, and special needs population. The first section discusses the different methods of retinoscopy: dry or static, cycloplegic, and near (Tables 14.1 and 14.2). Subjective refraction is summarized in the second section. The last section focuses on newer technologies such as visually evoked potentials, autorefraction, and photorefraction.

DRY RETINOSCOPY

Visual deprivation is the diffusion of an image on the retina. It can be caused by a number of processes, including uncorrected refractive error, which can result in amblyopia (1). The time of onset and duration of the deprivation have a profound effect on potential visual function (2–7). The earlier the deprivation occurs, the more profound the effect on the visual system (8). Early detection and prompt treatment is important to avoid lifelong visual impairment. Thus, it is imperative to evaluate infants and small children for refractive errors and to

TABLE 14.1 Common Cycloplegic Agents and Their Ocular and Systemic Side Effects

Medication	Side Effects: Ocular, Systemic	Dosage	Onset of Action	Duration of Action
Atropine	**Ocular:** allergic reaction, increased IOP, photophobia, decreased lacrimation **Systemic:** dryness of skin, mouth, and throat; restlessness; irritability or delirium; tachycardia; flushed skin; ataxia; convulsions; high fever; coma; and death from general central depression or respiratory failure	0.5% drops in lightly pigmented eyes; 1% drops in darkly pigmented eyes	3–6 hours	7–14 days
Cyclopentolate	**Ocular:** transient stinging, increased IOP angle closure, hyperemia **Systemic:** usually occur in 2% concentration or multiple doses of 1% and include central nervous system disturbances such as cerebellar dysfunction, or visual and tactile hallucinations; milder allergic drug reactions can also occur (e.g., localized rash); patients may also complain of weakness, dizziness, difficulty breathing, or a loss of consciousness	0.5% drops in infants younger than 3 months; 1% drops in infants older than 3 months	15–30 minutes	8–24 hours
Tropicamide	**Ocular:** increased IOP, transient stinging, blurred vision, photophobia with or without corneal staining **Systemic:** most common side effects are dryness of the mouth, tachycardia, headache, parasympathetic stimulation, or allergic reactions; others are less common (e.g., psychotic reactions, behavioral disturbances, and cardiorespiratory collapse).	0.5% drop in infants; 1.0% drop in children over the age of 1 year	15–30 minutes	4–6 hours

IOP, intraocular pressure.

TABLE 14.2 Methods of Refraction: Advantages, Disadvantages and Modifications

Methods	Advantages	Disadvantages	Modifications
Distance retinoscopy	Similar to refraction performed in adults	Can be difficult to perform in children younger than 2 years of age; difficult to control accommodation	Child-friendly distance targets (e.g., TV monitor with children's programming)
Cycloplegic retinoscopy	Increases accuracy of refraction; improved control of accommodation	Requires the use of drops, which can be stressful for children; increases examination time and potential side effects	Use of tropicamide in children with hypersensitivity to cyclopentolate or atropine
Mohindra near retinoscopy	Useful for young children because they tend to look at the light in a darkened room; does not require the use of cycloplegic agents and their potential side effects	Results are not as accurate as cycloplegic retinoscopy	Modify the fudge factor to +1.00 in preschool children and +0.75 to +0.50 in infants
Autorefraction	Can be performed by technician; can confirm traditional retinoscopy techniques	Can be difficult for children younger than 3 years of age; poor control of accommodation	
Photorefraction	Can be used to confirm traditional retinoscopy techniques; can be used as a screening method	Provides only an estimate of refractive error	
Visually evoked potential	Objective method of measuring visual improvement with spectacle correction	Extremely costly; not readily available; can be difficult to perform on a young child	

provide them with a clear retinal image, which can prevent or even reverse vision loss resulting from the child's earlier abnormal visual experiences (8–10).

In an adult or older child, refractive error is estimated objectively and verified by subjective refraction. In preverbal infants, young children, or children with special needs, however, limited verification can be obtained subjectively or reliably. As such, clinicians rely heavily on objective findings for the diagnosis and treatment of refractive errors. An accurate measure of refraction is necessary to yield appropriate correction, thereby enabling normal visual development, and clear and comfortable vision (11). The standard method by which objective refractive errors are assessed in adults and chil-

dren is retinoscopy (12). It is best to perform procedures when the child tends to be more cooperative, such as early in the morning or after a nap to achieve maximal results. Infants tend to be more alert during feedings; it is helpful to suggest that the parents bring a bottle for the child. It is imperative to obtain the maximal amount of information in the minimal amount of time when working with young children because they are easily distracted.

Retinoscopy can be performed in one of two fashions, each eliciting very different information. Practitioners can perform either *static retinoscopy* with accommodation relaxed for distance refractive error assessment, or *dynamic retinoscopy* to evaluate near accommodative abilities (13). The focus of this section is distance refraction evaluation and, as such, only *static retinoscopy* is discussed.

Instrumentation

In static retinoscopy, refractive error is assessed while the patient fixates a distant target in order to relax accommodation. Retinoscopes are electrically or battery powered handheld light sources that direct a beam of slightly divergent light (when the sleeve of the retinoscope is in the down position) into the patient's eye. The illumination of the retina is reflected back and the examiner can observe movements of the red reflex in the patient's pupil. The refractive status of the eye is determined by using appropriate correcting lenses to make the far point of the ametropic eye conjugate to the pupil of the examiner's eye. When this is achieved, the movement of the reflex will be neutralized and no movement will be observed.

Retinoscopes come in several basic styles. The most widely used scopes are the *streak* retinoscope, which reflects a rectangular beam from a line source, and the *spot* retinoscope, which reflects a round light from a circular source (13). Although clinically, streak retinoscopes have widely replaced spot retinoscopes because of their ease in viewing the axis of astigmatism, spot retinoscopes are an excellent choice while working with the pediatric population. The spot scope, based on the shape of the reflex, can help detect astigmatism quickly without the need to change the orientation of the light source. Moreover, the round spot enables better observation of pupillary reflex changes indicating fluctuations in accommodation. It is worthwhile for practitioners who service a large pediatric population to invest in pediatric trial frames. The glasses should be stylish to encourage children to keep the glasses on and with flexible hinges to prevent breakage (14). It would be helpful to show the children the trial frame before placing it on the child to acclimate the child to the device being used. For infants or young children who do not allow the placement of the pediatric trial frame, loose lenses or a lens rack may be a useful alternative. If a child is already wearing glasses, Halberg clips, or other trial lens clip holder that can be placed on the glasses so the practitioner can perform an over-refraction by adding standard trial lenses in the grooves (15). Begin by fitting the child in a pediatric trial frame (e.g., the Como Baby Pediatric Trial Frame) and, after a period of acclimation, begin testing for best success. The standard phoropter is cumbersome and impractical for young children for several reasons.

1. Infants and young children have small interpupillary distance that cannot be accommodated by the phoropter.
2. Children may be afraid of the phoropter's imposing size. This can be alleviated in slightly older children by allowing the child to sit on a parent's lap.
3. It is difficult for children to maintain proper fixation, which is critical for the accommodative control in static retinoscopy behind the phoropter.
4. It is difficult for the practitioner to determine the child's fixation.

Proper fogging of the patient is required before beginning retinoscopy. This can be done by placing fogging lenses in the trial frame, using loose lenses, or by positioning the lens rack horizontally when scoping the patient to ensure relaxation of accommodation.

Fixation Targets

Traditionally with adults, the standard target is a 20/400 projected letter with a bichrome red and green filter to minimize the brightness of the chart's reflection in the phoropter lenses. With infants and young children, however, creativity is required when devising a distance fixation target. The target must be capable of maintaining the child's interest for the entire procedure to ensure proper relaxation of accommodation. If no other target is available, it is possible to engage the child's attention by asking questions about the target: Which letter do you see? What colors do you see? How many lines does the letter have?

Better alternative targets are:

1. A picture slide projector
2. Blinking lights

3. Commercially available toys that can be remote activated with sound, music, or lights

4. A video recorder playing a child's favorite video, such as Barney or Sesame Street

5. An assistant or a parent making faces or noises to attract the child's attention (14)

Technique

After the fogging lens is in place and an appropriate target is displayed, the practitioner can begin the retinoscopy. First, the practitioner should work at a comfortable working distance. The most common test distances are 1 m (+1.00 D), 67 cm (+1.50 D), or 50 cm (+2.00 D). Turn the retinoscope to the sleeve-down position and begin scoping. Conventionally, examine the patient's right eye first with your right eye, after ensuring the patient's left eye is appropriately fogged by rapidly scoping the child's left eye to see *against* motion in all meridia.

Three possible movements are observed during retinoscopy: with, against, or neutral. *With* motion appears in hyperopic eyes or in eyes with a lesser degree of myopia than that of the practitioner's working distance. As the practitioner directs the streak or spot source of light into the eye and moves the light from side to side, the reflected image that appears in the patient's pupil will move in the same direction as the movement of the retinoscope. This is an indication to add plus or convex lenses. *Against* motion appears in myopic eyes that exceed the practitioner's working distance. As the practitioner directs and moves the light source from side to side in the eye, the reflex moves in the opposite direction to that of the retinoscope. This is an indication to add minus lenses. *Neutrality* is achieved when the patient's far point is conjugate with the practitioner's retinoscope and no movement is observed as the retinoscope is moved side to side. Astigmatic eyes have different powers in different meridia. When performing retinoscopy on an astigamatic eye, therefore, it is necessary to determine the refractive power of each principal meridian separately. Astigmatism should always be corrected with minus cylinders to facilitate accommodative control.

Neutralization should adhere to the following sequence:

1. Locate the two principal meridia in the right eye with the retinoscope in front of your right eye.

2. Determine the meridian that can be neutralized with the most plus or least minus lens.

3. Neutralize that meridian.

4. Confirm neutrality by either
   a. Moving the sleeve all the way up, creating a concave mirror; the reflex should appear neutralized.
   b. Moving in closer to the patient should cause the *with* motion to return; moving away should cause the *against* motion to appear.
   c. Place an extra +0.25 D sphere; an *against* motion should appear.

5. Repeat the neutralization in the meridian 90° away. This is accomplished by rotating the sleeve on the streak retinoscope. During spot retinoscopy, no need is seen to rotate the sleeve, just scope along the meridian.

6. Move across to the other side of the patient, being careful not to obscure the distant target. Neutralize the patients left eye with the retinoscope in front of your left eye. The patient's right eye will be fogged by an amount equivalent to the dioptric value of your working distances and no further fog is required.

7. Recheck both eyes again and record your results, taking the working distance into account.

8. Always record retinoscopy findings in terms of correcting lenses, not neutralizing lenses. Therefore, to make the subject emmetropic for optical infinity, the refractive correction needs to be reduced by an amount equal to the dioptric value of the working distance.

Undoubtedly, some children will not allow the placement of phoropter, loose lenses, lens racks, or trial frames during retinoscopy. In such cases, the practitioner can move closer to or further from the patient until a neutral reflex is achieved and then measure the distance at which neutrality was observed. Convert this distance into diopters.

Several sources of error in retinoscopy can yield inaccurate results and, thus, should be avoided:

1. Incorrect working distance: It may be helpful to attach a string the length of the desired working distance to the retinoscope that can be routinely used to verify working distance.

2. Scoping off the patient's visual axis: It is important that retinoscopy is performed as close as possible to the visual axis. Accordingly, use your right eye to examine the patient's right eye, and the left eye to examine the patient's left eye.

3. Patients failing to fixate the distance target: To mitigate this, routinely ask the patient questions about the target to ensure proper fixation. In addition, fluctuation observed in the patient's pupil size may be an indication of accommodative fluctuations. Measurements should be assessed when pupil size is at a maximum.

4. Failure to obtain reversal: This can result in over- or undercorrection.

5. Failure to locate the principal meridia: The axis of astigmatism can be determined by evaluating the break and width of the streak. When the streak is aligned with the principal meridian, the *break* effect disappears and the width of the reflex appears the narrowest and brightest. With spot retinoscopy, you should observe that both the patch of light and the reflex move along the same meridian. If the reflex does not move in the same meridian as the patch of light, this indicates that you are not working along one of the principal meridia.

CYCLOPLEGIC RETINOSCOPY

Medications

Medications are used to facilitate the determination of refractive status of the eye. Among them are *atropine, tropicamide,* and *cyclopentolate* (Table 14.1). They each function by decreasing ciliary muscle activity on the crystalline lens, thereby diminishing or eliminating fluctuations of accommodation. Thus, these cycloplegic agents improve the accuracy with which the refraction can be performed (17). Cycloplegic retinoscopy is a useful procedure when it is imperative to control the accommodation of the child. Most would argue that cycloplegic refraction is the standard of care in children who have high amounts of hyperopia, greater than 1.00 D of anisometropia, and strabismus, especially esotropia (16). It is not necessary, however, for most children being examined. In addition to cycloplegia, these medications are mydriatics and result in pupillary dilation, which facilitates the dilated fundus examination.

Atropine is an antimuscarinic drug that inhibits the action of acetylcholine. When applied topically to the eye in 1% concentration it produces mydriasis after 10 to 15 minutes, reaching optimal dilation and cycloplegia levels in 30 to 40 minutes (18) and can last up to 14 days. In children, atropine ointment (0.5% concentration in lightly pigmented eyes and 1% concentration in darkly pigmented eyes) (14) is instilled in both eyes twice daily for 3 days before the examination. Atropine provides the most complete cycloplegia of all the available agents. Ointment is the ideal preparation for use in children and can be easily administered while they sleep.

Atropine, however, has some significant ocular and systemic side effects. Ocular side effects include allergic reaction, increased intraocular pressure (IOP), photophobia, and decreased lacrimation. Systemic side effects include dryness of skin, mouth, and throat; restlessness, irritability, or delirium; tachycardia, flushed skin, ataxia, convulsions, high fever, coma, and death from general central depression, which causes decrease in blood pressure, circulator collapse, and respiratory failure. The estimated fatal dose in children is 10 mg; one drop of 1% atropine solution contains 0.5 mg. A fatal dose is 20 drops. In almost all the cases in the literature that resulted in death, the children were mentally or physically disabled. As such, caution should be used when dealing with the specials needs population (18).

Tropicamide is another antimuscarinic (parasympatholytic) drug (14). The onset of action of the drug begins in 15 to 30 minutes after instillation. Its duration of action is 4 to 6 hours, having the shortest half-life of all the drugs. Because it is eliminated quickly from the body, it is ideal for children with special needs and other instances of hypersensitivity to cholinergic agents (19). Tropicamide has fewer side effects then the other cycloplegics. Side effects include increased IOP, psychotic reactions, behavioral disturbances, and cardiorespiratory collapse in children and some adults More common side effects are transient stinging, dryness of the mouth, blurred vision, photophobia with or without corneal staining, tachycardia, headache, parasympathetic stimulation, or allergic reaction. Tropicamide has the most residual accommodation after maximal effect from all the cycloplegic agents; 40% to 60% of accommodation remaining in brown eyes and 20% to 40% residual accommodation in blue eyes (15,17). A 1% tropicamide solution is only 60% to 70% as effective as atropine in producing cycloplegia (20).

Cyclopentolate HCl is the drug of choice for cycloplegic refraction because of its rapid onset of action, minimal side effects, and minute residual accommodation (17). Cyclopentolate HCl is available in 0.5%, 1%, and 2% concentrations; however, 2% cyclopentolate HCl is rarely used because of its increased risk for significant side effects (11). One percent cyclopentolate does not yield significantly greater cycloplegia than 0.5%. Moreover, 0.5% cyclopentolate produces greater control of accommodation than 1% tropicamide and yields just less than 0.50 D hyperopia as compared with atropine (17,21). Cyclopentolate HCl is used in 0.5% concentration in infants under the age of 3 months and 1% concentration for children over the age of 3 months. Cycloplegia is maximal within 30 minutes and returns to normal in 24 hours with 80% of accommodative amplitude recovered after 7 hours (11,17). A reduced effect of cycloplegia was seen when comparing brown irises than blue irises; however, recovery from cycloplegia with cyclopentolate was slower for brown irises than blue irises (17,20).

The ocular side effects of cyclopentolate include transient stinging, increased IOP, the precipitation of angle closure, and hyperemia. The systemic side effects usually occur in 2% concentration or multiple doses of 1% and include central nervous system disturbances such as cerebellar dysfunction and visual and tactile hallucinations; milder allergic drug reactions can also occur and are usually manifested in a localized rash. Patients may also complain of weakness, dizziness, difficulty breathing, or a loss of consciousness (22,23).

Methods

Cycloplegic refraction is performed at the end of the examination just before fundus evaluation, but after completion of all binocular testing. Several methods of drop instillation are used with children: These include

1. One drop in each eye as quickly as possible. Wait 5 minutes and repeat. It is best with the child lying supine in a parent's lap with the head toward the parent's knees. If the parent needs to hold the child in the crook of an arm, instill the drop in the eye closer to the parent because once the drop is administered, most children will turn their heads toward the parent and then you can instill the drop in the eye closer to you.

2. Some advocate the use of proparacaine hydrochloride 0.5%. Proparacaine causes a deepening of cycloplegia in brown versus blue irises 20 minutes after the instillation of cyclopentolate. It does not have an impact on the recovery from cycloplegia in either cyclopentolate or tropicamide (17). Although proparacaine will reduce the intensity of the stinging sensation, the instillation of more drops than absolutely necessarily in small children is difficult and may prevent the instillation of the cycloplegic agent. If you can only get one application of solution in the eye, you would want it to be the cycloplegic drop.

3. An alternate method is to instill drops onto the closed lids of the child. Ask the child to tip the head back and close the eyes. Apply the cycloplegic solution to the nasal portion of the upper lid. When the child opens the eyes, the drop will drip into the eye. Do not give the child tissues, as they will wipe away the medication. No statistical difference was seen with this method when compared with that of instillation of drops to the open eye (23).

4. Spray is another option in the instillation of cylcoplegia in small children. Spray represents an alternative, less irritating and intimidating method of cycloplegia. The spray solution is a combined preparation of 3.75 mL of cyclopentolate 2%, 3.75 mL of phenylephrine 10%, and 7.5 mL tropicamide 1%, yielding a final concentration consisting of cyclopentolate 0.5%, phenylephrine 2.5%, and tropicamide 0.5%. The combination of agents produces adequate mydriasis for fundus evaluation and allows effective cycloplegia in 20 to 30 minutes. Studies have found that spray administered to the closed eyelid is as effective as an ophthalmic solution drop instilled to the open eye with no major side effect reported (23).

After the instillation of a cycloplegic agent, a second dose is usually advisable after 5 minutes. Punctal occlusion is recommended. Also, having the child close the eye will collapse the nasal lacrimal canal, reducing systemic absorption (15). No more than three doses of cyclopentolate should be used to avoid the risk of toxic reactions. Cycloplegic retinoscopy can be performed 30 minutes after instillation of cycloplentolate and should be completed approximately 40 minutes after installation of the cycloplegic agent. A nonvariable reflex observed during retinoscopy is a good indicator of cycloplegia. If variability is present, you can consider another drop of cyclopentolate, waiting a few more minutes or, if necessary, atropinization (14).

Instillation of cycloplegic agents does not assure precise refractive results and ultimately it is the responsibility of the practitioner to make a judgment call regarding objective findings. It is important to note that dilated pupils cause an increase in spherical aberration in the eye (25). Thus, only the central 4 mm should be observed during retinoscopy, ignoring the peripheral spherical aberration. Reducing the intensity of illumination can minimize spherical aberration (26). Oblique axis retinoscopy is another potential source of error in cycloplegic retinoscopy (25).

NEAR RETINOSCOPY

Near retinoscopy is another objective method of estimating refractive error in young children. The technique is valuable when children require frequent follow-up visits, when children are anxious about the instillation of drops, when parents refuse to consent to drops, or if the child has had or is at risk of adverse reaction to the drops.

Near retinoscopy was first described by Mohindra in 1977 (25). The procedure is described as being performed monocularly in a darkened room with the only target being the light of the retinoscope. The intensity of the light is set at a minimum. The child's eye is occluded either by a parent's hand, occluder, or patch. Some studies have shown that occlusion does not have an impact on the final results obtained via near retinoscopy (27,28). To ensure the appropriate working distance of 50 cm, Mohindra (25) recommends a string be tied to the retinoscope and measured to the patient. Sound projection (e.g., ring bells or making animal sounds) can enhance the attention of the child. Retinoscopy is performed, neutralizing each principal meridian separately, and then subtracting the empirically derived 1.25 D from the final spherical neutralizing lens (25,29). Mohindra reported good correlation between cycloplegic refraction and Mohindra's near retinoscopy technique in children and adults with the use of the empirically derived 1.25-D adjustment factor.

Borghi and Rouse (30) found that retinoscopy under cycloplegic conditions revealed an additional +0.50 D to +0.75 D of hyperopia as compared with Mohindra's findings. Less difference was observed as the amount of hyperopia increased. This difference in adjustment factors can be attributed to alternate cycloplegic agents used in the two studies. Mohindra used tropicamide 1% in conjunction with phenylephrine HCl 10% ophthalmic solution, whereas Borghi and Rouse used cyclopentolate 1%, which has a deeper level of cycloplegia than tropicamide. Studies have indicated that tropicamide can leave a residual of 3.5 D up to 6.25 D of hyperopia (15,17,20,31). Maino et al. (32) compared cycloplegia using tropicamide .075% and phenylephrine 2.5% in a hyperopic population aged 18 to 24 months. When comparing cycloplegic with near retinoscopy, they found only 35.7% of adjusted spherical findings were in agreement. Moreover, they could not find another adjusting factor that would yield a more reliable correlation between the two techniques. Thus, they recommend that Mohindra's near retinoscopy be used as a screening test (32). Review of the literature would suggest that the near retinoscopy technique is more closely related to cycloplegic findings in older children than in infants and that in infants the difference between near retinoscopy and the cycloplegic findings was 2.12 D. These studies, however, used cyclopentolate as the cycloplegic agent (28,30,32). It is important to be aware of the literature when evaluating the impact near retinoscopy has on the final prescription dispensed to the child.

SUBJECTIVE REFRACTION

Subjective refraction should be attempted whenever possible, after the retinoscopy technique is performed. Children, as young as 3 to 4 years of age, are capable of cooperating and providing valuable information during subjective refraction, whereas occasionally older children respond unreliably (12). The key to performing refraction is in listening to the response of the child. Some children may have difficulty in responding to "which is better—choice one or choice two," because they may be more inclined to listen to the examiner's tone and give the practitioner the response they think they want to hear. Ask the child to read the letters and then change the lenses and ask the child to read again, "which way is it easier to read the letters?" Over time, the practitioner will develop the skill in judging not the response, but the manner in which the response is rendered. Is the patient hesitant or confident, slow to answer, or rapid with assurance (33)? The key to evaluating the reliability of the child's responses is by how well the subjective refraction corresponds with objective findings and by entering visual acuity. If poor correlation is found, the examiner should immediately suspect one of the findings incorrect. If a child's entering visual acuity is 20/20 and retinoscopy findings is −2.00 D, something is clearly amiss. Another example is if +4.00 D of hyperopia is found in retinoscopy but the

child can only read 20/200, that is not an appropriate prescription and another assessment is necessary, perhaps even on another day. Some sources of error can include

1. Too large or too small a pupil
2. Desire of the child to avoid or obtain glasses

With experience, the practitioner will be able to better assess correspondence between all objective and subjective testing (33).

VISUALLY EVOKED POTENTIALS

Another method of completing refraction objectively is *visually evoked potentials* (VEP). In response to visual stimuli, the occipital cortex generates an electrical signal termed a *visually evoked response* (VER) (34). VEP is seldom done clinically but can be useful in determining the effects of corrective lenses in preverbal children to prevent amblyopia. A small region of the scalp is cleaned and an electroconductive gel is used to attach the electrode (34). VEP assesses foveal projections to the visual cortex and has been shown to be affected by the sharpness of retinal image focus, whereby the largest evoked potential is a result of the sharpest retinal image (35). Thus, by using various lenses after objective retinoscopy, the largest evoked potential will yield the best *objective* refraction and sharpest visual acuity but lacks information regarding the child's comfort with the prescription.

AUTOREFRACTION

Background

An autorefractor determines the refractive error of the eye without the need for subjective judgments by the clinician or the patient. The refractive error is determined by either monitoring the retinal image of the eye, measuring the vergence of ray bundles emerging from the eye, or obtaining wavefront analysis. One of the newest means of monitoring the retinal image includes using charge-coupled device imaging cameras. Instruments that measure the vergence of light use the principles of retinoscopy or the double pinhole principle of Scheiner.

Autorefraction is often used by technicians during pretesting in an ophthalmic office. The instrument, therefore, can save the clinician time in the examining room. Speed of testing and use by lay personnel offer significant benefits when examining the pediatric population in both office and screening settings. Adequate positioning and fixation of the child must be obtained, however, to ensure accurate measurements. Therefore, with young children, the instrument is usually confined to confirmation of retinoscopic results or use in a screening setting.

Features

Since the first autorefractor was introduced in the 1970s, many features have been added to the instruments. The most obvious change has been in testing time. The first autorefractors needed 1 minute per eye. Current autorefractors complete measurements in less than a second. The first additional tests included visual acuity and subjective refinement. Today's instruments can also incorporate interpupillary distance, keratometry, topography, and wavefront analysis. Instruments can include any combination of auto-alignment, auto-tracking, auto-fogging, and auto-measurement. Current instruments can obtain measurements through pupils just under 3 mm. The spherical range can be as high as ±25.00 D. And cylindrical range can be as high as ±10.00 D. In addition to interfacing with a printer, many autorefractors can interface with other examination equipment.

Types

Autorefractors can be table-top or handheld models. Currently, approximately 16 table-top models are available from a half dozen companies. This style of autorefractor is only beneficial in children 3 years of age and older when fixation and accommodation are easier to control. Studies on autorefractors no longer commercially available showed autorefraction is more useful in children aged 3 to 5 years than cycloplegic refraction so that the disadvantages of cycloplegia can be avoided (36,37). The only study of children on commercially available table-top autorefractors investigated the Humphrey HARK 599 (Carl Zeiss Meditec, Dublin, California) (38). This autorefractor has the

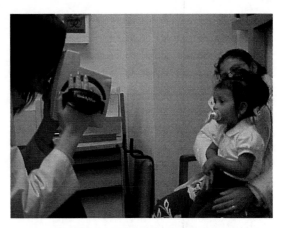

FIGURE 14.1. SureSight autorefractor.

capability of a subjective over-refraction following autorefraction and the determination of visual acuity using letters, numbers, or pictures. The investigators found that the HARK correlated well with cycloplegic retinoscopy in children 5 to 16 years of age. The accuracy of the instrument compared with subjective refraction improved, however, with cycloplegia (38).

Alignment is easier with handheld autorefractors because they have no chin rest. The instruments are also easily portable. These two features are beneficial when examining very young children as well as children with special needs. Three commercially available handheld autorefractors are available: Retinomax (Right Manufacturing, Virginia Beach, VA), SureSight (Fig. 14.1) (Welch Allyn, Skaneateles Falls, NY), and Palm AR (Marco, Jacksonville, FL).

Instruments

The Retinomax was the first available handheld autorefractor and, hence, has been the most widely studied with children. It is the only handheld instrument to date that has been investigated in children younger than 3 years of age. Autorefraction with the Retinomax has been completed in children as young at 5 months (39). Testability with the Retinomax is high, with recent studies indicating that greater than 99% of children could complete the procedure (40,41). The examiner places the instrument's headrest on the child's forehead while encouraging the child to fixate the internal target. The mire must be focused in the center of each pupil in turn. Refractive error is measured along two meridia and eight or more readings are taken automatically. If the reliability reading is less than eight the manufacturer recommends that the measurements be repeated. The instrument can be operated in three modes: automatic, continuous, or quick. The automatic and continuous modes both use a fogging system to minimize accommodation. The automatic mode responds to a shift of the instrument from right to left eye while the continuous mode takes readings until the operator indicates the set of readings are complete. The quick mode disables the fogging system and speeds the measurement process.

Some disagreement exists in the literature about the need for cycloplegia to obtain accurate Retinomax measurements. Most studies have found adequate to excellent results without cycloplegia (40–47). Some, however, found it to be inaccurate before cycloplegia (39,48) and one group cautioned use outside of screenings because of large individual variations even with cycloplegia (49). The most recent studies (40,41) showed a sensitivity of 63% to 78 % when specificity is set at 90%. Retinomax measurements are repeatable and show excellent discrimination for hyperopia and acceptable discrimination for cylinder (47).

The SureSight autorefractor is currently the only instrument to measure refractive error using wavefront technology. The measurements are taken monocularly in two meridia. Greater than 98% of preschool children can complete testing with the SureSight (40,50,51). Testing is performed at approximately 36 cm. The instrument is noncontact and, hence, is nonthreatening. The examiner looks through the viewfinder, instructs the child to fixate on the red lights of the instrument, and centers a crosshair on the pupil of the right eye. Testing distance is adjusted based on auditory cues. The procedure is repeated for the left eye. The refractive error and reliability rating can then be printed. If the reliability reading is less than six (the manufacturer's recommended minimal value) or the refractive error exceeds the SureSight normal bounds (indicated by an asterisk), the measurement should be repeated. Measurements can be performed in the child or adult

mode. The child mode attempts to compensate for the accommodation of the preschool child by adding +2.5 D to the measured value.

Accuracy of the SureSight autorefractor to determine spherical refractive error has differed in the literature. Many investigators found the instrument to overminus children (50–52). One study, however, found an overestimation of hyperopia using the child mode (45). Findings for cylinder power and axis are similar to cycloplegic retinoscopy. (50,51,53) Huffman et al. (47) found the SureSight to be slightly more accurate than the Retinomax, but accuracy was dependent on refractive error. The manufacturer's recommended referral criterion was associated with a sensitivity of 85% but a specificity of only 62%. When the referral criterion for hyperopia, astigmatism, and anisometropia were raised to create a specificity of 90%, sensitivity fell to 63% (40).

The largest study of young children that investigated autorefractors was the nationally funded Vision in Preschoolers Study (40). This group compared vision screening tests administered by eye care professionals in a large high-risk Head Start population. The two autorefractors investigated were the Retinomax and SureSight. Both were found to have performance similar to noncycloplegic retinoscopy when administered by a skilled doctor. Of the eleven screening tests investigated, the two autorefractors were found to be two of the four best tests to detect amblyopia, strabismus, significant refractive error, or unexplained reduced visual acuity. With 90% specificity, however, the four best tests only detected two thirds of children with one of the above conditions.

The newest handheld autorefractor is the Marco Palm AR. Only one investigation of the instrument has been done on young children to date (41). Testability was found to be greater than 99% (41). The Palm AR is the smallest and most lightweight of all the autorefractors. A headrest is placed on the child's forehead while the child is directed to look at a scenery chart. With a specificity of 90%, sensitivity was 74%, which is similar to the Retinomax (41). A high correlation was seen between the Palm AR and the Retinomax for both sphere and cylinder measurements (41).

PHOTOREFRACTION

Background

Eccentric photorefraction can determine the presence of significant refractive error, strabismus, and media opacity using a camera-based system. The technique offers the clinician many advantages when working with challenging populations such as infants, toddlers, and children with special needs. It is quick (usually <3 minutes), nonthreatening, noninvasive, and easy to use. A still or video camera captures an image of both the corneal and retinal reflexes of the child's eyes. The photo of an emmetropic eye will reveal a homogeneous red reflex that fills the pupil, whereas ametropia is evidenced by a whitish crescent.

Photorefraction has primarily been investigated as a tool for large-scale screenings for amblyogenic factors (40,54–60). The technique is objective and does not require cycloplegia. Because both eyes are imaged simultaneously, it is especially sensitive to anisometropia. In addition to its other benefits, newer models are portable and can be administered by lay personnel. The technique is not routinely used as an in-office procedure because results are not always immediately available and often only an estimated refractive error is determined.

Types

The camera systems can be set up on-axis (the optical axis of the camera and the flash are aligned) or off-axis. On-axis or isotropic photoscreening requires three photographs. The first is focused at the pupillary plane, the second is defocused in front of the pupillary plane, and the third is defocused an equal magnitude behind the pupillary plane. Comparison of the blur circles in the two defocused images determines the sign and magnitude of the refractive error. A blur ellipse indicates the presence of astigmatism. The elongated direction of the ellipse gives the axis of the minus cylinder correcting lens (61).

Many disadvantages are seen of on-axis photorefraction. The most obvious drawback is that three photographs are required, which introduces time as a variable and can produce changes in fixation and accommodation (62).

The need for pupillary dilation increases examination time as well as producing cycloplegic risks and side effects. The apparent size of the blur circle is influenced by fundus pigmentation, pupil size, and contrast between the subject's face and the blur circle (34). Interpreting the defocused images is difficult. Strabismus and media opacities cannot be detected with on-axis photorefraction. The range of refractive errors the camera can detect is narrow (4.00 D of hyperopia to 4.00 D of myopia) (60).

The first photorefractor to be investigated used an on-axis system but the light was captured through an array of wedge-shaped cylindrical lenses (63). This technique, orthogonal photorefraction, produces a star-shaped image. The length of the star arms is related to the refractive error in the vertical and horizontal meridian. Star arms of equal length indicate spherical refractive error, whereas different lengths indicate astigmatism. Anisometropia is detected by comparing the star arm lengths between eyes. The star arms do not differentiate between hyperopia and myopia. Orthogonal photorefraction is more difficult to set up, calibrate, and assess than isotropic or off-axis photorefraction (62).

Off-axis or eccentric photorefraction yields more easily interpreted images than on-axis systems. A focused image of the pupil, corneal reflex, and retinal reflex are captured. It is the most commonly used technique and the basis for commercially available instruments. The earliest description of the technique was by Kaakinen (64). The original "self-made" versions used a 35 mm camera, telephoto lens, and a strobe flash placed directly below the optical axis of the camera.

The image captured is a homogenous red reflex in the pupil if no refractive error is present. If ametropia is present, a whitish crescent will be captured within the red reflex. This is a picture of the reflected blur circle at the plane of the pupil. The size of the crescent is dependent on pupil size, eccentricity of the light source, camera-to-subject distance, and distance at which the eye is focused (62). Crescent size indicates the magnitude of the refractive error, whereas crescent location indicates the type of the ametropia. Hyperopic crescents are located on the opposite side of the camera flash and

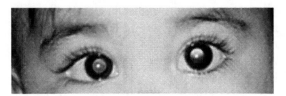

FIGURE 14.2. Off-axis photorefraction image. The crescent on the top (the same side as the flash) indicates myopia. The crescent is larger in the left eye than the right which indicates the infant has anisometropia. (See color well.)

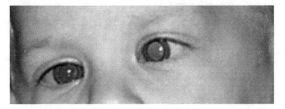

FIGURE 14.4. Off-axis photorefraction image. The corneal reflex is displaced temporally in the left eye indicating esotropia. The Bruckner reflex is also brighter in the left eye. (See color well.)

myopic crescents are on the same side of the camera flash (Fig. 14.2). Even with large refractive errors, when crescents fill the pupil, the direction of the ametropia can be determined by observing the attenuation of the crescent opposite the side from which the pupil filled (Fig. 14.3). Anisometropia is present when the crescent size is unequal in the two eyes. (Fig. 14.2)

Eccentric photorefraction can only detect astigmatism in a dual flash system or in two sequential photographs with the flash oriented in different directions. The 90° meridian is measured with the flash positioned either on the top or bottom of the lens and the 180° meridian is measured with the flash positioned either to the right or left of the lens. Comparison of the crescents size with the flash in different orientations demonstrates the presence of astigmatism. Systems that use two photographs introduce time as a variable, which can produce changes in fixation and accommodation.

Strabismus and media opacities can also be detected using eccentric photorefraction. The corneal (Hirshberg) reflex captured in the image can be measured to determine ocular alignment. Esotropia is present when the reflex is

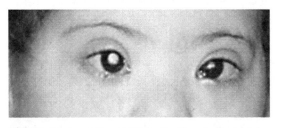

FIGURE 14.3. Off-axis photorefraction image. The attenuation of the crescent on the bottom of the pupil indicates high myopia in a child with Down syndrome. (See color well.)

displaced temporally in the deviating eye (Fig. 14.4). Exotropia is present if the reflex is displaced nasally. A unilateral brightening of the red reflex (positive Bruckner reflex) can indicate strabismus or anisometropia (Fig. 14.4). The clarity or color of the red reflex can reveal media opacities. A corneal opacity appears as a bluish haze obscuring the view of the iris, pupil, or both, whereas a lens opacity appears black or blue within the pupil margin.

Instruments

The Visiscreen ocular screening system (Vision Research Corporation, Birmingham, AL) was the first commercially available photorefractive instrument and is currently still in production. The system consists of two components, a camera station and a patient viewing station, which are separated by 6.5-foot rails. The rails fold, enabling portability. Before photographing, the room lights are dimmed for 30 seconds so that the pupils dilate. The child stands so that the eyes are centered in the cut-out of the viewing station. This eccentric photorefractor measures only the vertical meridian so neither with-the-rule or against-the-rule cylinder can be detected. Color images are produced after film development. The two studies of the Visiscreen (65,66) determined a sensitivity and specificity range of 65% to 91% and 74% to 87%, respectively.

The MTI Photoscreener (Medical Technologies, Inc., Riviera Beach, FL) has been the most widely investigated photorefractor (54,57,58,67–71). This is probably because of its portability (only 7 pounds and less than a foot long), on-site interpretation via Polaroid film, and low cost relative to other photorefractors.

It is also performed at 1 m without any physical contact with the child. The instrument is no longer in production, however. This eccentric photorefractor used a flash that rotated 90° to take two photographs with different flash orientations. Although both images were displayed on one photograph, time is a variable that can produce changes in fixation and/or accommodation. The reported sensitivity and specificity of the instrument has varied widely from 37% to 91% and 20% to 94%, respectively (40,57,58,67–70). This large range of sensitivity and specificity can be attributed to poor interobserver correlation (72), age of subjects studied, variable exclusion of unreadable photographs, and a lack of a standard pass or fail criterion.

The iScreen photoscreener (iScreen, Inc, Memphis, TN) is a commercially available off-axis photorefractor that attaches to a laptop computer. The digital image has the advantage of instantaneous result without the cost of film. It, however, measures only one meridian and eye alignment. Moreover, the child must rest the head against a headrest while fixating a red light. The examiner centers the child's eyes on the display and takes a binocular photograph. There is an automatic confirmation of good images. The image is then transmitted to a scoring center. The first study of the iScreen examined children age 3 to 12 years and showed much promise with a sensitivity of 92% and a specificity of 89% (56). The most recent study showed poorer sensitivity (37%) with a 94% specificity (40). This may be attributed to different subject ages and differing failure criteria.

One of the newest photoscreeners is a table-top infrared video-photorefractor. The Power Refractor (Plusoptix, Nuremberg, Germany) binocularly measures refractive error in eight meridia, as well as eye alignment. The child sits approximately 1 m from the instrument and fixates red and green lights. The screener repeats measurements for refractive error and eye alignment until the display turns green or the measurement is repeated monocularly. This on-site interpretation of photographs is especially beneficial for large-scale screenings. The sensitivity of the instrument was 54% when the specificity was set at 90% (40). The Power Refractor measurements were found to be repeatable and similar to a table-top autorefractor (73). The mean difference of Power Refractor measurements and cycloplegic retinoscopy, however, were significantly different (45). Disagreement is found in the literature about the effect of a viewing distance longer than 1 m on mean spherical equivalent measurements (45,73).

The most recent study investigating photoscreeners was the nationally funded Vision in Preschoolers Study (40). This group compared vision screening tests administered by eye care professionals in a large high-risk Head Start population. The three photoscreeners investigated were the MTI, iScreen, and Power Refractor. Almost all the children were able to complete the photoscreening. A significant percentage of the images were invalid or ungradeable, however. The Power Refractor yielded the highest percentage of one image set completed but the lowest mean image set. The specificity of the Power Refractor was set at 90% because there was no set failure criterion. The sensitivity and specificity of the MTI and iScreen were identical (Table 14.3). The study concluded that the MTI and iScreen photorefractors are not as accurate as noncycloplegic retinoscopy, Sure-Sight autorefractor, Retinomax autorefractor, or monocular Lea visual acuity in detecting amblyopia, strabismus, significant refractive error, or unexplained decreased acuity (40).

TABLE 14.3 Investigation of Photorefractors by the Vision in Preschoolers Study

	Not Testable (%)	Invalid or Ungradeable (%)	One Image Set (%)	Mean Image Set	Sensitivity	Specificity
MTI photoscreener	0	5.8	63.6	1.48	0.37	0.94
iScreen	0.1	2.6	70.3	1.37	0.37	0.94
Power refractor	1.5	2.2	90.5	1.14	0.54	0.90*

*Adapted from VIP 2004.

Although the sensitivity of the Power Refractor was lower than the other four tests, it was not statistically significant.

SUMMARY

Quantification of refractive error can be easily accomplished in the pediatric population with several standard tools readily available in most optometric offices. It is important for clinicians to recognize which instruments and techniques are most appropriate for the child's age and disposition as well as the advantages and disadvantages of each. New tools and methods of evaluating infant visual development provide support for early clinical assessment. The effective early diagnosis and treatment of refractive error, its associations, and consequences will reduce visual disability and improve the visual health of children.

REFERENCES

1. Daw NJ. *Visual Development.* Plenum Press. New York; 1995:193–200.
2. Moore BD. *Eye Care for Infants and Young Children.* Boston: Butterworth-Heinemann; 1997:26,155,220, 224,244.
3. Smith EL, III, Harwerth RS, Crawford ML, et al. Observations on the effects of form deprivation on the refractive status of the monkey. *Invest Ophthalmol Vis Sci* 1987;28:1236–1245.
4. Raviola E, Wiesel TN. An animal model of myopia. *N Engl J Med* 1985;312:1609–1615.
5. Wiesel TN, Raviola E. Myopia and eye enlargement after neonatal lid fusion in monkeys. *Nature* 1977;266:66–68.
6. Greene PR, Guyton DL. Time course of rhesus lid-suture myopia. *Exp Eye Res* 1986;42:529–354.
7. Smith EL, III. Spectacle lenses and emmetropization: the role of optical defocus in regulating ocular development. *Optom Vis Sci* 1998;75:388–398.
8. Press LJ. *Applied Concepts in Vision Therapy.* St. Louis: Mosby; 1997:76–79.
9. Held R. Binocular vision... behavioral and neuronal development. In: Mehler J, Fox R, eds. *Neonate Cognition: Beyond the Blooming, Buzzing Confusion.* Hillsdale, NJ: Erlbaum; 1984.
10. Mohindra I, Jacobson SG, Thomas J, et al. Development of amblyopia in infants. *Transactions of the Ophthalmic Society of the United Kingdom* 1979;99:344–346.
11. Ciner EB. Examination procedures for infants and young children. *Optometric Vision Development* 1996 27:54–67.
12. Moore A. Refraction of infants and young children. In: Taylor D, ed. *Pediatric Ophthalmology.* Boston: Blackwell Scientific Publications; 1990:65–70.
13. Campbell CE, Benjamin W J, Howland HC. Objective refraction: retinoscopy, autorefraction, and photorefraction. In: Benjamin WJ, ed. *Borish's Clinical Refraction.* Philadelphia: WB Saunders; 1998:559–628.
14. Ciner EB. Refractive error in young children. In: Moore B, ed. *Eye Care for Infants and Young Children.* Boston: Butterworth-Heinemann; 1997:47–74.
15. Leat SJ, Shute RH, Westall CA, eds. *Refraction in Assessing Children's Vision: A Handbook.* Oxford: Butterworth-Heinemann; 1998.
16. American Optometric Association. *Pediatric Eye and Vision Examination Optometric Clinical Practice Guidelines.* St. Louis: AOA;1994.
17. Lovasik JV. Pharmacokinetics of topically applied cyclopentolate HCL and tropicamide. *American Journal of Optometry and Physiological Optics* 1986;63(10):787–803.
18. North RV. A review of the uses and adverse effects of topical administration of atropine. *American Journal of Ophthalmology and Physiological Optics* 1987;7(2): 109–114.
19. Doughty MJ, Lyle WM. Ocular pharmacogenetics. In: Fatt HV, Griffing JR, Lyle WM, eds. *Genetics from Primary Eye Care Practitioners.* Boston: Butterworth-Heinemann; 1981.
20. Milder B. Tropicamide as a cycloplegic agent. *Arch Ophthalmol* 1961;66:70–72.
21. Rosenbaum AL, Bateman JB, Bremer DL. Cycloplegic refraction in esotropic children. *Ophthalmology* 1981;88:1031–1034
22. Vale J, Cox, B. *Drugs and the Eye.* London: Butterworth; 1978:21.
23. Jones LWJ, Hodes DT. Possible allergic reactions to cyclopentolate hydrochloride: case reports with literature review of uses and adverse reactions. *Journal of Ophthalmology and Physiological Optics* 1991;11:16–21.
24. Bartlett JD, Wesson MD, Swiatocha J, et al. Efficacy of a pediatric cycloplegic administered as a spray. *Journal of the American Optometric Associations* 1993;64(9):617–620.
25. Mohindra I. A non-cycloplegic refraction technique for infants and young children. *Journal of the American Optometric Association* 1977;48 (4):518–523.
26. Amos JF. Cycloplegic refraction. In: Bartlett JD, Janus SD, eds. *Clinical Ocular Pharmacology* Boston: Butterworth-Heinemann;1989:425–432.
27. Griffin JR. *Binocular Anomalies: Procedures for Vision Therapy,* 2nd ed. Chicago: Professional Press; 1982:436.
28. Wesson MD, Mann KR, Bray NW. A comparison of cycloplegic refraction to the near retinoscopy technique for refractive error determination. *Journal of the American Optometric Association* 1990;61:680–684.
29. Mohindra I, Molinari JF. Near retinoscopy and cycloplegic retinoscopy in early primary grade schoolchildren. *American Journal of Optometry and Physiological Optics* 1979;56(1):34–38.
30. Borghi RA, Rouse, MW, Comparison of refraction obtained by "near retinoscopy" and retinoscopy under cycloplegic. *American Journal of Optometry and Physiological Optics* 62(3):169–172.
31. Milder B. Tropicamide as a cycloplegic agent. *Arch Ophthalmol* 1961;66:70–72.
32. Maino JH, Gerhard W, Cibis MD, et al. Noncycloplegic vs cycloplegic retinoscopy in pre-school children. *Ann Ophthalmol* 1984;16(9):880–882.
33. Hirsch MJ. The refraction of children. In: Hirsch MJ, Wick RE, eds. *Vision of Children: An Optometric Symposium.* Philadelphia: Chilton Book Company 1963;158–165.
34. Orel-Bixler D. Electrodiagnostics, ultrasound, neuroimaging, and photorefraction in young children. In: Moore B., ed. *Eye Care for Infants and Young Children.* Boston: Butterworth-Heinemann; 1997:89–122.
35. Regan D. Rapid objective refraction using evoked brain potentials. *Invest Ophthalmol* 1975;12(9):669–679.

36. Aslin RN, Shea SL, Metz HS. Use of the Canon R-1 autorefractor to measure refractive errors and accommodative responses in infants. *Clinical Vision Science* 1990;5:61–70.

37. Evans E. Refraction in children using the Rx1 autorefractor. *Br Orthop J* 1984;41:46–52.

38. Isenberg SJ, Del Signore M, Madani-Becker G. Use of the HARK autorefractor in children. *Am J Ophthalmol* 2001;131:438–441.

39. el-Defrawy S, Clarke WN, Belec F, et al. Evaluation of a hand-held autorefractor in children younger than six. *J Pediatr Ophthalmol Strabismus* 1998;35(2):107–109.

40. The Vision in Preschooler Study Group. Comparison of preschool vision screening tests as administered by licensed eye care professionals in the Vision in Preschoolers Study. *Ophthalmology* 2004;111:637–650.

41. Carter A, Ciner E. A comparison of two autorefractors in the Vision in Preschoolers Study. *Optom Vis Sci* 2004;81(12s):44.

42. Wesemann W, Dick B. Erfahrungen mit dem handgehaltenen autorefraktometer ARetinomax bei erwachsenen und kindern. *Klin Monatsbl Augenheilkd* 1997;211:387–394.

43. Harvey EM, Miller JM, Wagner LK, et al. Reproducibility and accuracy of measurements with a hand held autorefractor in children. *Br J Ophthalmol* 1997;81(11):941–948.

44. Cordonnier M, Dramaix M. Screening for abnormal levels of hyperopia in children: a non-cyclopleplegic method with a hand held refractor. *Br J Ophthalmol* 1998;82(11):1260–1264.

45. Suryakumar R, Bobier WR. The manifestation of non-cycloplegic refractive state in pre-school children is dependent on autorefractor design. *Optom Vis Sci* 2003;80(8):578–86.

46. Cordonnier M, Dramaix M. Screening for refractive errors in children: accuracy of the hand held refractor Retinomax to screen for astigmatism. *Br J Ophthalmol* 1999;83:157–161.

47. Huffman S, Schimmoeller K, Mitchell L, et al. The accuracy of autorefractor measurements in young children. *Optom Vis Sci* 2004;81(12s):44.

48. Wesemann W, Dick B. Accuracy and accommodation capability of a hand held autorefractor. *J Cataract Refract Surg* 2000;26(1):62–70.

49. Steele G, Ireland D, Block S. Cycloplegic autorefraction results in pre-school children using the Nikon Retinomax Plus and the Welch Allyn SureSight. *Optom Vis Sci* 2003;80(8):573–577.

50. Buchner TF, Schnorbus U, Grenzebach UH, et al. [Examination of preschool children for refractive errors. First experience using a handheld autorefractor.] *Ophthalmologe* 2003;100(11):971–978.

51. Iuorno JD, Grant WD, Noel LP. Clinical comparison of the Welch Allyn SureSight handheld autorefractor versus cycloplegic autorefraction and retinoscopic refraction. *J AAPOS* 2004;8:123–127.

52. Schimitzek T, Wesemann W. Clinical evaluation of refraction using a handheld wavefront autorefractor in young and adult populations. *J Cataract Refract Surg* 2002;28:1655–1666.

53. Adams RJ, Dalton SM, Murphy AM, et al. Testing young infants with the Welch Allyn SureSight non-cycloplegic autorefractor. *Ophthalmic Physiol Opt* 2002;22:546–551.

54. Donahue SP, Johnson TM, Leonard-Martin TC. Screening for amblyogenic factors using a volunteer lay network and the MTI photoscreener. Initial results from 1,500 preschool children in a statewide effort. *Ophthalmology* 2000;107:1637–1644.

55. Arnold RW, Gionet EG, Jastrzebski AI, et al. The Alaska Blind Child Discovery project: rationale, methods and results of 4000 screenings. *Alaska Med* 2000;42:58–72.

56. Kennedy RA, Thomas DE. Evaluation of the iScreen digital screening system for amblyogenic factors. *Can J Ophthalmol* 2000;35:258–262.

57. Simons BD, Siatkowski RM, Schiffman JC, et al. Pediatric photoscreening for strabismus and refractive errors in high-risk populations. *Ophthalmology* 1999;106:1073–1080.

58. Tong PY, Enke-Miyazaki E, Bassin RE, et al. Screening for amblyopia in preverbal children with photoscreening photographs. National Children's Eye Foundation Vision Screening Study Group. *Ophthalmology* 1998;105:856–863.

59. Morris CE, Scott WE, Simon JW, et al. Photorefractive screening for amblyogenic factors: a three centre study. Transactions of the VIIth International Orthoptic Congress, Nuremberg, Germany 1991:243.

60. Atkinson J, Braddick OJ, Durden K, et al. Screening for refractive errors in 6–9 month old infants by photorefraction. *Br J Ophthalmol* 1984;68:105–112.

61. Howland HC. The optics of static photoskiascopy. *Acta Ophthalmol (Copenh)* 1980;58:221–227.

62. Duckman RH. Photorefraction: an update. *J Optom Vis Dev* 1996;27:68–79.

63. Howland H, Howland B. Photorefraction: a technique for study of refractive state at a distance. *Journal of the Optometric Society of America* 1974:64:240–249.

64. Kaakinen K. A Simple method for screening of children with strabismus, anisometropia or ametropia by simultaneous photography of the corneal and fundus reflexes. *Acta Ophthalmol (Copenh)* 1979;57:161–171.

65. Morgan KS, Johnson WD. Clinical evaluation of a commercial photrefractor. *Arch Ophthalmol* 1987;105:1528–1531.

66. Cogan MS, Ottemiller DE. Photorefractor for detection of treatable eye disorders in preverbal children. *Alaska Med* 1992;62:16–20.

67. Freedman HL, Preston KL. Polaroid photoscreening for amblyogenic factors: an improved methodology. *Ophthalmology* 1992;99(12):1785–1795.

68. Ottar WL, Scott WE, Holgado SI. Photoscreening for ablyogenic factors. *J Pediatr Ophthalmol Strabismus* 1995;32:289–295.

69. Tong PY, Bassin RE, Enke-Miyazaki E, et al. Screening for amblyopia in preverbal children with photoscreening photographs. II: Sensitivity and specificity of the MTI photoscreener. *Ophthalmology* 2000;107:1623–1629.

70. Cooper CD, Gole GA, Hall JE, et al. Evaluating photoscreeners II: MTI and Fortune. *Aust NZ Ophthalmol* 1999;27:387–398.

71. Donahue SP, Johnson TM, Ottar W, et al. Sensitivity of photoscreening to detect high-magnitude amblyogenic factors. *J AAPOS* 2002;6:86–91.

72. Lewis RC, Marsh-Tootle WL. The reliability of interpretation of photoscreening results with the MTI PS-100 in Head Start preschool children. *Journal of the American Optometric Association* 1995;66(7):429.

73. Choi M, Weiss S, Schaeffel F, et al. Laboratory, clinical, and kindergarten test of a new eccentric infrared photorefractor (Power Refractor). *Optom Vis Sci* 2000;77:537–548.

15 Pediatric and Adolescent Contact Lens Correction

David P. Libassi and Ralph E. Gundel

PEDIATRIC CONTACT LENS CORRECTION

Around the world, one of the most common causes of blindness in children is the presence of pediatric cataracts (1). By advancing pediatric vision care, we hope to improve early detection of lens opacities and provide enhanced postsurgical management of pediatric aphakia. Dense amblyopia that develops from an undetected cataract or undetected high myopia requires early intervention, early optical correction, and consistent patch therapy as the steps toward ensuring a future of clear functional vision. With better detection, we can significantly reduce the number of children who suffer a life of compromised vision.

Pediatric Aphakia and High Myopia

For the infant born with a congenital cataract, most pediatric ophthalmologists prefer to remove the opacified lens within the first 4 to 6 weeks of life. If cataract extraction is not performed by 6 months of age or if postsurgical correction is ignored, dense persistent amblyopia will develop. Ophthalmic literature, however, shows that children born with congenital cataracts or significant refractive error, who receive early surgical intervention followed by consistent optical correction and amblyopia treatment, can still have compromised vision simply because they may suffer from other ocular anomalies. Children who acquire a cataract

because of metabolic problems or secondary to trauma have a slightly lower risk of developing deep amblyopia. These children may have had longer visual stimulation and more normal neurologic development before cataract development (2).

Although universal agreement exists on the need for early surgical removal of the opacified lens, little agreement is seen on the best method of postoperative pediatric aphakic correction. Pediatric aphakic rehabilitation can currently be accomplished by a variety of surgical or optical devices. Epikeratophakia, and intraocular lens (IOL) implantation are two invasive surgical procedures for the correction of pediatric aphakia, whereas spectacle and contact lens correction are less-aggressive forms of optical correction for the child with significant refractive error.

Epikeratophakic procedures, once thought to be a safe and effective treatment for the child with aphakia, have largely been abandoned today. This refractive surgical correction requires removal of the corneal epithelial surface of the host eye and a lathe cut donor corneal button is sutured into place. This surgical process results in significant ocular pain, risk of epithelial in-growth, postoperative corneal inflammation, potential corneal scarring, and generally unpredictable refractive outcome (3). Epikeratophakia does not facilitate repeat procedures needed to correct for axial elongation and myopic shift as the infant eye matures through the toddler, young child, and young adult stages of life (4–6).

Implantation of an IOL for pediatric aphakic correction has been a controversial topic for many years. Although the age for IOL implantation has been decreasing in recent years, most surgeons are reluctant to suggest their use in patients less than 2 years of age (7). Perceived advantages are seen for the IOL for the pediatric patient. Children who receive an IOL theoretically have less uncorrected treatment time, and their parents avoid contact lens handling and lens loss problems. It is important that practitioners and parents realize that the use of an IOL presents additional risks to ocular health and vision development in the already compromised pediatric eye. These complications include possible postsurgical inflammation, possible IOL-induced iritis, and the potential side effects of the high doses of topical steroids needed to manage the postsurgical eye. The rough and tumble life of the toddler leads to additional concern about the possible subluxation of an IOL, iris capture of a displaced IOL, and the need for repeat surgeries to remove, replace, or reposition the IOL (7,8). During the first 2 years of life alone, the increasing axial length of the eye creates 2.00 to 3.00 D of change in refractive power, requiring repeat surgical procedures to exchange the IOL. The additional 1 to 2 mm of axial length known to be added during puberty further compounds the limitations of the pediatric IOL (9,10). Add to these problems, that we do not really know the effects on ocular tissue of long-term IOL presence in the eye (7). In addition to all the ocular health concerns listed, and because it is very difficult to accurately predict the final refractive error for these children, IOL implantation becomes a less than ideal approach to pediatric aphakic vision correction (11).

Aphakic and myopic spectacle correction have been and will continue to be a safe and successful means of providing vision correction. Both monocular and binocular spectacle correction, however, present a variety of optical problems (e.g., image distortion, limitations in peripheral vision, disparities in retinal image size, fluctuations in magnitude of optical correction because of changing vertex distance in the active child, and the challenge of frame

fitting with the pediatric patient) (3). Despite these problems, spectacle correction remains the least invasive form of pediatric aphakic or myopic correction.

For the pediatric patient, contact lens correction provides a means of precise refractive control with an acceptable level of ocular complications when compared with all other pediatric aphakic and myopic corrections. With a variety of contact lens materials and fitting parameters available, it is easy to find the right combination of lens material, permeability, lens parameters, and corrective power, to provide a safe and effective means of refractive correction. Clinical studies designed to compare the visual outcome of children who are pseudoaphakic with aphakic contact lens-corrected children have failed to exhibit a statistically significant difference in visual acuity 6 months following surgery (12). These studies have found that both parents and pediatric patients can do very well with aphakic or myopic contact lens correction when given adequate training and support.

Pediatric Contact Lens Materials

Contact lens options for the pediatric patient are similar to those of the adolescent or adult contact lens population. Lens material choices include silicone elastomer, spherical and toric hydrogel, and rigid gas permeable (RGP) lenses. The most frequently used contact lens for the correction of pediatric aphakia is the Silsoft lens (10). This 100% silicone lens, manufactured by Bausch & Lomb, is easy to handle, easy to maintain, and is extremely durable. The rubberlike silicone elastomer material provides high oxygen permeability with diffusion and solubility (Dk) of 340 (cm^2/sec) (mL O_2/mL × mm Hg), excellent thermal conductivity, and is approved for six consecutive nights of wear. The Pediatric Silsoft lens is available in an 11.3-mm diameter with steepest base curve of 7.5 mm radius followed by 7.7 mm and 7.9 mm. The lens power range starts at +20.00 D and increases in three diopter steps up to +32.00 D. The Adult Silsoft lens is available in the larger 12.5 mm diameter with base curves as steep as 7.5 mm and flattens by 0.2 mm up to an 8.3-mm radius. Because of the unique characteristics of the silicone elastomer material, the lens is easy to handle, and is capable of correcting up to 2.00 D of corneal astigmatism. Containing only 0.02% water, the fit of a Silsoft lens is evaluated with the use of fluorescein dye applied to the tear film (13). The cost per lens to the practitioner is approximately $120.00.

Custom-made pediatric aphakic hydrogel soft contact lenses are available from a number of specialty lens manufacturers such as Continental Soft Lens, Flexlens, Kontur Kontact Lens, Ocu-Ease Optical, and Optech Incorporated. On request, specialty laboratories will provide the fitter with a 12.0-mm diameter lens, with a base curve range from 6.8 mm to 8.0 mm, and lens power between +20.00 to +40.00 D. These pediatric lenses are manufactured in 53% to 55% water content lens materials having a relatively low Dk (14). With this wide range of lens parameters, fitting a well-centered lens with adequate movement on a blink can be successfully accomplished. Because of the characteristics of hydrogel lens materials used, careful monitoring of the lens surface condition and corneal health is required. The U.S. Food and Drug Administration (FDA) Group 4 hydrogel materials used for these lenses will attract tear mucin and protein deposits during months of lens wear, reducing lens comfort and optical quality, and increasing the possibility of bacterial contamination. In addition, the reduced oxygen transmission available through these thick hydrogel lenses raises concerns about possible corneal edema. A handheld slit lamp or white light view through the magnifying lens of the Burton lamp is helpful to assess hydrogel lens movement. The cost per lens of pediatric hydrogel lenses ranges from $50.00 to $100.00.

Although slightly more challenging to accomplish, RGP contact lenses provide several advantages over all other contact lenses for the pediatric patient. RGP lenses are known for their excellent optical quality, high oxygen permeability (Dk ranging from 50 to 151), and low risk of bacterial or protein contamination. When properly fitted, RGP lenses provide significant postlens tear film exchange with each blink. These benefits typically translate into fewer corneal complications and fewer days of nonlens wear. For pediatric patients who have had traumatic eye injuries, RGP lenses offer the added benefit of correcting for significant amounts of irregular corneal astigmatism (15). In addition, replacement RGP aphakic lenses can be one third to one half the cost of a replacement silicone or hydrogel lens. The underutilization of RGP pediatric lenses is likely related to practitioner inexperience, lack of fitting sets, and perceived lens intolerance. Those practitioners with RGP pediatric lens experience report that lens adaptation and success is much better than perceived (15).

Pediatric Prefitting Examination

Fitting the infant with a pediatric contact lens typically requires little cooperation from the patient and significant cooperation from the parents. When fitting toddlers with their first contact lens, although cooperation of the child would be greatly appreciated, a significant struggle is usually the reality. As is usually recommended for pediatric patient care, avoid wearing a white coat to help reduce the child's anxiety and enlist greater cooperation. During the first office visit, the parents must be educated about the risks and rewards of pediatric contact lens correction and their role in lens handling. These parents will be required to learn the technique for contact lens insertion, removal, and periodic eye lens evaluation. Parents will be asked to carefully study their child's ocular appearance several times each day to determine ocular health. Parents' willingness to learn lens handling and to be compliant with lens care and wearing instructions are critical for their child's success.

Before lens fitting, careful evaluation of the patient's lids, bulbar conjunctiva, and cornea are essential. Using an ultraviolet light of the handheld Burton lamp or handheld slit lamp with cobalt filter illumination, fluorescein dye can be applied to the corneal surface in an effort to identify areas of corneal compromise. If the keratometry readings taken in the operating room are unavailable, an attempt should be made to gather this information. Although keratometry is helpful, fitting without this information can proceed. It has been well established that infants and toddlers who are aphakic have steep corneal curvatures and high plus refractive errors (16,17). Selection of initial trial lens base curve is typically based on the patient's age. Careful observation of the trial lens centration, movement, and possible fluorescein pattern is critical for a successful fit. Retinoscopy, with handheld trial lenses, of the pediatric eye before lens fitting is helpful to determine a starting contact lens power.

For example: If neutrality in the vertical meridian is achieved with a + 18 D handheld lens, and in the horizontal meridian with + 20 D lens, these powers are averaged and then adjusted for vertex distance back to the corneal plane using the following relationship (assuming an 11-mm vertex distance): Contact lens Rx = Spectacle Rx/1 – vertex distance (in meters) × Spectacle Rx (10). This would result in the following calculated contact lens power: +19.00 D/1−[.011 (+19.00 D)] = +24.00 D.

Pediatric Contact Lens Selection

When planning to use a Silsoft pediatric lens, parameters of the initial fitting lens can be based on the age of the child. For children less than 2 years of age, start lens fitting with a 7.5-mm base curve, 11.3-mm diameter, + 32.00 D lens. As the toddler matures, it is expected that the child's corneal curvature will flatten, aperture will enlarge, and the prescription will require less plus power. The 7.7-mm base curve lens is the starting point for children between 2 and 4 years of age, whereas the 7.9-mm base curve is for the child older than 4 years of age (16).

Pediatric hydrogel lens use should be considered when the child is in need of lens parameters not available in the Silsoft lens. Hydrogel lenses are available in high minus lens corrections, high plus corrections above +32.00 D, or base curves steeper that 7.5 mm. The specific soft contact lens parameters available from a particular manufacturer can be provided by the manufacturer's consultation service. By providing the consultant with the on eye assessment of a pediatric diagnostic contact lens, or the age and approximate retinoscopy findings for the patient, new hydrogel lens parameters can be selected. Although the hydrogel lens insertion and removal technique is identical to the silicone soft lens technique, the inability to use fluorescein dye makes hydrogel lens fit assessment more challenging.

The use of RGP contact lenses for pediatric patients should not be overlooked. Because of their excellent safety profile, RGP lens application should be considered for children with high myopia or corneal pathology such as micro-ophthalmia or postcorneal ulcer (15,16). Although sometimes done in the operating room under general anesthesia, pediatric RGP contact lens fitting can certainly be performed in the office. The pediatric RGP trial lens set is typically composed of small (8.5 mm) diameter lenses, with base curves as steep as 5.0 mm as well as high plus and minus powers. Keratometry measurements, usually taken during the surgical procedure, can make the fitting process efficient but are not essential for fitting success. Before trial lens application, a drop of topical anesthetic should be applied to speed the trial lens process. The base curve of the first trial lens should be equal to the average of the flat and steep keratometry measurement or 7.5 mm when such measures are unknown.

Pediatric Contact Lens Insertion

Insertion of the initial pediatric aphakic trial contact lens can be one of the most challenging and rewarding contact lens procedures. A variety of methods exist to stabilize a child during the contact lens insertion and removal process. Contact lens insertion and removal during the infant stage is relatively easy and can often be done by one parent. For the completely cooperative infant, one parent may be able to hold the child and insert or remove the contact lens. The infant can be placed face up with its back on the parent's thighs and head positioned on the parent's knees. The infant's legs should be wrapped around the parent's waist (18). The parent's nondominant hand is used to stabilize the child's forehead while the dominant hand is used for lens insertion. When inserting a Silsoft or hydrogel lens, the thumb and forefinger of the dominant hand hold a partially pinched contact lens. The inferior one third of the lens is pinched closed, yet the top one third of the lens is completely open. As the palm of the nondominate hand stabilizes the forehead, the thumb of this hand is used to retract the upper eyelid allowing for the fanned out superior lens edge to rest on the superior bulbar conjunctiva. As the middle finger of the lens-holding hand retracts the lower eyelid, the inferior lens edge is allowed to unfold onto the inferior cornea. When inserting an RGP contact lens, the lens should be adhered to the tip of the pointer finger by a wetting agent, and then placed directly onto the corneal apex. The upper and lower lids are slowly released and the child is allowed to blink naturally. The parent is encouraged to comfort the child as we wait for the contact lens to equilibrate.

Contact lens fitting for the 2- or 3-year-old toddler can prove to be very challenging for the experienced fitter as well as the nervous parents. Toddlers have developed the muscle strength and coordination needed to demonstrate a significant struggle during the early stages of the patient's contact lens experience. When first introducing contact lenses to the toddler, two adults are usually needed for lens insertion and removal. One parent is needed to firmly secure the toddler while the second adult inserts or removes the contact lens. The toddler is cradled across the lap of one adult, with the toddler's head securely nestled in the angle of the adult's elbow. If the parent inserting the contact lens is right handed, it is helpful for the child to be secured in the angle of the holder's right elbow. Depending on the cooperation and age of the child, this parent must concentrate on securing the body, arms, and legs of the child while comforting the child throughout the lens insertion or removal process. The child's left arm is placed behind the holder's body while the child's right arm is held by the parent's right hand, which is wrapped around the child's head. The child's legs may need to be secured by the holder's left hand. Once secured, the second parent will focus on the actual lens insertion or removal process, as previously described. Releasing the child from the secure hold and comforting the child with a bottle or pacifier is recommended while waiting for the contact lens to settle down.

An alternative approach to stabilize the struggling toddler requires wrapping the child in a sheet or blanket to immobilize the child's arms and legs (10). Once tightly wrapped in the sheet, the child is placed across the lap of the holding adult with the child's head cradled in the angle of the right elbow. The adult manipulating the contact lens can then proceed with contact lens insertion or removal using the techniques previously described.

Parents benefit when having the complete cooperation of the infant, providing them with the best possible opportunity to learn lens handling despite the emotional challenges they may be experiencing. Starting aphakic contact lens wear as an infant gives the child the opportunity to gain comfort with the ritual of lens insertion, lens wear, and removal. Despite the formidable challenge put forth by the toddler, with determination, a firm grip, and loving care, these children learn to accept contact lens wear as part of their daily routine and demonstrate a high level of cooperation as they mature. Changes in contact lens parameters as the pediatric child matures are generally uncomplicated.

Pediatric Contact Lens Fit Assessment

The ability to use fluorescein dye to help evaluate the fit of a Silsoft pediatric aphakic contact lens is a great advantage. After 15 minutes of lens equilibration, fluorescein dye is instilled in the child's eye. The ultraviolet lights and magnification of the Burton lamp aid in determining the Silsoft lens centration, movement, and thickness of a post-lens tear film. The ideal Silsoft lens fluorescein pattern would exhibit minimal apical clearance, minimal bearing in the intermediate zone, and peripheral edge clearance to moderate nasal edge lift. Lens movement of 1 to 2 mm is expected on a normal blink (18). If the first fitting lens demonstrates no movement, the lens is too steep and a flatter base curve should be tried. A steep-fitting Silsoft lens would demonstrate no fluorescein exchange under the lens base curve and a flatter base curve should be tried. Conversely, a flat-fitting Silsoft lens exhibits significant edge lift and excessive movement, and is easily displaced off the cornea onto the conjunctiva. When such a flat-fitting Silsoft lens has the steepest (7.5 mm) base curve, transition to a hydrogel or RGP lens is required. Hydrogel lenses are available with base curves as steep as 6.8 mm, whereas RGP lenses can be made with base curves as steep as 5.0 mm.

Unlike the silicone lens, hydrogel lenses will readily absorb fluorescein dye if it is accidentally placed in the eye. Consequently, the fit assessment for pediatric hydrogel lenses is completed using the same observation skills needed to assess a conventional or disposable hydrogel lens. After allowing 15 minutes for lens equilibration, the white light from a handheld slit lamp or ophthalmoscope is used to illuminate the lens on the eye. The practitioner must determine if the diagnostic lens demonstrates complete corneal coverage and exhibits 1 to 2 mm of movement with a natural blink. The use of a push-up test or gentle manipulation of the upper or lower lids should help determine the amount of lens float on the eye. Hydrogel lenses that move more than 2 mm with the blink or easily shift off the cornea onto the temporal bulbar conjunctiva and do not return to center with a natural blink are considered flat fitting. The next steeper base curve or larger diameter hydrogel lens should be considered in an effort to provide a more stable lens fit. Those pediatric hydrogel lenses that do not appear to move with a blink or with lid manipulation are too steep in fit and require the use of a lens with a flatter base curve. When in doubt about which diagnostic lens to dispense for trial use, it is safer to release the flatter fitting lens for daily wear use. Because of the increased center thickness of pediatric aphakic hydrogel lenses, oxygen transmission through these pediatric lenses is less than the oxygen transmission through a myopic hydrogel lens of the same material. As a result, it is very important that pediatric lenses move adequately with a blink to allow for tear film exchange under the lens.

The RGP lens assessment is performed using fluorescein dye applied to the anterior surface of a diagnostic lens. Illumination of the eye with the handheld microscope and cobalt filter, or black light of the handheld Burton lamp, is undertaken to appreciate the tear exchange under the lens. Careful and critical assessment of the central and peripheral fluorescein pattern is paramount. Time should be taken to observe the on eye lens pattern as the child blinks naturally and looks around the room. Comforting the child with a bottle or pacifier will help provide the fitter with ample time to observe the lens position and tear exchange. The ideal fluorescein dye lens pattern would represent apical alignment surrounded by a mild amount of edge lift (17). Changes in trial lens parameters, namely base curve and diameter, are made until the well-fitted RGP lens centers over the apex of the cornea and demonstrates 1 to 2 mm of movement with a blink. Although an easily displaced lens is not desired, the successful lens base curve to cornea relationship should avoid a tight adherent lens relationship.

Once a trial lens with the most appropriate parameters is on the eye, an accurate over refraction must be determined. Using handheld trial lenses or lens rack, retinoscopy through the most appropriate trial lens should be completed to determine optical neutrality in each meridian. Before adding the over refraction lens power to the underlying trial lens power, vertex distance adjustment must be made to the corneal plane to determine the final contact lens power. A near vision correction of +2.50 to +3.00 D should be added to the calculated distance correction for children under the ages of 4 or 5 years. For these preschool children, most of their visual tasks are within arms reach. Once the child reaches the age of 5 years or begins to attend school, the near add correction and possible astigmatic correction should be placed in spectacles (6,18).

Pediatric Contact Lens Removal

Once the lens evaluation has been completed, the child needs to be held securely for the removal process. The child should be returned to the original secured position used for lens insertion. The same two-finger lens trapping technique is used when removing Silsoft, hydrogel, or RGP pediatric contact lenses. The thumb or pointer finger of the nondominant hand is placed at the midpoint of the upper eyelid margin, while the thumb or pointer finger of the dominant hand is placed at the midpoint of the lower lid margin. While keeping the eyelid margins in contact with the globe, the lid margins are retracted from the lens center. Once the superior and inferior lens edges are exposed, the lid margins are drawn toward the lens edges. The lens is trapped between the lid margins and is gently flexed, forcing the lens to pop off the eye.

Training Parents How to Handle Pediatric Contact Lenses

Once the appropriate contact lens parameters have been determined and the first lens order placed with a lens manufacturer, valuable time should be spent training the parents how to handle the contact lens. While awaiting delivery of the pediatric lens, an office visit should be scheduled for training the parent how to insert, remove, and care for the contact lens. The previously described techniques of lens insertion and removal should be demonstrated for the parents. As the parents practice holding the child and lens handling techniques, positive support and detailed guidance should be offered. The parents need to understand that, although the child may cry and strongly resist insertion or removal, if done carefully, they will do no harm. During this practice session, parents are informed that all pediatric contact lenses are to be worn on a daily wear schedule and that extended wear will be considered in time, depending on contact lens type and circumstances. Although some pediatric lenses are approved for extended wear, requiring daily wear of all pediatric lenses forces the parents to practice their new skills of lens handling. As the parents become more comfortable and successful with lens handling, their child becomes more familiar with the process as well, improving overall cooperation. In addition to lens handling, parents need to be trained as critical observers during lens wear. Parents should be taught how to identify the signs of ocular irritation, lens-induced discomfort, or simple contact lens displacement. Parents are asked to observe the appearance of the lens-wearing eye several times each day in an effort to avoid lens-related complications.

Pediatric Contact Lens Dispensing, Wear Schedule, Lens Care

The contact lens dispensing visit is an opportunity for the practitioner to reaffirm the appropriate fit and prescription of the lens to be dispensed, as well as the parents' lens-handling skills. After the practitioner has completed the on eye lens assessment, a review of the parents' ability to insert, remove, and care for the lens should completed. To take the lenses home, parents must be successful with lens insertion and removal while the practitioner is absent from the room. Parents are then reinforced that all lenses are for daily wear use. Infants are allowed to nap with their lenses in place, but both infants and toddlers should have their lenses removed before going to sleep for the night. Although the Silsoft pediatric aphakic contact lens is approved for extended wear, we prefer to have children wear these lenses on a daily wear schedule to ensure that the parents are skilled with lens handling, insertion, and removal. Once the child has been successful for a number of months, extended wear on a weekly basis can be considered.

Parents receive a chemical or multipurpose care system for soft lenses to which a separate daily surfactant lens cleaner is added. Parents are instructed to rub the lenses daily with the daily surfactant lens cleaner to aid in the removal of protein or mucin lens coatings, and to ensure the effectiveness of overnight chemical disinfection. In general, we avoid hydrogen peroxide solution systems for the pediatric patient because of their complexity and potential for creating ocular discomfort. Parents are warned not to change lens solution systems without checking with the provider. Parents are again asked to observe the lens-wearing eye several times a day to check for signs of redness, irritation, or lens displacement. If parents observe evidence of pain, redness, excessive tearing, or behavior that suggests discomfort, the lens should be removed and the practitioner should be called. Before leaving the office the child is scheduled for a follow-up office visit in 3 to 5 days.

Pediatric Contact Lens Follow-up Visits

All follow-up visits begin with a careful history about lens wear, lens wearing time at this visit as well as the maximal length of time the lens has been worn. The parents are asked if there are any problems with lens handling, insertion or removal. Parents are asked to report episodes of lens displacement during the day, ocular redness, tearing, or changes in the child's behavior that might suggest ocular discomfort. Each follow-up examination should include an assessment of lens fit, movement, retinoscopic over refraction, and visual acuity, if possible. Once the on eye lens assessment has been completed, the parents are asked to remove the lens as a means to evaluate their lens-handling skills. Once the lens is off the eye, microscopic examination of the cornea with fluorescein dye using a handheld microscope or Burton lamp is completed to assess the health of the epithelial tissue. The handheld microscope or Burton lamp can also be used to inspect the contact lens as well for any signs of compromise or damage. Changes in contact lens parameters are made if indicated. If the child and parents are content with lens wear, the next visit is scheduled to occur in 2 weeks. Once the success of contact lens wear has been established, follow-up visits occur every 3 months. Periodic changes in lens parameters are expected as the child grows and matures. Clinical studies suggest that after the first month of follow up, the next most common period for base curve and lens power change occurs between the second and third year of life (17).

Successful pediatric contact lens wear and vision development depends on multiple factors not always within the control of the practitioner or parents. Ophthalmic literature supports the fact that children born with congenital cataracts or significant refractive errors typically have abnormal eyes in other ways. Frequently, the presence of congenital cataracts can be associated with microcornea or micro-ophthalmus, both of which compromise ocular health as well as complicate contact lens wear (19). Some children born with cataracts have persistent hyperplastic primary vitreous reducing their potential for improved visual acuity. Patients with congenital cataracts are at higher risk for the development of secondary glaucoma because of the crowded nature of their ocular structure. If secondary glaucoma develops in a child, the medical or surgical treatment for glaucoma may require the suspension of contact lens wear until the condition is brought under control. Surgical or medical treatment for elevated intraocular pressure can change corneal shape or increase corneal sensitivity, making continued contact lens wear unlikely (5). During this non–lens-wearing period, occlusion therapy should be continued and spectacle correction should be substituted for contact lens wear.

As a group, children with acquired cataracts are generally more successful with aphakic contact lens wear and vision development than those with congenital cataracts. Excluding those children who have had severe intraocular trauma resulting in soft tissue injury beyond the cataract itself, those with acquired cataracts typically have had an opportunity to develop good visual acuity before cataract development. Because of this early visual stimulation, these children retain a greater potential to resume good vision once the lens opacity has been removed and optical correction provided. Children with a significant refractive error and their parents appreciate the cosmetic and optical benefits that go along with pediatric contact lens wear.

ADOLESCENT CONTACT LENS CORRECTION

Nontherapeutic reasons for considering contact lenses for the adolescent patient include cosmetic appearance and self-esteem, as well as minimizing the inconvenience or cost associated with lost, bent, or broken spectacles. Options for cosmetic contact lens use by adolescent patients include daily or extended wear RGP lenses, daily or extended wear soft lenses, or RGP lenses used as part of an orthokeratology program. Soft lens use can be further subdivided into conventional versus disposable or planned replacement modalities. Studies have shown children as young as 8 to 11 years of age can successfully master insertion and removal of either soft or rigid lenses and lens care, independent of parental involvement (20–22). Potential lens dislocation during wear, lost lenses, and reduced initial comfort of conventional RGP lenses places them at a disadvantage to soft lenses for the adolescent patient, especially given today's wide range of available soft lens parameters.

Although numerous reports suggest traditional RGP lenses can be used to slow the progression of myopia, no well controlled studies yet exist to support this common misconception (20). In the only well-controlled, randomized study to date, Katz et al. (23) failed to

TABLE 15.1 Daily Disposable Lens Parameters

Lens Name/Material	Diameters (mm)	Base Curves (mm)	Available Powers (D)
Softlens One Day/ hilafilcon A (70%)	14.2	8.6	+6.50 to −9.00
Focus Dailies/ nelfilcon A (69%)	13.8	8.6	+6.00 to −10.00
Focus Dailies Toric/ nelfilcon A (69%)	14.2	8.6	+4.00 to −8.00/0.75 cylinder (axis 90 and 180)
1 Day Acuvue/ etafilcon A (58%)	14.2	8.5, 9.0	+6.00 to −12.00

demonstrate any reduction in myopia progression over a 24-month period in a group of 400 children, aged 6 to 12 years. Regardless of the potential for controlling myopic progression, interest in providing cosmetic contact lens correction for this population is fueled by the high incidence, approximately 15%, of myopia among US teenagers (24). A related concern with soft lens use has been their potential contribution to myopic progression; however, at least one study has shown no significant progression as a result of 1 year of soft daily lens wear (22).

Of the various soft lens options currently available, daily disposable lenses would appear to be the most logical choice for the adolescent patient because they eliminate the risks associated with overnight soft lens wear and provide for optimal convenience and compliance by virtue of the elimination of the need for daily lens care (21). The selection of a daily disposable soft lens for the preteen or teenage patient is no different than for the adult, being based on central corneal curvature as determined by manual or video keratometry and refractive findings. Several daily disposable lenses are available (Table 15.1) such that the eye care practitioner can accommodate nearly all spherical as well as a limited range of astigmatic errors.

An alternative nontherapeutic contact lens modality for the myopic adolescent patient is the use of overnight orthokeratology lenses. Although conventional soft lenses may be the only current option for correcting hyperopia or high astigmats, overnight orthokeratology is possibly the most promising option available today for correcting low to moderate amounts of myopia in adolescents.

Adolescent Prefitting Examination

Common to all prospective contact lens wearers is the need to take a targeted case history along with an evaluation of the cornea, conjunctiva, lids, and the precorneal tear film. Key to history-taking for the prospective adolescent contact lens wearer is probing for any experiences of seasonal allergies or use of systemic medications that might have an adverse impact on contact lens use. The most likely drug-related interactions in the adolescent population would result from the use of antihistamines, dermatological preparations, or even antidepressants, all of which have been associated with causing dry eye symptoms that will likely compromise the individual's ability to wear either rigid or soft lenses. Other contraindications for lens wear include structural lid or lash abnormalities, active infection, corneal edema, and persistent corneal staining over grade 2 (mild). Individuals with a compromised precorneal tear film should be approached with caution as well. Common in the adolescent population is seborrheic or staphylococcal blepharitis. This should be addressed before initiating lens wear, with either lid scrubs or the use of ocular and systemic antibiotics as deemed appropriate based on the severity of presenting signs and symptoms.

History of Orthokeratology for Adolescents

The first published use of rigid lenses to control myopia dates back to the early 1960s (25). The effect, however, was both variable and unpredictable, required multiple lens changes, and effected only a minimal reduction in myopia.

Poor lens centering was possibly the single greatest problem seen with these flat-fitting lid attachment fits. The situation improved somewhat with the introduction of reverse geometry RGP lenses in the early 1990s, whereby with a single lens, myopia could be reduced from 1.00 to 3.00 D within as little as 1 month of lens wear (26,27). This advance in lens manufacturing technology enabled fitting-flat central curves for myopia reduction while maintaining good lens centering by using secondary curves 4.00 to 6.00 D steeper than the central base curve. Acceptance remained limited for pediatric patients, because up to 8 hours of daily "retainer lens" wear was required. The potential use of orthokeratology in adolescents became truly viable with the development of multiple reverse curve designs using high oxygen permeable (Dk) materials. These lenses enabled the "retainer lens" to be worn exclusively overnight, all but eliminating the need for adaptation to rigid lens wear, while also hastening the period required for myopia reduction to 7 days or less (28).

Orthokeratology: Lens Design and Fitting

The basic premise of orthokeratology is to bring about a flattening of the central 5 to 6 mm of the cornea (29). The most current *advanced ortho-K* RGP designs accomplish this by combining a flat, central base curve with a secondary *reverse curve* that can be as much as 12 D steeper than the base curve radius (28). These very steep secondary curves are intended to create a potential space toward which the central corneal tissue can be moved. In addition, these steep secondary curves ensure good lens centration that was not possible with traditional tricurve design RGP lenses. Near-perfect centration is needed to eliminate the possibility of an off-centered flattening effect that would result in unwanted, induced corneal astigmatism. Peripheral curves are then added to control edge lift for optimal tear exchange and also serving to bring the contact lens back into alignment with the mid-peripheral cornea.

Although subtle differences may exist between the various lenses available for orthokeratology, all share the same basic fitting approach. Lens diameter is generally more than 10 mm and is not generally used as a primary fitting variable. Using a table or nomogram, a base curve radius is selected that is flatter than the central flat keratometry value by an amount equal to the level of myopia to be reduced. Most practitioners would find it of value to flatten the base curve by 0.50 to 0.75 D to account for the expected amount of regression that occurs during the day following overnight lens wear. Once chosen, the central curve is only altered to increase or decrease the level of myopia reduction. Initial secondary and peripheral curves are specific to each design and not generally practitioner derived.

Evaluation of lens fit with fluorescein should reveal 3 to 5 mm of central touch, surrounded by 2 to 3 mm of pooling followed by mid-peripheral lens alignment beginning at a point approximately 6 to 7 mm from the lens center. In addition, 1 to 2 mm of lens movement should be present to ensure adequate tear exchange. Less than 3 to 5 mm of central touch, less than 1 to 2 mm of movement, or inferior decentration generally indicates a steep fit. A steep fit may also exhibit centrally entrapped air bubbles, debris entrapment, or central dimple veil. Any of these findings require flattening of the secondary reverse curve. Conversely, more than 3 to 5 mm of central touch, more than 1 to 2 mm of movement, or superior decentration generally indicate a flat fit that requires a steeper secondary reverse curve or, rarely, an increase in lens diameter. An excessively flat fit is also likely to cause excessive central superficial punctate staining. As with a standard RGP design, the outermost peripheral curve can be altered to control edge lift, thereby maximizing tear exchange.

Orthokeratology: Follow-up Care

The orthokeratology patient should be examined in the early morning after the first night of lens wear, primarily to ensure adequate corneal response to overnight lens use. Although unaided visual acuity and a manifest refraction are needed, it would be premature to make any changes based solely on these findings. Corneal topography, however, becomes essential even at this early point because lenses worn overnight can cause corneal distortion not easily realized even if the lenses are reinserted for evaluation during the day. The ideal topography pattern is one of symmetrical central flattening with a steep mid-periphery. Bow tie patterns are indicative of induced corneal astigmatism, the result of a decentered lens. It is possible for a lens that appears centered during waking evaluation to become decentered overnight as a result of eye movements during sleep. This can be resolved by a steeper secondary curve or larger lens diameter. Small central steep areas (*central islands*) indicate an inadequate treatment requiring further flattening of the central base curve.

Assuming an adequate physiologic response, the patient can continue with nightly lens wear and be re-evaluated after 1 week, 2 weeks, 1 month, and 3 months of wear. These subsequent evaluations are best scheduled late in the day so that the degree of myopic regression can be evaluated. At each visit, unaided acuity, a manifest refraction, and corneal topography, along with a slit lamp examination are repeated. The spherical component of the manifest refraction provides insight whether an over- or undercorrection exists, whereas any change in cylinder power or axis is indicative of unwanted induced astigmatism resulting from a decentered lens. Assuming a subjectively acceptable level of myopia reduction has been achieved, future visits can be scheduled at 6-month intervals.

Orthokeratology: Myopia Reduction and Daytime Regression

Few studies have methodically reported on the degree of myopia reduction or the time course for regression of the orthokeratology effect during the day following lens removal after overnight lens wear. Mountford (27) reported on 48 patients followed for at least 3 months of lens wear. From a baseline mean level of 2.27 D of myopia, he found an average of 1.93 D reduction in myopia on awakening by the seventh day of overnight lens wear, with only a slight increase in effect (2.23 D) after 1 month. Regression as measured 8 to 9 hours after awakening averaged approximately 0.50 D (27). Nichols et al. (30), working with a very limited sample size of eight subjects, found unaided acuity to improve from an average 20/66 to 20/39 after the first night of overnight orthokeratology, and further improve to 20/25 by the seventh day of lens wear, all as measured 4 hours following lens removal. They furthermore report stable vision up to 8 hours following lens removal (30). In possibly the largest study involving overnight orthokeratology to date, the LOOK pilot study reported a mean reduction of just over 2 D following 1 month of lens wear, with daytime regression averaging 0.25 to 0.50 D as measured 6 hours after lens removal (31). In Hong Kong where overnight orthokeratology is more widely utilized, Cho et al. (32) reported on 59 consecutively examined overnight orthokeratology patients with at least 1 month of lens wearing experience. Mean level of myopia before lens wear was −3.93 D (±2.30 D) with 10 subjects reporting the need for corrective spectacles at least occasionally because of residual myopia. They correlated this need for daytime corrective spectacles with higher levels of pretreatment myopia, although no specific cut-off values were reported (32).

Orthokeratology: Patient Selection and Problem Solving

It is reasonable to predict that for patients with 2 D of myopia or less, a nearly complete elimination of myopia with overnight orthokeratology is probable, and at least a partial effect will be seen for levels of myopia up to 4 D. Additionally, the target reduction is generally increased by about 0.50 D to ensure adequate late day vision (33). The assumption is that, in an adolescent population, the 0.50 D of overcorrection upon awakening can easily be overcome by accommodation.

In addition to considering the level of presenting myopia, corneal astigmatism, pupil size, and patient expectation factor into patient selection for overnight orthokeratology. Experience has indicated that higher levels of corneal astigmatism compromise both the ability to provide an adequate fit or acceptable visual outcome, with 1 to 1.50 D being considered a reasonable upper limit for patient selection (20,34). Because the orthokeratology effect is generally considered to be limited to the central 5 to 6 mm, pupil diameters in normal illumination that exceed this should be a contraindication (29). Even with pupil sizes below 6 mm, halos or ghosting, especially at night, are common initial complaints; however, by the end of the first 1 to 2 weeks of wear, this is less likely to continue to bother patients. Patients must be cautioned that regression following the first night often exceeds 50% of the initial level of myopia, with up to 1 week needed for the full orthokeratology effect to be appreciated. One way to handle this is to provide disposable lenses with one half the original prescription for the first 1 to 3 days, and then one fourth the original prescription for days 4 through 7 (35). It should be noted that, even in the absence of significant reduction in objectively measured myopia at the 1-week visit, subjective improvement is often sufficient to motivate patient continuation with the orthokeratology program. When no objective or subjective evidence is seen of significant myopia reduction after 2 to 4 weeks of lens wear, however, it is unlikely to expect further improvement.

Up to 75% of patients, at some point, demonstrate lens bind on awakening, hence it is essential to recommend using a lens lubricant before bed and again before morning lens removal. Although this cessation of lens movement often leads to superficial central punctate staining, it rarely requires clinical intervention (31,32,36). When faced with persistent or excessive central staining that cannot be attributed to central debris entrapment or to an excessively flat fit causing central corneal abrasion, check for the presence of back surface deposits. Not uncharacteristic of an adolescent population, lens care is often far from perfect. Using a cotton-tipped swab in conjunction with a RGP cleaning solution can minimize such back surface deposits.

Finally, although a pigmented ring similar to that seen in keratoconus has been reported in up to 50% of overnight orthokeratology patients after 12 months of wear, this change is not believed to be of clinical significance (37). Current thinking is that this ring represents mineral deposits in the superficial cornea caused by alterations in tear exchange dynamics.

Adolescent Soft Lens Selection

For individuals not interested in or outside the range for effective orthokeratology, soft lenses remain the modality of choice for the adolescent patient. As previously suggested, traditional RGP lenses worn during waking hours are more apt to dislocate, especially during contact sports; they can limit motivation because of greater initial lens awareness; they are more easily lost and they lack the convenience of current soft lens modalities. One potential concern with continuous overnight soft lens wear, especially with the novice wearer, is that, in the absence of repetitive daily lens insertion and removal, the adolescent patient may not develop the necessary lens handling dexterity needed during unanticipated emergencies (21). Among daily wear soft lens modalities, daily disposable lenses are associated with the lowest number of lens-related complications (38,39). Besides eliminating the need for routine lens care, daily disposable lenses mitigate concerns over lost lenses or the prolonged use of a lens damaged during handling. Where prescription requirements fall outside the range of available daily disposable lenses, 2-week to 1-month replacement lenses may be needed.

Base curve and diameter selection is no different for the adolescent versus adult patient because the most conservative reporting shows corneal size and radius to reach their adult proportions before age 5 years (40). The initial soft lens diameter should be approximately 2 mm larger than the measured horizontal visible iris diameter (HVID), and the initial base curve should be at least 0.8 to 1.0 mm flatter than the flat central corneal curvature value. An acceptable lens fit requires complete corneal coverage and at least .25 mm of lens movement on blink in primary gaze as viewed where the inferior nasal edge of the soft lens intersects the inferior lid margin. Incomplete corneal coverage and movement in excess of 1 mm require changing to a steeper base curve. Conversely, movement under .25 mm or entrapped air bubbles beneath the lens should prompt trial fitting with a flatter base curve. On occasion, the need to alter diameter or base curve will force a change in lens manufacturer, based on parameter availability.

Contact Lenses and Accommodative-Convergence Demand

Although moving the correction from the spectacle plane to the corneal plane will increase accommodative demand for the myope and decrease it for the hyperope, this effect is proportional to the lens power and remains under 0.50 D for corrections between +6.00 and −10.00 D (40). As such, this effect is unlikely to be of significance for the prepresbyopic adolescent patient. Spectacle lenses, however, produce a prismatic effect when an individual converges to read. Viewing inside the geometric center of a minus spectacle lens during reading creates a base-in effect, whereas for plus lenses the induced prism will be base-out. As such, the convergence demand is increased for those who are myopic when switching from spectacles to contact lenses, and decreased for those who are hyperopic. The magnitude of this prism (P) can be obtained from the formula $P = d\, F$, where d is the distance between the line of sight and optical center of the spectacle lens in mm, and F is the dioptric lens power (in the horizontal meridian). For example, a patient who is 5 D myopic reading 2 mm inside the optical center of spectacles, would experience a 1-D loss of effective base in prism for each eye when switching from spectacles to contact lenses. For the patient who is myopic with marginal base-out reserves, this can bring on symptoms of convergence insufficiency. Anytime an onset of near point symptoms occur, the practitioner should re-evaluate near point binocular skills through the contact lens correction.

Adolescent Soft Lens Follow-Up Care

We instruct novice wearers to initiate lens wear at home beginning with 2 to 4 hours of wear, increasing 2 to 3 hours per day to a maximum of 10 to 12 hours. This schedule should enable adolescents to wear their soft lenses to school by the second or third day after lens dispensing. Follow-up visits should be scheduled late enough in the day for the patient to be wearing the lenses for a minimum of 6 to 8 hours at the time of examination. Assuming adequate physiologic response, good lens fit, comfort, and vision, the patient with daily wear lens can be scheduled for a second follow-up 2 to 3 weeks later. During this time, wearing time should be increased to a maximum of 14 to 16 hours per day. Assuming no negative findings, a subsequent visit after 3 months of wear is suggested before placing the patient on a routine schedule of 6-month progress evaluations.

When electing non-daily wear disposable lenses, lens care should be initiated with a *no-rub* chemical care system, because their simplicity will serve to maximize lens care compliance. Hydrogen peroxide systems should be reserved for those instances where concern exists over allergic response because of an extensive history of atopic disease or, in the very rare case, when the patient develops a sensitivity reaction to the chemical care system. Regardless of system, proper lens handling needs to be reviewed at every follow-up or progress evaluation.

Contact lens wear success also depends largely on the adolescent's sense of responsibility and apparent level of maturity. Parent support is also essential but their direct involvement should be limited, because the adolescent must be able to handle his or her contact lenses independently. Practitioner patience and a positive attitude are also important to success. Care should be taken to fully explain all procedures before and while they are being carried out to avoid heightening patient anxiety over the unknown. The eye-care provider should also plan on a longer period of time for examination and fitting. Lens insertion and removal training can take more than twice as long as with the adult patient. If the adolescent cannot master lens handling within the first 30- to 45-minute training session, it is best to reschedule for a second session to avoid frustration and a sense of failure on the part of the patient. Most authorities report girls to mature at an earlier age than boys and they do make up a larger proportion of the preteen contact lens wearing population. Nevertheless, overall success fitting preteen patients under the age of 13 has been reported to be as high as 80% (5).

PEDIATRIC AND ADOLESCENT REFRACTIVE ANOMALIES

Accommodative Esotropia

Bifocal contact lenses have often been suggested as an alternative to spectacle bifocals for children with accommodative insufficiency or accommodative esotropia. Few studies, however, report of their success in a nonpresbyopic population. One evaluation involving aspheric design, multifocal soft lenses failed to demonstrate any positive effect among adolescent patients 12 to 17 years of age (41). One significant limitation to any nontranslating bifocal design in the patient who is not presbyopic is the lack of assurance that the near portion is actually being utilized for reading. Although this would favor the use of a translating bifocal design, such lenses are only available in RGP designs, which are more challenging for the practitioner to prescribe, and are associated with a longer adaptation period. An alternative is single-vision contact lenses for distance and the use of a near addition in spectacle form. Compliance with use of the reading correction may become a concern, however. Pending conclusive clinical studies to the contrary, spectacle bifocals remain the preferred modality for the patient with an accommodative insufficiency who is not presbyopic.

Anisometropia

When more than a 2- to 3-D difference exists in refractive error between the patient's two eyes, image size difference is often sufficient to interfere with binocular vision, resulting in asthenopia or the development of monocular amblyopia. Because individuals will present with as little as 1-D difference in refractive error who are symptomatic, and others with more than 4 D of refractive asymmetry who function without deficit, rely on history and binocular testing to determine who would benefit from contact lens correction. By moving the correction from the spectacle plane to the corneal plane, however, image size differences can be reduced to the point of being insignificant.

High Myopia

In the case of high myopia, the advantage of contact lens correction is more universally evident. Whereas spectacle magnification can be manipulated by controlling material index, base curve, thickness, and the selection of individual surface power, retinal image size can be reduced by more than 10%, even for a well-designed spectacle lens above 10 D (21). In addition to providing for a larger field of vision, the relative increase in image size can translate into a one- to three-line improvement in Snellen visual acuity for the patient who is highly myopic going from spectacle correction into contact lenses.

Nystagmus

The most recent evidence suggests that improvement in visual function secondary to contact lens use in nystagmus results from improved optical correction and not a true damping of the nystagmus (42). Although numerous anecdotal reports promote the use of RGP lenses for proprioceptive feedback aimed at reducing either the frequency or amplitude of the oscillations in nystagmus, no conclusive supportive research exist. Because nystagmus is often associated with significant levels of refractive error, however, contact lenses should be considered for both their potential enhancement of visual function as well as cosmetic appearance. Where the nystagmus is the result of ocular albinism, the eye-care provider should select an iris-tinted lens material that also filters ultraviolet (UV) light. Until conclusive evidence shows RGP lenses to provide any additional benefit in reducing nystagmus, soft lenses remain our primary mode of correction for nystagmus.

Amblyopia

Successful visual outcome is only partially related to early intervention and appropriate refractive correction. Attainment of good visual acuity in children with refractive anomalies is equally dependent on successful antiamblyopia treatment. Oftentimes, the critical difference between those children who develop good visual acuity and those who do not lies with the parent's ability to consistently apply patch therapy to the normal eye. As a result, the pediatric or adolescent vision care provider's role does not end with a successful contact lens correction, but continues with the possible application of occlusion contact lens therapy (19,44). Occlusion contact lens use can be considered as an alternative for those children who have become frustrated and noncompliant with conventional adhesive patch therapy. Before proceeding with an occluder lens for the child's better seeing eye, parents must understand the risks and rewards of occluder lens wear. If the parents wish to proceed, the previously described prefitting examination and lens fitting is completed on the preferred eye. Hydrogel lens parameters used in the eye with significant refractive error

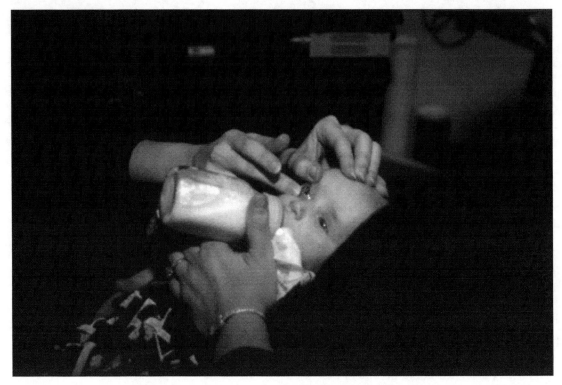

FIGURE 15.1. Insertion of pediatric aphakic contact lens.

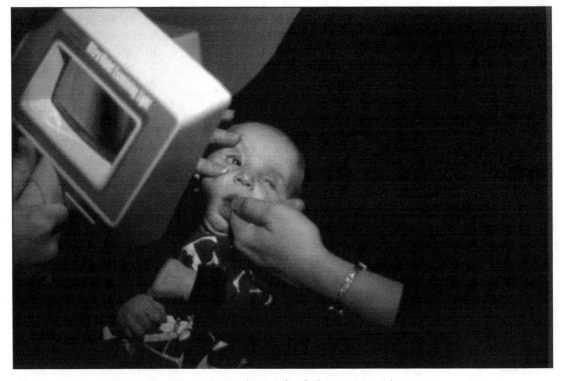

FIGURE 15.2. Evaluating fit of silicone contact lens.

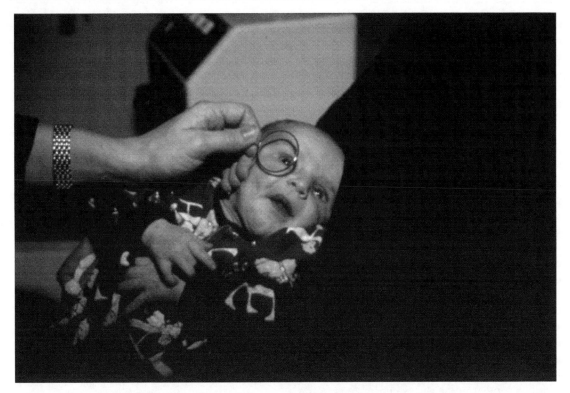

FIGURE 15.3. Determining appropriate contact lens prescription.

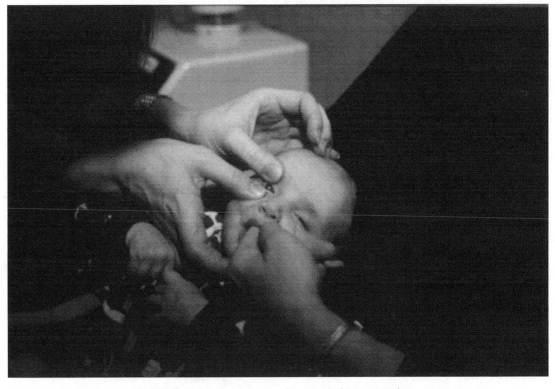

FIGURE 15.4. Removing pediatric aphakic contact lens.

are often successful in the better-seeing eye as well. After establishing successful daily wear of the clear lens for the preferred eye, an opaque-tinted occluder version of this lens is ordered from the manufacturer. If the original lens manufacturer cannot provide an opaque tinted lens, a number of soft lens custom tinting companies can place an opaque black center on the original clear lens at a cost of $50.00 (14). Although most available occluder contact lenses are opaque tinted hydrogel materials, opaque polymethyl methacrylate (PMMA) lenses can be provided through RGP lens manufacturers. A PMMA occluder lens could be used for patients who wear an RGP lens in the fellow eye. Silicone elastomer materials cannot be tinted, however. The number of hours an occluder lens should be worn depends on the patient's age, parental supervision, and the rate at which visual acuity improves. Because of concern for occlusion amblyopia, infants rarely wear occluder lenses more than three quarters of their waking hours. Owing to their increased rate of activity, toddlers tend to wear the occluder lens fewer hours because of additional concern about possible bodily injury. Parents must carefully supervise their child's play activities during occluder lens wear to avoid falls or trauma (4,44) (Figs. 15.1–15.4).

REFERENCES

1. Nelson LB. Diagnosis and management of cataract in infancy and childhood [review]. *Ophthalmic Surgery* 1984;15:688–697.
2. Davis LJ. Complex refractive errors in pediatric patients: cause, management, and criteria for success. *Optom Vis Sci* 1998;75(7):493–499.
3. Morgan KS, Stephenson GS, McDonald MB, Kaufman HE. Epikeratophakia in children. *Ophthalmology* 1984;91:780–784.
4. Moore BD. Pediatric aphakic contact lens wear: rates of successful wear. *J Pediatr Ophthalmol Strabismus* 1993;30:253–258.
5. Wright KW. Pediatric cataracts. *Curr Opin Ophthalmol* 1997;8:50–55.
6. Moore B. The fitting of contact lenses in aphakic infants. *Journal of the American Optometric Association* 1985;56:180:2–3.
7. Ma JJ, Morad Y, Mau E, et al. Contact lenses for the treatment of pediatric cataracts. *Ophthalmology* 2003;110:299–305.
8. Aasuri MK, Venkata N, Preetam P, et al. Management of pediatric aphakia with Silsoft contact lenses. CLAO J 1999;25(4):209–212.
9. Moore BD. Mensuration data in infant eyes with unilateral congenital cataracts. *American Journal of Optometry and Physiological Optics* 1987;64:204.
10. Zadnik K. Pediatric lenses. In: *Specialty Contact Lenses: A Fitter's Guide*. Philadelphia: WB Saunders; 1996:133–141.
11. McClatchey SK, Dahan E, Maselli E, et al. A comparison of the rate of refractive growth in pediatric aphakic and pseudophakic eyes. *Ophthalmology* 2000;107: 118–122.
12. Ainsworth JR, Cohen S, Levin AV, et al. Pediatric cataract management with variations in surgical technique and aphakic optical correction. *Ophthalmology* 1997;104:1096–101.
13. Bausch & Lomb Silsoft (elastofilcon A) contact lenses for aphakic daily and extended wear. Rochester NY, 1995.
14. Thompson TTT, ed. *Tyler's Quarterly* 2004;21(3):9–18.
15. Shaughnessy MP, Ellis FJ, Jeffery AR, et al. Rigid gas permeable contact lenses are a safe and effective means of treating refractive abnormalities in the pediatric population. *CLAO J* 2001;27(4):195–201.
16. Hill JF, Anderson FL, Johnson TK, et al. Eighteen-month clinical experience with extended wear silicone contact lenses on 400 patients. *American Journal of Optometry and Physiological Optics* 1983;60:578–581.
17. McQuaid K, Young T. Rigid gas permeable contact lenses in the aphakic infant. *CLAO J* 1998;24:36–40.
18. Nelson LB, Cutler SI, Calhoun JH, et al. Silsoft extended wear contact lenses in pediatric aphakia. *Ophthalmology* 1985;92(11):1529–1531.
19. Moore BD. Contact lens therapy for amblyopia. Robert Rutstein, ed. Vol. 3: *Problems in Optometry*. Philadelphia: JB Lippincott; 1991:355–368.
20. Walline JJ, Mutti DO, Jones LA, et al. The contact lens and myopia progression (CLAMP) study: design and baseline data. *Optom Vis Sci* 2001;78:223–233.
21. Walline JJ, Long S, Zadnik K. Daily disposable contact lens wear in myopic children. *Optom Vis Sci* 2004;81:255–259.
22. Horner DG, Soni PS, Salmon TO, et al. Myopic progression in adolescent wearers of soft contact lenses and spectacles. *Optom Vis Sci* 1999;76:474–479.
23. Katz J, Schein OD, Levy B, et al. A randomized trial of rigid gas permeable contact lenses to reduce progression of children's myopia. *Am J Ophthalmol* 2003;136:82–90.
24. Walline J. Children: an untapped population of contact lens wearers. *Contact Lens Spectrum* 2002;17(2):26–31.
25. Jessen GN. Orthofocus techniques. *Contacto* 1962;6: 200–204.
26. Harris DH, Stoyan N. A new approach to orthokeratology. *Contact Lens Spectrum* 1992;7(4):37–39.
27. Mountford J. An analysis of the changes in corneal shape and refractive error induced by accelerated orthokeratology. *ICLC* 1997;24:249–257.
28. Day JH, Reim T, Bard, RD, et al. Advance orthokeratology using custom lens design. *Contact Lens Spectrum* 1997;12(6):34–40.
29. Swarbrick HA, Wong G, O'Leary DJ. Corneal response to orthokeratology. *Optom Vis Sci* 1998;75:791–799.
30. Nichols JJ, Marsich, MM, Nguyen M, et al. Overnight orthokeratology. *Optom Vis Sci* 2000;77:252–259.
31. Rah MJ, Jackson JM, Jones LA, et al. Overnight orthokeratology: preliminary results of the lenses and overnight orthokeratology (LOOK) study. *Optom Vis Sci* 2002;79:598–605.

32. Cho P, Cheung SW, Edwards MH, et al. An assessment of consecutively presenting orthokeratology patients in a Hong Kong based private practice. *Clin Exp Optom* 2003;86:331–338.

33. Mountford J. Retention and regression of orthokeratology with time. *Int Contact Lens Clin* 1998;25:59–64.

34. Tahhan N, Toit RD, Papas E, et al. Comparison of reverse-geometry lens design for overnight orthokeratology. *Optom Vis Sci* 2003;80:796–804.

35. Marsden HJ. Clinical Orthokeratology. In: Scheid TR, ed. *Clinical Manual of Specialized Contact Lens Prescribing.* Woburn: Butterworth-Heinemann;2002; 185–199.

36. Lui WO, Edwards MH. Orthokeratology in low myopia. Part 2: Corneal topographical changes and safety over 100 days. *Contact Lens Anterior Eye* 2000;23:77–89.

37. Cheung SW, Cho P. Subjective and objective assessments of the effect of orthokeratology—a cross sectional study. *Curr Eye Res* 2004;28(2):121–127.

38. Suchecki JK, Ehlers WH, Donshik PC. A comparison of contact lens–related complications in various daily wear modalities. *CLAO* 2000;26:204–213.

39. Hamano H, Watanabe Ke, Hamano T, et al. A study of the complications induced by conventional and disposable contact lenses. *CLAO* 1994;20:103–108.

40. Borish IM. *Clinical Refraction,* 3rd ed. Chicago: The Professional Press, 1970.

41. Morton GV, Kushner BJ, Lucchese NJ, et al. The efficacy of SimulVue and Unilens RGP aspheric bifocal contact lenses in the treatment of esotropia associated with a high accommodative convergence ratio. *J AAPOS* 1998;2(2):108–112.

42. Biousse V, Tusa RJ, Rusell B, et al. The use of contact lenses to treat visually symptomatic congenital nystagmus. *J Neurol Neurosurg Psychiatry* 2004;75:314–316.

44. Elsas FJ. Visual acuity in monocular pediatric aphakia; does epikeratophakia facilitate occlusion therapy in children intolerant of contact lens or spectacle wear? *J Pediatric Ophthalmol Strabismus* 1990;27:304–309.

16 Evaluation of Ocular Motor Function

Richard London

Alignment of the eyes during early years of life is critical for the development of normal binocular vision and sensory fusion. Always determine alignment from the most natural condition to the less natural conditions. That is, start with the normal, undisrupted viewing conditions sometimes referred to as *associated viewing* conditions, where both eyes are allowed to take their natural alignment in an attempt to view an object of regard. Examples of tests under associated viewing conditions that detect the presence of an ocular deviation are observation, Hirschberg, Bruckner, and unilateral cover tests. When possible, the magnitude of the deviation can be confirmed by *dissociated viewing* conditions such as the neutralization of the angle with an alternate cover test. These tests prevent the eyes from seeing simultaneously and, thus, are less natural because this does not occur in the routine viewing of the world.

Assessment of ocular alignment begins with the first observation of the patient. Notice any assumed head postures. Head turns may be indicative of horizontal rectus palsy, a null point for nystagmus, or special conditions such as Duane retraction syndrome. Head tilts are suggestive of vertical deviations—usually superior oblique palsies (Fig. 16.1). It is also helpful to review old photos ("Fat scan" or *family album tomography*). The fact that a patient adopts an assumed head posture usually suggests fusion potential and should be viewed as a positive sign for future therapy.

The observation begins from the time the patient is greeted, and continues during the taking of history. The goal is to obtain an assessment of the patient's head posture under natural and un–self-conscious conditions. An estimate of the magnitude of the assumed head posture in degrees should be attempted.

Following observation, more objective measurements of the angle of deviation are accomplished by light reflex tests and cover tests. Whereas the light reflex tests are the simplest, quickest, and easiest to perform on infants and young children, they are not as sensitive as cover tests. All of these tests require controlling the patient's attention and accommodation.

All measurements of alignment should first be done with the patient allowed to manifest the assumed head posture, if any is present. This permits the clinician to judge the effectiveness of the attempted compensation. The head is then straightened to the *forced primary position* and the alignment remeasured to determine the actual magnitude of the deviation that the patient must overcome to maintain fusion.

LIGHT REFLEX TESTS

Bruckner

The least obtrusive measurements are those where the patient simply looks at a light source held by the examiner. These measurements are determined by the Hirschberg and Bruckner

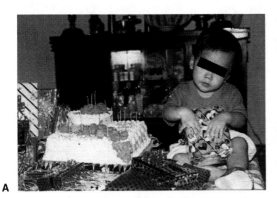
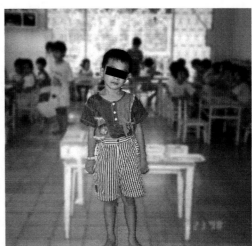

FIGURE 16.1. **A:** Infant manifests left head tilt resulting from a right superior oblique palsy. **B:** Same child manifesting same head tilt several years later.

tests. The Bruckner test permits a qualitative judgment regarding the alignment of the eyes and anisometropia (1,2). Suspicion of the presence of these two major contributors to the development of amblyopia, therefore, can be increased or decreased by a quick and simple screening test. Evidence suggests that the Bruckner test is more reliable when the patient is older than 8 months of age (3). The direct ophthalmoscope is used as the light source for testing. A +1.00 D lens is placed in the ophthalmoscope to partially compensate for working distance and the large circular target is aimed at bridge of nose of the patient from approximately 50 cm away. Both pupils are visualized simultaneously and the brightness of the red reflexes compared. The eye with the brighter reflex is presumed either strabismic or more anisometropic (4). Pathology that affects the normal red reflex will also be identified by this test. This includes retinal detachment, gross retinal pathology; corneal, lenticular, and media opacities; anisocoria can possibly confound the result as well. It is reported that the sensitivity of the Bruckner test is 3 to 4 prism diopters (5). This test is particularly useful support as part of a battery of tests to help compensate for inherent limitations of each individual test with young children (6–8).

A commercially available instrument that makes use of the Bruckner reflex is the MTI (Medical Technologies, Inc) photoscreener. A Polaroid photograph is taken that enhances the retinal reflex and allows a documented, simultaneous comparison between the eyes. The MTI is reported to be effective for children as young as 6 months of age. It is potentially useful as a screener for use by nurses and in schools. It has been reported easier for pediatric residents to interpret compared with direct viewing of the Bruckner reflex (9).

Hirschberg Test

The Hirschberg test is also performed at a distance of about 50 cm from the patient, with a light aimed directly at the bridge of the patient's nose. The light source should be sufficiently large to allow simultaneous viewing of both corneas, and is best done with a light of adjustable intensity to allow for patient comfort. The surrounding room should be sufficiently dark to reduce peripheral distracting elements. Various techniques to capture the child's attention at the light source must be used to complete the measurement. Depending on the clinician's talents, cooing, cat, bird, or dog sounds may be used. If using a transilluminator, it also helps to place the light source through a small toy to capture the child's attention.

The light source will produce light reflexes, the first Purkinje image, behind the patient's pupil (although we often use the misnomer *corneal light reflex*). The difference in the location of these reflexes between the corneas results from the magnitude of the ocular deviation. The accepted conversion is 1 mm of displacement equals 22 prism diopters of deviation (10–12), although for flatter corneas, a more accurate conversion may be 27 prism diopters (13). This may be relevant in infants because they tend to have flatter corneas.

It is important to estimate the location of the light reflexes from the center of the pupil. Because this point is not physically present, many clinicians attempt to estimate the location from the physical edge of the pupillary margin. This is subject to error because of the possibility of anisocoria and, therefore, unequal reference points. Some have suggested estimating from the limbus, but this is a relatively large distance. Additionally, the standard recording is based on distance from the center of the pupil. Use of any other reference point will necessitate an additional conversion.

With patients who have dark irides, it is often difficult to determine where the pupil ends and the iris begins. For these patients, using the direct ophthalmoscope as the light source facilitates the determination of the Hirschberg reflex. By placing a +1.00–D lens in the ophthalmoscope and viewing the corneas simultaneously, the pupils will show a red reflex used in the Bruckner assessment and a pinpoint of light in the background of the red reflex that is the reference for the Hirschberg test. This method is so quick and effective that I tend to use it regardless of iris color.

Determine the strabismic magnitude by estimating the position of the fixating eye's reflex compared with that of the deviating eye. By convention, a reflex located nasally to the center of the pupil is called *positive* (+), whereas that temporal to the center is called *negative* (–). Remember, a light in a nasal location on the cornea projects temporally in the retina, whereas a temporal corneal reflex projects nasally. The common position of the corneal light reflex is +0.5 mm, representing the slightly temporal location of the fovea. A range of normality exists, however, and small deviations from the accepted norm should not be viewed with concern.

The important factor for angular estimation is the difference between the reflexes. For example, if the right eye has a reflex of +0.5 mm and the left eye −1.0 mm, the difference between them is 1.5 mm. The accepted conversion into prism diopters is 22 prism diopters per millimeter. In the above example, the ocular deviation would be approximately 33 prism diopters left esotropia, with the right eye being the fixating eye and the left eye turned inward, yielding a temporal corneal reflex.

At times, the corneal light reflexes are so close to the expected norm that it is difficult to know which is the fixating and which is the turned eye. For instance, the right eye reflex is +0.5 mm and the left eye −0.5 mm. Which is the fixating eye? To be certain, look at the monocular corneal light reflexes. This monocular reflex is angle lambda, which is defined as the angle between the center of the entrance pupil and the visual axis. It is often misnamed *angle kappa*. Angle kappa, by definition, is measured at the nodal point of the eye. Because that point is not clinically accessible, the best we can do is assess angle lambda. In the example above, if we cover the left eye and the right eye moves so its angle lambda is now −0.5 mm, and we cover the right eye and the left eye maintains its −0.5 mm angle lambda, then we can state that this patient has a 22 prism diopter right exotropia. If it was the left eye that changed during angle lambda assessment, the patient has a 22 prism diopter left esotropia.

A potential misleading finding occurs in the rare case when a patient has unequal angle lambdas. In these cases, a unilateral cover test on either eye will result in no refixation movement and, therefore, no change in angle lambda in either eye .

Occasionally, a patient can have eccentric fixation sufficiently large to be seen on angle lambda testing. Most clinicians believe that a 0.5-mm deviation is the smallest that can be determined with good confidence. This translates into a minimal eccentric fixation of 11 prism diopters—a very large amount. When viewed binocularly as the Hirschberg test, however, eccentric fixation has no effect. In the very rare situation where the degree of eccentric fixation is equal to the angle of deviation and both are sufficiently large to be seen on these tests, no movement will be observed when one eye is covered. Although this provides a good academic exercise, its true occurrence is fleetingly rare.

Krimsky Test

To improve quantification of the Hirschberg test, a modification was made known as the *Krimsky test*. A prism is held before one eye until the light reflexes appear in the same location in each eye. The prism can be placed before either eye, and each method has its proponents. Remember, a prism placed before the fixating eye will result in a version movement of both eyes in the direction of the apex. Following insertion of the prism, the fixating eye sees a displaced image and refixates it. Because of Hering's Law, the deviating eye moves in the same direction. In comitant deviations, the eye will move a degree equal to stimulus prism. Prism is inserted until the light reflex in the deviating eye matches that of the fixating eye before prism insertion. Those who favor this method argue that it is easier to see the light reflex with no prism in front of the eye. Two potential problems exist with this technique, however: first, the clinician must remember the initial location of the fixating eye's reflex; and second, if the deviation is not comitant, the measured angle of deviation will be the secondary angle, often much larger than the primary angle, which is measured with the dominant eye fixating. For this reason, when incomitancy is suspected based on evaluation of ocular motilities (below), the Krimsky must be done with the measuring prism placed before the deviating eye. Thus, no version response is expected. This is the second method. In fact, this is the method I recommend being used exclusively. The criticism for this method is that the clinician must view the light reflex through a prism. I find this is easily done, and this method has the advantages of direct comparison of the light reflexes—no need to rely on memory—and it works with both comitant and incomitant deviations, with no need to change methods for different types of cases.

Prism position and orientation are always important during angle neutralization. The apex points to the direction of deviation of the eye.

Be sure to hold the base-apex line parallel to the cornea. Do not stack prism in the same direction. Horizontal prism can be stacked with vertical prism, but the stacking of prism in the same direction results in a greater magnitude deviation than indicated by the number written on the prisms. For instance, stacking a 40- and 16-prism diopters results in an angle of 76 prism diopters rather than the expected 56 prism diopters.

COVER TESTING

Unilateral Cover Testing

If the child is old enough to fixate accurately for cover testing, it is usually not necessary to perform the light reflex tests. The most natural of the cover tests is the unilateral cover test (UCT), also know as the cover-uncover test. The patient is allowed to view the fixation target without external barriers to fusion. One eye is then covered while the uncovered eye is observed to determine any movement toward refixation. The occluder, or examiner's thumb for infants, should be held in place for 1 to 2 seconds to allow time for a deviated eye to pick up fixation. An inward refixation movement occurs with exotropia, whereas an outward movement indicates esotropia, downward with hypertropia and upward with hypotropia. No movement means that the uncovered eye is showing no manifest deviation. Following the covering of the eye, the occluder is then removed and the patient is allowed to refixate on the target. Remember, the UCT is essentially just a probe of the habitual alignment of the eyes. Following each probe, allow the patient several seconds to return to habitual deviation. Then, the other eye is probed with occlusion. The results of this testing will be findings of orthotropia, esotropia, exotropia, hypertropia, hypotropia, or some combination.

Care must be taken not to *telegraph* which eye will be covered. If the patient can anticipate which eye will be occluded, those with small angle alternating strabismus will switch fixations so quickly as to not be observed to have movement on the actual cover test. Bring the occluder from a central location, in front of the nose or from the center of the forehead, so that the patient cannot anticipate which eye will be occluded. Vary the pattern of occlusion following the return to the habitual deviation so that the patient does not get into a rhythm.

The UCT is performed at distance and near. With young children, a distance target with color that produces sound is often required to hold the patient's attention. Videos can be useful for very young children, but are too large to allow accurate determination of small angle strabismus. A discrete target (e.g., an animated animal that makes noise) is preferred. If children are old enough, call their attention to specific markers on the target. For instance, ask the patient: "What color is the elephant's eye?" "His nose?" This allows for most accurate fixation. Following distance testing, the UCT should be repeated at near.

The accuracy of this test depends on accommodation being locked onto the target of regard. Small pictures on fixation sticks make good targets. Again, ensure fixation and accommodation by asking questions of the child regarding the fixated picture.

The three most common errors in performing an appropriate UCT at near are (a) telegraphing the eye to be occluded; (b) using a target that does not lock accommodation; and (c) holding the fixation target too far from the child. A young child does not hold objects at 40 cm. Testing a child who is routinely visually examining objects at 25 cm at the adult standard of 40 cm will almost guarantee missing many accommodative esotropic conditions.

Remember, a patient can have a strabismus at one distance or position of gaze and not another, or, a constant deviation can occur at one location and an intermittent one at another. To determine the impact of a strabismus on visual development, the results of the UCT must be viewed along with the monocular visual acuities and stereopsis and, if the child is old enough, status of correspondence. (see Chapters 2, 7, 10 and 17).

Alternate Cover Testing

Unlike the UCT, the alternate cover test (ACT) demands that no opportunity is provided for the eyes to fuse or return to their habitual state. The goal is to determine the magnitude of the full deviation of the eyes in a fusion-free state. Thus, the ACT alone cannot determine whether a phoria or strabismus is present. It does, however, allow measurement of the challenge to fusional vergence and how it changes at different distances and different positions of gaze.

To encourage full dissociation, the occluder should be held over one eye for several seconds, then rapidly moved to the other eye, allowing no opportunity for fusion. The movement should shift occlusion between the eyes like a toggle switch. One is covered, then the other, with no pause between. The uncovered eye is observed to determine refixation, and the direction of this refixation is interpreted as with the UCT.

Measurement of the dissociated deviation is accomplished by neutralizing the movement with prism. A prism bar or loose prism is held before the deviating eye for patients who are strabismic, or either eye for those who are phoric. To neutralize a deviation, the base is held in the direction that the eye moves to pick up fixation. Ideally, the prism is held behind the cover paddle so that one eye clearly provides a fixation and accommodative control. As the ACT continues, prism is increased or decreased until no refixation movement is seen in the eye under the prism. Note, at times, a rebound or redress occurs in the uncovered eye even when the deviation is totally neutralized by prism (14). Equality of this redress should be considered the neutral point.

Again, remember when neutralizing the deviation with prism, to resist the temptation to stack prism in the same direction. To do so yields a significantly greater power because of the artificially increased angle of combined prism. You can stack horizontal and vertical prism and maintain accurate readings.

If the eye under the prism is neutralized, but movement is still observed in the other eye, some additional conditions must be considered. Of most importance is a true incomitant deviation resulting from a palsy of an extraocular muscle. Accommodative differences between the two eyes resulting from residual hyperopia (natural or induced) can mimic this condition in primary gaze.

If a deviation is incomitant, it will be equal in the cardinal positions of gaze or with either

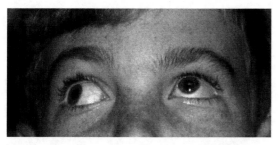

FIGURE 16.2. Importance of testing ocular deviation in different positions of gaze. This child is aligned in primary position, but note marked exotropia in upgaze.

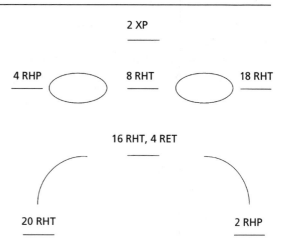

FIGURE 16.4. Sample of ocular deviations recorded in different positions of gaze.

eye fixating. With incomitant deviations, the deviation will change in different positions of gaze or in primary gaze when the fixating eye is changed, because of Hering's Law. In the latter case, the standard method of recording is OD fixating = 20 Δ ET; OS fixating = 35 Δ ET. After determining the magnitude of the eyes' deviation in primary gaze at distance, determine the angle in up, down, left, and right gazes (Fig. 16.2). This is accomplished by having the patient fixate an appropriate distance target as the clinician turns the patient's head to the right in the patient's left gaze; to the left, up in the patient's downgaze, all approximately 30°; and down in the patient's upgaze approximately 25° (15). This series is done at distance so accommodation should not influence the results. If a vertical deviation is noted, the ACT should also be done with the head tilted to each side approximately 30° looking for increase in hyperdeviation.

To record the angle of deviation in different positions of gaze the following diagram (Fig. 16.3) is very useful. It is also used later in this chapter to record ocular motilities.

The following diagram (Fig. 16.4) is an example of recording a patient with a right superior oblique palsy. Note, the diagram permits all the measurements needed to complete the Parks 3-Step Test. This test is designed to identify a paretic, vertically acting muscle by comparing the eye with the hyperdeviation in primary gaze, horizontal gazes, and on forced head tilt to the right and left. A convenient way to map these changes in clinic is through the use of the diagram using ovals. Ovals are placed over the potential pairs of muscles that might be responsible for the paretic vertical deviation. Following all three measurements, only one muscle will be circled three times; that is the affected muscle (16,17).

Although it is a commonly used method, the Park's 3-Step is really most accurate when diagnosing superior oblique palsy. Many of the other vertically acting muscles that might be identified by the test rarely occur, such as isolated inferior oblique palsy. In fact, what often presents on this test as an inferior oblique palsy is usually the result of a tight (contracted) contralateral superior rectus (18,19). The 3-Step Test does not account for overacting muscles, dissociated vertical deviation (DVD), restrictive changes (e.g., fibrosis), nor systemic conditions (e.g., myasthenia gravis) (20,21). Therefore, the 3-Step Test must be used along with the motility evaluation

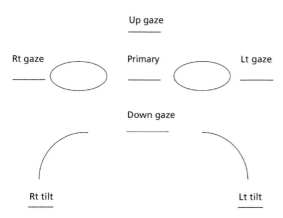

FIGURE 16.3. Positions to record ocular deviation of this diagram.

and observations of habitual head posture to arrive at the best diagnosis.

Superior oblique palsy occurs congenitally fairly frequently with no ominous consequence. Incomitancy caused by ominous factors tends to also demonstrate other evidence of *bad company*, that is, there tend to be additional signs or symptoms. Other causes are seen for incomitancy often seen in young children. Duane syndrome (Duane retraction syndrome) can present mimicking lateral rectus palsy, often leading to needless and expensive testing. Look for the globe retraction on adduction resulting from co-contraction of the lateral and medial rectus of the adducting eye. It is thought that the sixth nerve nucleus on one side fails to develop (22,23). The lateral rectus on that side is then innervated by a branch of the third nerve often intended for the ipsilateral medial rectus. Thus, when attempting to make the lateral rectus abduct, no signal is capable of being generated and no abduction occurs. On attempted adduction, both ipsilateral medial and lateral recti are stimulated. The degree of adduction probably depends on the number of nerve fibers innervating the medial versus lateral rectus. Likewise, the initial starting position of the eyes, esotropic, orthoropic, or exotropic probably depends on the distribution of fibers between the medial and lateral recti (24). Interestingly, regardless of the starting deviation of the eyes, if an ACT is done in the position of gaze opposite the effected eye (right gaze in a left Duane), a small exotropia deviation will usually be noted. Again, this is probably caused by a decreased number of fibers innervating the medial rectus. Duane syndrome is more common in females and in the left eye; however, males also can be affected as right eye or bilateral presentation (25). This condition occurs most frequently as a sporadic manifestation; therefore, it is rarely observed in family members. It is usually an isolated condition, but occasionally can be associated with several other conditions such as deafness, arteriovenous (A-V) malformations, and skeletal problems (26,27). Through a combination of head turn and good motility in one field of gaze, patients with Duane syndrome often exhibit excellent binocular vision. Treatment is usually recommended only in cases of a strabismus in primary gaze.

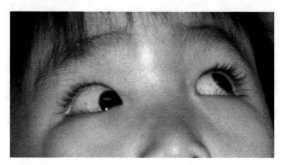

FIGURE 16.5. Brown syndrome of the right eye easily notice on attempted upgaze.

Brown syndrome, or superior oblique tendon sheath syndrome, is often noted by parents because it is most obvious when the child looks in upgaze. The adducting eye is unable to elevate, appearing as the rarely occurring inferior oblique palsy. Because children usually have to physically look up to their parents, this is an easily detected deviation (Fig. 16.5). Unlike patients with Duane syndrome, the right eye is more frequently affected, although the left eye or both eyes can be involved. The typical mechanism appears to be the thickening of the superior oblique tendon so that it does not easily slip through the trochlea. It is usually congenital, but can result from inflammation or trauma, or even be iatrogenic following aggressive superior oblique surgery or sinus surgery (28,29). In most cases, it is uncomfortable for patients to attempt to look into the affected field of gaze. Occasionally, in intermittent cases, a "click" or "pop" may be felt as the tendon clears the trochlea. Although many patients are binocular unless gaze is directed into the superior oblique field of action, a significant number of these patients are unable to compensate and have decreased binocularity (30). On motilities, patients with Brown syndrome may demonstrate a V pattern exodeviation in upgaze that might further differentiate it from the rare inferior oblique palsy that presents with an A pattern (31). Unless hypotropia is seen in primary gaze, most patients do not require treatment beyond assumed head postures.

Likewise, an esotropia more pronounced in upgaze, an A pattern, or an exotropia more obvious in upgaze, a V pattern, is frequently detected by parents. On the other hand, a V intermittent esotropia or an A intermittent exotropia can have more impact on everyday tasks, although they are not as cosmetically obvious.

Simultaneous Cover Test

At times, in the small angle strabismus known as monofixation syndrome (32,33), the observed movement on the UCT appears markedly less than on the ACT. This condition is usually conceived of having (a) a manifest deviation (the strabismus noted on UCT) that cannot be compensated by fusional vergence, and (b) a superimposed phoria that is compensated by fusional vergence and revealed only by the complete disruption of fusion during a test such as the ACT. A special cover test is useful in these cases. This test, known as the *simultaneous cover test* (SCT) allows measurement of the deviation observed on the UCT by simultaneously imposing a prism before the deviating eye and a cover paddle before the fixating eye. If no refixation of the eye occurs under the prism, this measurement represents the manifest deviation of the eyes. If a refixation movement does occur, the prism and paddle must be removed for several seconds to allow the patient an opportunity to regain fusion before reinserting a new prism.

CONFOUNDING FACTORS

Reliable assessment of ocular alignment and motility depends on being able to attract and maintain the child's attention. Frequent changing of toys of visual interest or sounds is often necessary. It often helps if the clinician is a bit uninhibited and practiced at making some animal sounds or singing to the infant or young child.

The single largest factor resulting in referral for presumed strabismus that turns out to be pseudostrabismus is epicanthal folds. This is especially confounding if the folds are unequal between the two eyes. Not only will this anatomic feature make many patients with orthophoria appear to have esotropia, but it also masks exotropia in other patients. Furthermore, it makes evaluation of ocular motilities very difficult on the medial side, often suggesting an overaction of the medial rectus or inferior oblique when none exists. For the clinician to be convinced and to convince the parents of the status of the patient's alignment and motilities, the clinician must become facile at pinching the folds to allow sclera to show on the medial side. The clinician must rely on the combined results of several tests (e.g., the Bruckner, Hirschberg, and UCT) to develop a preponderance of data suggesting a diagnosis.

VERSIONS AND DUCTIONS

Smooth pursuits develop very early in life; however, they are asymmetric for approximately the first 3 months of life. Although temporal to nasal movements are followed accurately, those from nasal to temporal that send neural connections ipsilaterally through the occipital cortex tend to be jerky during the first months of life. Between 4 and 6 weeks of age, they usually achieve symmetry.

Pursuits are slow (up to 30°/sec) movements, generated from the ipsilateral occipital parietal cortex that demand good fixation and feedback. Versions permit evaluation of conjugate movements into the nine cardinal positions of gaze, whereas ductions are monocular movements into these fields. The clinician can analyze these extraocular muscle movements to obtain an estimate of development and any obstacles to binocularity, including paresis, restrictions, or congenital anomalies. Additionally, the ability to fixate monocularly on and accurately follow small targets is an indication of relative visual acuity in very young children.

To obtain a child's attention, colorful toys should be used as fixation devices during version testing. Those with lights or that make sound are also desirable. Have several toys ready to allow rapid changing. Frequently, the best the clinician can obtain is "one toy, one look."

Several systems have been developed to judge the developmental aspects of the oculomotor system. Clinicians interested in the developmental aspects of eye movements often pay careful attention to movement across the midline. As children develop, they can visually follow an object smoothly as it crosses the midline. In earlier stages a *jump* is frequently observed as the eyes cross the midline. One attempt to quantify, uses a 1 to 4+ scale for pursuits and saccades. Smooth and accurate is rated as 4+. One fixation loss or slight overshoot is 3+. Two fixation losses or gross over- or undershoots is 2+. More than two fixation losses, increased latency, or inability to do the task is 1+ (34).

A popular test to judge the developmental age equivalent of pursuits and saccades is the NSUCO (Northeastern State University College of Optometry) oculomotor test. Norms are calculated from ages 5 to 14 (35). This test attempts to quantify observations related to eye movements, taking into account head and body movements during attempted ocular movements and over- and undershooting on saccades. Two types of observation are scored: the qualitative judgment of performance and the quantitative counting of the number of times the clinician observes a particular behavior. The testing is scored from 1 point (lowest) to 5 points (highest). Minimal acceptable values were developed for males and females performing pursuits and saccades. Each was judged in four categories: ability, accuracy, head movement, and body movement. The intention of this test is to look at patient's oculomotor skills and to predict certain aspects of reading readiness.

When the main concern in assessing versions and ductions is to determine over- or underacting muscles, a convenient system uses a 0 to 4 scale and the motility diagram introduced above. Pursuit movements can be used to determine the limits of ocular motility. The pursuit takes the muscles into the extreme positions of gaze. The challenge must extend beyond the usual fields of gaze. This permits determination of faulty action that starts at the extremes well before they manifest in the normal field of action. Overaction is rated as 0 to +4; underaction as 0 to −4. To aid in easy visual recognition, the underactions are also shaded in the diagram. Zero implies normal muscle action. Because the scale is a 4-point system, each number represents a change of 25%. Underactions are easiest to visualize. A −4 means the eye cannot pass the midline. Mentally divide the area between the midline and the canthus into three sections, each representing 25%.

The motilities should be consistent with the results from the ACT in different positions of gaze. A −3 underaction of the right lateral rectus with all other extraocular (EOM) being

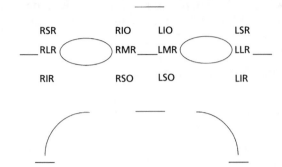

FIGURE 16.6. Diagnostic action fields of extraocular muscles.

normal should show a marked increase in esotropia on right gaze. If not, either the motility rating, the deviation measurement, or both require careful remeasurement.

Placing the motilities in the diagram presented above permits a good overview of the motoric challenge to the patient. First, a brief review of the diagnostic action fields of the muscles (Fig. 16.6): Placing all the findings together yields the following diagram (Fig. 16.7): From this diagram, we can immediately determine that the patient has a right superior oblique palsy (right hypertropia that increases on right gaze and with right head tilt) and, on motilities, the patient has an underacting right superior oblique and overacting right inferior oblique.

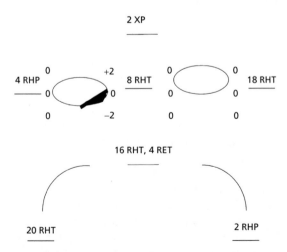

FIGURE 16.7. Sample of recording ocular alignment in seven positions of gaze along with rating of motilities.

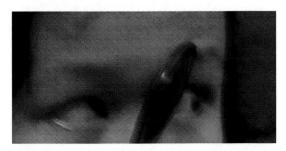

FIGURE 16.8. Use of an occluder to ensure that only the abducting eye is fixating the target. This facilitates evaluation of oblique function.

To determine more accurately the motility of the oblique muscles, it is often advisable to partially occlude the adducting eye by angling the thumb or occluder on the bridge of the nose to permit fixation only with the abducting eye (Fig. 16.8). Otherwise, the patient may fixate with the adducting eye, and the oblique action may be masked.

When an underaction is noted on version testing, a duction is performed to see if any further movement may be detected.

For some patients, underaction can best be determined by the oculocephalic maneuver (passive head-turning or the dolls-head maneuver). With young infants, it is possible to take advantage of the oculovestibular reflex by holding the infant facing you while you are seated in a chair capable of rotating. Rotate in complete circles, first clockwise, then counter clockwise while you observe the infant. The eyes are expected to deviate in the direction opposite to where the head is turned. When the deviation is full, nuclear and infranuclear pathways are intact. Full vertical movements indicate a normally functioning pretectal area, whereas full horizontal movements indicate patency of the pontine conjugate gaze centers (36).

Saccades

Saccades are rapid conjugate eye movements that quickly allow fixation to be moved from one target to another. Saccades are eye movements necessary to maintain fixation once a target demands eye movements faster than 30–40° per second. They are generated by the contralateral frontal lobe and are present from birth—often in response to sounds. Often referred to as *ballistic*, these movements start quickly and then brake to allow an accurate trajectory. The fastest eye movements, they have velocities approximately 10 times that of pursuits and can be generated by vision, sound, or memory. In response to head movements, an involuntary refixation saccade often occurs that serves to compensate and allow stability of fixation. Voluntary saccades permit fixation to rapidly change viewing targets without the need for head movements. This movement is the result of a signal generated from the retina to cerebral, collicular, and cerebellar processes to generate a final instruction through the brainstem (37). All this takes place with a latency of only 200 milliseconds. Disruption of mechanisms anywhere along this pathway will negatively affect saccadic speed or precision.

Visually driven saccades are predetermined, probably as a result of the angular distance from the fovea to the point of retinal stimulation. Most saccades that occur in the course of normal activities are less than 15° (38). Beyond that, a head movement usually accompanies the eye movement. During the actual eye movement, saccadic suppression prevents a perception of the world sweeping by (39). Saccades become increasingly important as children progress through the early grades in school. As with pursuits, dysfunctions can be a result of development (functional) or it can be caused by faulty neurologic control resulting from disease.

Many school-related and life skill problems are thought to be associated with ocular motility problems, particularly saccades. These include excessive head movement when reading, skipping lines or losing place while reading, omitting words or transposing words when reading, requiring the use of a finger or marker to stay on line when reading, reporting shifting of words on the page when reading, and difficulty with playing ball sports (40). This has led clinicians to seek office tests that might reveal saccadic dysfunction.

Testing of saccades can be divided into the evaluation of the fine saccades required in reading, and the larger gross saccades. The patient can be tested for gross saccades by the clinician holding two targets 25 to 40 cm apart at a 50 cm distance from the patient. With young children, the targets should be bright with different characteristics. Those that make noise can be beneficial. The patient's attention is drawn to first one, then the other target. The clinician should fixate on the bridge of the patient's nose. This allows simultaneous observation of the motion of both eyes. The goal is evaluate the accuracy and range of the movements. Hypermetric (overshoots) and hypometric (undershoots) movements should be noted, as well as corrective movements following fixation and ability to reach the target. The targets should then be held vertically and the procedure repeated evaluating vertical saccades.

Many systems have been designed to rate the developmental quality of gross saccades. Some specify the use of different targets. In general, the easiest is a 0 to 4+ scale that uses 4+ as the standard for accurate movements, 3+ for one inaccuracy, 2+ for two inaccuracies, and 1+ for more than two inaccuracies (40). The NSCUCO oculomotor test mentioned above also has criteria for evaluating saccadic eye movements.

For children who are old enough to read numbers, the developmental eye movement (DEM) test is very useful (41). This test is particularly useful for patients in the early grades in school where reading skill is often assessed by oral reading. The DEM attempts to separate out eye movement speed from naming speed. This permits the clinician to determine whether a patient has age-appropriate saccades, age-appropriate naming speed (automaticity), or deficiencies in one or both.

When the child can actually read words, the use of an infrared eye movement recorder (e.g., one of the Visagraph models) is my instrument of choice. This allows measurement of the number of fixations, regressions, average duration of fixation, and interactions between these variables to determine reading rates for a 100-word paragraph. I have recently been having young patients read one paragraph silently and another one orally, again trying to isolate specific reading-related eye movement dysfunctions from the problem of naming the words.

Inaccuracy in saccadic eye movements can be caused by the rapid pulse portion that initiates the saccade or drift at the end of the saccade. Normal asymptomatic patients may show small amounts of dysmetria. Infants tend to make several small saccades rather than one large saccade. The clinician, however, must be aware of pathologic conditions that can affect saccades. Be especially wary in cases of an asymmetry between opposing directions.

The cerebellum adjusts the *gain* of the saccade. If a lesion affects the cerebellar outflow, a hypermetric saccade is likely. Many lesions throughout the pathway, including cerebellum, brainstem, and cerebral lesions, can result in hypermetric or hypometric saccades. Vertical saccades can be skewed in the direction of a hemispheric lesion. Visual defects such as hemianopia or neglect may also affect saccades.

Vergence

Vergences are disjunctive eye movements that maintain fusion. They allow both foveae to be pointed at the target of regard. Vergences compensate for heterophoria and decreased vergence ranges can cause symptoms of fatigue and asthenopia.

Three types of vergence movements normally considered clinically are convergence, divergence, and vertical vergence. Additionally, cyclovergence can be a factor in some cases. Clinically, vergence dysfunctions are usually classified as excessive or deficient at distance or at near. This leads to the following categories of the Duane-White classification scheme: convergence insufficiency, convergence excess, divergence insufficiency, divergence excess (42). When a deviation is the same at distance and near, it is referred to as *basic*, as in a basic eso or basic exo.

Of the major Maddox vergence categories (fusional, accommodative, proximal and tonic), fusional and accommodative are most commonly evaluated clinically.

With young children, objective testing is always desired. Clinicians advocate several different methods of testing the near point of convergence (NPC). Many clinicians like a detailed target, demanding accommodative accuracy if the child is old enough to respond to verbal prompting. I am concerned that, although NPC provides a good overview, it combines both accommodative and convergence, therefore, precluding determination of each system's individual function. A useful alternative is to use the light of a transilluminator as the target. Make sure it is turned down to a comfortable level. The light as a target essentially neutralizes the accommodative response (43). It is relatively easy for both the clinician and the patient to observe when fusion is lost. A nice addition can be accomplished by remeasuring the NPC, this time with a red lens held before one eye (44,45). This lens embarrasses sensory fusion and demonstrates the ability of the visual system to overcome stress. A difference of more than 3 cm. between the two NPC measurements is thought to be suggestive of a potentially symptomatic patient (46). Very young children tend to be asymptomatic because of their visual demands, unless they are diplopic. Testing at this age is to rule out pathology and to alert the clinician to a potential problem area in need of regular monitoring.

The NPC can be repeated five times looking for fatigue effects. Most asymptomatic patients will maintain a consistent NPC measurement over this number of repeats.

If the measurements of the vergence ranges are deemed necessary, as in the case of high phoria or intermittent tropia where determination must be made regarding adequate compensation, out-of-instrument techniques are preferred so the clinician can monitor the child's eyes during testing.

Smoothly increasing prism demand, for instance with a prism bar, while a child fixates a distance or near target usually yields at least a break and recovery finding (47). The clinician must carefully observe the child's eye to determine bifixation. To estimate blur, an observant, cooperative, and communicative child is required.

Use of the random dot E as the fixation target eliminates some of the unreliability of reports of clarity. In this modification, the child must distinguish the random dot E from the *dummy* target following insertion of prism, thus indicating bifoveal fusion (48).

As children approach school age, jump vergence facility, which is essentially repeated fusional recovery, may be more valuable. Several standards are used for this testing. *Fusional reflex* uses a rating of the speed of response to 6 prism diopters inserted repeatedly in a base-in or base-out direction (48,49).

Expected readings for jump vergence facility of 12 prism diopters base-out, 6 prism diopters base-in at distance, and 15 prism diopters base-out, 12 base-in at near have been found to be useful. The prism is abruptly inserted before one eye of the patient as fixation is maintained on a 20/30 vertical line of letters. Both singleness (assessed by observation as well as subjective report when possible) and clarity of letters must be obtained. Then the prism is removed and the patient allowed to return to the ortho demand position. This procedure must be successfully repeated four times (cycles) to be considered passing. If the patient is unable to meet the demands listed above, the test should be repeated with 2 prism diopters less demand. This should be repeated until a passing level is determined. This provides both a guide of where to begin therapy and a gauge to judge post-therapy improvement.

SUMMARY

Evaluation of ocular motility allows the clinician to determine obstacles to the development of binocularity that might also have an impact on development of visual acuity. Motilities can be restricted because of paretic, restrictive, or congenital nerve misdirection. Being aware of the conditions that might impede normal development of binocularity and ocular motility guides the clinician during examination. The principal axiom being "you see what you look for, not what you look at."

REFERENCES

1. Bruckner R. Practical use of the illumination test in the early diagnosis of strabismus. *Ophthalmologica* 1965;149(6):497–503.
2. Tongue AC, Cibis GW. Bruckner test. *Ophthalmology* 1981;88(10):1041–1044.
3. Archer SM. Developmental aspects of the Bruckner test. *Ophthalmology* 1988;95(8):1098–101.
4. Roe LD, Guyton DL. The light that leaks: Bruckner and the red reflex. *Surv Ophthalmol* 1984;28(6):665–670.
5. Miller JM, Hall HL, GreivenKamp JE, Guyton DL. et al. Quantification of the Bruckner test for strabismus. *Invest Ophthalmol Vis Sci* 1995;36(5):897–905.
6. Gole GA, Douglas LM. Validity of the Bruckner reflex in the detection of amblyopia. *Aust N Z J Ophthalmol* 1995;23(4):281–285.
7. Griffin JR, Cotter SA. The Bruckner test: evaluation of clinical usefulness. *Am J Optom Physiol Opt* 1986;63(12):957–961.

8. Romano PE, von Nooden, GK. Limitations of cover test in detecting strabismus. *Am J Ophthalmol* 1971;2:10–12.

9. Paysse EA, Williams GC, Coats DK, et al. Detection of red reflex asymmetry by pediatric residents using the Bruckner reflex versus the MTI photoscreener. *Pediatrics* 2001;108(4):E74.

10. Jones R, Eskridge JB. The Hirschberg test—a reevaluation. *American Journal of Optometry and Archives of the American Academy of Optometry* 1970;47:105–114.

11. Wick B, London R. The Hirschberg test: analysis from birth to age 5. *Journal of the American Optometric Association* 1980;51:1009–1010.

12. Eskridge JB, Wick B, Perrigin D. The Hirschberg test: a double-masked clinical evaluation. *Am J Optom Physiol Opt* 1988;65(9):745–750.

13. Eskridge JB, Perrigin DM, Leach NE. The Hirschberg test: correlation with corneal radius and axial length. *Optom Vis Sci* 1990;67(4):243–247.

14. Mehdorn E, Kommerell G. 'Rebound-saccade' in the prism cover test. *Int Ophthalmol* 1978;1(1):63–66.

15. Caloroso EE, Rouse M. *Clinical Management of Strabismus.* Boston: Butterworth–Heinemann, 1993.

16. Koch P. An aid for the diagnosis of a vertical muscle paresis. *J Pediatric Ophthalmol Strabismus* 1980;17: 272–276.

17. London R. Strabismus. In: Barresi BJ, ed. *Ocular Assessment: The Manual of Diagnosis for Office Practice.* Boston: Butterworth-Heinemann, 1984.

18. Jampolsky A. Superior rectus revisited. *Trans Am Ophthalmol Soc* 1981:243–256.

19. London R. An alternative approach to interpretation of the vertically acting extraocular muscles: excerpts from the writings of Arthur Jampolsky. In: London R, ed. *Ocular Vertical and Cyclovertical Deviations.* Philadelphia: JB Lippincott; 1992:556–564.

20. Kushner B. Errors in the three-step test in the diagnosis of vertical strabismus. *Ophthalmology* 1989;96:127–132.

21. Jampolsky A. Management of vertical strabismus. *Transactions of the New Orleans Academy of Ophthalmology* 1986;34:141–171.

22. Hotchkiss MD, Miller NR, Clark A. et al. Bilateral Duane's retraction syndrome. A clinical-pathologic case report. *Arch Ophthalmol* 1980;98(5):870–874.

23. Miller NR, Kiel SM, Gree WR. et al. Unilateral Duane's retraction syndrome (type 1). *Arch Ophthalmol* 1982;100(9):1468–1472.

24. Alexandrakis G, Saunders RA. Duane retraction syndrome. *Ophthalmol Clin North Am* 2001;14(3):407–417.

25. Rutstein RP. Duane's retraction syndrome. *Journal of the American Optometric Association* 1992;63(6):419–429.

26. Terashima M, Hayasaka S. Multiple congenital anomalies associated with Duane's syndrome. *Ophthalmic Paediatr Genet* 1990;11(2):133–137.

27. Guirgis MF, Thorton SS, Tychsen L. et al. Cone-rod retinal dystrophy and Duane retraction syndrome in a patient with achondroplasia. *J AAPOS* 2002;6(6):400–401.

28. Hermann JS. Acquired Brown's syndrome of inflammatory origin. Response to locally injected steroids. *Arch Ophthalmol* 1978;96(7):1228–1232.

29. Wilson ME, Eustis Jr. HS, Parks MM. Brown's syndrome. *Surv Ophthalmol* 1989;34(3):153–172.

30. Clarke WN, Noel LP. Brown's syndrome: fusion status and amblyopia. *Can J Ophthalmol* 1983;18(3):118–123.

31. Rutstein RP, Daum KM. *Anomalies of Binocular Vision: Diagnosis and Management.* St. Louis: Mosby, 1998.

32. Parks MM. Th monofixation syndrome. *Trans Am Ophthalmol Soc* 1969;67:609–657.

33. Parks MM. Monofixation syndrome: a frequent end stage of strabismus surgery. *Trans Am Acad Ophthalmol Otolaryngol* 1975;79(5):733–735.

34. Hoffman, L., Rouse, MW, Referral recommendations for binocular function and/or developmental perceptual deficiencies. *J Am Optom Assoc,* 1980. 51:119–126.

35. Maples WC. *NSUCO Oculomotor Test.* Santa Ana, CA: Optometric Extension Program, 1995.

36. Gay AJ, Newman N, Keltner JL, Stroud MH. *Eye Movement Disorders.* St. Louis: CV Mosby, 1974.

37. Leigh RJ, Zee D. *The Neurology of Eye Movements.* Philadelphia: FA Davis, 1991.

38. Bahill AT, Adler D, Stark L. Most naturally occurring human saccades have magnitudes of 15 degrees or less. *Invest Ophthalmol* 1975;14(6):468–469.

39. Zuber BL, Stark L. Saccadic suppression: elevation of visual threshold associated with saccadic eye movements. *Exp Neurol* 1966;16(1):65–79.

40. Rouse M, London R. Development and perception. In: Barresi BJ, ed. *Ocular Assessment: The Manual of Diagnosis for Office Practice.* Boston: Butterworth-Heinemann, 1984.

41. Richman J, Garzia RP. *Developmental Eye Movement Test (DEM).* South Bend, IN: Bernell VTO, Mishawaka, Indiana.

42. Duane A. A new classification of the motor anomalies of the eye based upon physiological principles, together with their symptoms, diagnosis and treatment. *Ann Ophthalmol Otolaryngol* 1896;5:969–1008.

43. Owens DA, Mohindra I, Held R. The effectiveness of a retinoscope beam as an accommodative stimulus. *Invest Ophthalmol Vis Sci* 1980;19(8):942–949.

44. Capobianco NM. The subjective measurement of the nearpoint of convergence and its significance in the diagnosis of convergence insufficiency. *Am Orthopt J* 1952;2:40.

45. Capobianco NM. Symposium: convergence insufficiency; incidence and diagnosis. *Am Orthopt J* 1953;3: 13–17.

46. London R, Rouse MW. Predicting fusional vergence difficulties. Presented at American Academy of Optometry, Anaheim, California, 1979.

47. Scheiman M, et al. A normative study of step vergence in elementary school children. *Journal of the American Optometric Association* 1989;60(4):276–280.

48. Grisham JD, et al. Vergence orthoptics: validity and persistence of the training effect. *Optom Vis Sci* 1991;68(6):441–451.

49. Grisham JD. The dynamics of fusional vergence eye movements in binocular dysfunction. *American Journal of Optometry and Physiology Optics* 1980; 57:645–655.

Clinical Tests of Fusion and Stereopsis · 17

M. H. Esther Han and Robert H. Duckman

WHY TEST FOR FUSION AND STEREOPSIS IN INFANTS AND CHILDREN?

The purpose of testing fusion and stereopsis is to assess a patient's level of binocular function. The information a clinician expects and eventually obtains from the patient is often age dependent. The infant, preschooler, and school-aged child have different visual needs. Specific visual findings are necessary, therefore, to make a comprehensive binocular vision assessment with respect to the child's needs. This chapter discusses the clinical significance of testing and the considerations to be made when administering tests of fusion and stereopsis.

In infants and preschoolers, the main objective in testing fusion and stereopsis is to assess for the presence of strabismus and amblyopia. The earlier such conditions are treated, the greater the prognosis for maximizing visual function (1). Performance on stereo tests is influenced by such factors as equal visual acuity in each eye and on ocular alignment (2). Stereopsis testing also provides a means of documenting changes in visual function during treatment (1). One of the main difficulties in examining this age group is their limited cooperation and maturity level. Children under the age of 5 years, in general, do not provide reliable verbal responses and can be uncooperative in a clinical setting (2). Some children will not respond to specific examination procedures that require eye patching or special lenses or glasses. A study conducted by Shute et al. (3) compared the success rates in measuring monocular visual acuity and stereopsis in subjects aged 1 month to 53 months. They determined that 75% of the infants tested under the age of 6 months ($N = 15$) tolerated the use of a patch. Only 22% of those 12 to 24 months ($N = 18$) and 47% of those 24 to 36 months ($N = 15$), however, were able to wear the patch and successfully complete monocular visual acuities. Interestingly, they found an inverse relationship with respect to stereopsis testing using the Frisby and the Lang tests. They found that 74% of those 12 to 24 months, and 88% of those 24 to 36 months were able to undergo stereopsis testing. Therefore when monocular visual acuity assessment is unsuccessful, stereopsis testing will increase the probability of detecting a vision disorder.

Clinical evaluation of fusion and stereopsis in the school-aged child (ages 6 to 8 years) is completed to determine any binocular dysfunctions that can negatively affect their sensory and motor function. Such deficits can interfere with the child's visual efficiency in an academic setting. Limitations to testing a child can involve developmental delays in the gross motor or fine motor abilities; learning disabilities that can involve visual perceptual deficits and difficulty understanding instructional sets; attention-related deficits; and sensory integration deficits. The difficulty in examining this age group is that these conditions may have not yet been diagnosed. Instructions and procedures must be tailored to the abilities of the patient and, at times, objective testing may be required when examining children with special needs.

Older school-aged children (ages 9 years and up) are in the stage of "reading to learn" as opposed to "learning to read." The changes in the child's visual demands involve smaller print text with less spacing, copying from the board, and visual accuracy when playing sports, such as baseball, basketball, tennis, or soccer. There is an overall increase in their need to be more visually efficient, particularly during periods of sustained near work. Testing in this group would emphasize endurance and stability of binocular function over sustained periods.

CLINICAL TESTS OF STEREOPSIS

Stereopsis involves the perception of relative depth under binocular conditions resulting from a horizontal retinal disparity that exists within Panum's fusional area (4–6). Stereoacuity is a quantitative measure of stereopsis, which represents the smallest horizontal retinal image disparity that gives rise to a sensation of depth (7). Clinically normal stereoacuity should be less than 40 to 60 seconds of arc, depending on the test and the study cited (8). Age norms are 150 seconds of arc for ages 3 to 4 years, 70 seconds of arc for ages 4 to 5 years, and 40 seconds of arc for ages 5 to 8 years (9).

Stereoacuity depends on visual acuity or clarity of the retinal image, and ocular alignment (7). Even 1.00 D of uncorrected anisometropia can cause a reduction in stereoacuity (4). A study by Richardson et al. (10) in children ages 3 to 5 years also showed that refractive correction alone could improve stereoacuity to expected levels.

The main types of stereograms discussed in this chapter will be line or contour stereograms or global stereograms. Line stereograms involve the use of horizontal retinal image disparity to elicit the perception of stereopsis and global or random dot stereograms (RDS) which use computer-generated dot patterns that give rise to a central stereoscopic form when fused (11). In these patterns, some of the dots are displaced to one side for one of the eyes. When the two images are fused, the displaced dots appear to have depth (12).

A disadvantage of line stereograms is the presence of monocular cues that can be used to detect disparity (12). RDS tests do not have monocular cues and correct responses cannot be elicited unless there is bifoveation, and reasonably good visual acuity in each eye (12). Patients with a two-line difference in acuity can demonstrate considerably reduced stereoacuity (4). Given such stringent requirements to achieve RDS stereopsis, one study confirmed that local stereopsis is better than stereoacuity measured using RDS (13). Another advantage of RDS over the line stereogram is that those who are microtropic (whose objective angle of turn equals the amount of eccentric fixation) will not appreciate RDS stereopsis because, by definition, they are not bifoveal (11). Patients who are microtropic will appreciate gross stereopsis with line stereograms (>100 seconds) if peripheral targets are used.

Frisby Stereo Test

The *Frisby Test* (Fig. 17.1) uses global stereograms that do not require the use of special glasses. The test consists of three test plates of different thicknesses (6, 3, and 1 mm). Each plate has four squares, one of which has a circular pattern that must be detected by the patient. The 6-mm plate is tested first because it has the largest disparity. The disparity can be increased by using either a thicker plate or decreasing the test distance (7). When testing at 40 cm, the disparities range from 480 to 15 seconds of arc (5). Normal stereopsis is considered to be 50 seconds of arc or passing the 3-mm plate at 70 cm or the 1-mm plate tested at 40 cm (7).

While administering the test, reflections must be minimized, and the test plate should be placed perpendicular to the patient's visual axes. The clinician must also ensure that the patient does not make excessive head movements, because it will induce parallax (6,7). Three correct successive answers is the criterion used to determine the level of stereoacuity. Rosner and Rosner (7) also suggest placing a white sheet against the back surface to minimize background confusion. For testing children as young as 13 months of age, a forced-choice preferential looking (FPL) presentation can increase reliability of stereopsis responses.

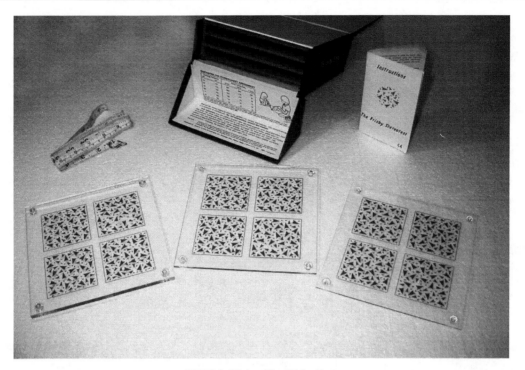

FIGURE 17.1. The Frisby Test.

This can be done by cutting the plates into quarters and placing them on a gray background (7). The clinician then presents two test plates, one with a stimulus and one blank. Broadbent and Westall (5) have shown that this test can be successfully administered to 65% of children under the age of 3 years. Saunders et al. (14) used a nonstereo practice plate with auditory reinforcement to first teach subjects how to perform the test. When administering the test with these modifications, they achieved a 64.7% success rate in infants aged 9 to 11 months, and 100% in children aged 18 to 23 months.

Lang Stereo Test I and II

The *Lang Stereo Tests* (Fig. 17.2) use RDS stimuli and do not require the use of special glasses. The Lang I card has pictures of a cat (1200 seconds), car (550 seconds), and a star (600 seconds) when used at 40 cm (7). The Lang II card has three pictures with smaller disparities (elephant with 600 seconds, car with 400 seconds, and a crescent moon with 200 seconds) and one nonstereo picture (star) that is seen by all patients (15). To reduce the disparity, Rosner and Rosner (7) stated that the test distance should be increased. Lam et al. (16) used 550 seconds of arc or better to define normal stereopsis in children 4 to 5 years of age. One disadvantage of the Lang test is that it does not measure stereoacuity but only screens for gross level stereopsis (17). As a screening tool, this test can successfully be used in children as young as 6 months and up to 4 years (5,7).

Random Dot E Test

The *Random Dot E (RDE) test* uses a global stereogram and also requires the use of polarized filters. It comes with a demonstration plate that has a raised "E" and two random dot stereogram plates; one is blank and the other has the stereoscopic "E." The test distances typically used are 0.5 m (504 seconds of disparity) and 1.0 m (252 seconds of disparity), but it is also recommended to use 1.5 m (168 seconds of disparity) because this distance is more sensitive to both visual acuity reductions and binocular vision deficits. The goal is to present the stereograms to the child and have the child choose the plate with the "E." Practicing with the demonstration plate ensures that the child understands the task. Rosner and Rosner (7)

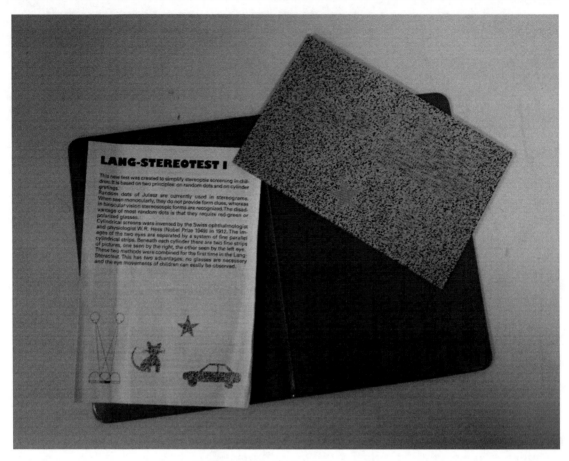

FIGURE 17.2.   The Lang Stereo Test.

stated that if the child is having difficulty understanding the task, try decreasing the working distance to 33 or 40 cm. In addition, they emphasized that the stereograms should be held slightly below eye level and slightly tilted so they are perpendicular to the patient's visual axes, thereby minimizing reflections. The test is complete when four successive correct responses occur or when six trials have been administered (7). This test can be performed in children as young as 3 years of age (7). Children with poor figure-ground abilities, however, may show inconsistent responses because they have difficulty discerning a target from a visually busy background (9).

Random Dot Stereo Test

The *Random Dot Stereo Test* (Fig. 17.3) consists of three subtests, with two tests using line stereograms and one using RDS. It also requires the use of polarized filters. The *randot forms* subtest is a pure RDS test with two disparity levels, 500 and 250 seconds. The *animals' subtest* (cat with 400 seconds, rabbit with 200 seconds, and monkey with 100 seconds), and the *circles subtest* (from 400 to 20 seconds) are line stereograms embedded within a random dot background to reduce the effects of monocular cue interpretation. The test is administered at 40 cm and excessive head movement and reflections must be minimized. Poor responses on this test may reflect language or communication difficulties. To reconfirm the patient's responses, present the plate upside-down so the patient sees the stereograms in uncrossed disparity with the forms appearing to go into the page. The child can also point to reduce the need to communicate verbally. Rosner and Rosner (7) suggested that, when performing the circles subtest, running a finger across all three circles often helps the child appreciate stereopsis. The

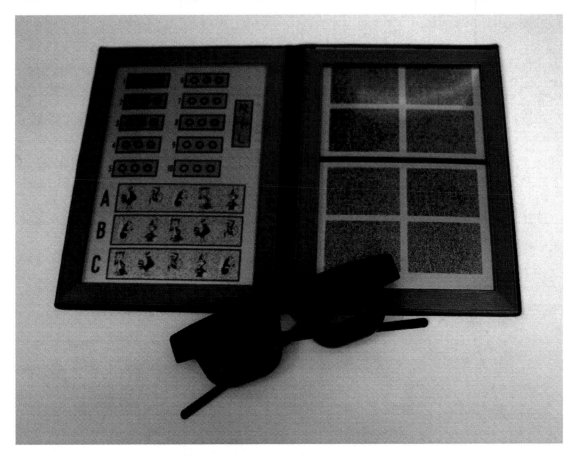

FIGURE 17.3. The Random Dot Stereo Test.

randot forms and the *animals subtest* can be performed by 4 year olds and the *circles subtest* by 5 year olds (7). The mean stereoacuity achieved by age 6 years is 30 seconds, which is shown to improve to 20 seconds by age 11 years (10).

Random Dot Preschool Stereoacuity Test

The *Random Dot Preschool Stereoacuity* test uses RDS stimuli and requires polarizing filters. It consists of three books developed by Birch et al. (18). The left-hand side of each book contains two-dimensional black and white illustrations of four test shapes in random order on the page. The right-hand page contains two sets of four random dot patterns with matching shapes, including three stimuli and one blank. Book 1 is made up of shapes with intermediate disparities (200 and 100 seconds); book 2 is made up of figures with fine disparities (60 to 40 seconds); and book 3 uses figures with course disparities

(800 and 400 seconds). At each level, the child must identify two of the three stereoscopic stimuli present. If the child passes book 1, then book 2 is administered. If book 1 is not passed, then book 3 is administered. A child should not view all three books when performing this test.

Success rates determined by Birch et al. (18) were 89% to 95% in children ages 3 to 5 years, and 70% in children 2 years of age. These success rates were higher than the rates seen for the *Titmus* (see below) and the *Randot Stereo Tests* in children ages 2 to 5 years. Its efficacy was determined to be high with respect to stereoacuity measurement and as a screening tool. Lam et al. (16), however, found that randot stereoacuity was not a measure of biological function as a result of the random distribution of stereoacuity findings seen in normal children 4.5 to 5.5 years of age. They stated that a measure of biological function should show a Gaussian rather than a random distribution.

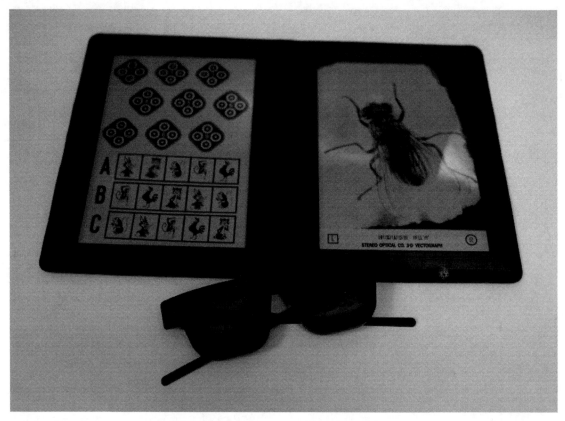

FIGURE 17.4.   The Titmus Stereo Fly Test.

Titmus Stereo Fly Test

All three subtests of the *Titmus Stereo Fly Test* use line stereograms and require the use of polarizing filters (Fig. 17.4). The *house fly subtest* is a gross disparity target (3000 seconds), the *animals subtest* ranges from 400 to 100 seconds, and the *circles subtest* ranges from 400 to 40 seconds. To ensure a true stereopsis response, the *house fly subtest* can be repeated to depict uncrossed disparity by turning the test upside-down. The child will then attempt to point into the page when asked to touch the wings. These subtests are initially performed at 40 cm but, if the child is having difficulty discerning stereopsis, try decreasing the working distance (7). The *house fly subtest* can be used on children as young as 3 years, the *animals subtest* as young as 4 years, and the *circles subtest* as young as 5 years of age. The main disadvantage of this subtest is the presence of monocular cues, although Rosner and Rosner (7) indicate that the *animals subtest* has fewer cues, whereas the first

five of the nine circles have strong monocular cues.

TNO Stereo Test

The TNO (Fig. 17.5) is the only stereo test that uses anaglyphic random dot stereograms and the only test that requires red-green filters. The screening subtest consists of three plates made of disparities ranging from 2000 seconds of arc when administered at 40 cm (7). The second subtest is the suppression subtest and the last is the graded stereoacuity subtest. This last test consists of 12 items divided over three pages. The disparities range from 480 to 15 seconds at 40 cm (13). Each page is divided into four squares with a random dot stereogram of a circle of which a 60° wedge has been removed. Each stereogram has a wedge missing at a different orientation. A main disadvantage of the TNO is that the red-green filters have been shown to cause more binocular dissociation as compared with polarized filters, which often results in

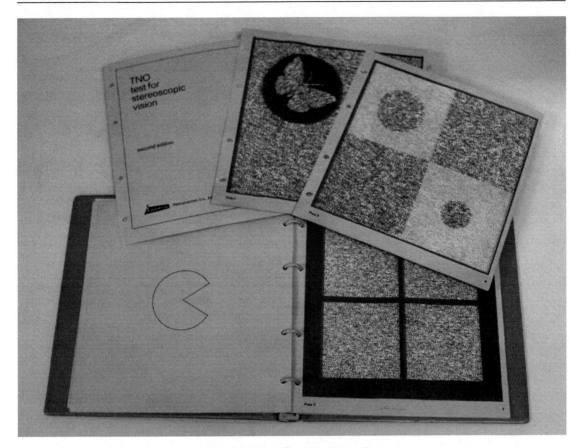

FIGURE 17.5. The TNO Stereo Test.

the underestimation of stereoacuity (6). Larson (13) suggested that red-green filters induce rivalry, suppression, and other binocular interactions that also lead to reduced stereoacuity measurements. Cooper (4) stated that chromatic aberrations could lead to different accommodative demands for each eye, which can also reduce stereoacuity. Finally, studies conducted by Simons and Elhatton (19) found that the green filter increases the contrast in the amblyopic eye, thereby artificially improving stereoacuity findings with the TNO.

The screening subtest can be administered to children ages 2.5 to 3 years, whereas the graded stereoacuity test is successfully used in children ages 6 years and older (7). Broadbent and Westall (5) found that the graded stereoacuity subtest is an excellent screening device for amblyopia. They also suggested that children under the age of 2 years do not appear to understand the task. Williams et al. (20) found the prevalence of stereoscopic defects to

be 2.1% to 3.2% in children ages 7 to 11 years when using the TNO.

CLINICAL CONSIDERATIONS

Filter Considerations

Frantz et al. (21) found that certain plastic prisms, but not glass prisms, cause a reduction in stereoacuity or an apparent failure to perceive stereopsis using tests requiring polarizing filters. Some specific observations noted were that the eye behind the prism may see both eyes' targets or see only the fellow eye's target, rather than its own. A thickness-dependent relationship exists that alters the polarization of the light as it passes through the prism. The polymerization process that occurs when manufacturing the plastic prisms creates polymer chains in an orientation that can cause the birefringence of light, which will polarize light as it passes through the plastic. This birefringent property of the plastic is known to be dependent on the material's thickness and on the angle the light enters the material. This polarization effect of the plastic prisms can be avoided by placing the prism behind the filter rather than in front of the filter, but this is not clinically practical. The clinician must be aware when using a prism with polarized vectographic materials to view the suppression controls monocularly through the prism at various angles of tilt to ensure that the prism is not affecting the polarization.

Some stereo tests have polarized-free versions (Titmus Stereo, Stereo Reindeer, Random Dot Butterfly, Random Dot Figures, and the Random Dot E, Circle, Square). Hatch and Richman (1) compared the validity of the polarized-free tests with their polarized counterparts. They found no statistical difference in the stereoacuity attained with each version. Proper administration, however, is critical with the polarized-free tests. A small amount of tilt can prevent one image from being seen. Proper placement is ensured when suppression controls are seen equally in each eye. This is an important consideration when testing younger and more restless children.

Age Considerations

The sensitive period for binocular development is the time when binocular neurons are plastic, which Broadbent and Westall (5) describe as beginning a few months after birth and peak between 1 to 3 years of age. They also stated that neural development, rather than the development of accurate vergence, limits a child's performance on stereoacuity tests. Clinically, cognitive factors also affect the measurement of stereoacuity. Studies have concluded that the apparent age-related improvement in stereoacuity is attributable to a child's cognitive maturation rather than to the completed development of the visual system (22).

Different methods of obtaining responses from children, who are not cognitively mature enough to understand a test's instructional set, have been investigated. Several authors have stated that operant preferential looking (OPL) presentation provides more reliable stereopsis findings in very young children (11,22,23).

TABLE 17.1 Operant Preferential Looking Stereoacuity Age Norms

Age (months)	Stereoacuity (seconds of arc)
18–23	250
24–29	225
30–35	125
36–53	100
54–65	60

From Ciner EB, Schanel-Klitsch E, Scheiman M. Stereoacuity development in young children. *Optom Vis Sc* 1991;68(7):533–536, with permission.

Based on OPL, Ciner et al. (22) developed clinical guidelines for stereoacuity as listed in Table 17.1. These values are consistent with the idea that adultlike stereopsis is present at earlier ages in childhood. This study clearly showed that the method of administrating the test is key to accurately assessing stereopsis in younger patients.

Screening Considerations

The literature emphasizes the screening role of stereoacuity tests, particularly for the Lang II, Frisby, Randot, Titmus, and TNO tests (15). High under-referral rates, however, were found in a study done by Ohlsson et al. (15) using these tests in children ages 12 to 13 years. They found under-referral rates as high as 54% to 88% for amblyopia, and 25% to 67% for strabismus. Patients who were amblyopic without strabismus were more likely to be missed using these tests. Richardson et al. (10) also showed that stereoacuity testing using the *Randot test*, in children ages 3 to 5 years, did not provide additional information regarding visual function, particularly for unilateral reductions in vision.

In children ages 2 to 3 years, RDE reliability was shown by Schmidt (24) to be greater than other screening modalities such as visual acuity and refractive error. It was determined to be a fast test and also sensitive to uncorrected refractive error, strabismus, and amblyopia. No conclusive evidence appears to exist on the role of stereo tests as an effective vision screening tool. In preschool children (ages 2 to 4 years), however, stereopsis testing may be the only method of screening for vision disorders given their poor cooperation with monocular vision acuity assessment. Thus, the practical use of stereopsis testing as a screening method ultimately depends on the judgment of the clinician conducting the screening.

Strabismus and Amblyopia Considerations

Cooper (11) stated that RDS stimuli should not be used to screen for amblyopia but are effective when screening for those who are amblyopic with microtropia. Manny et al. (17) indicated that neither the Frisby nor the Lang "is appropriate to rule out, with certainty, the presence of amblyopia or anisometropia in the absence of strabismus." Richardson et al. (10) stated that refractive correction alone can improve stereoacuity to expected levels. Their study in a preschool population (ages 3 to 5 years) also found that stereoacuity is mainly affected by refractive blur. They also found that delaying correction of refractive error and delaying active amblyopia treatment does not result in poorer stereoacuity outcomes when reassessed 12 months later.

Stereopsis testing can be used to determine the prognosis in maintaining visual acuity improvement in amblyopic patients after vision therapy. Patients who achieve some degree of RDS stereopsis or better than 70 seconds of arc on a line stereogram test (e.g., the Titmus stereo test) are expected to maintain their visual acuity gains after the completion of therapy (25).

CLINICAL TESTS OF FUSION

Fusion involves the interaction between the motor and sensory systems. The motor fusion system involves all the vergence components (disparity, accommodative, proximal, and tonic) required to bifixate an object of interest and stimulate corresponding retinal points in each eye (26,27). When this occurs, the sensory fusion system acts by integrating two slightly disparate retinal images into the perception of a single object (27). Disorders of motor fusion can lead to sensory fusion disorders that can include adaptations such as suppression, amblyopia, and anomalous retinal correspondence (ARC) (27). Such adaptations evolve in response to long-standing motor fusion disorders.

Motor fusion can be evaluated by measuring the near point of convergence (NPC), vergence ranges, fixation disparity, and the efficiency of vergence–accommodative interactions. Tests that evaluate binocular function in the patient who is not strabismic will be emphasized in this section. Many of these tests of motor fusion provide insight into the inefficiencies and inaccuracies of the motor fusion system. Commonly used tests of sensory fusion in the nonstrabismic pediatric population are the *Worth-4-Dot* (W4D) and the *Keystone Visual Skills Cards* (KVS).

With multiple methods for evaluating fusion, questions arise. The first involves the need to perform several different tests that appear to measure the same function, and the second asks whether these tests can be used interchangeably when monitoring the progress of treatment. Birnbaum (8) answered the first question by discussing the need to evaluate the binocular system using both *weak* and *strong* stimuli to fusion. Weak stimuli to fusion are small, nonstereoscopic targets that stimulate central retina and do not have peripheral cues to fusion. Targets used to assess phorometric ranges constitute weak stimuli to fusion. In contrast, strong stimuli are detailed, stereoscopic, larger targets that stimulate both the central and peripheral retina. Patients who have difficulty (i.e., restricted ranges, suppression, or poor stereopsis) with strong stimuli often have severe binocular deficits and are considerably more symptomatic. To answer the second question, Feldman et al. (28) studied and compared vergence ranges measured with Risley prisms, vectograms, and the computer orthopter. They concluded that each method provided different kinds of information and, therefore, cannot be used interchangeably. Hence, several methods of evaluating fusion should be administered to adequately assess binocular function and monitor progress in vision therapy.

TESTS MEASURING VERGENCE RANGES

Risley Prism or Phorometric Ranges

Scheiman and Wick (29) stated that *Risley prism ranges* measure smooth vergence abilities, as opposed to step vergence abilities used when measuring prism bar ranges. Risley prisms are typically attached to all phoropters but also come in a handheld version (30). The prisms should be smoothly increased in the same direction by the same degree in both eyes and turned slowly enough to allow the child to respond. The blur, break, and recovery values are recorded. The blur value relates to the status of the vergence–accommodative system; the break value is a descriptor of the quality of binocular function; and the recovery value describes how effectively the system is able to restore fusion (8). In the younger child, the blur response may be the most difficult one to elicit (9). Typically, base-in (BI) ranges are measured before base-out (BO) ranges (30). Vergence ranges should also be repeated to assess for consistency and fatigueability, particularly in asthenopic patients with high phorias. Scheiman and Wick (29) stated that measuring vergence ranges a single time is sufficient because it is important to observe how a patient performs over time. In addition, measuring only the compensating ranges or only the near ranges does not constitute an adequate assessment of binocular function in a symptomatic patient.

The most commonly used norms are Morgan's, which are listed below in Table 17.2. As a guideline, Sheard's criterion states that the compensating vergence range should be at least twice as large as the heterophoria value for comfortable vision. Daum (30) summarized that this is incorrect only about 25% of the time.

Prism Bar Ranges

Prism bar ranges uses step-wise increases in BI or BO prism. Typically, BI ranges are measured before BO ranges (30). The prism bar technique is used when the clinician has prejudged that the child may be unable to provide reliable subjective responses. The examiner will then rely on objective observation of ocular alignment when assessing ranges. Ocular misalignment occurs when the child begins to fixate alternately from one image to the other. At this point, the examiner asks the child how many images are seen. Fixation must be closely monitored throughout this procedure and not wait for subjective responses from the child. Again, the blur, break, and recovery values are recorded. Some norms for the break and recovery values in children ages 4 to 12 years are listed in the Table 17.3.

Vectograms: Clown

Vectograms (Fig. 17.6) are a strong stimulus to fusion, because the format is large, detailed, and stereoscopic by design. Polarizing filters are needed when administering this test. It is usually performed at 16 inches (or 40 cm) and, at that distance, each number or letter corresponds to 1 prism diopter (8). In children younger than the age of 5 years, vectogram ranges should be measured in free space so the examiner can objectively observe ocular alignment. The vectogram can also be performed at distance using an overhead projector when a need exists to assess peripheral fusion abilities. The image must be displayed on an aluminum screen to maintain the polarization of light.

Several observations should be made when measuring vectogram ranges, as described by Birnbaum (8). One observation is the perception of SILO or SOLI. This refers to the patient's ability to perceive the image becoming smaller and closer (small-in or "SI") as the BO

TABLE 17.2 Morgan's Norms for Vergence Ranges

	Base-in		Base-out	
	Mean	SD	Mean	SD
Distance (6 m)	×/7/4	×/3/2	9/19/10	4/8/4
Near (40 cms)	13/21/13	4/4/5	17/21/11	5/6/7

SD, standard deviation.

From Daum KM. Vergence amplitude. In: Eskridge JB, Amos JA, Bartlett JD, eds. *Clinical Procedures in Optometry.* Philadelphia: JB Lippincott; 1991:91–98, with permission.

TABLE 17.3 Age Norms for Prism Bar Vergence Ranges

	Base-in				Base-out			
	Ages 4.5–5.5 y		Ages 7–12 y		Ages 4.5–5.5 y		Ages 7–12 y	
	Mean	SD	Mean	Mean	Mean	SD	Mean	SD
Distance (6 m)	8.9/5.7	2.7/2.9	—	—	14.5/10.6	5.5/5.2	—	—
Near (40 cms)	15.5/12.3	4.5/4.3	X/12/7	X/5/4	28.9/23.4	5.6/5.1	X/23/16	X/8/6

SD, standard deviation.

From Lam SR, LaRooche GR, De Becker I, et al. The range and variability of ophthalmological parameters in normal children aged 4½ to 5½ years. *J Pediatr Ophthalmol Strabismus* 1996;33:251–625; and Scheiman M, Wick B. *Clinical Management of Binocular Vision: Heterophoric, Accommodative, and Eye Movement Disorders.* Philadelphia: Lippincott Williams & Wilkins, 1994, with permission.

demand is increased. Conversely, the image will get larger and appear further away (large-out or "LO") when measuring BI ranges. This phenomenon gives an indication what visual cues the patient uses to make visual spatial judgments. An individual reporting SILO (SI, LO) responses uses the vergence angle of the eyes to determine object localization, whereas the SOLI (SO, LI) responder uses the apparent size of the image to determine localization (31). The latter individual understands that objects that are further away will be smaller, and objects that are closer will be larger. SOLI responders are more experiential in their perception of

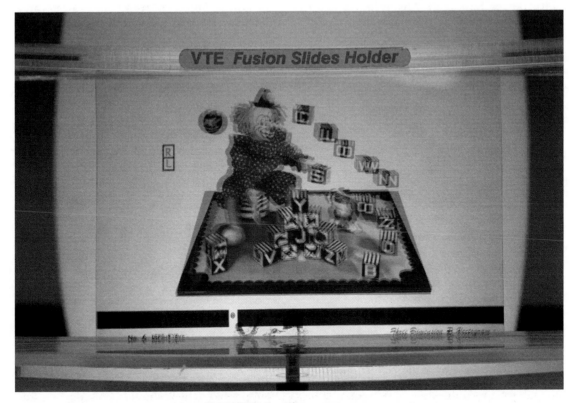

FIGURE 17.6. Clown vectogram.

TABLE 17.4 Age Norms for Accommodative Facility

	6 y	7 y	8–12 y	Young Adults
Monocular	5.5 cpm	6.5 cpm	7 cpm	10–17 cpm
Binocular	3 cpm	3.5 cpm	5 cpm	7–13 cpm (6–8 cpm w/supp check)

From Birnbaum MH. *Optometric Management of Nearpoint Vision Disorders.* Boston: Butterworth-Heinemann, 1993; and Press LJ, Moore BD. *Clinical Pediatric Optometry.* Boston: Butterworth-Heinemann, 1993, with permission.

visual space and have a tendency to rely on prior knowledge. Another observation is the patient's perception of parallax, in which the image moves in the same direction as the patient moves when set at BO position, or in the opposite direction when the vectogram is in a BI setting. Such observations help the clinician to determine what areas need to be emphasized when planning a vision therapy program for the child.

Some patients with restricted phorometric ranges have adequate vergence ranges with the *clown vectogram.* Other patients who have poor vectogram ranges in addition to poor phorometric ranges, however, will likely have a severe binocular dysfunction. The greatest advantage of measuring ranges using a vectogram is the ability to observe how a patient makes visual spatial judgments under more natural viewing conditions (8).

Major Amblyopscope and Synoptophore

The major amblyoscope (Fig. 17.7) is primarily used in the binocular assessment of strabismic patients. In such patients, the amblyoscope is used to assess the objective and subjective angles of deviation, as well as motor and sensory fusion abilities (6,32). The level of sensory fusion (first, second, and third degree fusion) can be determined using different slides that come with the instrument. In addition, stability of fusion and suppression can be noted when administering the test. Braddick slides, the stereopsis slides that can quantify stereopsis ranging from 90 to 720 seconds of arc, use RDS stimuli (6).

A patient must remain relatively stationary throughout the procedure, which should be administered to children who are cooperative and can give reliable responses. When setting up the instrument, it is important to adjust the instrument for the child's pupillary distance and the chinrest for the height of the child. Using the first-degree fusion slides, the objective angle is measured using the alternate cover test. If the amblyopic patient has eccentric fixation, this amount must be added to determine the total objective angle. Then, the subjective angle is measured by asking when the two different images are aligned. For instance, one slide can be a picture of a birdcage and the other slide a picture of a bird. The child is asked to say when the bird is inside the birdcage. Patients with horror fusionalis are unable to fuse and will not see the bird inside the cage but, rather, may see the bird disappear and then reappear on the other side of the cage (32). The angle of anomaly is equal to the difference between the objective and subjective angles, and is an indication that the patient has abnormal retinal correspondence when the value is greater than zero (32). Motor fusion ranges can also be measured with slides using different size targets that stimulate different parts of the retina (foveal, central, or peripheral).

TESTS MEASURING DIFFERENT LEVELS OF FUSION

Binocular Accommodative Facility

Binocular accommodative facility using ±2.00 D flippers is a procedure used to assess the ability of the patient to shift accommodation closer or further than the plane of the target, while maintaining vergence alignment. Binocular facility is measured in cycles per minute (cpm). A suppression check should be used when this is performed binocularly. Press and Moore (9)

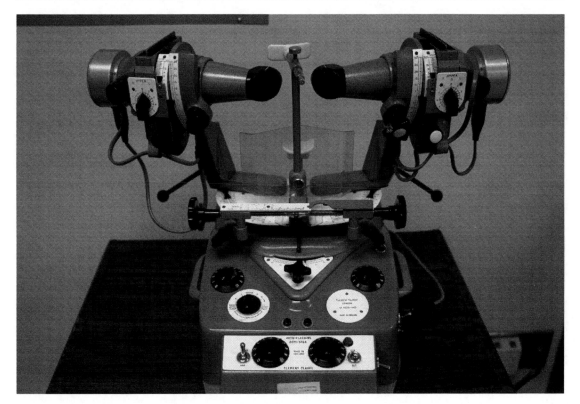

FIGURE 17.7. Major amblyoscope/synoptophore.

use the Bernell no. 9 acuity suppression slide. Alternatively, a polarized bar strip can be used over the target. Press and Moore (9) stated that the frequent flipping of the lenses can distract children during the test, and would affect the interpretation of the results (9). Behaviors (e.g., grimacing, squinting, straining, or attempting to change working distance) should also be observed as it is an indication that the child is having difficulty with the task (8).

Cheiroscopic Tracing

Cheiroscopic tracing, which is used to evaluate interocular transfer abilities, uses the *Keystone Correct-Eye-Scope* (Fig. 17.8) or Titmus biopter (9). When the instrument is set at optical infinity, 87 mm between the test pattern and the tracing would be considered orthophoria—the lines of sight are parallel based on the optics of the instrument. Birnbaum (8) stated that 68 mm should be the orthophoric reference point because of the proximal vergence cues from a target that is physically 8 inches (20.3 cm)

away. Less than 68 mm is considered eso posture, whereas greater than 68 mm is considered exo posture. Most patients exhibit a slight eso-posture when performing this test.

The oculars are set at optical infinity with the test pattern placed on the side opposite the dominant hand, and the patient is asked to trace the target while keeping both eyes open. Several observations should be made while administering this test as described by several authors (8,32). The separation between the tracing and the test pattern is measured to determine binocular posture (eso-, exo-, hyper-, ortho-). The quality of the tracing is evaluated by noting the presence of a shift in the tracing, with most patients exhibiting an eso shift. An increase in accommodative effort may lead to a gradual eso shift in the tracing, with a marked eso shift suggesting the presence of a near point, stress-induced vision disorder. Suppression is noted if the patient crosses over and traces directly on the test pattern. If part of the test pattern or the pencil point disappears, the patient is exhibiting intermittent central

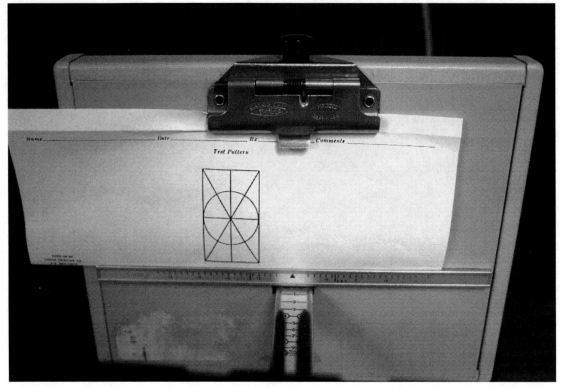

FIGURE 17.8.   Keystone Correct-Eye-Scope with cheiroscopic tracing test pattern.

suppression. The presence of hyperphoria is noted when the tracing is higher or lower than the test pattern.

FIXATION DISPARITY

Steinman et al. (12) defines fixation disparity (FD) as a small and persistent error in vergence in which the visual axes are not intersecting exactly at the target of interest. The images may not lie precisely on corresponding retinal points, but are still within Panum's fusional areas, so that the object is perceived as being single when viewed under binocular conditions (12,33). FD is usually measured in minutes of arc. Measuring FD is useful in older and more cooperative school-aged children, particularly when the severity of the child's symptoms do not match the binocular visual findings.

A forced vergence FD curve is generated to further assess binocular stability by measuring FD using different amounts of prism. The unit can be placed on the reading rod on the phoropter, as seen in Figure 17.9, or can be held by the patient. The patient is asked to determine

if the vertical lines are aligned, one above the other. First, FD without prism is measured. Then prism is placed before the eyes beginning with 3Δ and increasing the amount of prism in 3Δ steps until the patient is diplopic or suppressing. The prism can be either increased gradually or its directions can be alternated. To prevent prism adaptation, patients should close their eyes between measurements (33). Then graph the points with the x-axis being the amount of prism. The BI prism is to the left of the y-axis and BO to the right of the y-axis. The y-axis is the FD, with eso FD above the x-axis and exo below the x-axis. The x-intercept is the associated phoria (AP: the amount of prism necessary to neutralize the fixation disparity), whereas the y-intercept is the FD. The four types of curves (Fig. 17.10) that patients can exhibit are described in Table 17.5.

Two instruments that measure near FD are the *Sheedy disparometer* (Fig. 17.9) and the *Wesson FD card*. The Sheedy disparometer is calibrated for 40 cm, whereas the Wesson is calibrated for both 25 cm and 40 cm. Both instruments require polarizing filters. These two instruments

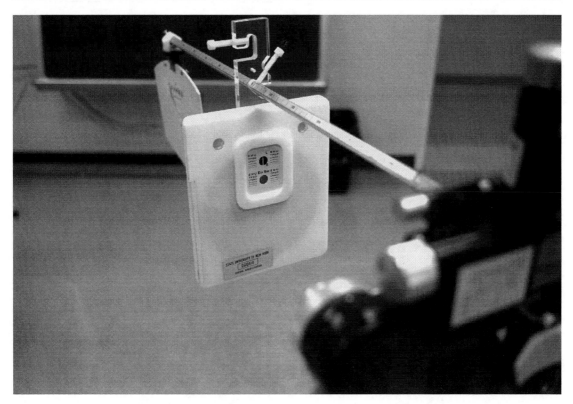

FIGURE 17.9. Sheedy disparometer.

TABLE 17.5 Four Fixation Disparity (FD) Curve Characteristics

FD Curve	Frequency in Population (%)	Associated Vision Findings	Recommended Treatment Options
Type I	60	These patients are typically asymptomatic. Symptomatic patients have a curve with a steeper slope, indicating poor prism adaptation. The flatter the curve, the better the prism adaptation.	Patients respond very well to vision therapy.
Type II	25	Patients tend to be esophoric.	Patients respond better to prisms and plus lenses at near.
Type III	10	Patients tend to be exophoric.	Patients can be trained with vision therapy, but not as easily as those who are type I. Prism can also be prescribed with an amount that correlates to the flattest central portion of the curve.
Type IV	5		General treatment options for this group have not been agreed on in the optometric literature.

From Goss DA. Fixation disparity. In: Eskridge JB, Amos JA, Bartlett JD, eds. *Clinical Procedures in Optometry*. Philadelphia: JB Lippincott; 1991:716–726, with permission.

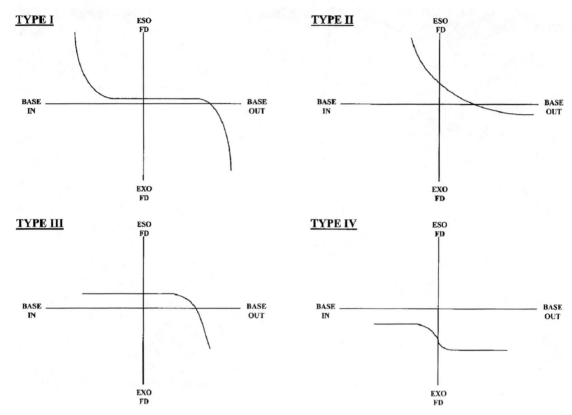

FIGURE 17.10. Four types of fixation disparity graphs.

can be used to generate a FD curve. In general, FD curves generated using the Wesson card results in more type I and II curves, and shows more exo findings and steeper slopes, when compared with curves generated using the Sheedy disparometer (33).

In general, the FD curve provides information about binocular status as it is relates to the patient's symptoms, as well as the prognosis for vision therapy as a treatment option (33). Good correlation is seen between forced vergence curves and patient's symptoms (29). For instance, a patient with eso FD tends to be more symptomatic, and irregular FD curves are indicative of an accommodative dysfunction. Weak correlations are found when comparing dissociated phorias (von Graefe phorias) with FD, and yet many binocular dysfunctions are diagnosed based mainly upon findings that include the dissociated phoria (33).

The instruments listed in Table 17.6 measure AP, which is the amount of prism required to reduce the FD to zero (33). To measure the

AP, the patient is asked to view the target and state whether the two lines are aligned. If they are aligned, the AP is zero. If not aligned, prism is added until the lines are one above the other. The two units measuring distance AP, as well as the three near point instruments, show good correlation in findings (33). The Sheedy AP, as extrapolated from the FD curve, determines a

TABLE 17.6 Instruments Measuring Associated Phoria

Distance	Near
American Optical (AO) vectographic slide	Bernell test lantern
Mallet box	Borish near card
	Mallet box for near

From Goss DA. Fixation disparity. In: Eskridge JB, Amos JA, Bartlett JD, eds. *Clinical Procedures in Optometry.* Philadelphia: JB Lippincott; 1991:716–726, with permission.

higher AP than the three instruments listed in Table 17.6.

Vertical AP can be measured by simply rotating the units. Some units also have horizontal lines that are used to make the vertical AP measurements. AP measurements are effective when evaluating and managing vertical deviations. Studies have shown that the amount of vertical prism to prescribe should be equal to the AP, which should be carefully measured at distance and near (33).

Jiménez et al. (34) studied the relationship between AP (as measured using the Mallet box) and global stereopsis. Subjects with high AP showed poor stereopsis responses. In addition, they found that the direction of the AP (i.e., exo vs. eso) did not affect stereopsis as much as the size of the AP.

Keystone Visual Skills Cards

The *KVS cards* are a series of cards that screen for the presence of acuity reductions, binocular anomalies, stereopsis defects, and color vision defects. Cards no. 1,2,3,4,6,10, and 11 are the cards most commonly administered during a binocular vision assessment. These cards are placed in the Keystone telebinocular (Fig. 17.11). The complete series, as described by Birnbaum (8), has 15 cards with 10 tested at distance and 5 at near. Card 1 is a test of simultaneous perception; card 2 grossly measures a vertical imbalance; cards 3 and 9 measure lateral imbalance at distance (card 3) and at near (card 9); cards 4 and 10 tests fusion at distance (card 4) and at near (card 10); and card 6 measures stereoacuity using line stereograms, with disparities ranging from 1103 seconds to 82.5 seconds. KVS cards 3 and 9 also provide an indication of phoria and fusional stability at distance and near, respectively (8).

While administering each card, the stability of the target should be monitored by asking the child if the target is moving. This test can be effectively performed on children as young as 4 years of age based on my clinical experience. Asking the patient to point to a picture that lies

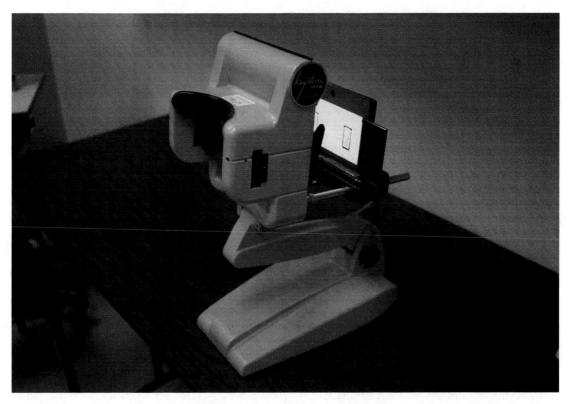

FIGURE 17.11. Keystone telebinocular.

in front of the eye that is opposite the hand that is pointing adds motor reinforcement to the task. This modification also eliminates the need for the young child to verbally communicate answers.

Near Point of Convergence

Near point of convergence (NPC) is a procedure that measures the amplitude of convergence—the closest distance that fusion is maintained (26,29). A break of 3 inches (7 cm) with a recovery at 6 inches (15 cm) is the expected NPC finding. NPC can be measured accurately in children as young as 2 years of age. NPC findings are well developed and adultlike by the age of 6 years (8). With an accommodative target, the expected NPC is 2.5 cm/4.5 cm, and 3 cm/5 cm when measured with red-green glasses and a penlight (29).

Very colorful and interesting targets need to be selected when examining younger patients because they will lose interest very quickly. Beginning at 16 to 20 inches (40–50 cm) away, move the target toward the patient along the midline toward the patient's nose. The break point occurs when either the patient reports double or when the examiner objectively sees one of the eyes turn out or in. Birnbaum (8) stated that the distance is measured from the bridge of the nose. If the pen appears single up to the nose, the finding is recorded as to the nose (TTN). The recovery point is the distance where the target is single again or the examiner observes ocular alignment of the eyes.

Observations to be noted when measuring NPC include reach (R), the ability of the patient to localize the target; grasp (G), the ability to sustain convergence while the target is moving; release (R), the ability to look away from the target; and regrasp (RG), the ability to look from a distant point back to the target (32). In addition, facial expressions made during convergence (grimacing, tensed and furrowed eye brows, discomfort during testing, and redness or tearing of the eyes), and whether the patient moves back as the target moves closer should also be noted and recorded as behavioral indicators of the difficulty of the task (8). Children are very good at avoiding tasks that induce

discomfort and such observations provide the examiner with an idea of how the child performs near vision tasks for sustained periods. The NPC should be repeated several times, because the NPC can recede with fatigue. The NPC recedes on repeat testing in both patients who are normal and patients diagnosed with convergence insufficiency (29). The NPC was found to recede less than 1 cm in normal patients, but in the convergence insufficiency group, the NPC was shown to recede by 1.5 cm after five repetitions and about 4 cm after ten repetitions. Therefore, the NPC worsens with repetitions and because most patients also have an accommodative dysfunction in addition to a binocular dysfunction, the NPC may be noted to significantly recede in under five repetitions.

Birnbaum (8) also suggested varying test conditions to determine if the NPC finding improves. Some examples include having the patient touch the target for motor reinforcement, using an accommodative target, or using the appropriate near-point prescription. Such findings will provide an indication of the treatment options most appropriate for the patient. For instance, a patient may require a combination of lenses and vision therapy, or only a near-point lens prescription.

Another modification is the use of a red lens and a penlight to measure the NPC. Some individuals who show a significantly receded NPC with a red lens over one eye have a fragile binocular system. A significant difference exists in the NPC measurement with convergence insufficiency patients when the NPC is measured with an accommodative target as compared to using red-green filters and a penlight (29). The mean NPC with the accommodative target was found to be 9.3/12.2 cm and 14.8/17.6 cm using the red-green filters and the penlight. No difference was found in patients with normal binocular vision.

Van Orden Star

The *Van Orden Star Test* investigates binocular posture and visual–motor integration abilities when performing a bilateral motor task (9,32). The test pattern presents a vertical row of figures at each edge and is placed at the far point setting on the *Correct-Eye-Scope* or a stereoscope

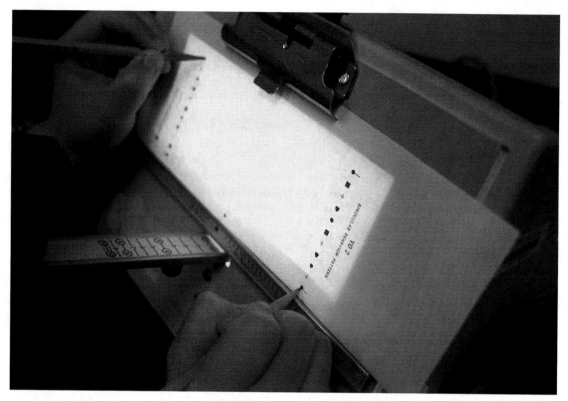

FIGURE 17.12. Van Orden Star.

(Fig. 17.12). The patient holds a pencil in each hand. The dominant hand's pencil is placed on the lowest shape while the nondominant hand is placed on the highest shape on the opposite side of the test form. The patient is asked to draw a line toward the other pencil at the same speed and at the same time, then to stop drawing when the pencils look as though they are touching, not when the patient feels the pencil points physically touching. The pencils are placed on the next shape and the process is repeated until all the shapes have been done. The completed tracing looks like two triangles. The separation between the apices of the triangles is measured and 68 mm is considered to be ortho-posture. A distance of less than 68 mm is eso-posture, and greater than 68 mm is considered exo-posture. If one apex is higher than the other, a hyperphoria is present. Observations to note during this test include binocular posture, stability, and quality of the final drawing. Central suppression is present when one of the apices of the triangles is missing and the apex of the other triangle is overextended.

VERGENCE FACILITY

Daum (35) stated that horizontal vergence facility is tested to assess the quality of a patient's vergence response. Some parameters to note when testing vergence facility with respect to the quality of fusion include the response latency, velocity, accuracy, and fatigue (8). The norms range from 5 to 7cpm, but a standard is lacking for age norms and for agreement on which prism powers should be used (35). Norms for school-aged children using 4BI/16BO are 7 cpm at age 5 years, and to 11 cpm by age 13 years (8).

The total amount of prism should be split between the two eyes and Daum (35) suggested using 6BI/6BO or 8BI/8BO. It may not be possible to test amblyopic patients or patients with deep suppression. If a suppression check in the form of an anaglyphic or polarized stimulus is used, facility findings can be reduced by about 2 cpm (35). The patient is first asked whether the target is single with the BI and then with the BO prism. The patient is then instructed to indicate when the target is single after each prism flip. This is performed for a minute and the number of cycles per minute is recorded. The number of cycles is determined to be half the number of flips of the prism. If the patient cannot fuse the target on either side, the test is discontinued.

Daum (35) reported that patients with poor vergence facility have poor binocular findings and are asthenopic. Patients with normal vergence ranges can demonstrate poor vergence facility, indicating that patients with inadequate binocular function may go undetected when only smooth vergence is assessed (29). Studies also show that vergence facility should be used to monitor the progress of vision therapy because of the positive correlation between post-therapy improvement in both vergence facility and vergence amplitude findings (35).

Worth-4-Dot: Red-Green

The *W4D Test* requires the use of red-green glasses and determines a patient's level of sensory fusion (simultaneous perception, flat fusion, or suppression). The typical responses include (a) four lights (one red, two green, and one with red-green luster), which indicate flat fusion; (b) two red lights or three green lights, which indicate suppression; and (c) five lights (2 red and 3 green), which indicate simultaneous perception (32). In general, peripheral fusion is being assessed when testing at near, and central fusion is tested when W4D is performed at distance (36).

If suppression is present at different test distances, the size of the suppression scotoma can be estimated (7,29,36). Suppression scotomas are larger when noted at near with W4D testing, and smaller when detected at distance. The image of a dot on the W4D will subtend a larger angle on the retina at near rather than at distance. Larger suppression scotomas are also associated with reduced stereopsis, suggesting poorer prognosis when considering treatment options (29). Arthur and Keech (37) emphasized the importance of central suppression responses with W4D testing to support the diagnosis of amblyopia in a patient with a microtropia.

As described in the stereopsis section, the disadvantage of the red-green filters is the phenomenon of binocular dissociation. Stud-

ies comparing a polarized version of the W4D with the red-green version found a higher frequency of fusion responses and a lower frequency of suppression responses using the polarized W4D (37). Another study by Simons and Elhatton (19) found that the filters do not perfectly match the color of the light emitted from the W4D. In addition, they also found illuminance differences between the green and red dots. They suggested repeating the test with the filters reversed to confirm the patient's responses before making conclusions regarding the patient's binocular status.

Morale et al. (36) found that the W4D can be used in a child as young as 3 years, but also found the mean age of failing the test was 8.2 years. Children under the age of 5 years are rarely tested with the W4D because they are not cognitively mature enough to understand the instructions. For instance, they may not be able to count or correctly name colors. The literature states that, in children aged 42 months, 90% are able to name colors and to count objects sequentially, and 15% were able to do so at age 29 months. At 31 months, 90% can name pictures, whereas 15% can do so at 20 months. Using this information, Morale et al. (36) studied the effectiveness of a preschool version they constructed called the *Worth 4-Shape Test*. They concluded that this version has (a) higher success rate in children younger than 4 years of age, (b) equivalent accuracy, and (c) high test-retest reliability, and therefore is a valid test for young children.

SUMMARY

Clinical Relevance of Stereopsis Testing

The advantages of stereopsis testing in children under the age of 6 years include the following: (a) tests are administered quickly, (b) results provide objective data when assessing the progression of treatment, and (c) tests can be used as an effective screening device (to detect constant strabismus or refractive amblyopia) when used in conjunction with some form of visual acuity assessment. The disadvantages associated with stereopsis testing relate to the limited information regarding binocular efficiency, the need for specialized glasses, and the difficulty in testing children under the age of 3 years. A

TABLE 17.7 Summary of Stereopsis Tests

Stereo Test	Requires Special Glasses	Disparity Range	Age Group	Type of Stereogram
Frisby	No	480–15 sec at 40 cm	Ages 3 y and up	RDS
Lang	No	Lang I: 1200–600 sec Lang II: 600–200 sec	Ages 4 y and up	RDS
Random dot E	Polarized filters	168 sec of arc at 1.5 m	Ages 3 y and up	RDS

Random dot	Polarized filters	Randot subtest:
		  500–250 sec
		Animals subtest:
		  400–100 sec
		Circles: 400–20 sec
			Randot and animals:
			  Ages 4 y and up
			Circles: 5 y and up
				RDS and line stereograms

Randot preschool stereoacuity	Polarized filters	800–40 sec	Ages 2 y and up	RDS
Titmus stereo fly	Polarized filters	Fly: 3000 sec Animals: 400–100 sec Circles: 400–40 sec	Fly: Ages 3 years and up Animals: Ages 4 y and up Circles: Ages 5 y and up	Line stereograms
TNO	Red-green filters	Screening: 2000 sec Graded stereoacuity: 480–15 sec at 40 cm	Screening: Ages 2.5 y and up Graded stereoacuity: Ages 6 y and up	RDS

RDS, random-dot stereograms; RDE, random dot E.

summary of the characteristics of the tests discussed in this chapter can be found in Table 17.7.

Normal or adequate binocular function should not be concluded on the basis of an age-appropriate stereoacuity finding, particularly because intermittent strabismic patients perform well on stereopsis tests (8). Birnbaum (8) also suggested "there is an uncertain correlation between stereopsis and visual spatial function in real, physical space." The significance of stereoacuity assessment is apparent, however, when a patient needs to make instantaneous spatial judgments (e.g., in sports or when viewing under unusual conditions, such as driving when it is snowing or when it is dark).

Clinical Relevance of Fusion Testing

The advantages of fusion testing in children are most evident in the school-age population. As noted above, fusion is the result of a com-plex and dynamic process that involves motor and sensory fusion. Different types of vergence (smooth, step, and jump), integration of accommodation and vergence abilities, and integration of visual–motor abilities, can all be readily evaluated in this population. The job of the pediatric optometrist is to translate the binocular findings into a picture of how effectively and comfortably the child visually functions throughout the day. In recognizing and remediating vision disorders, clinicians can significantly maximize a child's vision efficiency in an academic environment.

APPENDIX: SOURCE LIST

Bernell: 4016 N. Home Street, Mishawaka, IN 46545. 1-800-348-2225. www.bernell.com

Frisby Stereo Test: 137 Brookhouse Hill Sheffield, S10 3TE, UK 0114-230-7819. www.frisbystereotest.co.uk

Keystone View: Nevada Capital Group, Inc. 2200 Dickerson Road, Reno, Nevada 89503. 1-866-574-6360. www.keystoneview.com

Optometric Extension Program (OEP): 1921 E. Carnegie Ave., Suite 3-L, Santa Ana, CA 92705-5510. 949-250-8070. www.oep.org

Richmond Products: 4400 Silver Ave SE, Albuquerque, NM 87108. 505-275-2406. www.richmondproducts.com

Stereo Optical Co, Inc: 3539 N. Kenton Avenue, Chicago, IL 60641. 1-800-344-9500. www.stereooptical.com

Veatch Ophthalmic Instruments: 1-800-447-7511. www.veatchinstruments.com

REFERENCES

1. Hatch SW, Richman JE. Stereopsis testing without polarized glasses: a comparison study on five new stereoacuity tests. *Journal of the American Optometric Association* 1994;65(9):637–641.
2. Fawcett SL, Birch EE. Validity of the Titmus and Randot Circles tasks in children with known binocular vision disorders. *J AAPOS* 2003;7:333–338.
3. Shute R, Candy R, Westall C, et al. Success rates in testing monocular acuity and stereopsis in infants and young children. *Ophthalmic Physiol Opt* 1990;10:133–136.
4. Cooper J. Stereopsis. In: Eskridge JB, Amos JA, Bartlett JD, eds. *Clinical Procedures in Optometry.* Philadelphia: JB Lippincott; 1991:121–134.
5. Broadbent H, Westall C. An evaluation of techniques for measuring stereopsis in infants and young children. *Ophthalmic Physiol Opt* 1990;10:3–7.
6. Lee J, McIntyre A. Clinical tests for binocular vision. *Eye* 1996;10:282–285.
7. Rosner J, Rosner J. Question #6: What is the patient's binocular status? In: *Pediatric Optometry.* Boston: Butterworth-Heinemann 1990;175–260.
8. Birnbaum MH. *Optometric Management of Nearpoint Vision Disorders.* Boston: Butterworth-Heinemann, 1993.
9. Press LJ, Moore BD. *Clinical Pediatric Optometry.* Boston: Butterworth-Heinemann, 1993.
10. Richardson SR, Wright CM, Hrisos S, et al. Stereoacuity in unilateral visual impairment detected at preschool screening: outcomes from a randomized controlled trial. *Invest Ophthalmol Vis Sci* 2005;46:150–154.
11. Cooper J. Clinical stereopsis in testing: contour and random dot stereograms. *Journal of the American Optometric Association* 1979;50(1):41–46.
12. Steinman SB, Steinman BA, Garzia RP. *Foundations of Binocular Vision: A Clinical Perspective.* New York: McGraw–Hill, 2000.
13. Larson WL. Effect of TNO red-green glasses on local stereoacuity. *Am J Optom Physiol Optics* 1988;65(12):946–950.
14. Saunders KJ, Woodhouse JM, Westall CA. The modified Frisby Stereotest. *J Pediatr Ophthalmol Strabismus* 1996;33:323–327.
15. Ohlsson J, Villarreal G, Abrahamsson M, et al. Screening merits of the Lang II, Frisby, Randot, Titmus, and TNO stereo tests. *J AAPOS* 2001;5:316–322.
16. Lam SR, LaRooche GR, De Becker I, et al. The range and variability of ophthalmological parameters in normal children aged 4 1/2 to 5 1/2 years. *J Pediatr Ophthalmol Strabismus* 1996;33:251–625.
17. Manny RE, Martinez AT, Fern KD. Testing stereopsis in the preschool child: is it clinically useful? *J Pediatr Ophthalmol Strabismus* 1991;28(4):223–231.
18. Birch E, Williams C, Hunter J, et al., and the ALSPAC "Children in Focus" Study Team. Random dot stereoacuity of preschool children. *J Pediatr Ophthalmol Strabismus* 1997;34:217–222.
19. Simons K, Elhatton K. Artifacts in fusion and stereopsis testing based on red/green dichoptic image separation. *J Pediatr Ophthalmol Strabismus* 1994;31:290–297.
20. Williams S, Simpson A, Silva PA. Stereoacuity levels and vision problems in children from 7 to 11 years. *Ophthalmic Physiol Opt* 1988;8:386–389.
21. Frantz, K.A., Cotter, S.A., Brown, W.L, and Motameni, M. Erroneous findings in polarized testing caused by plastic prisms. *J Pediatr Ophthalmol Strabismus.* 1990;27(5):259–264.
22. Ciner EB, Schanel-Klitsch E, Scheiman M. Stereoacuity development in young children. *Optom Vis Sc* 1991;68(7):533–536.
23. Ciner EB, Scheiman MM, Schanel-Klitsch E, et al. Stereopsis testing the 18- to 35-month-old children using operant preferential looking. *Optom Vis Sci* 1989;66(11):782–787.
24. Schmidt PP. Vision screening with the RDE stereotest in pediatric populations. *Optom Vis Sci* 1994;71(4):273–281.
25. Ciuffreda KJ, Levi DM, Selenow A. *Amblyopia: Basic and Clinical Aspects.* Boston: Butterworth-Heinemann, 1992.
26. Ciuffreda KJ. Components of clinical near vergence testing. *J Behav Optom* 1992:3(1);3–13.
27. Caloroso EE, Rouse MW. *Clinical Management of Strabismus.* Boston: Butterworth-Heinemann, 1993.
28. Feldman JM, Cooper J, Carniglia P, et al. Comparison of fusional ranges measured by risley prisms, vectograms, and computer orthopter. *Optom Vis Sci* 1989;66(6):375–382.
29. Scheiman M, Wick B. *Clinical Management of Binocular Vision: Heterophoric, Accommodative, and Eye Movement Disorders.* Philadelphia: Lippincott Williams & Wilkins, 1994.
30. Daum KM. Vergence amplitude. In: Eskridge JB, Amos JA, Bartlett JD, eds. *Clinical Procedures in Optometry.* Philadelphia: JB Lippincott; 1991:91–98.
31. Alexander KR. The foundations of the SILO response. *Optometric Weekly* May 19, 1994;22–26.
32. Gruning CF, Hong C, Wong LC, eds. *Vision Therapy Diagnostic Procedures Laboratory Manual.* New York: SUNY State College of Optometry, 1993.
33. Goss DA. Fixation disparity. In: Eskridge JB, Amos JA, Bartlett JD, eds. *Clinical Procedures in Optometry.* Philadelphia: JB Lippincott; 1991:716–726.
34. Jiménez JR, Olivares JL, Pérez-Ocón F, et al. Associated phoria in relation to stereopsis with random-dot stereograms. *Optom Vis Sci* 2000;77(1):47–50.
35. Daum KM. Vergence facility. In: Eskridge JB, Amos JA, Bartlett, JD, eds. *Clinical Procedures in Optometry.* Philadelphia: JB Lippincott; 1991:671–676.
36. Morale SE, Jeffrey BG, Fawcett SL, et al. Preschool Worth 4-shape test: testability, reliability, and validity. *J AAPOS* 2002;6:247–251.
37. Arthur BW, Keech RV. The polarized three-dot test. *J Pediatr Ophthalmol Strabismus* 1987;24(6):305–308.

Evaluation of Accommodation

18

Ida Chung-Lock

IMPORTANCE OF EVALUATING ACCOMMODATION

The evaluation of accommodation as part of a comprehensive eye examination is the standard of eye care for pediatric patients, because not only are accommodative deficiencies and inefficiencies associated with poor academic performance, but they can also signify a neuropathy or systemic abnormality. Accommodative problems have been linked to reading problems and learning disabilities in children (1). Studies note that 61% to 85% of children with learning problems (2,3) and 88% of those with diagnosed learning disabilities (4) have accommodative disorders of amplitude or facility. Accommodative deficiencies reported in healthy young individuals can be associated with convergence insufficiency, altitude changes, emotional stress, and refractive errors (2,5–8). Accommodative dysfunctions have been found to be associated with a wide variety of pathologic conditions. Ocular conditions include intraocular inflammation and premature sclerosis of the crystalline lens (8,9). Neurologic conditions affecting accommodation include those secondary to head trauma, neuralgic disease affecting the third cranial nerve, pharmacologic agents primarily parasympathetic, and encephalitis (9,10). Systemic conditions that have an impact on accommodation include myasthenia gravis, botulism, diphtheria, diabetes mellitus, Wilson's disease, vascular hypertension,

Guillian-Barré syndrome, chicken pox, tuberculosis, influenza, whooping cough, measles, dental caries or infections, endocrine disorders, anemia, arteriosclerosis, tonsillar infections, infectious mononucleosis, syphilis, and food poisoning (8–13). The varied causes of accommodative dysfunction make it essential for the clinician to evaluate accommodative function and interpret the findings in the context of the patient's history and other clinical findings to reach an appropriate management plan.

ASPECTS OF ACCOMMODATIVE FUNCTION TO EVALUATE

The exact prevalence of accommodative dysfunction is not well documented. The prevalence of accommodative dysfunction is reported to be present in 60% to 80% of patients with binocular dysfunction, but less than in 10% of an optometric clinic population (1,2).

Accommodative insufficiency, by far the most common of the accommodative disorders, is diagnosed primarily with the amplitude test. The other two aspects of accommodative function frequently tested clinically are accommodative response and accommodative facility. To separate the accommodative system from the binocular system and thereby remove possible contamination of the accommodative findings secondary to inefficiencies of binocularity, testing should be carried out under monocular conditions. Clinical tests are available to evaluate the various aspects of accommodative function: push-up, pull-away, minus lens, dynamic retinoscopy, and visually evoked potentials to evaluate amplitude; monocular estimate method, Nott retinoscopy, fused cross-cylinder, book retinoscopy, bell retinoscopy, and photorefraction to evaluate accommodative response; plus and minus flipper lenses, and distance rock test to evaluate facility; and plus and minus added lenses to evaluate range of relative accommodation. Monocular accommodative facility and monocular amplitude tests give accommodative findings without interference from the binocular system, whereas the monocular estimate method, fused cross-cylinder, binocular accommodative facility test, and negative and positive relative accommodation tests results are derived under binocular conditions.

CLINICAL TESTS

Accommodative Amplitude

The amplitude of accommodation can be measured monocularly or binocularly. Measured monocularly, it is the maximal dioptric value produced by the accommodative system. Measured binocularly, it is the maximal dioptric value produced in the presence of convergence. Binocular measures are usually higher than monocular measures by 0.20 to 0.60 D because of convergence accommodation, although the measures can vary on repeated measurements and among different patients (6). Accommodative amplitude can be measured subjectively with the push-up method, the pull-away method, or the minus lens technique, and objectively using dynamic retinoscopy.

Push-up Method

PROCEDURE

With one eye occluded, move the target, generally a 20/20 to 20/30 letter or detailed picture, toward the patient's unoccluded eye at a rate of 5 cm/s (1). Encourage the patient to keep the target clear and to report when the target first starts to blur. The inverse of the measured distance in meters from the near point of accommodation (defined as the first sustained blur) to the patient's spectacle plane is the maximal amplitude of accommodation expressed in diopters (15). This should be repeated with the other eye, and can be performed binocularly with presentation of the target along the midline. Patients should be wearing their distance manifest refraction and ambient lighting should provide sufficient illumination on the target as it approaches the patient's eyes, but not so bright as to cause abnormal pupillary constriction. The push-up method has been shown to be reliable (16).

Pull-away Method

PROCEDURE

The pull-away or push-away method involves moving a 20/20 to 20/30 letter target away from the patient's spectacle plane until the patient can identify the stimulus (15) (Fig. 18.1). A variation of the push-up method, it is performed under similar conditions, except the target is initially presented directly in front of the unoccluded eye and is then moved away from the patient. The inverse of the measured distance at which the patient can correctly identify the target from the spectacle plane is the monocular amplitude of accommodation. The pull-away method is advantageous over the push-up method because the correct identification of the target gives a more reliable finding of the minimal amplitude of accommodation in patients with questionable subjective responses. The amplitude obtained with the pull-away method is comparable with the conventional push-up method (15,17–19).

Minus Lens Method

PROCEDURE

The minus lens method is performed at 40 cm through the distance manifest refraction with a 20/30 target or, if the visual acuity is less than 20/20, choose a target that is two lines below the best acuity. The test is performed monocularly with the addition of lenses in −0.25-D steps until the patient reports first sustained blur. The absolute value of the lens addition +2.50 D for the working distance compensation is the total amplitude of accommodation for that eye.

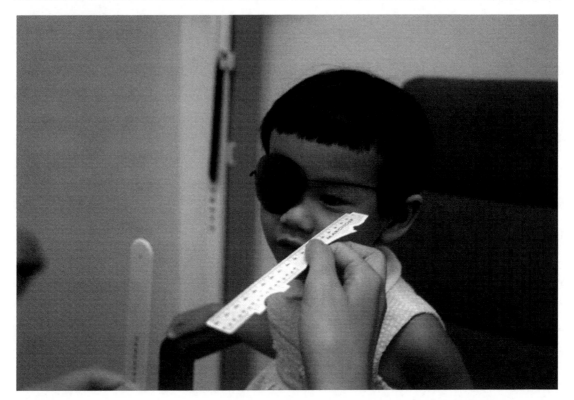

FIGURE 18.1. Procedure for pull-away method to measure monocular amplitude of accommodation.

Dynamic Retinoscopy

PROCEDURE

Dynamic retinoscopy gives an objective measure of accommodative amplitude (20). While the patient is viewing a near target, a 20/20 to 20/30 letter or picture equivalent, the clinician moves the retinoscope and the target together toward the patient. A change in reflex from a broad, bright and fast with motion reflex (indicating a normal lag of accommodation) to a narrow, dimmer and slower reflex, indicates focusing is lost and the amplitude of accommodation is exceeded (21,22).

Visually Evoked Potentials

PROCEDURE

Visually evoked potentials (VEP) can be used to objectively measure accommodative amplitude. While viewing a phase-alternated checkerboard pattern, the amplitude is determined by having the patient view the stimulus through decreasing plus power lenses and then minus lenses until the measured VEP response produces a nearly constant value (23). Although VEP is a feasible method to determine amplitude of accommodation, the time and equipment involved limits its clinical utility, particularly when other methods are available.

Accommodative Response

Accommodative response is the actual amount of accommodation generated in response to a stimulus. Because of depth of focus, the accommodative response does not have to equal the stimulus demand exactly, and is usually less than the accommodative stimulus (24). The difference between the accommodative stimulus and accommodative response is the lead or lag of accommodation. Accommodative response is clinically most commonly measured objectively with the monocular estimate method (MEM) or without lenses using Nott retinoscopy. Using Nott retinoscopy, accommodative responses in children as young as 3 years of age was measured to be accurate to within 0.50 D (25).

Subjectively, it is most commonly measured using the fused cross-cylinder method (FCC).

Monocular Estimate Method

PROCEDURE

The MEM is performed with age-appropriate reading material at the plane of the retinoscope light held at the patient's habitual near working distance (as determined by asking the patient to hold reading material) or at the patient's Harmon distance (the distance from the patient's elbow to the third knuckle) (21) (Fig. 18.2). This distance is often approximately 20 to 25 cm (8–10 inches) for a young child. For infants or toddlers, a detailed toy or shiny object is a suitable target (21). The patient's eyes should be in down-gaze when viewing the target, similar to a normal reading posture. Room illumination should be such that the reading target is adequately illuminated while allowing the clinician to easily view the retinoscopic reflex. The patient wears the appropriate lenses, such as a dis-

tance correction, a tentative near prescription, or no lenses. With both eyes open, lenses are quickly interposed monocularly, plus lenses for *with* motion and minus lenses for *against* motion, to neutralize the reflex, leaving the lens in place no longer than half a second in order not to change the accommodative response or binocular fixation (26). The lens that neutralizes the reflex is the measured accommodative response. If astigmatism is present, the two major meridians can be neutralized separately. It is important to measure the response only when the patient is actively viewing the target presented. The use of magnetic fixation cards with premanufactured square cut-outs attached to the Welch Allyn retinoscope facilitates the MEM technique (Fig. 18.3).

Nott Retinoscopy

PROCEDURE

Nott retinoscopy is similar to MEM, except that to neutralize the reflex, the retinoscope

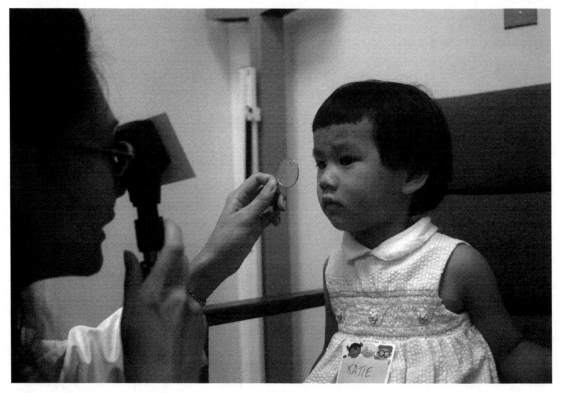

FIGURE 18.2. Procedure for monocular estimate method (MEM) retinoscopy to measure accommodative response.

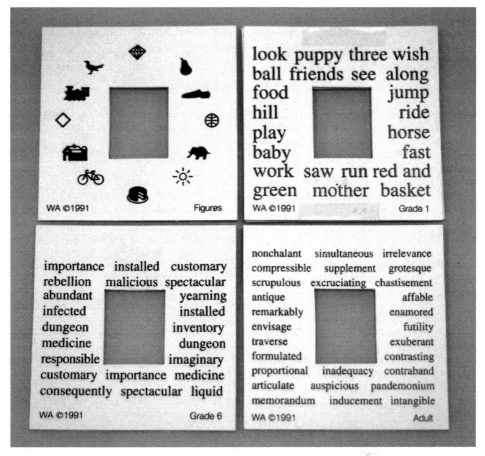

FIGURE 18.3. Set of magnetic fixation cards for patient fixation during monocular estimate method (MEM) retinoscopy. Available from Lombart Instrument Co., 5358 Robin Hood Road, Norfolk, VA 23513.

is moved closer or further from the patient while the target remains at a fixed distance (27,28). Thus, the target cannot be affixed to the retinoscope. The test is performed with the fixation distance at 40 cm and initial observation through the retinoscope at 50 cm. The retinoscope is then moved away from the patient if *with* motion is seen, and closer if *against* motion is seen until the reflex is neutral. The dioptric difference between the target and the position of the retinoscope at the point of neutrality is the measured accommodative response. When performing Nott retinoscopy, definite fixation, active accommodation, and alignment of the target and retinoscope beam within 10°, are important in order not to induce erroneous findings (29,30). Nott retinoscopy is said to be superior to MEM because it does not present the possible contamination of results

from the neutralizing lens itself (27,31). Nott retinoscopy has been shown to be a repeatable and valid objective technique for assessing accommodative lag (32).

Bell Retinoscopy

PROCEDURE

Bell retinoscopy is an objective test of accommodative response using a silver chrome bell attached to a thin metal rod as a target (33). With the retinoscope at 50 cm from the patient, the bell is held at the clinician's forehead, and the clinician observes the retinoscopic reflex while the patient views his or her own image reflected off the bell's surface. The bell is then moved either closer to the patient, if *with* motion is initially seen, or away from the patient, if *against* motion is initially seen, until the reflex appears neutral. The dioptric difference between the bell and the retinoscope at the point a neutral reflex is observed is the accommodative lag. Bell retinoscopy was found to be incomparable to results of MEM (34), but it can provide the clinician with a qualitative assessment of patients' ability to focus and align their eyes in free space (35). The bell target is particularly effective for the preverbal child.

Book Retinoscopy

PROCEDURE

Book retinoscopy is performed with the patient reading grade-appropriate text paragraphs, while the clinician views the reflex of a retinoscope held directly above the reading material (36). The clinician is able to interpret the patient's interest and comprehension of the reading material by noting the color and motion of the reflex (i.e., the quality of the accommodative response). A bright and pink reflex with neutral to *with* motion indicates free and easy reading, a bright and pink reflex with varying fast *against* motion indicates reading with comprehension under stress, and a dull brick red reflex with a slow *against* motion indicates frustration reading (37,38). Some clinicians prefer book retinoscopy to other dynamic retinoscopy procedures because this objective method mimics a more natural reading environment (37).

Photorefraction

PROCEDURE

A less-common method of assessing accommodative response that is mainly used in research is photorefraction. Photorefraction can determine the point of accommodation from the camera plane, which when compared to a known refractive status for a patient, an accommodative response can be calculated (39,40).

Fused Cross-Cylinder

PROCEDURE

Fused cross-cylinder is performed in the phoropter with the ±0.37 D cylinder lenses and

the cross-cylinder grid target composed of vertical and horizontal sets of lines presented at 40 cm in dim room illumination (41). With the patient's distance correction in place, lenses are added binocularly +0.25 D at a time until the patient reports the vertical lines are sharper. It is recommended to start the test with added plus lenses and binocularly reducing the plus lenses a 0.25 D at a time until equality of the lines are achieved, or when the patient reports that the horizontal lines are sharper. The added lenses that gives this endpoint response is the measured accommodative response. A response of vertical lines being sharper before any lenses are added indicates a lead of accommodation. The FCC test can also be performed monocularly. The FCC test is not as repeatable as MEM (42) and relies on subjective responses, making MEM a preferred method of testing accommodative response in children.

Accommodative Facility

Accommodative facility is the ability to stimulate and inhibit accommodation. It is a measure of accommodative flexibility and stamina.

Lens Flipper

PROCEDURE

The lens flipper test uses ±2.00 D lenses and a 20/30 letter target at 40 cm (Fig. 18.4). The lenses are presented binocularly or monocularly with one eye occluded to measure binocular and monocular facility, respectively. The patient is asked to report when the letters are clear as +2.00 lenses and −2.00 lenses are alternately presented. Once the patient reports the letters are clear and single, the lenses are flipped (43). Accommodative facility is measured as the number of cycles of plus and minus lenses the patient is able to clear within 1 minute (cpm). One cycle is clearing one set of plus and minus lenses.

A suppression check is necessary for accurate testing under binocular conditions (44). The norms for accommodative facility were derived from studies using the *SOV9 acuity suppression vectogram* (Fig. 18.5) and is the recommended target for clinical testing (42). The patient wears Polaroid glasses and is asked to keep

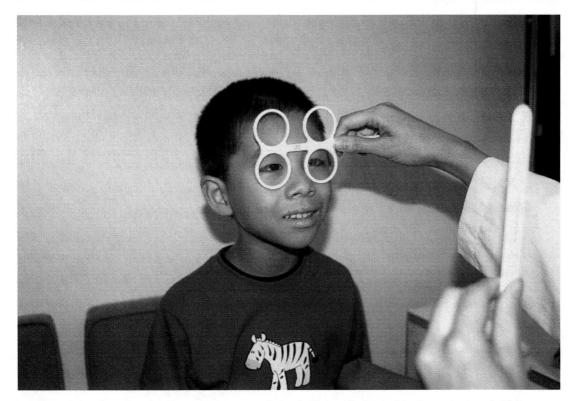

FIGURE 18.4. Procedure for binocular accommodative facility performed with plus and minus 2.00-D flipper lenses.

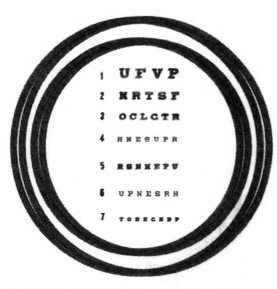

FIGURE 18.5. SOV9 acuity suppression vectogram. Available from Bernell/USO, 4016 N. Home Street, Mishawaka, IN 46545.

the letters clear and to report if the letters disappear, indicating suppression. The target consists of seven lines, with line no. 4 seen by the left eye only, line no. 6 seen by the right eye only, and all other lines are seen binocularly. For younger children, whose responses are questionable, the test can be modified by asking the child to say aloud the letters or words on the target rather than simply reporting whether the letters are clear. Suppression can also be monitored by the physiologic diplopia technique, which requires the placement of a pen or pencil halfway between the patient and the reading sample. The patient should see two pen tips throughout the testing if no suppression exists (45).

An objective measure of accommodative facility using ±2.00 D lenses and MEM was described by Gallaway and Scheiman (46). They predetermined the lens value that would indicate blur through the flipper lenses by first performing negative and positive relative accommodation, and then performing MEM to measure the accommodative responses through these lens values. The two lag findings would then be used to judge when and if the patient is able to clear the lens flippers. They found an agreement in 86% of the subjects. The drawbacks of this technique are that validity has not been established and the premise of this objective test still requires a subjective determination of the lens values that indicate blur.

LENS POWER

The choice of ±2.00 D lenses at 40 cm as the standard for accommodative facility testing appears to be chosen by consensus. No particular reasons have been given, except these powers are similar to the expected negative or positive relative accommodation (NRA/PRA) norms and 40 cm is the typical test distance for many optometric procedures (47). Authors who investigated the use of a certain percentage of an individual's accommodative amplitude for testing distance and lens power range to more accurately differentiate symptomatic and asymptomatic patients, found a higher level of sensitivity, but similar specificity compared with the ±2.00 D standard lenses (48). The authors suggest, however, that the differences do not warrant a change in clinical practice for testing accommodative facility.

Distance Rock

PROCEDURE

Accommodative facility can also be tested using the distance rock method (9,49). The test involves measuring the cycles per minute the patient is able to alternately clear a distance target and a 40-cm near test target. The distance rock test has not gained clinical acceptance, partially because performance is substantially influenced by a patient's ability to shift eye fixation and validated norms are not available.

Vision Therapy Assessment Program

PROCEDURE

The Vision Therapy Assessment (VTA)* is a computer-based program that uses red-green

*Available from HTS, Inc. PO Box 6028, Apache Junction, AZ 85278; www.visiontherapysolutions.net.

glasses and ±2.00 D lenses to test accommodative facility. The test requires the patient to indicate the correct responses by viewing a computer screen and moving a joystick in the direction of the correct answer. This can negatively influence the results for those patients who have difficulties with directional and visual–motor discrimination tasks. At this writing, the program has been shown not to be a valid method of diagnosing accommodative facility deficiencies (50).

Relative Accommodation

Relative accommodation is a measure of the patient's ability to relax or stimulate accommodation to a fixed vergence target. This gives the clinician insight into the patient's accommodative–convergence system interaction, and its relative flexibility.

PROCEDURE

The measure of relative accommodation is usually performed in a phoropter through the distance manifest refraction or a tentative near prescription. Negative relative accommodation is a measure of the patient's ability to relax accommodation with a fixed vergence demand. Positive relative accommodation is a measure of the ability of the patient to stimulate accommodation with a fixed vergence demand. Usually, the target is a 20/30 line of letters at 40 cm. Lenses in the magnitude of +0.25-D steps are added binocularly until the patient reports first sustained blur for the NRA value, and lenses in the magnitude of −0.25-D steps are added binocularly until the patient reports first sustained blur for the PRA value.

NORMS FOR CLINICAL TESTS OF ACCOMMODATION AND DIAGNOSTIC CRITERIA FOR ACCOMMODATIVE ANOMALIES

The three measures of accommodation commonly used in the diagnosis of accommodative function include monocular amplitude, facility, and lag (51). Indirect measures of accommodation that assist in the diagnosis of accommodative dysfunction include accommodative

TABLE 18.1 Summary of Accommodative Test Normative Data

Aspect of Accommodation	Norm	Failure	Method
Amplitude	15 – ¼ (age)	Less than calculated	Push-up or pull-away minus lens
Lag	+0.25 ± 0.75	≥1.00 or <plano	MEM
			Nott retinoscopy
			Fused cross-cylinder
Facility	8 cpm bino	<8 cpm bino	± 2.00 D flipper with
	11 cpm mono	<11 cpm mono	suppression monitor
	Age 8–12:		
	5 cpm bino	≤2.5 cpm bino	
	7 cpm mono	≤4.5 cpm mono	
	Age 7:		
	3.5 cpm bino	≤1 cpm bino	
	6.5 cpm mono	≤4.5 cpm mono	
	Age 6:		
	3 cpm bino	≤0.5 cpm bino	
	5.5 cpm mono	≤3 cpm mono	

MEM, Monocular Estimate Method; cpm, cycles per minute; bino, binocularly; mono, monocularly.

convergence/accommodation ratio (AC/A) blur vergence findings, and positive and negative relative accommodation (52,53). The diagnosis of accommodative function is done by comparing the clinical finding with established norms. Validated tests, which include the push-up method for accommodative amplitude, MEM for accommodative response, and ±2.00-D lens flipper for accommodative facility, are preferred for the diagnosis of accommodative dysfunction. It is important to keep in mind that the published norms for the various accommodative tests are valid under the same test conditions from which they were derived (54). Variations in test parameters can result in erroneous conclusions. For example, accommodative facility testing is one area that has been shown to produce very different norms when conducted on children than on adults (42). Table 18.1 summarizes test normative data for accommodative amplitude, lag, and facility.

Accommodative Amplitude

Normal

The amplitude of accommodation is known to decrease with age. Data on accommodation amplitudes of children show a decrease starting at the age of 2 years (55). The accommo-

dation tables of age-expected amplitudes originated from Donder and were subsequently revised by Duane (56) (Table 18.2). Their data were derived from performing the push-up method on subjects 8 to 72 years of age. Eames subsequently published norms for children from 5 through 7 years of age (57). Based on these age-expected norms, Hofstetter derived mathematical formulas to calculate the minimal, average, and maximal amplitudes of accommodation (58). Based on his calculations, the formulas for the minimal amplitude is 15.00 D – ¼ (age), the average amplitude is 18.50 D – ⅓ (age), and the maximal

TABLE 18.2 Donder's Table of Age-Expected Amplitude of Accommodation

Age	Amplitude	Age	Amplitude
10	14.00	45	3.50
15	12.00	50	2.50
20	10.00	55	1.75
25	8.50	60	1.00
30	7.00	65	0.50
35	5.50	70	0.25
40	4.50	75	0.00

Modified from Carlson NB. *Clinical Procedures for Ocular Examination.* Norwalk: Appleton & Lange, 1996.

amplitude is 25.00 D – $\frac{1}{4}$ (age). The age is generally expressed in years of the past birthday.

Abnormal

A deficiency in accommodation is suspected if the patient's amplitude is less than the minimal calculated using Hofstetter's formula or if it is 2.00 D below the age-expected based on Duane's table of amplitude of accommodation expected (59). A difference of more than 0.50 D between the eyes is suggestive of a unilateral accommodative insufficiency.

Comparison of Test Methods

Push-up and pull-away comparison studies show they are highly correlated (15,17–19). Minus lens amplitude values are expected to be about 1.25 D (60) to 2.00 D (41,61) less than with push-up. The reasons cited for this are twofold: the minification of the target when viewed through minus lenses (41,61) and children show poorer accommodative responses to a negative lens stimulus compared with a free space target (62). Dynamic retinoscopy measures of accommodative amplitude, on average, were 2.70 D higher than with push-up method (22). The preferred methods of measuring accommodative amplitudes in amblyopic patients are dynamic retinoscopy or minus lens methods over the push-up technique, which tends to overestimate amplitudes (63).

Repeat Testing

A change of at least 1.50 D is needed to be considered a significant variation on repeated measurements of accommodative amplitude (64). Smaller changes are accepted as expected variations. Reduced amplitudes measured on repeated push-up testing can indicate a poor quality of accommodative response (i.e., poor sustaining ability) (65).

Socioeconomic Status

Children from lower socioeconomic status living in urban areas showed lower accommodative amplitudes than suburban children; on average, they have been reported to be 5.10 D less (55,57). This finding suggests that children living in poverty may be subjected to negative prenatal and environmental factors of malnutrition and undernutrition, which can result in decreased nervous system function.

Refractive Status

Nonamblyopic, uncorrected hypermetropes with and without strabismus show reduced amplitudes of accommodation, and it is speculated that these patients may have reduced amplitudes secondary to a longstanding hypoaccommodative state (66).

Accommodative Response

A normal accommodative response is a lag of 0.25 to 0.75 D. The most common finding on MEM testing is a lag of 0.50 to 0.75 D (21,67). The norm for the fused cross-cylinder test is +0.50 D with a SD of ± 0.50 D (68). A finding of below plano or above +0.75 D is considered abnormal (42).

Test Parameters

The accommodative state can be influenced by test target contrast, cognitive demand, and volitional effort (49,69). A blurred target, such as under conditions of reduced illumination, results in an increased accommodative response to low stimulus levels and a decreased accommodative response to higher stimulus levels (70). A reduction in pupil size also results in a reduced accommodative response (71). Anxiety and increased cognitive demand results in increased sympathetic innervation and, thus, can induce a decreased accommodative response in the order of 0.25 to 0.75 D (72). Target letter size, however, had little influence on the accommodative lag measured in patients with normal accommodative and binocular function (73).

The accommodative responses to a printed text target versus a computer-generated target (Gaussian image) have been studied and findings lack consistency. The PRIO Vision Tester[*] is based on the premise that the relatively poorer, sinusoidal-wave quality of computer print

---

[*] Available from PRIO Corporation, 8285 SW Nimbus Ave, Suite 148, Beaverton, OR 97008.

results in less-accurate accommodative responses (i.e., a greater lag of accommodation and a higher add acceptance for near). Some authors have reported results to support PRIO's finding (74,75). Other authors who have studied this have found either no difference in measured accommodative responses to either target type or have found small differences only (76,77).

Refractive Status

Patients with different refractive statuses give different accommodative responses: patients who are hyperopic accommodate more than those who are emmetropic, and those who are myopic accommodating less than patients who are emmetropic for a given stimulus (62,78,79). Those who are myopic, compared with emmetropic, show decreased accommodative response to negative lenses on the average of 0.90 D for a 3.00-D stimulus. No such difference was demonstrated for relaxation of accommodation through plus lenses. It is postulated that myopic patients may have a decreased sensitivity to blur (80).

Accommodative Facility

Normal

Accommodative facility is traditionally evaluated over a 1-minute period using plus and minus 2.00-D lens flippers (81). Normal is usually considered 8 cpm binocularly and 11 cpm monocularly (82). These norms were generated from the responses of adult subjects aged 18 to 30 years using the SOV9 acuity suppression vectogram.

Abnormal

Failure is usually considered less than 8 cpm binocularly and less than 11 cpm monocularly, and a difference of 4 cpm between the eyes is suggestive of accommodative dysfunction (82). Using a failure criterion of 3 cpm or less binocularly on accommodative facility testing has been shown to differentiate symptomatic from asymptomatic patients (83). Performance between 3 and 8 cpm is suggests binocular vision-related symptoms (83,84). For vision screening purposes, to minimize possible over referral, the recommended failure criterion is less than 3 cpm binocularly and less than 6 cpm monocularly, which is one standard deviation below the means (81).

Failures of accommodative facility testing can be categorized as *high fails* and *low fails* (81,85). For monocular testing, high fails is greater than 6 cpm but less than 11 cpm and low fails is less than 6 cpm. For binocular testing, high fails is greater than 3 cpm but less than 8 cpm and low fails is less than 3 cpm. Categorization in this way is useful when consideration is given to performing an extended facility testing beyond the 1-minute test time. Rouse et al. (81,85) showed that if accommodative facility testing is extended from 1 minute to 3 minutes, an improvement is expected more for the high fail group than low fail group for both monocular and binocular conditions. From the findings, they recommend performing extended facility testing of an additional 1 or 2 minutes in asymptomatic patients with initial monocular facility findings of between 6 and 11 cpm or binocular facility findings of between 3 and 8 cpm to arrive at an accurate diagnosis.

Children versus Adults

It is clear that children do not perform as many cpm on facility testing as do adults. Patients 6 and 7 years of age have been shown to perform fewer cpm on facility testing, partially attributed to their slower responses (48). Norms established for children 12 years and under are from a study by Scheiman et al. (86). This study suggested using a failure criterion monocularly of less than 4.5 cpm for children 8 to 12 years of age, and below 3 cpm for those who are 6 years of age.

Test Parameters

A number of factors inherent in the testing protocol can influence the facility results. These include the manual manipulation of the lens flippers, the involvement of saccadic eye movements, and the minification and magnification of the target by the lenses (87). Lower lens powers, larger target size, and shorter test distance results in higher accommodative facility (88). These variables stress the importance of using the same testing conditions in a clinical situation as those used to derive the norms. Prior to the Zellers et al. (82) study, a variety of lens powers and arbitrary failure rates were used to evaluate accommodative dysfunction in various populations (45). Setting a pass criterion of a high number of cpm with high-powered lenses will result in a higher failure rate for accommodative facility.

Suppression Control

The use of a suppression check and the type of suppression monitoring method used results in different facility findings. Facility testing performed with or without suppression check results in very different findings, with differences in the magnitude of 2.5 cpm higher (44) to 7 cpm higher (47) without suppression control. Additionally, the type of suppression control target can substantially influence the outcome (89). Commercially available vectographic targets are the Polaroid bar reader, which is a vectographic sheet with alternate Polaroid and clear bars, and the SOV9 acuity suppression vectogram. Accommodative facility rate using the Polaroid bar reader was lower than with the SOV9 acuity suppression vectogram of 8.56 cpm versus 11.02 cpm, respectively. More significantly, more than 40% of the subjects were unable to complete the Polaroid bar reader for 1 minute because of suppression or diplopia, compared with less than 2% of the same subjects unable to complete testing with the SOV9 acuity suppression vectogram (89). Anaglyph suppression control targets result in an even higher percentage of individuals unable to complete facility testing compared to Polaroid targets (90).

Testing Duration

Repetition of accommodative facility testing over time, such as repeat testing over a 3-week period, can result in significant increases in passing rates, particularly for those patients who are considered *high fails* (91). No significant diurnal variations have been observed, however (92). Variability on repeat testing is more likely in symptomatic patients. Performing the test for 30 seconds compared with 1 minute may not make a difference in the assessment of accommodative facility (88).

Learning Disabled

It has been suggested that one reason why the learning disabled population has such a high prevalence of accommodative infacility is because of verbal response delays in reporting clarity (45).

Relative Accommodation

The norm values for prepresbyopic patients are 2.00 ±0.50 D for NRA and 2.37 ±1.00 D for PRA (93). Less than 1.50 D for NRA or PRA, or a difference of 1.00 D are indications of possible inadequate accommodation function (5).

DIAGNOSIS OF ACCOMMODATIVE DYSFUNCTION

Case History

The symptoms related to nonpresbyopic accommodative dysfunction are consistent in presentation and include reduced visual efficiency; headaches, particularly a dull brow ache; asthenopia related to near work; avoidance of near work; blur at near; fatigue with reading; adaptation of a close working distance; and temporary blurring of vision when shifting from near to distance or vice versa. Therefore, pointed case history questions can give the clinician information early on in the examination to whether an accommodative disorder may exist (5,7,59,94,95). Ask the parents if the child has difficulty with concentration and attention with near work. How long can the child read or do near work before symptoms of blurred vision, headaches, or eyestrain develop? Ask the child if his or her eyes feel tired or hurt, or if his or her head hurts after reading for a little while. If the child avoids reading or extensive near work, there may be no symptoms.

Classification

Anomalies of accommodation can be separated into five distinct categories: (a) insufficiency of accommodation, (b) ill-sustained accommodation, (c) infacility of accommodation,

TABLE 18.3 Summary of Accommodative Anomalies and Their Associated Clinical Findings

Accommodative insufficiency	Low accommodative amplitude
	Low PRA
	Fails monocular and binocular accommodative facility with minus lenses
	Esophoria at near
	High lag of accommodation
Ill-sustained accommodation	Initial normal amplitude of accommodation, decreases with repeated attempts
	Low PRA
	Fails monocular and binocular accommodative facility, decreased performance over time
	Esophoria at near
	High lag of accommodation
Accommodative infacility	Fails monocular and binocular accommodative facility with plus and minus lenses, with equal difficulty through plus and minus
	Low PRA and NRA
Accommodative spasm or excess	Fails monocular and binocular accommodative facility with plus lenses
	Lead of accommodation
	Esophoria at near and distance
	Low PRA
Accommodative paresis or paralysis	Considerable reduction in accommodative amplitude monocular or binocular not improved with rest
	High lag of accommodation
	Reduced near acuity
	Dilated pupil

PRA, positive relative accommodation; NRA, negative relative accommodation.

(d) spasm or excess accommodation, and (e) paresis or paralysis of accommodation (9). This is known as the Duke-Elder classification (94). Table 18.3 provides a summary of the associated clinical findings for these anomalies of accommodation. More than one area of accommodative function should be tested in patients to achieve a more accurate clinical diagnosis. Wick and Hall (84) found only 4% of patients with accommodative deficiencies in accommodative facility, lag, or amplitude had failures on all three functions. Furthermore, accommodative findings should be evaluated in relation to other findings, including symptoms and additional binocular tests. A properly working accommodative system is particularly important for binocular function, especially when one is reminded that accommodative convergence usually contributes about two thirds of the convergence necessary, with the other one third supplied by fusional convergence, for clear, single binocular vision (96).

Accommodative Insufficiency

Diagnosis

Accommodative insufficiency is by far the most frequently reported of the accommodative dysfunctions (95). Decreased amplitude of accommodation of at least 2.00 D below the minimal age-appropriate amplitude is usually an essential single clinical finding to diagnose accommodative insufficiency (97). Other authors have offered a multiple sign criteria, but without consensus (42,63,98). Additional clinical signs include a positive relative accommodation less than or equal to 1.25 D, greater than +0.75 D lag on MEM, failure on monocular accommodative facility, or failure on binocular accommodative facility. Cacho et al. (97), the only ones who have attempted to determine the most sensitive test(s) for diagnosis of accommodative insufficiency, concluded that an abnormal monocular accommodative facility (not MEM, binocular accommodative facility, or positive relative accommodation) test finding is most associated with reduced accommodative amplitudes in symptomatic patients.

Association with Binocular Dysfunction

An excessive lag of accommodation can indicate latent hyperopia, accommodative insufficiency, esophoria, or other disorders of binocular function (24). This underaccommodation can be secondary to a decreased negative fusional vergence ability, particularly in the case of overconvergence.

Association with Strabismus

Reduced accommodation amplitudes and poor sustaining ability have been associated with strabismus (99). In cases where accommodation dysfunction is primary and the strabismus is secondary, a patient may exhibit esotropia because of excessive accommodative convergence, and a patient with exophoria may experience an increase in the frequency of exotropia secondary to decreased accommodative convergence as well as reduced fusional abilities secondary to poor focus.

Special Population

Children with Down syndrome consistently show reduced accommodation that can be as large as 5.00 D for a target at 25 cm (~10 inches) (100). It is believed that the reduced accommodative response is neural in origin and does not appear to improve with lens correction. This poses a difficult clinical management situation for these children who are functioning with decreased near visual acuities in a learning environment.

Children with cerebral palsy have a much higher prevalence of accommodative disorders. Leat (101) found 42% of her subjects had reduced accommodative responses, with 29% having accommodative amplitudes of 4.00 D or less.

Dyslexics may have accommodative dysfunction that is not a cause of their dyslexia, but it may coexist and potentially contribute to reading asthenopia. Evans et al. (102) found dyslexics have lower amplitudes of accommodation than the control group. Others have found that reading disabled children have a larger lag of

accommodation (103). Thus, treatment of identified accommodative dysfunction in these individuals will enhance near task performance.

Ill-Sustained Accommodation

Diagnosis

Ill-sustained accommodation is a reduction in accommodative function with extended accommodative use, despite normal accommodative amplitudes (1,94). If the accommodative amplitude test is repeated at the end of the examination or the test is performed three or four times, the clinician gains insight into the patient's ability to sustain accommodation. Performing dynamic retinoscopy and having the child maintain attention and focus on the near target for more than a few seconds can also provide a measure of a patient's ability to sustain accommodation (104).

Accommodative Excess or Accommodative Spasm

Diagnosis

Accommodative spasm is often used interchangeably with accommodative excess, a condition whereby accommodation is maintained in the absence of a stimulus or the accommodative response to a near stimulus demand is excessive (96,105). Accommodative spasm can be unilateral or bilateral and can be constant or intermittent. A lead of accommodation is the hallmark finding in the diagnosis of accommodative spasm, often with blurred distance vision (1). Scheiman and Wick (42) differentiate accommodative excess from accommodative spasm. They describe accommodative excess as a much milder form of accommodative spasm, more commonly seen clinically with signs of reduced lag of accommodation, difficulty clearing +2.00 D monocularly, and reduced negative relative accommodation. A more extreme form of accommodative spasm is found along with overconvergence and pupillary miosis, and is called spasm of the near reflex (SNR) (105).

Etiology

The etiology of accommodative spasm and accommodative excess is associated with uncorrected refractive errors, extensive near work, vergence problems, latent hyperopia, and psychogenic factors (105). Many of the true accommodative spasm cases are psychogenic in origin. Other causes include cholinergic drug side effects and myasthenia gravis (1). SNR is usually psychogenic in origin, but has been documented in patients with organic disease (e.g., cerebellar and pituitary tumors) and after head trauma (105). Accommodative excess is more associated with symptoms related to prolonged near tasks, and binocular ineffi-ciencies that affect accommodative function as the patient strives to maintain clear, single and comfortable vision (42). Thus, a finding of overaccommodation may be secondary to the presence of exophoria and low positive fusional vergence ability.

Accommodative Infacility

Diagnosis

Accommodative facility tested under monocu-lar conditions is the primary method of diagnos-ing accommodative infacility. If the patient has equal difficulty clearing plus and minus lenses, this is an indication of infacility. If a patient passes the monocular accommodative facility test, it is unlikely an accommodative problem exists (106). Ease in clearing the plus lens and failure with the minus lens is indicative of dif-ficulty with stimulation of accommodation and points to an accommodative insufficiency, par-ticularly with the presence of reduced accom-modative amplitudes. A patient with a quick re-sponse in clearing the minus lens but slow with clearing the plus lens is consistent with accom-modative excess tendencies (45).

Relationship to Learning

Although a high prevalence of accommodative dysfunction has been reported in the learn-ing disabled population, failure of accommoda-tive facility testing alone is not predictive of academic performance in the areas of writing, mathematics, reading, or gymnastics (107). Be-cause of the possible variability in patient re-sponses, facility test results should be correlated to symptoms and other binocular test findings to determine the relevance of the test find-

ings in the overall management of the patient's condition.

Paresis or Paralysis of Accommodation

Diagnosis

Paresis of accommodation is a considerable de-gree of insufficiency, usually of sudden onset and having an organic cause (9). The failure of the accommodative system to respond to any stimulus is called *paralysis of accommodation*, a very rare condition (52).

Etiology

Etiologic factors of accommodative paresis in-clude infectious conditions, food poisoning, and diabetes. Paralysis of the ciliary muscles can cause paralysis of accommodation, despite a physically normal crystalline lens (94). The cause of such a paralysis can be a congenital anomaly, secondary to drugs with cycloplegic ef-fects, infective, toxic, traumatic, or neurologic. Conditions that cause generalized body weak-ness (e.g., malnutrition, anemia, diabetes, en-docrine anomalies, and infectious diseases) can also affect the ciliary muscles (94). Paralysis of accommodation can be bilateral or unilateral (1). Unequal accommodation in the two eyes seems to be caused by unequal rigidity of the crystalline lens and its existence supports testing accommodative amplitude monocularly (6).

TREATMENT OF ACCOMMODATIVE DISORDERS

The two most common treatments for ac-commodative dysfunction are the prescription of nearpoint lenses and vision therapy. Be-fore treatment of accommodative disorders with lenses or therapy, it is imperative to de-termine that no underlying systemic disease or drug-induced effects exist. Successful treat-ment, with at least partial relief of accommoda-tive symptoms and improvement in objective findings, with lenses and therapy are docu-mented (45,98,108,109). Nearpoint lenses are indicated for patients with findings of a large lag of accommodation, very low positive relative accommodation, and failure on ±2.00 D binoc-ular facility test. The correction of refractive errors alone after 1 month of spectacle wear can result in a passive improvement of accommodative lag, facility, and amplitude (110).

Accommodative dysfunction can be found in association with other binocular anomalies, including convergence insufficiency and reduced stereopsis (9). When other anomalies coexist, therapy rather than lenses may be more effective (52,98,111). Reported treatment successes do not always include the percentage of patients who were fully treated or whether all aspects of accommodation were remedied (i.e., response, facility, and amplitude). Differences in treatment successes can be attributed to different therapies (home vs. office), the duration of therapy, as well as the pretherapy statuses of their accommodative systems. Most documented vision therapy success case studies have only involved small samples, highlighting the need for additional documentation on the effectivity of lenses, including prisms, and therapy in the remediation of functional accommodative dysfunction.

SUMMARY

A complete examination of a child's accommodative system should include tests for accommodative amplitude, response, and facility. Accommodative dysfunction can present in a child with a range of symptoms from blurred vision and headaches, to motion sickness and avoidance of near work. These symptoms can interfere with a child's academic performance and result in a decreased quality of life. Reduced accommodative function can also be secondary to a variety of ocular, neurologic, and systemic conditions. Thus, a thorough review of symptoms, ocular and medical histories, together with clinical findings are necessary to reach an accurate diagnosis and prescribe an appropriate management plan.

REFERENCES

1. AOA. *Optometric Clinical Practice Guideline Care of the Patient with Accommodative and Vergence Dysfunction.* St. Louis: AOA, 2001.
2. Bennett GR, Blondin M, Ruskiewicz J. Incidence and prevalence of selected visual conditions. *Journal of the American Optometric Association* 1982;53(8):647–656.
3. Chernick B. Profile of peripheral visual anomalies in the disabled reader. *Journal of the American Optometric Association* 1978;49(10):1117–1118.
4. Sherman A. Relating vision disorders to learning disability. *Journal of the American Optometric Association* 1973;44(2):140–141.
5. Weisz CL. How to find and treat accommodative disorders. *Review of Optometry* 1983;120(1):48–54.
6. Duane A. Studies in monocular and binocular accommodation with their clinical applications. *Am J Ophthalmol* 1922;5:865–877.
7. Mazow ML, France TD, Finkleman S, et al. Acute accommodative and convergence insufficiency. *Trans Am Ophthalmol Soc* 1989;87:158–173.
8. Chrousos GA, O'Neill JF, Lueth BD, et al. Accommodation deficiency in healthy young individuals. *J Pediatr Ophthalmol Strabismus* 1988;25(4):176–179.
9. Daum KM. Accommodative dysfunction. *Doc Ophthalmol* 1983;55:177–198.
10. Hofstetter HW. Factors involved in low amplitude cases. *American Journal of Optometry and Physiological Optics* 1942;19(7):279–289.
11. Cooper J, Kruger P, Panariello GF. The pathognomonic pattern of accommodative fatigue in myasthenia gravis. *Binocul Vis Strabismus Q* 1988;3(3):141–148.
12. Moss SE, Klein R, Klein BEK. Accommodative ability in younger-onset diabetes. *Arch Ophthalmol* 1987;105:508–512.
13. DeRespinis PA, Shen JJ, Wagner RS. Guillain-Barré syndrome presenting as a paralysis of accommodation. *Arch Ophthalmol* 1989;107:1282.
14. AOA. *Pediatric Eye and Vision Examination. Optometric Clinical Practice Guideline.* St. Louis: AOA, 2002.
15. Woehrle MB, Peters RJ, Frantz KA. Accommodative amplitude determination: can we substitute the pull-away for the push-up method? *Journal of Optometric Vision Development* 1997;28:246–249.
16. Yothers T, Wick B, Morse SE. Clinical testing of accommodative facility. Part II. Development of an amplitude-scaled test. *Optometry* 2002;73(2):91–101.
17. Atchison DA, Capper CJ, McCabe KL. Critical subjective measurement of amplitude of accommodation. *Optom Vis Sci* 1994;71:699–706.
18. Chen AH, O'Leary DJ. Validity and repeatability of the modified push-up method for measuring the amplitude of accommodation. *Clinical and Experimental Optometry* 1998;81(2):63–71.
19. Pollock J. Accommodation measurement-clear or blurred? *Australian Orthoptic Journal* 1989;25:20–22.
20. Eskridge JB. Clinical objective assessment of the accommodative response. *Journal of the American Optometric Association* 1989;60(11):272–275.
21. Bieber JC. Why nearpoint retinoscopy with children? *Optometric Weekly* 1974;65(3):23–26.
22. Rutstein RP, Fuhr PD, Swiatocha J. Comparing the amplitude of accommodation determined objectively and subjectively. *Optom Vis Sci* 1993;70(6):496–500.
23. Millodot M, Newton I. VEP measurement of the amplitude of accommodation. *Br J Ophthalmol* 1981;65:294–298.
24. Tassinari JT. Monocular estimate method retinoscopy: central tendency measures and relationship to refractive status and heterophoria. *Optom Vis Sci* 2002;79(11):708–714.
25. Leat SJ, Gargon JL. Accommodative response in children and young adults using dynamic retinoscopy. *Ophthalmic Physiol Opt* 1996;16(5):375–384.
26. Moses RA. *Adler's Physiology of the Eye,.* 5th ed. St. Louis: CV Mosby; 1970:366.
27. Daum KM. Accommodative response. In: Eskridge JB, Amos JF, Bartlett JD, eds. *Clinical Procedures in Optometry.* Philadelphia: JB Lippincott; 1991:677–686.

28. Nott IS. Dynamic skiametry, accommodation and convergence. *American Journal of Optometry and Psyological Optics* 1920;6:490–503.

29. Wolffsohn JS, Gilmartin B, Mallen EAH, et al. Continuous recording of accommodation and pupil size using the Shin-Nippon SRW-5000 autorefractor. *Ophthalmic Physiol Opt* 2001;21(2):108–113.

30. Haynes HM. Clinical approaches to nearpoint lens power determination. *American Journal of Optometry and Psyological Optics* 1985;62(6):375–385.

31. Rosenfield M, Portello JK, Blustein GH, et al. Comparison of clinical techniques to assess the near accommodative response. *Optom Vision Sci* 1996;73(6): 382–388.

32. McClelland JF, Saunders KJ. The repeatability and validity of dynamic retinoscopy in assessing the accommodative response. *Ophthalmic Physiol Opt* 2003;23:243–250.

33. Locke LC, Somers W. A comparison study of dynamic retinoscopy techniques. *Optom Vis Sci* 1989;66:540–544.

34. Cacho MP, Munoz AG, Garcia-Bernabeu JR, et al. Comparison between MEM and Nott dynamic retinoscopy. *Optom Vis Sci* 1999;76(9):650–655.

35. Apell RJ. Clinical application of Bell retinoscopy. *Journal of the American Optometric Association* 1975;46(10):1023–1027.

36. Pheiffer CH. Book retinoscopy. *Am J Optom Am Acad Optom* 1955;32(10):540–545.

37. Getman GN. Techniques and diagnostic criteria for the optometric care of children's vision. Santa Ana, Ca.: Optometric Extension Program, 1960.

38. Press LJ. Examination of the school-aged child. In: Press LJ, Moore BD, ed. *Clinical Pediatric Optometry.* Boston: Butterworth-Heinemann; 1993:63–80.

39. Howland HC, Howland B. Photorefraction: a technique for study of refractive state at a distance. *J Opt Soc Am* 1974;64:240–249.

40. Seidemann A, Schaeffel F. An evaluation of the lag of accommodation using photorefraction. *Vision Res* 2003;43:419–430.

41. Carlson NB. *Clinical Procedures for Ocular Examination.* Norwalk: Appleton & Lange, 1996.

42. Scheiman M, Wick B. Accommodative techniques. In: Scheiman M, Wick B, eds. *Clinical Management of Binocular Vision.* Philadelphia: JB Lippincott; 1994:199–210.

43. Rosner J. *Pediatric Optometry.* Boston: Butterworth-Heinemann; 1990:256–269.

44. Burge S. Suppression during binocular accommodative rock. *Optometric Monthly* 1979;79:867–872.

45. Garzia RP, Richman JE. Accommodative facility: a study of young adults. *Journal of the American Optometric Association* 1982;53(10):821–825.

46. Gallaway M, Scheiman M. Assessment of accommodative facility using MEM retinoscopy. *Journal of the American Optometric Association* 1990;61:36–39.

47. Wick B, Yothers TL, Jiang B. Clinical testing of accommodative facility. Part I. A critical appraisal of the literature. *Optometry* 2002;73(1):11–23.

48. Wick B, Gall R, Yothers T. Clinical testing of accommodative facility. Part III. Masked assessment of the relation between visual symptoms and binocular test results in school children and adults. *Optometry* 2002;73:173–181.

49. Haynes HM. The distance rock test-a preliminary report. *Journal of the American Optometric Association* 1979;50(6):707–713.

50. Rouse MW, Freestone GM, Weiner BA. Comparative study of computer-based and standard clinical accommodative facility testing methods. *Optom Vis Sci* 1991;68(2):88–95.

51. Goss DA. Clinical accommodation testing. *Curr Opin Ophthalmol* 1992;3:78–82.

52. Cooper J. Accommodative dysfunction. In: Amos JF, ed. *Diagnosis and Management in Vision Care.* Boston: Butterworth-Heineman; 1987:431–459.

53. Goss DA. Effects of lag of accommodation and proximal convergence on zone of clear single binocular vision. In: Goss DA, ed. *Ocular Accommodation, Convergence, and Fixation Disparity: A Manual of Clinical Analysis.* New York: Professional Press; 1986:35 and 39.

54. Jackson TW, Goss DA. Variation and correlation of clinical tests of accommodative function in a sample of school-age children. *Journal of the American Optometric Association* 1991;62(11):857–866.

55. Chen AH, O'Leary DJ, Howell ER. Near visual function in young children. Part I: near point of convergence. Part II: Amplitude of accommodation. Part III: Near heterophoria. *Ophthalmic Physiol Opt* 2000;20(3):185–198.

56. Duane A. Normal values of the accommodation at all ages. *JAMA* 1912;59:1010–1013.

57. Eames TH. Accommodation in school children, aged five, six, seven and eight years. *Am J Ophthalmol* 1961;51:1255–1257.

58. Hoffstetter HW. Useful age-amplitude formula. *Optometric World* 1950;38(11):42–45.

59. Hoffman LG, Rouse M. Referral recommendations for binocular function and/or developmental perceptual deficiencies. *Journal of the American Optometric Association* 1980;51:119–125.

60. Kragha IKOK. Measurement of amplitude of accommodation. *Ophthalmic Physiol Opt* 1989;9:342–343.

61. Rutstein RA, Daum K. Anomalies of accommodation. In: Rutstein RA, ed. *Anomalies of Binocular Vision: Diagnosis and Management.* St. Louis: CV Mosby, 1998.

62. Gwiazda J, Thorn F, Bauer J, et al. Myopic children show insufficient accommodative response to blur. *Invest Ophthalmol Vis Sci* 1993;34(3):690–694.

63. Hokoda SC, Ciuffreda KJ. Measurement of accommodative amplitude in amblyopia. *Ophthalmic Physiol Opt* 1982;2(3):205–212.

64. Rosenfield M, Cohen AS. Repeatability of clinical measurements of the amplitude of accommodation. *Ophthalmic Physiol Opt* 1996;16:247–249.

65. London R. Amplitude of accommodation. In: Eskridge JB, Amos JF, Bartlett JD, eds. *Clinical Procedures in Optometry.* Philadelphia: JB Lippincott; 1991:69–71.

66. von Noorden GK, Avilla CW. Accommodative convergence in hypermetropia. *Am J Ophthalmol* 1990;110:287–292.

67. Rouse MW, London R, Allen DC. An evaluation of the monocular estimate method of dynamic retinoscopy. *American Journal of Optometry and Psyological Optics* 1982;59(3):234–239.

68. Morgan MW. The clinical aspects of accommodation and convergence. *American Journal of Optometry and Archives of the American Academy of Optometry* 1944;21:301–313.

69. Ciuffreda K. The Glenn A. Fry invited lecture. Accommodation to gratings and more naturalistic stimuli. *Optom Vis Sci* 1991;68:243–260.

70. Heath GG. The influence of visual acuity on accommodative responses of the eye. *American Journal of Optometry and Archives of the American Academy of Optometry* 1956;33(10):513–524.

71. Hennessy RT, Iida T, Shina K. The effect of pupil size on accommodation. *Vision Res* 1975;16:587–589.

72. Gilmartin B. A review of the role of sympathetic innervation of the ciliary muscle in ocular accommodation. *Ophthalmic Physiol Opt* 1986;6(1):23–37.

73. Lovasik JV, Kergoat H, Kothe AC. The influence of letter size on the focusing response of the eye. *Journal of the American Optometric Association* 1987;58(8):631–639.

74. Salibello C. Comparing a printed image and a Gaussian image diagnostic system for prescribing VDT eyewear. *Journal of Behavioral Optometry* 1994;5:59–61.

75. Kolker D, Hutchinson R, Nilsen E. Comparison of tests of accommodation for computer users. *Optometry* 2002;73(4):212–220.

76. Penisten DK, Goss DA, Philpott GP, et al. Comparisons of dynamic retinoscopy measurements with a print card, a video display terminal, and a PRIO system tester as test targets. *Optometry* 2004;75(4):231–240.

77. Sorkin RE, Reich LN, Pizzimenti J. Accommodative response to PRIO computer vision tester versus printed text. *Optometry* 2003;74(12):782–786.

78. McBrien NA, Millodot. The effect of refractive error on the accommodative response gradient. *Ophthalmic Physiol Opt* 1986;6(2):145–149.

79. O'Leary DJ, Allen PM. Facility of accommodation in myopia. *Ophthalmic Physiol Opt* 2001;21(5):352–355.

80. Radhakrishnan H, Pardhan S, Calver RI, et al. Unequal reduction in visual acuity with positive and negative defocusing lenses in myopes. *Optom Vis Sci* 2004;81(1):14–17.

81. Rouse MW, Deland PN, Chous R. Monocular accommodative facility testing reliability. *Optom Vis Sci* 1989;66(2):72–77.

82. Zellers JA, Alpert TL, Rouse MW. A review of the literature and a normative study of accommodative facility. *Journal of the American Optometric Association* 1984;55(1):31–37.

83. Hennessey D, Iosue R, Rouse M. Relation of symptoms to accommodative facility of school-aged children. *American Journal of Optometry and Physiological Optics* 1984;61:177–183.

84. Wick B, Hall P. Relation among accommodative facility, lag, and amplitude in elementary school children. *American Journal of Optometry and Physiological Optics* 1987;64(8):593–598.

85. Rouse MW, Deland PN, Mozayani S. Binocular accommodative facility testing reliability. *Optom Vis Sci* 1992;69:314–319.

86. Scheiman M, Herzberg H, Frantz K, et al. Normative study of accommodative facility in elementary school children. *American Journal of Optometry and Physiological Optics* 1988;65:127–134.

87. Kedzia B, Pieczyrak D, Tondel G, et al. Factors affecting the clinical testing of accommodative facility. *Ophthalmic Physiol Opt* 1999;19(1):12–21.

88. Siderov J, Johnston AW. The importance of the test parameters in the clinical assessment of accommodative facility. *Optom Vis Sci* 1990;67:551–557.

89. Zost MG, Hogan CL, Sakihara DT. Binocular facility of accommodation testing: comparison of the vectogram #9 target/method vs. the Polaroid bar reader/rock card method. *J Behav Optom* 1998;9(5):121–125.

90. Pica M, Redmond M, Zost M. Polarized versus anaglyphic materials for suppression control in binocular accommodative facility testing. *Journal of Behavioral Optometry* 1996;7(2):43–45.

91. McKenzie KM, Kerr SR, Rouse MW. Study of accommodative facility testing reliability. *American Journal of Optometry and Psyological Optics* 1987;64(3):186–194.

92. Levine S, Ciuffreda KJ, Selenow A. Clinical assessment of accommodative facility in symptomatic and asymptomatic individuals. *Journal of the American Optometric Association* 1985;56(4):286–290.

93. Borish IM. Phorometry. In: Borish IM, ed. *Clinical Refraction*, 3rd ed. Chicago: Professional Press, 1970:843–845.

94. Duke-Elder S, Abrams D. Ophthalmic optics and refraction. In: Duke-Elder S, ed. *System of Ophthalmology*, Vol 5. St Louis: CV Mosby; 1970:451–486.

95. Daum KM. Accommodative insufficiency. *American Journal of Optometry and Physiological Optics* 1983;60(5):352–359.

96. Nott IS. Dynamic skiametry. Accommodative convergence and fusion convergence. *Am J Physiol Opt* 1920;7:366–374.

97. Cacho P, Garcia A, Francisco L. Diagnostic signs of accommodative insufficiency. *Optom Vis Sci* 2002;79(9):614–620.

98. Rouse MW. Management of binocular anomalies: efficacy of vision therapy in the treatment of accommodative deficiencies. *American Journal of Optometry and Psyological Optics* 1987;64:415–420.

99. Rutstein RP, Daum KM. Exotropia associated with defective accommodation. *Journal of the American Optometric Association* 1987;58(7):548–554.

100. Cregg M, Woodhouse JM, Pakeman VH, et al. Accommodation and refractive error in children with Down syndrome: cross-sectional and longitudinal studies. *Invest Ophthalmol Vis Sci* 2001;42:55–63.

101. Leat SJ. Reduced accommodation in children with cerebral palsy. *Ophthalmic Physiol Opt* 1996;16:375–384.

102. Evans BJW, Drasdo N, Richards IL. Investigation of accommodative and binocular function in dyslexia. *Opthalmic Physiol Opt* 1994;14:5–19.

103. Poynter H, Schor C, Haynes H, et al. Oculomotor functions in reading disability. *American Journal of Optometry and Psyological Optics* 1982;59:116–127.

104. Hunter DG. Dynamic retinoscopy: the missing data. *Surv Opthalmol* 2001;46(3):269–274.

105. Rutstein, RP, Daum KM, Amos JF. Accommodative spasm: a study of 17 cases. *Journal of the American Optometric Association* 1988;59(7):527–538.

106. Garcia A, Cacho P, Lara F, et al. The relation between accommodative facility and general binocular dysfunction. *Ophthalmic Physiol Opt* 2000;20(2):98–104.

107. Kedzia, B, Tondel G, Pieczyrak D, et al. Accommodative facility test results and academic success in Polish second graders. *Journal of the American Optometric Association* 1999;70(2):110–116.

108. Cooper J, Feldman J, Selenow A, et al. Reduction of asthenopia after accommodative facility training. *American Journal of Optometry and Physiological Optics* 1987;64:430–436.

109. Wold RM, Pierce JR, Keddington J. Effectiveness of optometric vision therapy. *Journal of the American Optometric Association* 1978;49(9):1047–1054.

110. Dwyer P, Wick B. The influence of refractive correction upon disorders of vergence and accommodation. *Optom Vis Sci* 1995;72(4):224–232.

111. Bobier WR, Sivak JG. Orthoptic treatment of subjects showing slow accommodative responses. *American Journal of Optometry and Physiological Optics* 1983;60:678–687.

Pediatric Color Vision Testing

19

Jay M. Cohen

This chapter, written for the clinician, is intended to be a practical and realistic clinical guide for the color vision testing of the pediatric patient. Discussion is limited mostly to color vision tests that are widely used and accepted, and are currently commercially available. The physiology and development of color vision and color deficiency is covered elsewhere in the text (see Chapter 8).

Color is an attribute of human vision that adds aesthetics and diversity to the visual percept. It provides unique and characteristic information about the world and the objects in it, and it is often used as the primary descriptor for identifying specific items (e.g. "the blue one over there").

Many people, however, have abnormal color vision and are unable to utilize color information with the same efficiency or surety as the rest of the population at large. These individuals, mostly males, are at a distinct disadvantage or are incapacitated when faced with performing activities based heavily on color information. The seriousness of the consequences of this handicap can range from merely inconvenient to life threatening.

Although patients are often labeled by the term *color blind*, this is a misnomer. These patients do perceive color, albeit differently than those with normal color vision. For the purposes of this chapter, the term *color deficiency*, a more apt description, is used in place of color blindness.

Most persons with color deficiencies are unaware, or at best minimally aware, of their problem, and it behooves the conscientious eye care practitioner to identify and educate these patients about the implications of their condition, both for their own personal safety and knowledge as well as for the safety of the general public.

Because color is such a vital part of the preschool and elementary school experience, it is especially important to identify children with color deficits at the earliest possible age. The rationale for early identification is twofold. First, short-term implications involve the need to isolate those children with the potential for academic difficulties because of their inability to respond to color-based curricular items and, if necessary, to plan appropriate interventions via altered curricula. Second, long-term implications are concerned with career counseling and the discussion of realistic options and goals for higher education and employment.

The main emphasis of this chapter is on the diagnosis and classification of hereditary red-green color vision defects, the overwhelming bulk of color anomalies. Hereditary blue-yellow defects are so rare that few color vision tests bother to check for them. Likewise, acquired color defects are not common in a normal pediatric population, especially without other more serious and obvious visual signs and symptoms.

COLOR VISION HISTORY

As with most aspects of health care, the first step in assessing color vision begins with a good case history. Hereditary red-green color vision defects, which affect approximately 8% of males and 0.5% of females, are transmitted in a predictable manner via the x-chromosome. A positive history of color vision problems on the maternal line (grandfather, sibling, or cousin) places a child, particularly males, in a high-risk category and warrants more aggressive screening protocol. A positive history from both parents should *red flag* even females for careful scrutiny.

It should be appreciated, however, that taking a family history for color vision anomalies has its limitations. Accurate information on lineage is often lacking because many affected family members may be unaware of a problem, or they may actively hide its presence. Therefore, although a positive history is helpful, a negative history is of uncertain value.

Another aspect of the case history for children is the parents' report of color vision performance problems. When questioning parents about their child's color ability, it is important to distinguish between color confusions and color naming skills. Color discrimination is present by 2 to 3 months of age (1), whereas accurate color naming may not develop until a child is 4 to 6 years of age (2). A child who is unable to discriminate between different confusion colors is likely to have a color deficiency, whereas a child who is unable to consistently name colors may be perfectly normal.

As noted earlier regarding lineage, parental observation of color vision performance can be misleading because of the child's desire to conform and the natural coping strategies used by color-deficient children. For example, many of my adult color-deficient patients report that, as children, they would only color with whole crayons so that they could read the color name on the wrapper. Another patient, who was deuteranopic, recounted how his family car appeared brown to him, however, he called it green because everybody else did.

Although adult patients may deny or trivialize their color defect, on careful questioning, those with significant anomalies will usually be-grudgingly admit to some difficulties and to an awareness of their variance from the color normal population. Thus, despite its shortcomings a good case history still remains one of the key factors in identifying potential color vision abnormality.

SIGNIFICANCE OF TEST DESIGN

The actual determination of color deficiency, however, is based on the results of clinically administered color vision tests. A wide assortment of color vision tests has evolved over the years. Many tests were never commercially available or are no longer available, and many tests have been shown to be unreliable. Our discussion will be limited to those tests with established reliability that are commonly available and used in the United States.

Doctors use many types of tests for assessing color vision. They are designed for a variety of purposes and measure different aspects of the color sense. Therefore, the proper administration of a color test requires a basic understanding of the test's design and strategy to ensure that it is appropriate for the age of the patient as well as the color function it is presumed to be measuring.

No single color vision test can provide complete information about a patient's color vision status. Instead, a battery of tests is selected to separate those with normal color vision from those who are color defective and then to further classify and grade the severity of any defects. Additional tests can be given to rate the patient's color discrimination abilities to determine that patient's aptitude for performing color-based activities.

The design of a color vision test will usually be influenced by its intended function. Screening tests are meant to be short, sensitive, and easily administered tests that differentiate patients with normal color vision from color-deficient patients, or those with generally good color skills from those with problematic color skills. They can also include provisions for classifying the type and severity of the defect.

Performance tests are designed to evaluate the level of some aspect of color ability. These tests are usually lengthier and broader in scope than screening tests. Tests that utilize color from the entire color circle give a better indication of real world function than those that use only a narrow range of colors along the red-green confusion axes.

Performance tests, such as lantern tests, attempt to simulate or duplicate color conditions of a particular task to predict those patients who will successfully manage the activity and those who will not.

Differences in design between tests can lead to differences in results. This is not unexpected and gives some balance to the testing process. Keep in mind when evaluating the results of any color vision test or tests is that they present a narrow, unnatural, preselected set of parameters that capitalize on the known vulnerable portions of the color circle. Be cautious not to overstep the bounds of the test design and to make unwarranted generalizations about a patient's color skills in the uncontrolled natural environment where a host of additional cues and adaptive behaviors may improve performance.

COLOR VISION TESTS

Color vision tests are made using a variety of strategies and tasks for measuring color vision and can be categorized by their strategy design. Test design strategies include aspects of color mixing, color matching, color discrimination, color arrangement, color naming, and color confusion.

Tests within a particular category are generally very similar and, within reason, will yield similar outcomes. Tests in different categories, however, do not necessarily measure the same color attributes and can produce differing results. When constructing a color vision test battery it is best, therefore, to use test probes with a variety of designs to gain information on the different aspects of the patient's color vision and to develop a fuller understanding of that patient's color abilities and limitations.

Anomaloscopy

The anomaloscope presents the patient with the task of mixing a spectrally pure red light with a spectrally pure green light to match a spectrally pure yellow light. It is the gold standard

of color vision testing, and it is the only test that will definitively identify the abnormal retinal pigment (protan vs. deutan) and determine the number of functioning pigments (dichromacy vs. anomalous trichromacy).

The anomaloscope, however, is not a clinical office test, and it is not a pediatric test. It is an expensive instrument requiring a sophisticated tester to administer it, and it is rarely found outside of a teaching or research institution. The testing protocol is relatively complex and is usually beyond the attentional and cognitive capabilities of most young children. If anomaloscopy is deemed necessary, it is best to wait until the child is older (at least 8 years old) and to refer to a clinic providing the test.

Pseudoisochromatic Plates

Pseudoisochromatic plates (PIP) are the major clinical test of color vision. They are relatively inexpensive, need short administration time and have low cognitive demands. On the other hand, PIP tests require good attentional and fixation skills, as well as good contrast and figure-ground capability.

The PIP are screening tests, in that they differentiate color normalcy from color variants. They do not determine the type of defect nor grade the severity of the defect. Only those tests incorporating additional plates especially designed for that purpose could be used to classify and grade the color vision defect. The common clinical practice of the using the number of screening plates correctly identified as a means of gauging severity of a color vision defect has no scientific basis.

The test plates consist of a mosaiclike array of colored dots which, when viewed under the proper light source, presents letters, lines, or geometric shapes constructed of confusion colors paired to the background. Those with normal color vision will see a particular target, whereas color-deficient patients will see a different target or nothing at all.

The two major plate types are the *vanishing plate* and the *transformation plate*. Vanishing plates are made so that people with normal color vision will see a target and those with color deficiency will not see a target. This design is very frustrating for the color-deficient patients because they are aware they are doing poorly, and the frustration and disbelief builds with each additional missed plate.

Transformation plates are constructed so that the person with normal color vision sees one target and the color-deficient patient sees a different one. This is a much less stressful condition than the vanishing plate because, by seeing a target, the patient is unaware of the poor showing.

Classification plates are a variation of the vanishing plates. They present two targets, one of which is more visible to patients with protan defects and the other of which is more visible to patients with deutan defects. The differential response determines the patient's classification. An estimate of severity can be made as well by using plates with different color saturations.

Although classification plates are useful, keep in mind that their results are not conclusive. Results of classification plate tests are not always in agreement with anomaloscopic findings and frequently do not agree with the results of other plate tests or arrangement tests. The reason it is necessary to perform a battery with multiple color tests is to establish a consensus of the findings. For a pediatric population, the most useful PIP are the Ishihara plates, the Hardy-Rand-Rittler plates, and Color Vision Testing Made Easy plates.

Ishihara Plates

The *Ishihara Pseudoisochromatic Plate Test* is the most widely used and accepted clinical color vision test. It is an unrivaled screening test for red-green color deficiencies with basic classification capability. The most appropriate test versions for the pediatric practice are the concise edition and the *Test for Unlettered Persons*.

The concise edition is a quick and efficient test with a total of 14 plates. The first 11 plates are for screening (1 demonstration plate, 9 number plates, and 1 wiggly line plate), and the last 3 are for classification (2 with numbers and 1 with wiggly lines). The wiggly line plates are intended for use by children (or adults) who may have difficulty with numbers (Fig. 19.1).

The *Ishihara Test for Unlettered Persons* uses only a circle, a square, and wiggly lines as targets. It works well with younger patients who may not respond well to numbers. It consists of

8 plates, including three-demonstration plates (circle, square, and wiggly line), 4 screening plates (circle, square, and two wiggly lines), and 1 wiggly line classification plate (Fig. 19.2). It is easy to administer and I have gotten responses on children as young as 2 years of age, although it is better suited for those 3 to 5 years.

Hardy-Rand-Rittler Test

After the Ishihara plates, the *Hardy-Rand-Rittler Test* (HRR) is the second-most widely accepted plate test. Screening sensitivity is less effective than the Ishihara plates, and a small number of patients who pass the HRR will fail the Ishihara test. The HRR, however, does have a more detailed classification capability.

The HRR is also one of the few plate tests that tests for blue-yellow color vision defects. The original test was produced by the American Optical Company as the AO-HRR Test and has been unavailable for more than 30 years. The test was recently re-engineered and is distributed by Richmond Products as the fourth edition of the HRR. Preliminary results indicate that the new edition has improved performance relative to the original (3).

The test consists of 24 plates (4 demonstration plates, 2 blue-yellow screening plates, 4 red-green screening plates, 10 red-green classifications plates, and 4 blue-yellow classification plates) using geometric shapes (a circle, a triangle, and a letter x) as targets (Fig. 19.3).

Each plate contains either one or two shapes and a patient must correctly identify each shape and its location on the page to gain credit. The shapes are familiar to even very young children and, by modifying test protocol by permitting shape matching and shape tracing, the age range over which children respond to the test can be expanded.

The four red-green screening plates use low color saturation and may present a challenge to even normal younger patients because of attentional factors. A clinical trick for the classification plates is to present them in reverse order (from highest saturation to lowest) as a hook to ensure maximal interest in the proceedings.

One of the nice features of the HRR is that the demonstration plates include a blank plate so that patients know that not seeing any target is an acceptable response option. This takes a lot

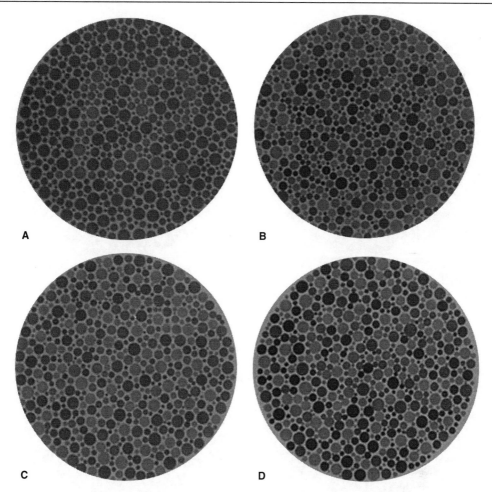

FIGURE 19.1. Concise edition of the Ishihara Pseudoisochromatic Plates. **A:** Demonstration plate: The 12 is seen by all viewers. **B:** Transformation plate: Color normal viewers see the 74, whereas red-green color-deficient viewers see the 21. **C:** Vanishing plate: Color normal viewers see the 45, whereas red-green color-deficient viewers see a blank plate. **D:** Classification plate: Mild protan (red pigment) color-deficient viewers see the 96, with the 6 seen more prominently than the 9. Strong protan color-deficient viewers see the 6 only. Mild deutan (green pigment) color-deficient viewers see the 96, with the 9 seen more prominently than the 6. Strong deutan color-deficient viewers see the 9 only. (See color well.)

of pressure off of the patient during the testing process.

Most children 5 to 6 years of age should be able to give valid responses on the HRR test and with patient, modified administration it may be possible to obtain responses from patients as young as 3 or 4 years of age.

Color Vision Testing Made Easy

The *Color Vision Testing Made Easy* (CVTME) test is a red-green color deficiency screener only. It has no classification capabilities. As an interest-

ing sidebar, the CVTME was reportedly developed by an optometrist whose son is color deficient and who was frustrated by the lack of any decent pediatric-friendly color vision tests.

The CVTME is designed for children and uses geometric shapes (a star, a circle, and a square) and simple line pictures (boat, balloon, and dog) as targets. The test consists of two parts. Part 1 has 10 plates using geometric targets (1 demonstration plate, 9 screening plates), and part 2 has 3 plates using pictures (Fig. 19.4).

One of the nicest features of this test is the placement of targets seen by all patients, both

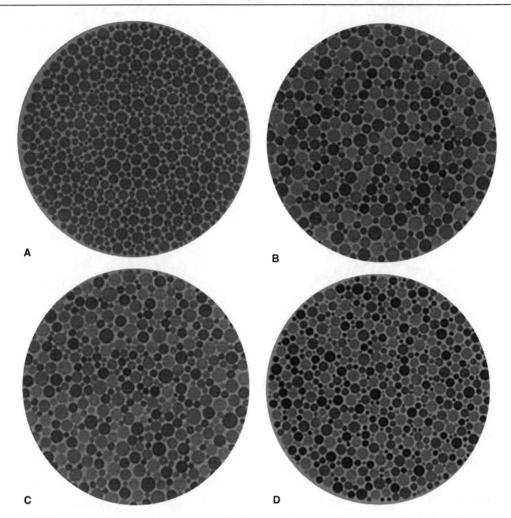

FIGURE 19.2. Ishihara Pseudoisochromatic Plates for Unlettered Persons. **A:** Demonstration plate: The circle is seen by all viewers. **B:** Transformation plate: Color normal viewers see a square, whereas red-green color-deficient viewers see a circle. **C:** Transformation plate: Color normal viewers see a wiggly line with a large loop, whereas red-green color-deficient viewers see a nearly straight line. **D:** Classification plate: Mild protan color-deficient viewers see two wiggly lines, with the purple-pink line seen more prominently than the red-pink line. Strong protan color-deficient patients see the lower purple-pink line only. Mild deutan color-deficient viewers see two wiggly lines, with the red-pink line seen more prominently than the purple-pink line. Strong deutan color-deficient viewers see the upper red-pink line only. (See color well.)

those with normal vision and those who are color deficient, on the first six plates of part 1. This not only confirms the child's ability to respond to the test, but also prevents the stigma of failure that most patients feel when every single test plate appears blank. Parts 1 and 2 are stand-alone tests. Part 1 is the basic test and part 2 is for younger patients with more limited responsiveness. The screening power of both parts compares favorably with the Ishihara plates (4).

Arrangement Tests

Arrangement tests involve the free placement of colored chips in a gradually transitional color sequence from a pre-set reference chip. The patient is assigned the basic task of ordering a series of color chips of equal brightness and saturation by color similarity. The chips are chosen to vary only by hue in fairly equal steps along the color circle.

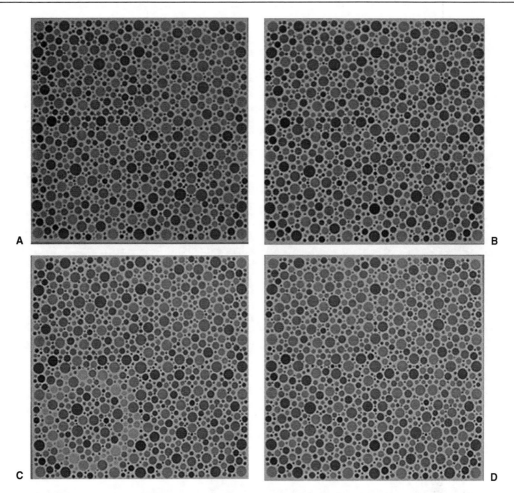

FIGURE 19.3.   Fourth edition of the HRR Pseudoisochromatic Plates. **A:** Demonstration plate: The circle and X are seen by all viewers. **B:** Red-green screening plate: Color normal viewers see a circle and triangle, whereas red-green color-deficient viewers see a blank plate. **C:** Strong red-green classification plate: Mild and moderate red-green color-deficient viewers see a circle and an X, whereas strong protan viewers see the circle and strong deutan viewers see the X. **D:** Strong blue-yellow classification plate: Mild and moderate blue-yellow color-deficient viewers see a circle and triangle, whereas a strong blue-yellow color-deficient viewer sees only one figure. (See color well.)

Arrangement tests, therefore, assess the level of color discrimination skills and the extent of color confusions. They do not determine the presence or absence of color vision *per se*, but rather reflect the characteristics of any defects. Free placement of chips allows detection of errors on both the blue-yellow and the red-green confusion axes as well as irregular errors often found in acquired defects. The task requires somewhat high-level concentration and cognitive development and may be difficult for the very young patient. The two major clinically used arrangement tests are the *Farnsworth Panel*

D-15 Test and the *Farnsworth Munsell 100 Hue Color Vision Test.*

Farnsworth Panel D-15 Test

The D-15 is a short, functional performance test of color discrimination that was designed for industrial classification purposes. The D of the Panel D-15 title stands for dichotomous, as the purpose of the test is to divide patients in to two groups; those with adequate color skills and those with inadequate color skills.

Patients who have normal color vision or who have mild color deficiencies will pass the

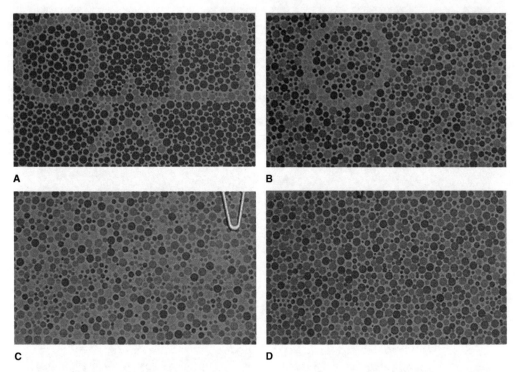

FIGURE 19.4. Color Vision Testing Made Easy. **A:** Demonstration plate: The circle, star, and square are seen by all viewers. **B:** Part 1 screening plate with control: Color normal viewers see a circle and square, whereas red-green color-deficient viewers see a circle only. **C:** Part 1 screening plate without control: Color normal viewers see a star and circle, whereas red-green color-deficient viewers see a blank plate. **D:** Part 2 screening plate: Color normal viewers see a sailboat, whereas red-green color-deficient viewers see a blank plate. (See color well.)

test, whereas patients with moderate to severe color deficiencies will fail the test. It is important to remember that the D-15 is not a screening test for color deficiency, and a passing performance does not guarantee that the patient has normal color vision.

The major clinical appeal of this test is its ability to quickly classify the type and severity of the color deficiency. Color confusion errors made by the patient will reflect the confusion axis of the defective retinal pigment. Because the patient has the freedom to arrange the colors in any sequence, the test identifies red-green color vision defects (protan and deutan) and blue-yellow ones (tritan) as well. The number of confusion errors and the magnitude of the errors will indicate the severity of the color vision defect.

The test consists of 16 color chips (1 anchored reference chip and 15 loose chips) covering the full color circle. The patient chooses from among the 15 free chips, the 1 chip that

most closely matches the reference chip and places it next to the reference chip in its wooden tray. Then, the patient chooses from the remaining 14 free chips the chip most closely resembling the latest positioned chip and places that one next to it in the tray. This process is continued until all 15 chips are in place in the tray. Final adjustments are then allowed so the linear array of chips has the appearance to the patient of a smooth colored transition from the reference chip to the end of the tray. Each chip is numbered and the order of the patient placement is recorded and transcribed on a color circle diagram for grading purposes (Fig. 19.5).

A sequential task such as this is difficult for younger patients and it has been recorded that the D-15 is inappropriate for children under 8 years of age (5). My own clinical experience is that with patiently individualized patient test administration and gentle prompting, many who are 6 years of age can give usable clinical results.

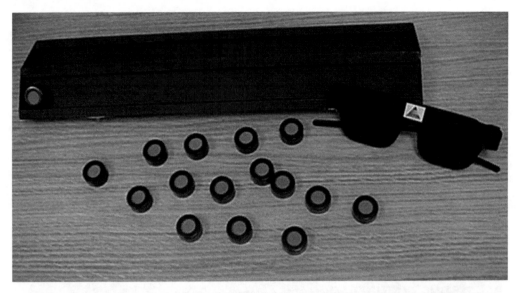

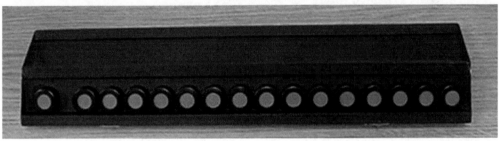

FIGURE 19.5. Farnsworth Panel D-15 Test. *Top*: D-15 prepared for test administration. Reference chip is mounted on the left side of the tray with the 15 loose chips mixed up on desktop. C-Daylite glasses are shown on the right side of the tray. *Bottom*: D-15 with chips arranged in the correct color sequence. (See color well.)

If the reliability of the results is suspect, simply look at the confusion error pattern. Color vision defects have predictable confusion axes. If no errors are seen, then near normal color vision is present. If the errors fall on one of the confusion axes, then a color vision defect is present. If the errors are random or chaotic, then the responses are not reliable and no definitive conclusion can be made regarding the patient's color vision status and the test should be repeated when the child is older.

Always keep in mind that chaotic errors can also be indicative of an acquired color defect; however, the discussion here assumes normal healthy ocular structure. The same logic applies to the plate tests. The scoring sheets provide appropriate responses for those with normal color vision and color-deficient patients. If the child gives inappropriate or nonsensical answers, it means that the results are not valid, rather than the presence of a color vision defect. Try a different test with simpler targets or wait until the child is older.

Farnsworth Munsell 100 Hue Color Vision Test

The *Farnsworth Munsell 100 Hue Color Vision Test* (FM100) is an industrial color vision test designed for rating color discrimination skills and is not particularly useful for a pediatric population. Despite its name, the FM100 contains of only 85 chips that are divided among 4 trays, each covering one fourth of the color circle. The testing procedure is similar to the D15, but it is much lengthier and more demanding. The D15 represents approximately every fifth chip in the FM100, so a much finer level of color discrimination is demanded for this test. Testing time runs between 15 and 30 minutes per administration, which is unmanageable for most younger patients.

The scoring protocol is complex and the FM100 does not distinguish those with normal color vision from those who are color deficient very well, nor does it isolate confusion axes well because of the wide overlap of scoring ranges. The information obtained from the test is mostly helpful for vocational counseling and, therefore, should not be given until the child reaches the junior high school or high school level. At that time, the child will be old enough to give useable responses and the test outcome will have some purposeful application.

GENERAL TESTING CONSIDERATIONS

Color vision tests are designed to be given under very specific testing conditions for the results to be valid. When working with children, it may be difficult to adhere to all of the protocols; however, every attempt should be made to follow the standards described in the instruction manual as closely as possible. Most of the errors induced by improper testing conditions are the passing of color variants as normals, although too low luminance levels can lead to an increase in the number of false positive findings on the screening tests. The key features to maintain are lighting (illumination level and color), test distance, and time exposure.

Lighting

All of the tests described are designed for an illuminant C light source. This requires a special lamp, which few clinics or private practices have. A practice should consider purchasing an illuminant C light source if specialty color vision testing is offered as a service. Otherwise, the easiest option for the general practice is to use a pair of C-Daylite glasses (available from Gulden Ophthalmics) with a standard 75- to 100-W tungsten incandescent bulb in the examination lamp or with a reflecting hood desk lamp. The C-Daylite glasses contain a blue filter in a fit-over frame (identical to the frame used with red-green anaglyph and Polaroid filters). The blue filter has the same transmission as the filter on the MacBeth lamp that converts the tungsten light bulb into an illuminant C light source. True color fluorescent bulbs (Color Rendering Index (CRI) > 90) can also be used as an acceptable substitute for an illuminant C light source (6).

Test Distance

Most color vision tests measure central vision and are designed for a 50- to 75-cm (19.6 to 29.5 inches) test distance. The test distance maintains the fixed visual angle for which the test is standardized. Color vision will improve with improved field size and may lead to misclassification of color defects. The instruction manual for each test will specify its required test distance.

Time Exposure

Plate tests should have a maximal exposure time of 3 seconds per plate. If no response is elicited after that time period, record the response as no target seen and move onto the next plate. If the patient sees a target but has difficulty discerning the shape, ask the patient to try to trace the figure and make a best guess of the shape. Excessive viewing time may allow mild color defectives to pass the plate tests.

Arrangement tests do not have time limits; however, adult patients who need unusually long test times are clearly demonstrating difficulty with the task even if their final ordering sequence is correct. Children generally will need more time on arrangement tests because of the increased cognitive demands of the test.

TEST BATTERIES

Selection of the right tests for assessing color vision of pediatric patients will vary with the age of the patient and the information desired from the patient. The task is somewhat simplified by the limited number of age-appropriate tests and the attentional limits imposed by age. Besides the use of formal color vision tests, it is a good idea to keep some real world color materials on hand for less-threatening, informal assessment of color identification skills. I have sets of watercolors, colored markers, crayons, colored light-emitting diodes (LED), colored

TABLE 19.1 Color Vision Test Batteries for Pediatric Patients

Age Group	Goal of Testing	Test Battery
Birth to 2 y	None	Color vision testing is not indicated
3–5 y	Detection of color vision deficiency	Ishihara Test for Unlettered Persons, or Color Vision Testing Made Easy
	Preliminary classification	HRR in reverse order
6–8 y	Detection	Ishihara Concise Edition
	Classification and rating of color deficiency	HRR and Farnsworth Panel D-15
9 y and older	Detection	Ishihara Concise Edition
	Classification and rating	HRR and Farnsworth Panel D-15
	Counseling	Anomaloscope and FM100 Hue Test as needed

HRR, Hardy-Rand-Rittler.

transparencies, and small colored toys in the office to see the true level of the handicap the patient exhibits when "playing" with them. The extent of intervention recommended might be more realistic based on performance with the real world materials than on the actual color vision tests.

The following is a guide for clinical color vision testing (Table 19.1). The age categories are general and should be modified based on the maturity of the child. Testing should be done binocularly unless some disease process is suspected, in which case testing must be done monocularly.

Birth to Two Years

Literature reports various techniques for assessing the color vision of infants. These techniques include visually evoked potential testing (7), preferential viewing (8), optokinetic nystagmus (9), and even gene analysis of the retinal pigments (10). These are research-based techniques, however, and none of these tests are commercially available or accessible to the public. I can think of no reason why testing the color vision of infants has any practical value in the management of their eye care.

Three Years to Five Years

At 3 to 5 years of age, the major concern is if a color defect is present or not. A positive family history of color vision problems makes the need

for testing more urgent. Information on the classification of the severity of any color vision defect is nice to have, but at this age is not essential. Screening tests, therefore, are the primary emphasis in the testing of this age group. The Ishihara Test for Unlettered Persons or CVTME test should both work well for detecting color deficiencies, although the Ishihara test has the advantage of also having a classification plate. If a defect is detected on the screening plates, the classification plates of the HRR test presented in reverse order should be useful in estimating the severity of the defect.

Six Years to Eight Years

At 6 to 8 years of age, the child is in elementary school and more information about the type and severity of any color vision defects is needed for educational counseling and intervention planning. The child is older and is capable of more sophisticated responses. Screening and classification testing should be done, using both the regular Ishihara plates and the HRR plates. The D-15 test should be attempted to corroborate the results of the plate tests, even though a significant number of the patients in this age group will not be able to complete the task.

Parents, the school principal and teachers should be alerted to the presence of any significant color vision defects, along with recommendations for modifications to any color-based items in the school curriculum.

Nine Years and Above

At 9 years of age and older, the child should be capable of responding to most color vision tests with the exception of the FM100. The standard battery remains the Ishihara and HRR plate tests and the D-15. If more detailed analysis is necessary, the child can be referred for anomaloscope testing, although it may be better to wait a few more years to ensure more reliable results.

Occupational testing should include the FM100 when the child is old enough to perform the test. Career options that require good levels of color vision should be discouraged early on, and consultation with the school guidance counselor may be helpful to avoid the bitter disappointment of being locked out of one's chosen profession because of strict color vision standards. Among the professions that have mandatory color vision standards include the military, law enforcement, transportation industries (aviation, maritime, rail and trucking), gemology, and uniformed services.

COUNSELING

The family of any child found to be color deficient should be informed of the findings and counseled on the consequences of the condition. They should be assured that the color defect is not a disease process but rather a variation of normal and is a stable, nonprogressive finding.

In the counseling session, I review the anatomy of the color vision system and the basics of the x-linked genetic transmission pattern. I also discuss the concept of confusion color pairs and provide a list of likely confusion colors based on their diagnosis of protan or deutan. Based on the test findings I will also relate whether I feel the color defect will manifest prominently in the daily world, or if it will only be of minor importance. I try to ascertain if any school subjects are utilizing color coding that may be problematic for the patient and demonstrate red and magenta color filters as a means of differentiating confusion colors and discuss the strategy of their use. A report detailing the clinical findings is provided for the patient's school file, which alerts the school authorities of the potential academic problems and sensitizes them to this nonvisible handicap.

TINTS FOR COLOR DEFICIENCY

Over the years there have been reports on the use of color altering tints as a means of compensating for color deficiencies (11). No system has had major success. The only system with any significant longevity has been the X-chrome lens, a deep red contact lens fitted monocularly over the non-dominant eye (12). The X-chrome lens creates a scintillating, lustrous appearance for colored objects secondary to a retinal rivalry effect.

The monocular fitting approach of the X-chrome lens can be troublesome for some patients by destabilizing their binocular posture. The temporal transmission lag induced by the dark red lens can lead to warpage of spatial perception by inducing Pulfrich Phenomenon-like effects. Binocular filters can be prescribed instead and are usually better tolerated.

Tints work because confusion colors can be differentiated by the luminous differences induced by the filter's selective absorption. For a pair of confusion colors, the color with a greater proportion of red appears brighter through the filter than the color with a lesser amount of red. Thus, the use of tinted lenses negates the design of PIP tests by created luminous differences between the target and the background. Previously unseen targets are now visible with the filters, although the reason is luminous cues rather than chromatic ones.

The boost in "correct" responses on the PIP tests leads to the misperception that color vision performance is actually improved with the lens. However, arrangement tests tell a different story. The colored filter does not improve performance, but merely shifts the confusion axis to a different area of the color circle. Arrangement tests are often *more* difficult because of the introduction of luminance cues and the elimination of chromaticity cues. The color deficient patient's well-developed adaptations are nullified by the tint, leading to performance breakdown.

For these reasons I find that most patients reject colored filters for general use, although admittedly there is a small number who do respond very positively to them and report increased range of subjective color appreciation.

While filters are not usually helpful for general use, they can be very helpful for specific conditions such as when a fixed color array is being used for identification purposes. An example is a student studying colored maps in geography class. Certain color pairs may look nearly identical, but if viewed through an appropriate tinted lens will clearly appear different. By alternating between normal vision without the tint and altered vision through the tint, most patients can learn to accurately distinguish the full set of colors and apply the correct color appeliations.

Red and magenta seem to be the two most effective colors for this purpose. Some relatively inexpensive aids assisting color deficient patients are the U90 (red), and U70 (magenta) UVShield fit-over specs available from NoIR. Gulden Ophthalmics produces a red folding pocket lens for portability and unobtrusive use. I often use small squares cut from a sheet of red acetate for home trial with patients. The red acetate sheets are available from Vision Training supply catalogs and photographic supply stores.

Computer technology is also emerging as a source of assistance for color deficient patients. There are several small hand-held color analyzers with voice synthesis available from adaptive device catalogs for the visually impaired. The probe is placed on an item and it will announce the name of the color. I have little personal experience with these devices, but I imagine they could be very helpful for the more severely affected color deficient patients, particularly for activities such as clothing shopping.

CONCLUSIONS

Color vision testing of the full range of pediatric patients can be achieved with a battery of only three or four simple clinical tests, all of which can also be used for adult patients. Testing time is short and no valid excuse exists for neglecting to screen all pediatric patients for hereditary color deficiency.

ACKNOWLEDGMENTS

The author recognizes and thanks Ms. Meira Cohen for the creation of the digital images and table used in this chapter.

Photographs of the color vision test plates are reproduced through the courtesy of Graham-Field Health Products (Ishihara Plates), Richmond Products (4th Edition of HRR Test), and Dr. Terrace L. Waggoner (Color Vision Testing Made Easy).

REFERENCES

1. Adams RJ, Courage ML. A psychophysical test of early maturation of infant's mid- and long-wavelength retinal cones. *Infant Behavior and Development* 2002;25:247–254.
2. Pitchford NJ. Conceptualization of perceptual attributes: a special case for color. *J Exp Child Psychol* 2001;80:289–314.
3. Bailey JE, Neitz M, Tait DM, et al. Evaluation of an updated HRR color vision test. *Vis Neurosci* 2004;21:431–436.
4. Cotter SA, Lee DY, French AL. Evaluation of a new color vision test: 'Color Vision Testing Made Easy.' *Optom Vis Sci* 1999;76:631–636.
5. Adams AJ, Balliet R, McAdams M. Color vision: blue deficiencies in children? *Invest Ophthalmol* 1975;14:620–625.
6. Hovis JK, Neumann P. Colorimetric analyses of various light sources for the D-15 color vision test. *Optom Vis Sci* 1995;72:667–678.
7. Ver Hoeve JN. A sweep VEP test for color vision deficits in infants and young children. *J Pediatr Ophthalmol Strabismus* 1996;33:298–302.
8. Pease P, Allen J. A new test for screening color vision: concurrent validity and utility. *Am J Optom Physiol Opt* 1988;65:729–738.
9. Cavanaugh P, Antis S, Mather G. Screening for color blindness using optokinetic nystagmus *Invest Ophthalmol Vis Sci* 1984;25:463–466.
10. Bieber ML, Werner JS, Knoblauch K, et al. M- and L-cones in early infancy. III. Comparison of genotypic and phenotypic markers of color vision in infants and adults. *Vision Res* 1998;38:3293–3297.
11. Horis JK. Long wavelength pass filters designed for the management of color vision deficiencies. *Optom Vis Sci* 1997;74:222–230.
12. Zeltzer HI. The X-chrome lens. *J Amer Optom Assoc* 1971;42:933–939.

PART 3

Treatment Strategies in the Pediatric Patient

Prescribing Lenses for the Pediatric Patient

20

Robert H. Duckman

No hard and fast rules govern the prescribing of lenses for the pediatric patient, particularly when dealing with an infant or toddler. We have not been doing it for a long time, especially when it comes to these younger children. General consensus is that an infant is born with low myopia (approx. $-0.75\,\mathrm{D}$) when measured without cycloplegia, and low hyperopia ($\sim +2.00\,\mathrm{D}$) when cycloplegia is used. This would be the norm of the infant and when prescribing lenses for them, we are interested in sharp variances from this *normal* refraction and not subtle differences. I often tell my students that we are not interested in a refraction of $-0.25\ -0.25 \times 180$ in a toddler. We are looking for the child who is $-15.00\ -3.00 \times 180$. We will not prescribe lenses for the first child, but will, in some form, prescribe for the patient with high myopia, a child who obviously needs a lens correction. The big question is: "What lens do you prescribe?" The answer depends on many things and will vary with various ages and developmental status. *What, when, and how* do you prescribe are all questions that will be answered in this chapter. Also discussed are special lenses such as bifocals, progressive addition lenses (PAL), and prisms. And the whole process of emmetropization will be considered as yet another variable. This chapter offers *guidelines* to the clinician, but not formularies.

Before proceeding remember, it is so easy to forget when you are running a busy private practice that *CHILDREN ARE PEOPLE!* Never forget this! In discussing clinical findings and the need for glasses, the clinician should address the parent(s), and the child. Too often, clinicians talk to the parents and totally exclude the child. This omission is acceptable when dealing with an infant, but do not underestimate the cognitive abilities of a child. It is a mistake to do this. Involve the child as much as possible, because the child is the one who is going to have to wear the glasses and needs to know why. This is especially true when the glasses are being used to correct posture or accommodative problems where acuity is not going to be any better with the glasses. From extensive experience with children, I have had many come in with plus lenses to be used for near work who say they do not need them because, "I see as good with them off as I do with them on." They need to understand that the glasses are not meant to make things clearer, but rather make them easier to see. This is just one good example to demonstrate the importance of involving the child. Another place it is very important to get the child involved is in frame selection. Children usually have strong opinions when it comes to things they like or dislike. It is very important for the *child* to like the frame, not the parent. My experience has taught me that if a child does not like the frame, the child is not going to wear the glasses. I always stress to parents the importance of allowing the child to choose the frame. (This is obviously not the case with infants.) Allow the child to choose the frame and hope that it is somewhat to the liking of the parents. Children who need glasses have many other reasons why they will not wear glasses. Parents can help with some of these problems, and some they cannot. One of the foremost reasons a child does not want to wear glasses is the ridicule from other children who call them names such as "four eyes." It is helpful to discuss the child's newly acquired glasses with teacher or day care individuals and allow this person to introduce this new element about the child to the other children in the group. It is very helpful in minimizing the *ridicule* factor. Another reason children will not wear glasses is lowered self-esteem. Children feel poorly about the fact that they need glasses. They therefore do such things as "lose" them, hide them, and throw them away. Children can be highly inventive when they do not want to wear glasses. It is necessary for parents to assure their children that they are loved as much, cared for as much, and of no lesser value than before they needed glasses. Some excellent books and videos explain the need for glasses to children and explain the importance of wearing the glasses that have been prescribed. My favorite is *Arthur's Eyes* by Marc Brown. It comes in book format from Little, Brown and Co. and a DVD or video format from Sony Wonder. Both formats show, in a very amusing way, how much Arthur is missing by not using his newly prescribed glasses. Arthur needs glasses, gets ridiculed in school when he wears them, and tries to lose them. This leads to embarrassing situations (e.g., going into the girl's bathroom by mistake). This is a difficult topic that is handled well and gently.

Uncorrected refractive errors are by far the most common cause of poor vision. Rehabilitation of such defects has probably added as much to the quality of life and extended its usefulness to society as any advance in biology. Indeed, optical correction safely restores serviceable and comfortable vision to a greater proportion of patients than any other form of ophthalmic therapy (1). Ophthalmic lenses, when

necessary, can significantly bring the child (or the adult for that matter) into conjugacy with the child's spatial environment. It is through the sensory modality of vision that a child learns about space and about movement through the environment, first crawling then toddling and finally walking and running. Without the vision and visual stimulation, motor development would be slow and delayed. As an example, a newborn baby, unbeknownst to her parents, is 20.00 D myopia OU. This child can see things clearly at 2 inches with everything beyond that point being increasingly blurred. Therefore distance objects are totally blurred. As the child grows she starts lifting her head and trunk to look at objects outside the crib. However, she cannot get any understanding of distant objects because of the extreme blur. Because the distant objects are the stimulation for trunk or head lifting, this child will quickly stop lifting herself up to look at distance. She will spend the time fixating at near. This will delay her gross motor development (trunk and neck) and all milestones from that point on will be delayed. This is a simple, straightforward example of how vision can have an impact on development. Many more subtle ones will be discussed in this chapter.

In Chapter 4, FitzGerald discusses the process of emmetropization, which is the tendency for refractive error to move toward plano from myopia, hyperopia and/or astigmatism. Most emmetropization occurs in the first 18 months of life (2). This does not mean the process is over at 18 months, but rather any changes from that point on will be small and gradual. It is important to consider emmetropization when selecting a correcting lens for an infant or toddler.

For example, in a 6-month-old infant with 12.00 D myopia OU requires a strong prescription and this needs to be addressed. It can be handled one of two ways:

1. The child can wear a pair of glasses with headstrap with a -8.00 D sphere. This is an undercorrection of the refractive error, but an intended one. The infant's world is not at optical infinity. It is at arm's length and closer. Therefore, the undercorrection provides the child with a clear retinal image at near and without accommodative effort. As

the child gets older, the distance correction will become more important.

2. The child can be fit with pediatric contact lenses (see Chapter 15).

At about 12 to 16 months, when the child starts walking, distance vision becomes more important. Children at this age are still centered at near, but they need the visual acuity to see the world around them to move through it. If the child's vision is uncorrected or significantly under corrected at distance, the blur may diminish the child's interest in distance targets, thus limiting mobility toward them.

A child with significant astigmatism needs correction, but the correction depends on age. It is well known that astigmatism in infants is prevalent and generally decreases with age (3). It has also been shown (4) that meridional amblyopia does not occur until about 2 years of age. No need, therefore, is seen to correct the astigmatism until the child is approaching 2 years of age. At that point, it becomes essential and important. Other signs indicate that correction should be applied. For example, in examining a child at 9 months, findings are OU plano -4.00 D $\times$ 90. You recheck the refractive error 3 months later and find the same correction. Another follow-up at 15 months reveals the exact same -4.00×90 cylinder. This is a cylinder that is not changing and correction should be given. Conversely, if this child comes to the first visit demonstrating -4.00×90 cylinder, 3 months later measures -3.00×90, and 3 months after that measures -2.00×90, continue to watch this child until the astigmatism becomes *stable* and then consider prescribing, if necessary. Another factor to consider is visual acuity—both uncorrected acuity and best corrected acuity. If, as you monitor your patient, the best corrected visual acuity is decreasing, consider prescribing lenses for the toddler patient. If the best corrected acuity remains the same, consider delaying spectacle correction.

These are just a few examples of the consideration of age and refractive error in prescribing lenses. With the information in this chapter, it should become clear when and how to prescribe for infants, toddlers, and children.

In all instances the operative word is *stability*. Whether talking about myopia, hyperopia,

astigmatism, or anisometropia, watch for stability of the refractive error.

Children who wear glasses do so because of necessity, although many children who *fake* needing glasses want them despite a lack of need. Children who *need* glasses and who have to wear them, despite what their peers do and say, need to feel good about their glasses. They need to like them and they need to feel comfortable wearing them. Rule number one, therefore, is that children who are going to wear glasses have to pick out their own frame. This is so important, much to the chagrin of the parents, family, and friends of the child. *If the child does not like the glasses, the child is not going to wear them.* This is a lesson I have learned over time. It is a problem because some parents feel they know better and do not support the child's choice of a frame. The child picks a frame, the parents are appalled by the choice and immediately participate in picking out what they like. This is not about the parents, it is about what the child wants. I agree that children's tastes often run askew of what I would consider tasteful, but these children have real tastes that are their own. A parent may not like it when their 5-year-old puts on a pink and yellow polka dot shirt with a brown and green plaid skirt. This is what the child wants and that child's choices should be supported despite what the parents feel about it. When my daughter was 3 years of age, she used to pick out her clothes every day and had definite feelings about what she wanted to wear. I have to confess that some of her combinations were nauseating. But we let her wear whatever she would pick out. No permanent damage was done and today she is a teenager who has excellent taste in putting outfits together. So too with glasses, children have to pick out the frame they want for the glasses they will wear.

I'll relate the story of a child I once examined who, at the age of 6 years, measured 8.50 D of myopia OU. Her parents picked out her frames for her continuously telling her how beautiful she looked in them and how much she was going to like them. The glasses were ordered and dispensed and acuity increased from 20/1200 to 20/30. Her parents called back within a week and reported that the child had flushed her glasses down the toilet. The glasses were replaced, redispensed, and within a week they had *fallen* out of the school bus. Then I again suggested letting the child pick out the frames and the parents finally acquiesced. This time the child picked the frames she wanted the first time and strangely enough nothing happened to the glasses after they were dispensed. They were worn full time without incident. It is not that the child was a *brat*, but rather just wanted to feel good about herself and her glasses. I may be belaboring this point, but it is extremely important.

Another practical issue is to make sure that a child is fitted with an appropriate *pediatric* frame. Not so many years ago, finding decent pediatric frames was not easy. Today, however, a wide range of products are available through many companies; frames are easy to find and the child has a good choice from which to make a selection. Avoid at all costs someone trying to adjust a small adult frame to fit the child. It does not work and it is not necessary.

MYOPIA

Family history of high myopia on the degree and onset of myopia is strong. Liang et al. (3) investigated the impact of a positive family history of high myopia on the level and onset of myopia and found a very strong association between parental myopia and the offspring's myopia. A very strong association was seen between the parental myopic status and the child's axial length. No statistical relationship was noted between anterior chamber depth and corneal curvature. Liang et al. (3) demonstrated a strong familial effect on the level and onset of myopia even after adjusting for environmental factors. Ben-Simon et al. (4) believe that the development of myopia is influenced by hereditary factors, environmental factors, and gene-environment interactions. His group studied 917 third grade students with an average age of 8.5 years (range 7–10 years). They found that reading and near work activity are associated with myopia and myopia progression. Studying students in three different school environments in Israel, they found that the more rigorous the academic demands, the faster the progression of the myopia. The three settings were: (a) secular, (b) orthodox, and (c) ultraorthodox. Children in the ultraorthodox group begin studying

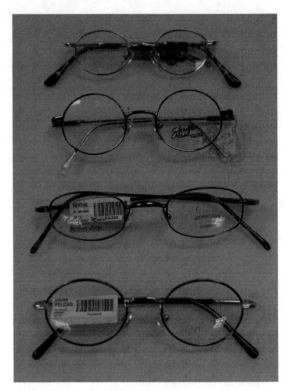

FIGURE 20.1. A sampling of frames available for very young children. (See color well.)

at the age of 3 years and their daily reading involves sustained near work with increased accommodative and head-rocking movements. Blurred vision at distance was used to indicate the likely development of, or an increase, in the degree of myopia. They found that males from ultraorthodox settings had the highest rate of reduced unaided vision (72.5%) compared with males from secular settings (27.3%), males from orthodox schools (59.3%), or with females from all three groups (34.8%). The authors conclude that the study habits of young children, including exposure to prolonged near tasks, high accommodative demands, and possibly optical defocus induced by body sway, can contribute to development of myopia.

Myopia will have a significant effect on the child in the acquisition of visual information at distance. With the blur induced by the focus of the distance objects falling in front of the retina, clear images are not possible uncorrected. The child can tolerate a certain degree of blur, but that is unique to the child and definitely not a specific dioptric power. To restore clarity of vision, concave lenses need to be prescribed. How

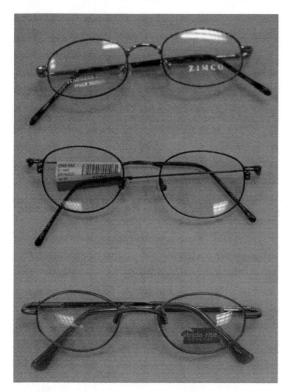

FIGURE 20.2. A sampling of frames available for very young children. (See color well.)

much to prescribe depends on age, posture, development, needs, and mobility. A very young child does not need 20/20 acuity and developmentally is not expected to have it. Therefore, the degree of myopia a child under 2 years of age needs to warrant the prescription of lenses is significant. The infant's total spatial world is at near. These children certainly look out at distance and see things in the distance, but spend most of their time in near space. The myopic child sees clearly in near space at some dis-

tance, depending on the degree of myopia. Of course, in considering a highly myopic child, we need to be concerned about blur at distance, but also at near. Infants who are 15.00 D myopic can only see things clearly that are less than 3 inches from their face. Visual acuity must be monitored in such a child for the development of amblyopia. Until the child starts walking and moving around in space, it is not essential for the child to have a perfectly clear focus. Therefore, for the first 12 to 18 months not correcting or undercorrecting as much as 4.00 D of myopia is reasonable. Once the child begins to walk and move around the environment, it becomes more important for the child to have access to single, clear, binocular vision. At that point, 4.00 D of blur is not acceptable. Toddlers and older children need lenses that will more closely bring them into conjugacy with the distance. This does not mean they require *full* correction, but rather a 4.00 D blur is no longer acceptable. These children need to be examined frequently (every 3–4 months) to monitor acuity, refractive error, and emmetropization. A 6-month-old who is 20.00 D of myopia is very unlikely to emmetropize, but still requires frequent examination to monitor acuities, retinas, and the prescription. The 20.00 D myopic 6-month-old, with compliant parents, would be a good candidate for contact lens wear, an option that should be offered.

Once the child has entered preschool, accurate myopic prescribing is necessary. This is usually in the child aged 3 to 4 years. Up to this point, myopia greater than 3.00 to 4.00 D is required before correction. Now, myopia of 2.00 D or greater requires correction. The clinician can still prescribe an undercorrection, but should

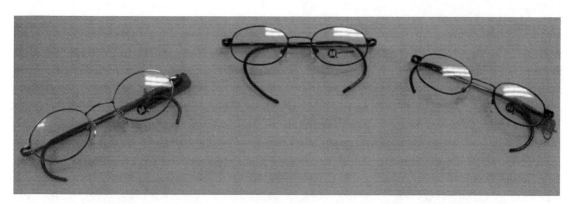

FIGURE 20.3. A sampling of frames available for very young children. (See color well.)

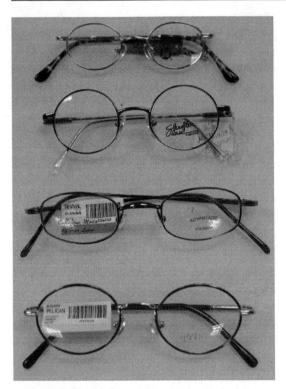

FIGURE 20.4. A sampling of frames available for very young children. (See color well.)

not leave the patient's vision significantly uncorrected. Once the child enters kindergarten (about 5 years), full correction of myopia should occur because, although most of the child's activities will be at near, some academic topics are taught off the blackboard. The myopic child whose vision is under- or uncorrected will miss information during these activities even if seated close to the blackboard. From this age on, blackboard work will increase, so distance

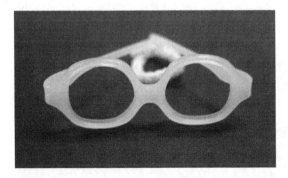

FIGURE 20.5. Solo Bambini soft plastic frames for young children. All frames come with straps to keep the glasses on. (See color well.)

correction is important. During the early years, myopic blur is tolerated well, but once school work becomes more demanding, blur is a problem and can impede a student's progress. When prescribing for any patient, consider binocularity. When it comes to the myopic patient, if the patient is esophoric, a mild undercorrection will help binocular posture by decreasing divergence demand. If the child is exophoric, full minus should be given to maintain ocular alignment by increasing convergence demand for the patient. My position is not to increase minus over and above the full minus prescription to facilitate alignment, although this has been done by some authors (5–8).

With the exception of pathologic myopia, which starts out as very high bilateral (usually) myopia, the young child who manifests low degrees of myopia will usually increase myopic correction throughout the school years. This is a direct effect of extended near work, genetics, or both. Whatever the cause, eye practitioners have been trying for decades to slow down the progression of this school year myopia. Attempts have included such minimal approaches as visual hygiene (e.g., taking breaks from extended near point task, good lighting, high-contrast text) to moderate approaches (e.g., undercorrecting distance prescriptions), to utilization of bifocal adds to decrease the accommodative demand of near work, to a more extreme form of therapy having bifocal lenses with atropine to eliminate accommodative effort.

Parssinen et al. (9) looked at myopia progression over a period of 3 years in schoolchildren 9 to 11 years of age. Three treatment groups consisted of (a) minus lenses, full correction to be used for continuous wear; (b) full correction of minus lenses to be used for distance only; and (c) full minus lenses for distance with a +1.75 D bifocal add OU. They retrieved 3-year refraction values from 237 children. They found no statistical correlation between the sphero-equivalent refraction and its increase in the right eye, but found a negative correlation in the left eye (i.e., the change in the continuous wear group—increased −1.46 D) that was less than the distance vision only group (increased −1.87 D). They noted no differences between the groups in school performance or accidents. It was interesting, however, that no

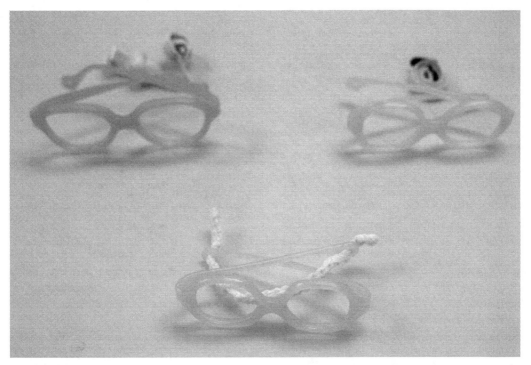

FIGURE 20.6. Solo Bambini soft plastic frames for young children. All frames come with straps to keep the glasses on. (See color well.)

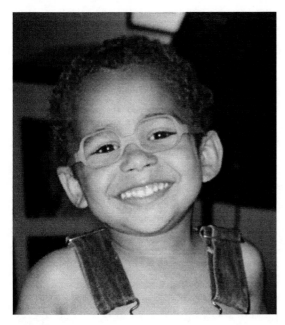

FIGURE 20.7. Logan wearing Solo Bambini frame with lenses. (See color well.)

matter what group was examined, the greater the daily close work done, the faster the rate of myopic progression and the shorter the average reading distance, the faster the myopic progression. Despite these findings, they found no relationship of myopia progression to accommodation. A significant amount of evidence disagrees with this conclusion.

Fulk et al. (10) looked at whether bifocals had any effect on the progression of myopia in children *with esophoria*. They had two groups of children: single-vision glasses use and a bifocals group with a +1.50 D add. These children were followed for 2.5 years after which time myopia progression was evaluated. Seven children were lost to follow-up but, of those who completed the study, a slightly slower progression was noted for the bifocal group (0.99 D) versus the single vision group (1.24 D).

Goss (11), in a literature review, found that when the near point phoria is eso, greater rates of progression occur, and that some degree of myopia control can be established by shifting the phoria into the normal range by spectacle corrections such as bifocals. Fulk et al. (12), in a 4.5 year study, looked at the effects of bifocal lenses on the progression of myopia. During the first 24 months, they found a significant difference between the children who wore single vision glasses and those who wore bifocals, with myopia in the latter group progressing more slowly than the single vision lens group. They also found a similar trend in vitreous chamber growth. During the last 2.5 years of the study, however, the difference in the degree of myopia was maintained, but did not increase. Fulk et al. (13), in an earlier paper, found that bifocal lenses slowed the progression of myopia in those children with near point esophoria. They also found, not surprisingly, that myopia progressed more rapidly during the school year than during summer vacation.

Ong et al. (14) look at the effects of spectacle intervention on the progression of myopia in children over a period of 3 years. They studied four groups of children: (a) full-time wearers; (b) myopic patients who started as distance only and shifted to full-time wear; (c) distance wearers; and (d) nonwearers. The progression of myopia for the four groups, when age-adjusted, was not significantly different. The study failed to show any overall effect of spectacle intervention on the progression of myopia.

Gwiazda et al. (15) in the Correction of Myopia Evaluation Trial (COMET) found that myopic children given bifocals for accommodative lags and or esophoria had an additional benefit of slowed myopia progression. Their results supported the COMET model that myopia progression is caused by retinal defocus. Results of the study suggest that children with large lags of accommodation and near esophoria can experience slowed progression of myopia.

Evidence suggests that some of the aforementioned therapies may slow the progression of myopia. One therapy, however, seems to guarantee it—atropine use with bifocals. Whether the results warrant the use of atropine is questionable. Nonetheless, it is effective in slowing down myopia.

In 1999, Shih et al. (16) examined the effectiveness of different concentrations of atropine on controlling the progression of myopia. It was known that 1% atropine effectively slows myopia progression, but the authors acknowledged its use was associated with adverse side effects including photophobia, blurred vision, and poor compliance. Therefore, they looked at whether lower concentrations of the drug would control myopia progression. They treated their sample (ranging in age from 6 to 13 years) with nightly drops of atropine of various concentrations ranging from 0.5% to 0.1% or a control treatment. After 2 years, they found that all groups showed significantly less myopic progression than the control group and many (61% of the students in the 0.5% group) had no myopic progression. Of the children in the 0.5% atropine group 4% had fast myopic progression as did 17% in the 0.25% group and 33% in the 0.1% group. Of the control group, 40% had fast myopic corrections. The authors concluded that all three concentrations of atropine had significant effects on controlling myopia, with 0.5% atropine being the most effective. Romano and Donovan (17) examined the effects of atropine and photochromic bifocal lenses on the progression of school myopia. They used full myopic correction with a +3.00 D add OU with photochromic gray extra lenses and 1% atropine OU. They found the mean refractive change was +.07 D for the "always compliant group" (i.e., a decrease in myopia). The "sometimes compliant group" increased on average −0.18 D per year and the "never compliant group" increased −0.17 D per year. The mean change in the refractive error of a similar cohort aged 8 to 15 years was −0.24 D per year. Romano and Donovan concluded that use of atropine and bifocals was an appropriate, effective, and safe management for progressive school myopia and also, probably for pathologic myopia. They made no assessment of symptoms during the period of bifocal wear with atropine. Another effort to show the effectiveness of atropine on the progression of myopia was done through a literature review (18). The authors reviewed records from 1968–2000. They reviewed ten clinical trials of different interventions to retard myopia progression, which included three atropine eye drops (0.5%) studies, bifocal studies, and a soft contact lens study. They concluded from their review that sufficient information did not exist to support interventions to prevent the progression of myopia.

Kennedy et al. (19), in a long term, cohort study, looked at the effects of atropine in reducing the progression of myopia. They looked at 214 children ranging in age from 6 to 15 years with a median age of 11 years. They all received atropine for myopia from 1967 to 1974. Control subjects were matched by age, sex, and refraction. The duration of treatment with atropine ranged from 18 weeks to 11.5 years (median, 3.5 years). Negative side effects included photophobia and blurred vision, but no serious adverse effects were associated with atropine therapy. During atropine therapy, subjects increased myopia of 0.05 D per year, whereas the controls increased 0.36 D per year. The data support the view that utilization of atropine slows the progression of myopia. Syniuta and Isenberg (20), using 1% atropine with bifocals, found that myopia progression for the atropine–bifocal group was 0.05 D per year, whereas the progression for the control group was 0.84 D per year. Shih et al. (21) performed a similar experiment with a much larger population. They used myopic patients and assigned them to one of three treatment groups: 0.5% atropine with multifocal glasses, multifocal glasses alone, and single vision spectacles. Follow-up was for at least 18 months. The experimenters found that the 0.5% atropine with multifocal lenses can slow the progression rate of myopia. Multifocal lenses alone, however, showed no difference in effect.

Atropine use consistently seems to have an ability to decrease myopia progression, either alone or in combination with multifocal lenses. The only question to answer then is, is it worth the risk and the potential side effects of blur, photophobia, and retinal light toxicity which the use of atropine carries. Many feel it is, and many feel it is not, so the matter is one of professional opinion and philosophy. I feel atropine's use is not worth the risk to decrease the degree of myopia. The myopia on which it is effective is moderate myopia. The myopia is not eliminated in most cases and glasses still have to be worn. Progressive myopia, of which we are speaking, rarely increases to a degree to which we would have to be concerned about the retinal integrity. (My opinion about using atropine in penalization therapy for amblyopia differs).

Because it is believed that excessive accommodation can lead to increased myopia, many people utilize bifocal prescriptions or undercor-

rect the myopia in an attempt to slow down the progression of the refractive error. Many have supported this with research. For instance, Fulk et al. (10,13) found a decrease in myopia progression in children who wore bifocals as compared with single vision glasses. In 2002, Chung et al. (22) did a prospective study of 94 myopic children aged 9 to 14 years over a period of 2 years. The children were allocated into two groups: one undercorrected by +0.75 D and the other fully corrected. They reported that the undercorrected group had a more rapid progression of myopia than the fully corrected group. They concluded that the myopic defocus (undercorrected group) speeds up myopia development. This study does not negate the use of bifocals for near vision to slow the progression of myopia, it merely says that when distance vision is blurred, myopia progresses more quickly. Chiang et al. (23) looked at a very large sample of children ranging in age from 6 to 16. All the children were initially myopic and all were prescribed full cycloplegic refraction with photochromic lenses and a +2.25 D add. In addition, both eyes were treated with 1% atropine (one drop per day). The results were consistent: full compliance with all aspects of the therapy was associated with decreased progression of myopia compared with the *partial* compliance group. The mean rate of myopic progression was significantly less than that of the normal pediatric population.

HYPEROPIA

Hyperopia is the refractive condition in which light is not refracted sufficiently to form a focused image on the retina. Instead, it is focused beyond the retina. Because of the pediatric patient's enormously competent ability to focus the crystalline lens, add convexity to the system, and focus the image, hyperopia is *self-correcting*. Hyperopia is self-correcting until a significant degree is present, an accommodative problem such as an accommodative insufficiency or infacility presents, or a very high accommodation: convergence accommodation (A:CA) ratio is found. The greatest concern with a hyperopic patient is a resultant accommodative esotropia. An accommodative esotropia is often a direct result of uncorrected hyperopia and often the correction of that hyperopia is sufficient to resolve the strabismus. The child must, however, wear the convex lens power to keep the eyes aligned. Compliance with these patients is usually good. When you give a child with an accommodative esotropia a pair of glasses, tell the patient *before hand* that the glasses will keep the eyes straight. When the child takes the glasses off, however, the eyes might not only turn, but might turn *more than* they had before the glasses were applied. Parents of many patients tell me their child's eyes have gotten worse with the glasses only to find out that the only time the eyes turn is when the glasses are off. The reason they turn more without the glasses is that once children start wearing the glasses and see how clear it can be, they try to replicate that clarity when the glasses are off by pulling in more accommodation and more convergence.

Correcting hyperopia is more difficult than correcting myopia. Often, myopia patients are given full correction to produce the best acuity. The hyperopic patient can often get the best acuity without correction. So how much hyper-

opic correction do you give? The answer to this question lies with the consideration of two factors: acuity and posture. A child with a low hyperopia (OU +0.75 D) who has 20/20, 20/20, 20/20, and orthophoria at distance and 4 exophoria at near does not need corrective lenses unless some significant accommodative problem manifests. On the other hand, a child with +2.00 D OU with an 8 esophoria at distance and an intermittent alternate esotropia at near would benefit from and should have a prescription for near vision at the very least. In cases of strabismus (accommodative esotropia) secondary to uncorrected refractive error, a lens prescription is indicated. This does not mean full correction is necessary or advised, although it often is. The main objective is to get the child seeing clearly and performing as a binocular individual.

Prescribing lenses is easy when symptoms are present, but what about when there are none. This occurs frequently with hyperopia. The child comes in seeing clearly, no headaches, blurred vision, or complaints of any kind. You examine such a child and find OU +4.00 D

PATIENT: SARA G.

Sara G. presented at age 2.5 years with the following case history. No problems present until the eyes started crossing a few weeks ago. No history in the family of a crossed eye or any other serious eye problem. Sara had no complaints except for the recent onset of diplopia. She reported that her vision was clear at distance and near and she had no symptoms. Sara was examined and all findings were normal except for (a) blur or diplopia on binocular acuity; (b) alternating esotropia at distance and near when encouraged to accommodate; (c) dry retinoscopy OU +4.50 D sphere. Various lenses were attempted and a prescription of OU +3.00 D was derived, which accomplished three things: (a) gave Sara clear single vision at distance and near; (b) maintained ocular alignment at distance; (c) allowed her definite random dot stereo with the Lang 2 stereo test. Sara G. returned after 3 months and all reports indicated the lens prescription was working (i.e., eyes were straight, Sara wore the glasses, and vision was clear).

This case is a simple example of how to deal with an accommodative esotropia. Often, it is that simple, but at times it is not. Take for example Dorina L., a child 3.5 years of age, who presented with a strabismus at distance (25 pd) and near (35 pd). Her refraction was OU +2.50 D the application of which decreased the distance deviation to 10 pd esophoria and the near deviation to 18 pd alternating esotropia. A near add of +2.00 D was attempted, which reduced the near deviation to 10 pd esophoria. Neither the near or distance deviation could be diminished further. Dorina was followed periodically and, because she wore the glasses, the plus did not change, but her deviation did. By the time she was 5.5 years of age, she was wearing the same prescription, but her eyes were essentially aligned and binocular at distance and near.

with no esophoria or esotropia and all findings within normal. What do you do? I strongly believe that 4.00 D uncorrected hyperopia must be taking a toll on the child's performance. Therefore, I will prescribe lenses for near work, at the very least, and preferably for full time in school and home. This is the child who is going to be problematic when it comes to compliance in wearing the glasses. The child, as far as he or she is concerned, has no visual problem. This is the child to whom you must explain the "ease of seeing clearly" and not the clarity itself.

For a preschooler with low to moderate hyperopia, *without* signs or symptoms, monitor this child and hold off on prescribing glasses. But, again, *once posture is involved, application of lenses must be considered.*

When moderate to high hyperopia is present, lenses should be considered even if no symptoms or signs are present. I have a child, Barbara D., I am treating who came in at the age of 5 years, symptom-free. Her visual acuity was 20/20, 20/20, 20/20, at distance *and* at near. Cover test revealed orthophoria at distance and at near with an accommodative target. When I finally got to retinoscopy, this girl was OU +8.00 D sphere. Despite the lack of signs and symptoms, this girl required a lens prescription. I chose a +5.00 D sphere OU to start and had her return in 3 months. On follow-up, she had done well with the lenses, tolerated them without problems, and was doing much better at all near work tasks, including reading and book work. No reports of near point difficulties were stated at the initial examination, but the mother had noticed how much better the child was able to do with the lenses. Depending on the child, the lenses might or might not be increased on subsequent visits. Barbara D. did not need to have her lenses increased because she was doing well with the initial prescription.

Edelman and Borchert (24) examined outcomes of children with high hyperopia (≥ 5 D). The age at which correction was applied ranged from 8 to 141 months. They examined visual acuity before application of lenses. Final visual acuity was taken after lenses were applied. Final visual acuity was 20/30 or better in 104 of 109 children. No relationship was found between final visual acuity and the age that the spectacles were applied. However, 84% ($N = 80$) of the original population ($N = 95$) had esotropia with or without the glasses and six had final visual acuity less than 20/30. The authors conclude that visual acuity outcome in children with high hyperopia is good regardless of age at initial optical correction or in the presence of strabismus.

Atkinson et al. (25) explored the effect of correcting hyperopia on the process of emmetropization. They took children who had significant hyperopia at 8 to 9 months and they were assigned to either a treated (partial lens prescription) group or an untreated group (no lens prescription). In addition, a control group was recruited who had no refractive error. By the age of 36 months in 148 children, they found that hyperopia shifted toward low hyperopia between 9 and 36 months regardless of group. The authors conclude that the benefits of spectacle correction for infants with hyperopia can be achieved without impairing the normal developmental process of emmetropization.

One of the biggest problems in young children with uncorrected refractive hyperopia is accommodative esotropia. Although it can occur earlier, accommodative esotropia generally appears for the first time between the ages of 18 and 36 months with a classic history. The parents will report that the eye never turned before and then about 2 to 3 weeks ago the eye started to turn. This history should point to an accommodative esotropia, and the application of lenses will generally be sufficient to solve the problem, unless the strabismus is long standing. Coats et al. (26) looked at refractive accommodative esotropia and found that it was diagnosed as early as 4 months. Prematurity is a risk factor and, to treat, they fully prescribed the hyperopic spectacle correction, which led to long-term alignment with relatively few patients requiring surgery.

Often, the accommodative esotropia is purely caused by uncorrected refractive error. Frequently, full hypermetropic correction, however, leaves a residual deviation, although it reduces much of the strabismic angle. Surgery results in a large number of under corrections. Therefore Wright and Bruce-Lyle (27) devised a formula for augmentation of the amount the rectus resection should be to achieve more appropriate alignment. They compared augmented surgery with standard surgery in patients who had bilateral medial rectus surgery for residual accommodative esotropia after full correction of hyperopia. A total of 70 patients were compared of whom 30 had standard surgery and the other 40 had augmented surgery. The success rate of the augmented surgery group was 98% compared with 74% for the standard surgery group. One patient whose surgery was not considered successful had a consecutive exotropia and remained exotropic even after removal of the hyperopic correction.

Berk et al. (28) examined the clinical features and functional outcomes in patients with accommodative esotropia who received conventional management and any amblyopia that developed in this group. At onset, they found that 87 of 147 (59%) were amblyopic and anisometropic, the latter anomaly being the sole significant risk factor for the amblyopia. They found that a minority of their subjects (24.2%) had stereo acuity between 40 and 100 seconds of arc, and 32.8% had no stereo acuity at all. Interestingly, the authors found no difference between early onset (<1 year) and typical onset (2 to 3 years) age groups.

Watanabe-Numata et al. (29) examined the changes in deviation following the correction of hyperopia in children with accommodative esotropia. Their population consisted of 49 children who were diagnosed as fully accommodative esotropia at the age of 4 years. All children were given full prescriptions for full-time spectacle wear. These children were re-evaluated at 10 or 11 years of age. At that time, 28 (57.1%) of the children had good alignment, 12 (24.5%) developed a partial accommodative esotropia, and 9 (18.4%) developed consecutive exotropia. The age of onset of the accommodative esotropia, age of initial visit, and refraction were similar for the three groups. The only *difference* finding was that the amblyopia in the consecutive exotropia group was higher (89%) than the amblyopia in the good alignment group (50%). These authors concluded that some purely accommodative esotropic patients are predisposed to developing consecutive exotropia.

A question that frequently arises when plus lenses are necessary for ocular alignment is: "Will my child have to wear these glasses forever?" The answer is not simple and cannot be made with assurance. Lambert et al. (30), however, looked at the ability to predict whether a child could be weaned from spectacles in the case of a fully accommodative esotropia. They took those with fully accommodative esotropia with refractive errors ranging from +1.50 to +5.00 D. They gradually weaned these children in half diopter steps until spectacles could be discontinued or they developed esotropia, asthenopia, or decreased visual acuity. They were able to wean 12 of 20 children (60%) from spectacles. The glasses were originally prescribed at 4.2 years and weaning was initiated at 8 years. The clinical characteristic most clearly identifiable with success with weaning from the glasses was the refractive error at the time the glasses were prescribed. The authors concluded that it is possible to wean children from spectacles in fully accommodative esotropia in the grade school years.

Prescribing lenses is fairly straightforward in those with high hyperopia or hyperopic patients with an accommodative esotropia. But what about the moderate to high hyperopic patient without anisometropia? These children, according to Klimek et al. (31), are at increased risk for isoametropic amblyopia. They looked at healthy children with greater or equal to 4.5 D hyperopia sphero-equivalent with anisometropia of no greater than 1.5 D. Children in the study had an increased risk of both isoametropic amblyopia and strabismus. The authors concluded that lenses should be prescribed for these children even in cases of no strabismus or fixation preference. It is very important to prescribe lenses for this type of child, not necessarily full plus, but a significant percentage of it.

ASTIGMATISM

It has been observed and known for several decades that infants have a very high incidence of astigmatism. It is also known that this astigmatism decreases in degree and in incidence with increasing age. Compared with school age children, infants, however, show ten times more incidence and considerably greater degrees of clinically significant astigmatism than older cohorts, according to Mohindra et al. (32). The degree of astigmatism, they find, begins to decrease in the second year, and the incidence declines during the third year. The same group.

(33) find that, in the presence of the astigmatism, infants and possibly toddlers do not develop meridional amblyopia. Their data show that infants with optical correction in place, appear like those who are not astigmatic. They conclude that no meridional amblyopia occurs in at least the first year of life in the presence of significant astigmatism. In a subsequent paper, Gwiazda et al. (34) measured visual acuity in 77 infants with astigmatism using a forced preferential looking procedure. The authors found similar acuity between infants who had astigmatism and those who did not. Acuity developed more quickly for vertical and horizontal gratings than it did for oblique gratings, but was similar for both groups. With the exception of infants with a strong myopic focus and one infant with a strong hyperopic focus, none of the infants showed acuity reductions. In addition, the acuity of the myopic and extremely hyperopic infants improved to normal levels when correction was applied.

When is a prescription required for cylindrical refractive error? The factors to consider are age, acuity, and stability. If an infant comes in with significant astigmatism (>3.00 D), certainly consider prescribing corrective lenses. Before giving the prescription, however, monitor the child carefully and often. At the beginning of the chapter, I gave an example of an infant with astigmatism who maintained the same astigmatic refraction across successive visits. Such a child needs vision correction to obtain good visual acuity development. The second child I gave as an example at the beginning was equally astigmatic who decreased in astigmatic correction with each subsequent visit. The first child has a stable refractive (astigmatic) error, whereas that in the second child is not stable and changing. Until the astigmatism shows stability, it should be monitored. That astigmatism decreases over time and meridional amblyopia does not seem to be an issue for the first 18 months or longer. Therefore, the astigmatism can be monitored and evaluated every 3 months until stability is reached or the refractive error is no longer present. When the astigmatic error stabilizes, if correction is needed, full correction or mild undercorrection of 0.5 D is advised. This must be considered within the context of the cylinder axis. Slight undercorrection for $-\times180$ and $-\times90$ cylinder is appropriate. Oblique cylinders should be corrected fully, however.

In 2005 a survey of pediatric ophthalmologists was conducted (35) regarding prescribing practices for astigmatism in infancy and early childhood with the objective to determine prescribing practices of these clinicians for astigmatism and astigmatic anisometropia. The survey was sent to 700 practitioners and 412 (59%) were returned. As expected, prescribing practices depended on age and degree of astigmatism. Considerable variability was seen to the responses, so a response rate at which 50% of the respondents would prescribe was considered normal practice. Agreement was that they would prescribe glasses for an infant with astigmatism if the astigmatism was equal to or greater than 4.00 D from birth to 6 months. This number decreased to greater than or equal to 2.00 D by 2 to less than 3 years of age. Of the respondents, 20% indicated that they would not prescribe glasses for any amount of astigmatism in infants under 6 months of age. The prescribing guidelines for astigmatic anisometropia were somewhat less variable, with 50% of the practitioners prescribing eyeglasses for astigmatic anisometropia greater than or equal to 3.00 D from birth to less than 6 months and greater than or equal to 1.50 D by 2 to less than 3 years.

ANISOMETROPIA

Anisometropia is the most insidious refractive condition because it is most often totally asymptomatic. Both the child and the parent are unaware of any problem. Unlike when a child is myopic, the parents notice the child bringing everything up close or the child gets close to everything. If the child is significantly hyperopic, generally an associated accommodative esotropia or an active avoidance of near work is seen, either of which is a sign of a visual problem. Anisometropia, especially if one eye is plano and the other is significantly myopic, hyperopic, or astigmatic, will not reveal itself. It is easily diagnosed in the course of an eye examination. But most children are not visually evaluated until they enter school or even later. The child's anisometropia, therefore, will go undetected and untreated until the child is school-aged and has a first eye examination. By this time, the child will surely be amblyopic. This amblyopia will then have to be dealt with along with the anisometropia. With preventive and early vision evaluations, this particular problem can be averted. Anisometropia is an amblyogenic factor that needs to be identified as early as possible and treated early so that a deep amblyopia will not develop. The key, as with many visual anomalies, is early detection and intervention. Vital-Durand and Ayzac (36) studied 2143 infants aged 5 to 15 months to see what risk factors there were for amblyopia. The single risk factor with the highest predisposition for amblyopia is anisometropia. The authors conclude that their results support screening of refractive and resolution defects in the entire population. Sen (37) reported on 172 pure anisometropic amblyopic patients of whom 167 were anisohypermetropic and 5 of them were anisomyopic. He found that amblyopia was dense and fixation was foveal in most of these cases, and the larger the anisometropia the deeper the amblyopia. No relationship was noted, however, between the age at presentation and the degree of anisometropia. Again, this is because this problem is asymptomatic. deVries (38) studied a hospital population of children to look at the incidence of anisometropia. He examined 1356 children and found 64 (4.7%) with anisometropia of at least 2.00 D of difference in spherical or cylindrical power. He eliminated 11 children with ocular lesions and considered the remaining 53 children. Of those, 27 had strabismus, which seemed to be caused by accommodative imbalances rather than the degree of anisometropia. deVries reported that amblyopia was present in 53% of the patients with orthotropic anisometropia. The greater the anisometropia, the deeper was the amblyopia. Therapy for this group was spectacle correction and part-time occlusion, which proved successful for 47% of the patients.

The literature (39–42) is clear in identifying anisometropia and strabismus as amblyogenic. No disagreement exists concerning this point. Anisometropia is strongly related to amblyopia. Hypermetropic anisometropia is more problematic and amblyogenic than myopic anisometropia because the more hyperopic eye is not used at any distance because it is easier for the child to accommodate to the lesser degree at both distance and near. In myopic anisometropia, again depending on the difference between the eyes, it is possible to use the less-myopic eye to look at distance and the more myopic eye to look at near. If the difference between the eyes is not more than 3.00 to 4.00 D of myopia, the latter scenario can play out. If the difference between the eyes is greater than 4.00 D, however, it is more likely that the lesser myopic eye will be used for distance and near.

Levartovsky et al. (43) looked at hypermetropic anisometropes to study the effects of the anisometropia on visual acuity development of treated patients 6 years after cessation of treatment (occlusion of the nonamblyopic eye). They divided patients into two groups: those where the difference between the eyes was small less than or equal to +1.50 D and those where the difference was greater than +1.50 D. All patients were followed up to at least 9 years of age. At the examinations done 6 years after cessation of therapy, they found that acuity had deteriorated in 51% of the lower anisometropia group and in 75% of the patients in the higher anisometropia group. At the time treatment was stopped, the average acuity of the amblyopic eye was 20/40+ in both groups. In the long-term follow-up, however, the average visual acuity was 20/40- in the group with lesser anisometropia and 20/70 in the group with a greater degree of anisometropia. They concluded that, even with diagnosis and treatment, anisohypermetropia of greater than +1.50 D can be a risk factor for acuity deterioration long term.

Aside from the effect anisometropia has on acuity development, it also interferes—sometimes very significantly—with the development of binocularity. The difference in refraction between the two eyes can create significant differences in acuity and image size between the two eyes. Weakley et al. (44) examined 345 patients with a refractive error of +2.00 D or more mean spherical equivalent (MSE) to look at what effect a difference of +1.00 D or greater had on ocular alignment. They clearly showed that anisometropia of more than or equal to 1.00 D is a significant risk factor for the development of accommodative esotropia, especially in patients with lower overall hypermetropia. Anisometropia additionally increases the risk that an accommodative esotropia will not be satisfactorily aligned with glasses. Tomac and Birdal (45) studied the effects of anisometropia on binocularity. They looked at 25 patients with anisometropia corrected by spectacles. They evaluated binocularity using Bagolini glasses, 4 prism diopter test, TNO stereotest, and Worth four dot tests. Acuity of each eye was recorded. Although they all demonstrated fusion by Bagolini glasses, most showed deficits or absence of response on the other testing. These authors found that the depth of amblyopia is more effective than the degree of anisometropia in causing a breakdown in binocularity. They found that all of their patients demonstrated bifoveal fusion. The TNO stereo test was the most sensitive test to binocularity deficits and the authors feel, therefore, that it is an effective way to detect anisometropic amblyopia. Weakley (46) studied 411 children with various levels of anisometropia, no previous therapy, and no ocular pathology. He looked at the effect of anisometropia (both corrected and uncorrected) on monocular acuity and binocular function. He found that spherical myopic anisometropia of greater than 2.00 D or spherical hyperopic anisometropia of greater than 1.00 D results in a statistically greater number of amblyopic patients and binocular dysfunctions when compared to those who are not anisometropic. With increasing differences between the two eyes is seen an associated increase in the depth of the amblyopia and a decrease in binocular function. Weakley concludes that the guidelines for treatment considered when there is a difference greater than 2.00 D of myopia or 1.00 D of hyperopia (46).

Prescribing spectacle lenses for the anisometropic patient is urgently important to establish equal acuity in the two eyes. Discussions in the literature indicate that great degrees of anisometropia, which are corrected by spectacle lenses, produce differences in image size that preclude binocularity. Many reports in the same literature, however, show that children with large anisometropic corrections adapt to the lenses very well with none of the expected negative effects.

As with all other refractive errors in very young children, it is important to watch for stability to occur. Anisometropia can change over the course of time in infants and toddlers. Therefore, if you identify an anisometropia and you can demonstrate equal acuities in the two eyes, you can monitor the refraction. As soon as acuity is compromised or the refractive error appears stable, a lens prescription should be given. It is not as important to give full correction as to give the full difference. Suppose a 9-month-old child on a first visit had a refraction of R +2.00 D sphere L +6.00 D sphere and acuities were normal. Have the child return for a recheck in 3 months, stressing the importance of follow-up. In 3 months, the same child comes in with normal and equal acuities and now the refraction is R +2.00 D sphere L +4.00 D sphere. Again, monitor the child and recheck in 3 months. On the third visit, the acuities are not equal with the left eye mildly worse (1 Cardiff card difference) and the refraction R +2.00 D sphere L +4.00 D sphere. At this point, glasses are indicated because of the inequality of monocular acuities and stability of the anisometropic difference over 3 months. Now the question is, "What do you prescribe?" Nothing is wrong with prescribing R +2.00 D sphere L +4.00 D sphere. Another option, however, is to underprescribe the plus, but maintain the full anisometropic difference. Therefore, another perfectly acceptable option would be R +1.00 D sphere L +3.00 D sphere. This will maintain equal clarity of the images to the two eyes and equal accommodation. Follow-up should be in 3 months. As the child gets older, it will be vitally important to monitor binocularity as well.

Roberts and Adams (48) reported on treating high anisometropia with amblyopia with contact lenses. Their anisometropic differences ranged from 6.00 D to 18.4 D (mean = 10.4 D) Their patients' ages at presentation ranged from 3.5 to 6 years. They reported modest success with corrected acuities in the amblyopic eye starting at from 20/60 to 20/1200 and after from 5 months to 4 years of wear ended at 20/40 to 20/1200. Two of their myopic patients improved four Snellen lines, but three with greater than 10.00 D difference did not improve at all. One of the problems with Roberts and Adams sample was the age at presentation. The mean age was 4.5 years. Again, the issue of early identification and intervention raises its head. When anisometropic differences are great (e.g. R +16.00 L plano, it is best to use a monocular contact lens. To do so, however, parents must be very compliant. (See Chapter 15). Using contact lenses for mild to moderate refractive differences may be taking unnecessary risks. The myopic anisometropic patient may be handled somewhat differently. Anisometropic differences do not have to be prescribed for smaller differences. Start prescribing for 2.00 D and greater differences. Undercorrecting the myopia is not recommended because good and equal acuities are desired in both eyes. Therefore, the myopic patient who measures R −4.00 and L −7.00 D should get that prescription without modification. Prescriptions should be given for full-time wear. If you prescribe the R −4.00 and the L −7.00 and the child has a significant esophoria at near, it is wise to consider undercutting the myopic lenses at near by use of a bifocal prescription (See below). Another option would be to undercorrect the more myopic eye by up to, but not greater than, 2.00 D. All of this must be done within the context of binocularity.

Another method of dealing with anisometropia being used increasingly is photorefractive surgery, both photorefractive keratectomy (PRK) and laser *in situ* keratomileusis (LASIK). The reasons for using photorefractive surgery vary from large anisometropia in noncompliant children, to children who have successfully brought acuity in the anisometropic amblyopic eye to a normal level (usually 20/30 or better) through treatment and the surgery is done to keep acuity stable.

Rashad (49) studied 14 children with myopic anisometropia and amblyopia, whose ages ranged from 7 to 12 years. LASIK was done in the more myopic eye in all 14 children. Preoperative spherical equivalent differences (SED) ranged from −4.62 to −12.50 D and best spectacle corrected visual acuity was 20/40 to 20/100. All patients completed at least 1 year of follow-up. One year after LASIK, the spherical equivalent manifest refraction of the eyes ranged from plano to −1.50. Spectacle-corrected visual acuity ranged from 20/20 to 20/40. All eyes improved in visual acuity and six eyes (42.9%) had a postoperative acuity of 20/20 in the amblyopic eye. Rashad concluded that LASIK was effective and safe for correction of myopic anisometropia and reversed anisometropic

amblyopia. Alio et al. (50) used PRK to treat pediatric patients with amblyopic myopic anisometropia in whom conventional amblyopia treatment had failed. The sample size was six patients aged 5 to 7 years. PRK was performed on the more myopic eye. Preoperatively, the refraction of the more myopic eye ranged from −4.00 to −13.00 D, with best corrected visual acuity ranging from 20/40 to 20/400. All six children were followed a minimum of 2 years postoperatively. After PRK, preoperative best-corrected visual acuity was maintained without optical correction and, with optical correction, 100% of the amblyopic eyes showed improvement. One child developed a severe haze after surgery. The authors use their data to support the use of PRK in pediatric anisomyopic patients where traditional therapies have failed. Phillips et al. (51) looked at the safety and efficacy of LASIK in pediatric and adolescent patients with anisometropic amblyopia. They had a cohort of 19 patients ranging in age from 8 to 19 years (mean age, 13.14 years). This group consisted of both hyperopic and myopic anisometropias. Seventeen patients had LASIK performed on the eye with the higher refraction and two who were older than 18 years had both eyes done. The percentage deviation from the attempted correction in the myopic group was 4%, whereas for the hyperopic group, it was 38%. Anisometropia decreased uniformly, however, to less than 2.00 D in all patients. The percentage of patients who had stereoacuity increased from 63% presurgically to 84% postoperatively. The authors propose LASIK to be a safe and effective means of reducing anisometropia in this population and note that stereoacuity, even if not present preoperatively, can be obtained postoperatively. Nassarella and Nassarella (52), Rybintseva and Sheludchenko (53), among many others, report on the success, safety, and effectiveness of LASIK on clinically managing pediatric patients with anisometropia to deal with acuity issues as well as binocularity. Others (54,55) praise the virtues of PRK procedures in dealing with pediatric patients with anisometopic amblyopia. Paysse (54) concludes that PRK can be safely performed on children with anisometropic amblyopia; and that visual acuity and stereopsis improved even in the older children. He contends, therefore, that PRK may have an important role in the management of anisometropic amblyopia in noncompliant children.

Although it is an aggressive therapy, photorefractive surgery may be a viable alternative for anisometropic patients when conventional therapies do not work to preserve visual acuity and establish or maintain binocularity.

CHILDREN AND BIFOCAL LENSES

Children wear bifocal lenses? That seems silly; bifocals are for old people. That is often the reaction when the clinician suggests a bifocal lens for a child. Although bifocal lens use for children is becoming increasingly common, parents may not be exposed to them. Bifocals should be considered anytime the child demonstrates a moderate to high eso posture, an esotropia at near (intermittent or constant), and accommodative insufficiency or excess. Bifocals should not be given until the child has reasonably good head and neck control and ocular motility. Otherwise, the child will have difficulty walking or moving about and the parent will not be able to observe the child carefully. If children are given the bifocal lens before good ocular motor skills are developed, they are likely to move their head and neck rather than their eyes and use only the top portion of the bifocal lens. The proper use of bifocal segments mandates good ocular motor control. If the child is very young (up to about 15 months), it is better to *overplus* the distance prescription than to give bifocal lenses. Again, the infant's world is within arm's reach, near will be clear with overplus lenses and it is hoped will control the binocular anomaly. When the child is old enough, a change to a bifocal lens would be appropriate. Use of bifocal lenses for toddlers, preschool, and school-aged children is becoming commonplace. Some parents come in expecting that their children may need bifocals to alleviate symptoms and problems at near point. It may not be necessary to explain why you are prescribing bifocals to some parents.

Bifocals are used for such things as:

1. Accommodative esotropia
2. Accommodative infacility or insufficiency
3. Moderate to high esodeviation at near
4. Myopia control

Bifocal use depends on three main factors: distance prescription, posture or tropia at near, and age. School-aged children with mild to moderate distance hypermetropia who maintain alignment without the bifocal (despite having esophoria) should use their glasses in school and for all school and near work activities. Younger children and school-aged children who manifest a high esophoria or an esotropia without the glasses should wear their prescription full time. Myopic patients who have eso at near (phoria or tropia), who wears a bifocal add to manage posture, should wear their glasses full time. And the myopic patient who wears a bifocal in an attempt to slow down the progression of myopia should wear the glasses full time. Some practitioners tell their mild to moderate myopic patients to wear their glasses for distance, but to take them off for any near activity. Most children will not adhere to that type of utilization and will leave the glasses on all the time. Therefore, a bifocal add would be a preferred option. Much has been written about bifocals and the progression of myopia, with little compelling data. Fulk et al. (56) reported a slight decrease occurs in progression of myopia when bifocals are used for near work instead of single vision glasses. Fulk and Cylert (57) looked at 32 children with near point esophoria who were randomly divided into correction with single vision glasses and bifocals containing a +1.25 D add. For the first 12 months, myopia progression was the same for both groups. Progression was much faster during the first 6 months, which coincided with the school year, than during the second 6 months, which included the summer vacation. During the last 6 months of the 18-month follow-up, the myopia in children with single vision progressed rapidly, but it progressed only half as much for the bifocal cohort. The authors conclude that, overall, myopia progressed more slowly in the bifocal group than in the single vision group. They also noted that myopia progressed more rapidly during the school year than during summer vacation. Parssinen et al. (58,59) studied the effect of spectacle use and accommodation on the progression of myopia in a 3-year clinical trial among school children aged 9 to 11 years. They allocated these children to one of three groups: (a) minus lenses with full correction for full-time wear; (b) minus lenses with full correction to be used for distance only; and (c) minus lenses with full correction with a +1.75 D add OU. Of 240 children, they followed 237 children for 3 years. The progression of the myopia was not significant for the right eye, but it increased significantly more in the left eye of the distance only group than in the other groups. No differences were seen in school performance between groups. In all three groups, the more close work the children did, the faster the myopia progressed. Myopic progression did not correlate with accommodation, but rather with the shorter average working distance. Parsinnen et al., therefore, feel that myopia progression cannot be related to accommodation and the utilization of accommodative adds and distance vision correction for distance only is not effective in slowing myopia. Fulk et al. (60), continuing the study mentioned above, followed up the children in their study after 4.5 years (54 months) and found that wearing bifocals instead of single vision glasses slowed the progression of myopia over the first 2 years; after that, although the difference in degree of myopia was sustained, it did not increase. This suggests that bifocals are effective in slowing the progression of myopia, but after a time they are at the apex of what they can facilitate.

Bifocals can be used successfully in the management of accommodative problems, particularly accommodative insufficiency. Chrousos et al. (61) examined patients between the ages of 10 to 19 years with accommodative insufficiency. In all these patients, the amplitudes of accommodation were significantly below age expected (average amplitude, 6.00 D). All of these cases were successfully managed with bifocal lenses or reading glasses eliminating complaints of near vision problems.

Saw et al. (62) found no conclusive evidence that use of bifocals, alterations of spectacle wear, ocular hypotensive medications, or contact lenses can change the pattern of myopia progression. The only proven treatment is the use of atropine eye drops in children and that myopia in these children progresses more slowly than in groups given placebo drops. Again, the negative side effects of atropine are raised (i.e., photophobia, light-induced retinal damage, and cataract formation). They suggest that other antimuscarinic agents (e.g., pirenzepine) might accomplish the same effects, but with lesser side effects.

Progressive addition lenses (PAL) are suggested for use in the effective treatment of accommodative esotropia. Smith (63) treated 32 children (age, 1.5 to 16 years) with accommodative esotropia with PALs. The advantages are the cosmesis and the more natural progression of accommodation. The big disadvantage was the difficulty in fitting these children with the lenses. He found, however, that if he could keep the add high enough, the children did well and none would return to the executive bifocals they had been wearing. Jacob et al. (64) corrected vision in 25 children with accommodative esotropia with PALs. Of these children, 25 had previously been wearing executive bifocals. The other 13 were fitted with PALs for the first time. Jacob et al. found that the strabismus was managed well and most of the children were able to demonstrate stereopsis. The children had no difficulty adapting to the PALs.

One more important lens application in the pediatric patient must be mentioned here: use of yoked prisms to stabilize head posture in children with nystagmus who distort posture to get to their null point. It is not a simple matter and no one-to-one relationship exists between the child's posture and that child's null point. For example, a 4-year-old boy (Christopher) presents with aniridia and vision impairment with nystagmus. The chief entering complaint was that he was photophobic and looked at everything with his head pointed downward. His physical therapist had grave concerns about the long-term effect on his posture. On examination, he had large amplitude, low-frequency pendular nystagmus that nulled when he looked into superior gaze. At the time, the boy had no communication skills except for a yes or no response. His visual acuity (VA) was 20/200, 200, 200 using Baylor Visual Acuity Tester (BVAT) Picture Optotype matching. Aniridia was complete and ocular health (including intraocular pressure) was normal. No significant refractive error was found. To get the boy to keep his head straight, we decided to use base down (BD) prism OU so that he would have to look upward to see things straight in front of him. But, how much prism should we give? There is no formula. It is strictly a matter of trial and error. We started with 8 BD OU, but worked up to 16 BD OU before Christopher's head appeared straight. We prescribed the prism for full-time wear and checked the boy in 3 months. At the time of the recheck examination, it was reported that Christopher had no difficulty with the prism; he seemed to see better and his head was straight most of the time. His physical therapist was very pleased with the change. Another child with the same symptoms might only need 10 BD OU to effect the same postural change. Therefore, it is necessary to try the prism on the patient to find the appropriate amount to prescribe. The appropriate amount is the least prism needed to effect the desired result (i.e., moving the child to the null point). These children should be monitored closely every 3 to 6 months. Over time, it is possible to decrease the amount of prism and maintain the posture.

REFERENCES

1. Michaels DD. Indications for prescribing spectacles. *Surv Ophthalmol* 1981;26(2):55–74.
2. Saunders KJ, Woodhouse JM, Westall CA. Emmetropisation in human infancy: rate of change is related to initial refractive error. *Vision Res* 1995;35(9):1325–1328.
3. Liang CL, Ye E, Su JY, et al. Impact of family history of high myopia on level and onset of myopia. *Invest Ophthalmol Vis Sci* 2004;45(10):3446–3452.
4. Ben Simon GJ, Peiss M, Anis E, et al. Spectacle use and reduced unaided vision in third grade students: a comparative study in different educational settings. *Clin Exp Optom* 2004;87(3):175–179.
5. Caltrider N, Jampolsky A. Overcorrecting minus lens therapy for treatment of intermittent exotropia. *Ophthalmology* 1983;90(10):1160–1165.
6. Rutstein RP, Marsh-Tootle W, London R. Changes in refractive error for exotropes treated with overminus lenses. *Optom Vis Sci* 1989;66(8):487–491.
7. Coffey B, Wick B, Cotter S, et al. Treatment options in intermittent exotropia: a critical appraisal. *Optom Vis Sci* 1992;69:(5):386–404.
8. Iacobucci IL, Martonyi EJ, Giles CL. Results of overminus lens therapy on postoperative exodeviations. 1986;23(6):287–291.
9. Parssinen O, Hemminki E, Klemetti A. Effect of spectacle use and accommodation on myopic progression: final results of a three-year randomised clinical trial among schoolchildren. *Br J Ophthalmol* 1989;73(7):547–551.
10. Fulk GW, Cyert LA, Parker DE. A randomized trial of effect of single-vision vs. bifocal lenses on myopia progression in children with esophoria. *Optom Vis Sci* 2000;77(8):395–401.
11. Goss DA. Effect of spectacle correction on the progression of myopia in children—a literature review. *Journal of the American Optometric Association* 1994;65(2):117–128.
12. Fulk GW, Cyert LA, Parker DE. A randomized clinical trial of bifocal glasses for myopic children with esophoria: results after 54 months. *Optometry* 2002;73(8):470–476.
13. Fulk, GW, Cyert LA. Can bifocals slow myopic progression? *Journal of the American Optometric Association* 1996;67(12):749–754.
14. Ong E, Grice K, Held R, et al. Effects of spectacle intervention on the progression of myopia in children. *Optom Vis Sci* 1999;76(6):341–342.
15. Gwiazda JE, Hyman L, Norton TT, et al; COMET Group. Accommodation related risk factors associated with myopia progression and their interaction with treatment in COMET children. *Invest Ophthalmol Vis Sci* 2004;45(7):2143–2151.
16. Shih YF, Chen CH, Chou AC, et al. Effects of different concentrations of atropine on controlling myopia in myopic children. *J Ocul Pharmacol Ther* 1999;156(1):85–90.
17. Romano PE, Donovan JP. Management of progressive school myopia with topical atropin eyedrops and photochromic bifocal spectacles. *Binocular Vision and Strabismus Quarterly* 2000;15(30):257–260.
18. Saw SM, Shih-Yen EC, Koh A, et al. Interventions to retard myopia progression in children: an evidence based update. *Ophthalmology* 2002;109(3):415–421.
19. Kennedy RH, Dyer JA, Kennedy MA, et al. Reducing the progression in myopia with atropine: a long term cohort study of Olmsted County students. *Binocul Vis Strabismus Q* 2000;15[3 Suppl]:281–284.
20. Syniuta LA, Isenberg. Atropine and bifocals can slow the progression of myopia in children. *Binocul Vis Strabismus Q* 2001;16(3):203–208.
21. Shih YF, Hsaio CK, Chen CJ, et al. An intervention trial on efficacy of atropine and multi-focal glasses in controlling myopic progression. *ACTA Opthalmologica Scandanavia* 2001;79(3):233–236.
22. Chung K, Mohidin N, O'Leary DJ. Undercorrection of myopia enhances rather than inhibits myopia progression. *Vision Res* 2002;42(22):2555–2559.
23. Chiang MF, Kouzis A, Pointer RW, et al. Treatment of childhood myopia with atropine eyedrops and bifocal spectacles. *Binocul Vis Strabismus Q* 2001;16(3):209–215.
24. Edelman PM, Borchert MS. Visual outcome in high hypermetropia. *J AAPOS* 1997;1(3):147–150.
25. Atkinson J, Anker S, Bobier W, et al. Normal emmetropization in infants with spectacle correction for hyperopia. *Invest Ophthalmol Vis Sci* 2000;41(12):3726–3731.
26. Coats DK, Avilla CW, Paysse EA, et al. Early-onset refractive accommodative estropia. *J AAPOS* 1998;2(5):275–278.
27. Wright KW, Bruce-Lyle L. Augmented surgery for esotropia associated with hypermetropia. *J Pediatr Ophthalmol Strabismus* 1993;30(3):167–170.
28. Berk AT, Kocak N, Ellidokuz H. Treatment outcomes in refractive accommodative esotropia. *J AAPOS* 2004;8(4):384–388.
29. Watanabe-Numata K, Hayasaka S, Watanabe K, et al. Changes in deviation following correction of hyperopia in children with fully refractive accommodative esotropia. *Ophthalmologica* 2000;214(5):309–311.
30. Lambert SR, Lynn M, Sramek J, Hutcheson KA. Clinical features predictive of successfully weaning from spectacles those children with accommodative esotropia. *J AAPOS* 2003;7(1):7–13.

31. Klimek DL, Cruz OA, Scott WE, et al. Isoametropic amblyopia due to high hyperopia in children. *J AAPOS* 2004;8(4):310–313.

32. Mohindra I, Held R, Gwiazda J, et al. Astigmatism in infants. *Science* 1978;202(4365):329–331.

33. Gwiazda J, Mohindra I, Brill S, et al. Infant astigmatism and meridional amblyopia. *Vision Res* 1985;25(9):1269–1276.

34. Gwiazda J, Mohindra I, Brill S, et al. The development of visual acuity in infant astigmats. *Invest Ophthalmol Vis Sci* 1985;26(12):1717–1723.

35. Harvey EM, Miller JM, Dobson V, et al. Prescribing eyeglass correction for astigmatism in infancy and early childhood: a survey of AAPOS members. *J AAPOS* 2005;9(2):189–191.

36. Vital-Durand F, Ayzac L. Tackling amblyopia in human infants. *Eye* 1996;10(Pt2):239–244.

37. Sen DK. Anisometropic amblyopia. *J Pediatr Ophthalmol Strabismus* 1980;17(3):180–184.

38. de Vries J. Anisometropia in children: analysis of a hospital population. *Br J Ophthalmol* 1985;69(7):504–507.

39. Cobb DJ, Russell K, Cox A, et al. Factors influencing visual outcome in anisometropic amblyopes. *Br J Ophthalmol* 2002;86:1278–1281.

40. Hardman Lea SJ, Loades J, et al. The sensitive period for anisometropic amblyopia. *Eye* 1989;3(Pt. 6):783–790.

41. Klimek DL, Cruz OA, Scott WE, et al. Isoametropic amblyopia due to high hyperopia in children. *J AAPOS* 2004;8(4):310–313.

42. Woodruff G, Hiscox F, Thompson JR, et al. The presentation of children with amblyopia. *Eye* 1994;8(Pt. 6):623–626.

43. Levartovsky S, Oliver M, Gottesman N, et al. Long-term effect of hypermetropic anisometropia on the visual acuity of treated amblyopic eyes. *Br J Ophthalmol* 1998;82(1):55–58.

44. Weakley DR Jr, Birch E, Kip K. The role of anisometropia in the development of accommodative esotropia. *J AAPOS* 2001;5(3):153–157.

45. Tomac S, Birdal E. Effects of anisometropia on binocularity. *J Pediatr Ophthalmol Strabismus* 2001;38(1):27–33.

46. Weeakley DR. The association between anisometropia, amblyopia and binocularity in the absence of strabismus. *Trans Am Ophthalmol Soc* 1999;97:987–1021.

47. Rutstein RP, Corliss D. Relationship between anisometropia, amblyopia and binocularity. *Optom Vis Sci* 1999;76(4):229–233.

48. Roberts CJ, Adams GG. Contact lenses in the management of high anisometropic amblyopia. *Eye* 2002;16(5):577–579.

49. Rashad KM. Laser in situ keratomileusis for myopic anisometropia in children. *J Refract Surg* 1999;15(4):429–435.

50. Alio JL, Artola A, Claramonte P, et al. Photorefractive keratectomy for pediatric myopic anisometropia. *J Cataract Refract Surg* 1998;24(3):327–330.

51. Phillips CB, Prager TC, McClellan G, et al. Laser in situ keratomileusis for treated anisometropic amblyopia in awake, auto-fixating pediatric and adolescent patients. *J Cataract Refract Surg* 2004;30(12):2522–2528.

52. Nassarella BR, Nassarella JJ Jr. Laser in situ keratomileusis in children 8 to 15 years old. *J Refract Surg* 2001;17(5):519–524.

53. Rybintseva LV, Sheludchenko VM. Effectiveness of laser in situ keratomileusis with the Nidek EC-5000 excimer laser for pediatric correction of spherical anisometropia. *J Refract Surg* 2001;17[2 Suppl]:S224–S228.

54. Paysse EA. Photorefractive keratectomy for anisometropic amblyopia in children. *Trans Am Opthalmol Soc* 2004;102;341–371.

55. Autrata R, Rehurek J. Clinical results of excimer laser photorefractive keratectomy for high myopic anisometropia in children: four-year follow-up. *J Cataract Refract Surg* 2003;29(4):694–702.

56. Fulk GW, Cyert LA, Parker DE. A randomized trial of the effect of single-vision vs. bifocal lenses on myopia progression in children with esophoria. *Optom Vis Sci* 2000;77(8):395–401.

57. Fulk GW, Cyert LA. Can bifocals slow myopia progression? *Journal of the American Optometric Association* 1997;67(12):749–754.

58. Parssinen O, Hemminki E. Spectacle-use, bifocals and prevention of myopic progression. The two-years results of a randomized trial among schoolchildren. *Acta Ophthalmol Suppl* 1988;185:156–161.

59. Parssinen O, Hemminki E, Klemetti A. Effect of spectacle use and accommodation on myopic progression: final results of a three-year randomized clinical trial among schoolchildren. *Br J Ophthalmol* 1989;73:547–551.

60. Fulk GW, Cyert LA, Parker DE. A randomized clinical trial of bifocal glasses for myopic children with esophoria: results after 54 months. *Optometry* 2002;73(8):470–476.

61. Chrousos GA, O'Neill JF, Lueth BD, et al. Accommodation deficiency in healthy young individuals. *J Pediatr Ophthalmol Strabismus* 1988;27(6):176–179.

62. Saw SM, Gazzard G, Au Eong KG, et al. Myopia: attempts to arrest progression. *Br. J Ophthalmol* 2002;86(11):1306–1311.

63. Smith JB. Progressive-addition lenses in the treatment of accommodative esotropia. *Am J Ophthalmol* 1985;99(1):56–62.

64. Jacob JL, Beaulieu Y, Brunet E. Progressive-addition lenses in the management of esotropia with a high accommodation/convergence ratio. *Can J Ophthalmol* 1980;15(4):166–169.

Options in Strabismus

21

Valerie M. Kattouf

Treatment of strabismus in the pediatric population requires a careful analysis of the diagnostic data. Consideration of the patient's age at presentation, age of onset of strabismus, refractive error, magnitude of deviation, and fusional ability will aid in determining the best treatment option for the patient. Multiple options are available for treating strabismus in the pediatric population. This chapter reviews the most commonly used methods of treatment including surgical referrals, spectacle options, orthoptic treatment, and occlusion.

As with all diagnoses, it is important to determine the goal of the patient and parent in regard to treatment. When treating strabismus in the pediatric population, the greatest concern is often the improvement of the cosmetic nature of the strabismus. The cosmesis of a strabismic deviation has a very significant role in the psychological and motor development of a child. A literature review by Groffman (1) revealed that the face and eyes are the most important parts of the body in revealing personality. A strabismic deviation makes a child feel abnormal or different. The recognition of the strabismus by other children usually occurs around the age of 3 years. The negative attention often causes the child's personality to adjust by either becoming shy and withdrawn or acting out to attract attention. A study by Fletcher and Silverman (2) revealed that, in strabismic patients, different personality characteristics and developmental issues arise at different stages of development.

From 6 months to 5 years, behavioral problems and gross and fine motor delays are often evident. From 5 to 10 years of age, learning and attention issues often present. The cosmesis of a strabismus often causes a reaction in parents as well. Mothers often respond with an anxiety that may often be communicated to the child. For these reasons, we must address the cosmetic as well as the functional cure of strabismus at the appropriate age.

TREATMENT OPTIONS

Stabismus Surgery

Strabismus surgery is a medical treatment modality that often leaves optometrists fearful and suspicious. When the proper comanagement relationship is developed with a pediatric ophthalmologist, strabismus surgery is a valid and useful treatment option for young patients with the proper diagnostic and clinical characteristics. Strabismus surgery is often considered when the deviation is cosmetically apparent and not manageable by optical or orthoptic treatment. Strabismus surgery is also used if the patient is too immature for treatment with nonsurgical methods, or if the deviation is very large.

Strabismus surgery usually entails an extraocular muscle recession, resection, or a combination of procedures. The decision to perform the surgery unilaterally or bilaterally depends on the nature of the deviation and the

TABLE 21.1 Strabismus Surgery Key Words

Recession	Causes weakening of the muscle. This procedure disinserts the eye muscle and reattaches it further back on the globe.
Resection	Causes strengthening of the eye muscle. This procedure excises a portion of the distal end of the muscle and then reattaches this to the globe.
Myectomy	Weakens the muscle by excising a portion of the muscle belly.

associated conditions. The three most common surgical procedures are extraocular muscle recessions, resections, and myectomies. A muscle recession weakens the muscle. This procedure disinserts the extraocular muscle and reattaches it further back on the globe. A resection strengthens the eye muscle. This procedure excises a portion of the distal end of the muscle and then reattaches it to the globe. A myectomy is also a weakening of the muscle. The procedure produces a weakening effect by excising a portion of the muscle belly. These terms are summarized in Table 21.1 (3). Common strabismic diagnoses and the most utilized surgical techniques for each are listed in Table 21.2 (2).

Determination of which extraocular muscles are to be operated upon and the age at which the surgery is performed is made on a case-by-case basis. The two most common clinical characteristics of strabismus that require surgical correction are deviations with a large magnitude and high frequency. Caloroso and Rouse (4) developed guidelines regarding the need for surgical correction in strabismic patients. They determined that when a patient's deviation measured with best correction is greater than 20 prism diopters of esotropia, 25 prism diopters of exotropia, and 10 prism diopters of vertical tropia, surgical treatment should be considered (Table 21.3). Associated conditions (e.g., amblyopia, central nervous system disorders) and previous treatment history all affect the decisions made by the referring optometrist and the operating ophthalmologist. Young patients are often excellent candidates for a surgical correction. The goal of strabismus surgery in an infant or toddler is to

TABLE 21.2 Strabismus Causes and Surgical Techniques

Etiology of Strabismus	Most Common Surgical Procedure
Partially accommodative esotropia with amblyopia	MR recession + LR resection
Partially accommodative esotropia without amblyopia	Bilateral MR recession
Infantile esotropia	Bilateral MR recession
Infantile exotropia	Bilateral LR recession
Intermittent exotropia/divergence excess	Bilateral LR recession
Intermittent exotropia/basic	MR resection + Ipsilateral LR recession
Superior oblique palsy magnitude <15Δ	Recession of antagonist IO muscles
Superior oblique palsy magnitude >15Δ	Ipsilateral LR recession + Recession of the contralateral IR muscle

MR, medial rectus muscle; LR, lateral rectus muscle; IO, inferior oblique muscle; IR, inferior rectus muscle.

maximize the patient's potential for sensory fusion development and to improve the motor fusion for a cosmetic cure.

When determining the success of a strabismus surgery, two different criteria are evaluated, the cosmetic versus the functional cure. Cosmetic cures can most easily be defined as a strabismus that is undetectable to the untrained eye. A recent study defined a strabismic angle evident to lay observers to be 8 to 12 prism diopters in exotropia and 12 to 15 prism diopters in esotropia (5). Determination of a functional cure

TABLE 21.3 Magnitude of Strabismus Deviation Necessary for Surgical Correction

Type of Deviation	Magnitude
Exotropia	>20Δ
Esotropia	>25Δ
Vertical	>10Δ

TABLE 21.4 Summary of Postsurgical Cures for Strabismus

Type of Deviation	Cosmetic Cure Magnitude	Functional Cure 3-Part Definition
Exotropia	>20Δ	No strabismus at any distance by cover test
Esotropia	>25Δ	Motor fusion ranges demonstrated
Summary of literature	>10Δ	Sensory fusion demonstrated

in strabismus varies throughout the literature. The most frequently used criteria include no strabismus at any distance by cover test, presence of motor fusion ranges at distance and near, and demonstration of sensory fusion (6). Table 21.4 contains a summary of cosmetic and functional cures.

In infantile strabismus, the practitioner and the parent must address specific goals to determine the need for a strabismus surgery. For example, a low percentage of infants with esotropia have a functional cure, whereas a high percentage will have a cosmetic cure (7) The longer the misalignment is left untreated, less is the chance for development of sensory fusion in a very young patient. In the infant and toddler population, surgical candidates fall into three main categories.

- Patients with early onset, large-angle, constant deviations with a significant cosmesis that is not improved by refractive correction and may put the child at risk for amblyopia development.
- Patients with large-angle, intermittent deviations with whom motor and sensory fusion is present when the patient is aligned. Surgical correction allows a higher frequency of fusion. These patients are excellent candidates for a surgical correction that can be followed with orthoptic training and prism correction as the child matures.
- Patients whose parents have the sole goal of improving cosmesis.

The greatest concerns of a parent in regard to a child having strabismus surgery are the health risks. The highest level of concern in the pediatric population is that of the anesthesia risk. Although minimal, the risk in children under the age of 7 years is greater than in adults. The overall mortality rate of strabismus surgery is 1.4 per 10,000 (8). Other possible, but extremely rare, complications from strabismus surgery include vomiting, orbital cellulitis, suture abscess, transient changes in refractive error, and diplopia.

Relieving Prism Treatment

Relieving prism is a treatment option to consider for pediatric patients with strabismus. Successful use of prism involves selection of the patient with the proper diagnostic criteria. Patients who are the most successful with prism are those who are capable of central fusion. For example, a very early onset, constant strabismic deviation develops significant sensory anomalies that do not permit central fusion. These patients are not proper candidates for relieving prism treatment. Patients with intermittent deviations, adequate sensory fusion, and poor motor control are aided by relieving prism treatment. The goal of such treatment is to reduce, not to eliminate, the motor fusional demand. The residual deviation that a practitioner hopes to create when using relieving prism differs with the direction of the deviation. For an esotropia, it is 4 to 6Δ eso; for exotropia, 10 to 15Δ exo; and for vertical deviations, it is 2 to 4Δ hyper (9).

In a pediatric population, the examiner may have to make prism prescribing decisions without the aid of subjective testing. In addition to a lack of testing choices, a young patient may not be capable of maintaining fixation that can be held through multiple cover testing procedures. In these instances, the amount of relieving prism is chosen with the goal of decreasing the frequency of the deviation and improving motor control for the patient. For example, a patient 1 year of age presents with a history of an intermittent exotropia noted by the parents for the past 3 months. The parents claim the deviation is noticed 25% of the time and report that the frequency is increasing. Examination by Krimsky testing reveals a 25-prism diopter intermittent alternating exotropia present 50% of the time. Trial framing a prismatic correction of

5Δ base in the right eye (*oculis dexter*, OD), 5Δ base in left eye (*oculis sinister*, OS) revealed a decreased frequency of the exotropia. The patient is now responsible for only 15 prism diopters of convergence with the relieving prism versus the full 25 prism diopters. As stated, the goal of relieving prism is to reduce but not eliminate the motor fusional demand. This is an example of how a prism prescription aids in achieving that goal.

If a pediatric patient can maintain fixation for cover testing and participate in fusion testing, then the prescribing of relieving prism may take into consideration Sheard's criteria. Sheard's criteria state that, to achieve visual comfort, the compensating fusional vergence should equal to twice the patient's phoria. Below is a case example using Sheard's criteria to prescribe prism for a patient with intermittent exotropia (10).

CASE EXAMPLE

- 6-year-old patient
- Distance cover test (CT): 10Δ exophoria
- Near cover test: 15Δ intermittent alternating exotropia (30% frequency)
- Near base-out (BO) ranges (prism bar):14/6 (break/recovery)
- Interpretation
  - Convergence insufficiency type exotropia
  - Does not meet Sheard's criteria (compensating vergence: 2 × phoria)
  - To meet Sheard's criteria, BO vergence break point (14) would need to be ≥30 (15 × 2)
  - Prism prescription of 8Δ base-in (BI) (4Δ BI OD, 4Δ BI OS) will allow the patient to meet Sheard's criteria
- Decreases exo deviation to 7Δ and allows break point of 14Δ to meet Sheard's criteria

The prescribing of prism in the pediatric population is a useful tool in treating strabismus. It is often necessary for the practitioner to determine the amount of prism without relying on the more commonly used methods of testing (e.g., Maddox Rod, Worth 4-dot, fixation disparity). Relieving prism is also a superb treatment modality when used in conjunction with other strabismus treatment options. Prism often makes orthoptic treatment progress faster and result in higher rates of success; it can be used before and after surgery to maintain fusion in a strabismic patient.

Orthoptic Vision Therapy Treatment for Strabismus

The goal of orthoptic training for a strabismic patient varies according to the patient's age and maturity level. In infants, the main goal is to preserve binocularity. The implementation of vision therapy in infants is typically home based. Use of occlusion techniques for amblyopia and strabismus will aid in improving acuity and avoiding the development of suppression. Gross vision therapy techniques can be used to improve motility, fixation, and vergence skills. Many orthoptic activities performed in infancy are done to avoid the development of anomalous sensory adaptations.

Use of large toys with varying amounts of contrast will encourage the infant to fixate and track an object that commands the child's attention. Suggestions include using a face target (Mom's face, baby doll face) to encourage fixation and tracking and using a toy to perform a near point of convergence push-up (11). Scheduling of these activities must avoid sleeping and feeding times for the infant. Parents are instructed to perform the suggested techniques daily for 5 to 10 minutes. Multiple vision therapy sessions can be done throughout the day.

In the toddler and preschool strabismic patient, the goal of orthoptic training is similar to that of an infant. Again, the techniques can be performed at home but with a bit more sophistication. The goals of vision therapy in this age range are to improve motility and depth perception; avoid the development of suppression; and to perform gross vergence activities (12). Motility and vergence activities can be done in free space with an age-appropriate target or can be computer based. Antisuppression activities with red-green anaglyphs and filters are often implemented for a preschool patient with strabismus. Depth perception activities often involve eye–hand coordination and visually directed reaching or pointing (e.g., placing stick in a straw).

As with all treatment options discussed, a weekly in-office vision therapy program is a viable option for the strabismic patient meeting the appropriate diagnostic and maturity criteria. Most children 5 or more years of age can be considered for structured orthoptic training. The orthoptic treatment of strabismus focuses on the motor vergence skills. Improving the compensating vergences of a strabismic patient can aid in increasing the frequency of fusion. Training the base-out (convergence) amplitudes for the exotrope and base-in (divergence) amplitudes for the esotropic patient aims to decrease how often the strabismic deviation manifests. In addition to vergence therapy, it is desirable to implement antisuppression tasks and normalize accommodative and ocular motor skills in all strabismic patients. The skills needed to perform orthoptic techniques require a certain level of cognitive ability and maturity. If the pediatric patient with strabismus is unable to perform the techniques, the practitioner may have to look to alternative methods of treatment to maintain fusion and consider vision therapy at a later time.

The orthoptic training of the motor vergence skills in a patient with a horizontal strabismus focuses on divergence (base-in) skills for an esotropic patient and convergence (base-out) skills for those who are exotropic. Motor training begins with smooth vergence activities (convergence only or divergence only) and eventually progress to jump vergence techniques (alternating between divergence and convergence in a step-by-step fashion). Motor vergence

activities include techniques such as Brock string, vectograms, or computer orthoptic programs. As the patient's motor vergences and fusional skills improve, the techniques progress to free space and utilize eccentric circle and lifesaver cards. Once motor vergences have reached the desired levels, the practitioner can begin techniques to integrate the vergence and accommodative systems (e.g., vectograms with ±0.75 D flippers). A successful orthoptic program for a strabismic patient with fusion typically takes 12 to 24 sessions.

TREATMENT FOR HORIZONTAL AND VERTICAL STABISMUS

Commonly encountered presentations of strabismic deviations in the pediatric population include infantile esotropia, accommodative esotropia, intermittent exotropia, and hypertropia. The practitioner is presented with the challenge of considering each treatment option available to the patient and parent. The most efficacious treatment decisions for these strabismic diagnoses are reviewed and summarized below.

TREATMENT OF INFANTILE AND ACCOMMODATIVE ESOTROPIA

Infantile Esotropia

Treatment Options

- Refractive error correction: if refractive error is out of age-appropriate range, if an accommodative component to the esotropia is suspected
- Prism: rarely effective secondary to lack of sensorimotor fusion in most patients
- Orthoptic training: rarely effective secondary to lack of fusion and immature age of many patients
- Occlusion: for amblyopia as necessary
- Surgery: most common treatment option

The clinical characteristics of infantile esotropia include an age of onset at 6 to 12 months, a constant deviation (13) of great magnitude, and a refractive error that is typically within the age-appropriate range. If the cycloplegic refractive error is greater than +2.00 to +2.50 D, the examiner must rule out the possibility of an accommodative component to the esotropia. The most common differential diagnosis for infantile esotropia is *accommodative esotropia*. The onset of accommodative esotropia can be as early as 4 months of age. Other differential diagnoses include pseudostrabismus, cranial nerve VI palsy, Duane's retraction syndrome, and an underlying organic cause (14).

As with any strabismic deviation, the proper refractive error correction, when appropriate, is the starting point of the treatment plan. The early age of onset and the constant frequency of an infantile esotropia predispose the patient to the development of associated conditions, such as amblyopia (when the esotropia is constant and unilateral), cross-fixation, and anomalous correspondence (15). If the risk of amblyopia is present, the patient must be treated appropriately before further treatment is initiated or referral made. The presence of central fusion in infantile esotropia at any point in life is a very rare occurrence. The lack of central fusion development and limited existence of peripheral fusion predispose prism and orthoptics to be unsuccessful treatment choices.

The most common treatment for infantile esotropia is strabismus surgery. If the onset of the strabismus is before 6 months of age, clinically significant refractive error has been prescribed, amblyopia risk has been treated, nonsurgical treatment options have been unsuccessful, and the cosmesis of the deviation is unacceptable, then a surgical correction should be considered as a treatment option. The referring optometrist must educate the parents on success rates, risks, and complications of surgery, as well as at what age surgical intervention for infantile esotropia is most appropriate. Scheiman et al. (16) reviewed the literature to assess the success rates of surgical treatment in infantile esotropia. The results of the study revealed that surgery plays a large role in the cosmetic cure of infantile esotropia. Better results are typically achieved when the surgical procedure is performed before, rather than after, the child is 2 years of age. Table 21.5 lists the percentages for success of surgical intervention for infantile esotropia in patients at varying ages. Even the early initiation of treatment, however,

TABLE 21.5 Surgical Success Rates for Infantile Esotopia

Age of Patient (Month)	Surgical Success Rates of Infantile Esotropia (%)
<12	71
13–24	43
>24	12

rarely restores bifoveal fixation and full binocular function. Most surgeons are hesitant to operate on a child younger than 6 months secondary to the higher risk of anesthesia in younger patients as well as the possibility of spontaneous resolution of the esotropia.

An optometrist should follow a young patient with infantile esotropia for two to three consecutive visits to check the stability of the strabismic deviation and allow the practitioner to elicit the possible existence of overacting inferior oblique muscles, a dissociated vertical deviation, or a nonconcomitant nature of the deviation (an A or V pattern esotropia) (13). The existence of any or all of these variables affect the type of strabismus surgery the surgeon will perform. The constant, unilateral infantile esotrope should be treated for amblyopia before a surgical consult. The occlusion treatment will improve both acuity and fixation ability in the amblyopic eye, thus creating a higher likelihood of surgical success.

Postsurgical follow-up visits for an infantile esotrope will include a measurement of the strabismic angle and close monitoring of visual acuity (VA). An expected outcome is the reduction of the strabismic angle to a small-angle esotropia ($\approx$8–10Δ) and a significant improvement in cosmesis. The optometrist must also carefully monitor and initiate treatment for amblyopia that may present postsurgically. A deviation that may have presented as a large-angle, constant, alternating esotropia can become a small-angle esotropia with a unilateral presentation after surgery (15). As the magnitude of the deviation has no effect on the development of amblyopia, a constant, unilateral esotropia of any size can cause amblyopia. Occlusion therapy must be initiated if this occurs after surgery. A

TABLE 21.6 Infantile Esotropia Treatment Summary

Proper diagnosis of cause of esotropia
Refractive error correction, as needed
Amblyopia/occlusion treatment, as needed
Follow-up visits, to determine stability of deviation and associated conditions
Surgical consultation, as warranted by cosmesis and fusional development
Postsurgical treatment, Occlusion treatment Orthoptic training

summary of the treatment of infantile esotropia is seen in Table 21.6.

Accommodative Esotropia

Treatment Options

- Refractive error correction: all patients
  - Bifocal: consider when the residual deviation with full hyperopic correction equals 9 to 16 prism diopters
- Prism: consider when fusion is present, a residual eso deviation exists at distance and near
- Orthoptic training: may be effective to improve accommodative skills and motor vergences in a patient with fusion
- Occlusion: for amblyopia, as necessary
- Surgery: only an option in partially accommodative esotropia (a large residual esotropia noted with the full cycloplegic correction)

The clinical characteristics of accommodative esotropia include an age of onset as early as 4 months and as late as 7 years. The mean age of onset is 2.5 years of age (17). The deviation typically presents gradually and is intermittent. The frequency of the esotropia increases the longer it is left untreated. The gradual onset and intermittent nature of this deviation make amblyopia and anomalous correspondence less frequently associated conditions than seen in infantile esotropia. Refractive error is typically moderate to high hyperopia (+2.00 to +7.00 D). The lower amounts of hyperopia are usually associated with high accommodative convergence to accommodation ratios

(AC:A ratio). Differential diagnosis for accommodative esotropia includes infantile esotropia, pseudostrabismus, and an underlying organic etiology.

The time course in the identification and initiation of treatment in accommodative esotropia is crucial. The longer the misalignment is left untreated, the poorer the prognosis for maintaining fusion. Other risk factors that affect the development of fusion in accommodative esotropia are high AC:A ratio and anisometropia (18). The proper refractive error correction is the most crucial step in the treatment of accommodative esotropia. The first goal of spectacle correction is to maximize the degree of hyperopia in order to decrease the magnitude of the accommodative esotropia (or maintain a phoric posture), and attain fusion. The second goal of the refractive error correction is to provide functional visual acuity.

The full amount of hyperopia must be identified by a cycloplegic refraction in any pediatric patient with an esotropia. Several steps are taken to determine the appropriate refractive error correction for an accommodative esotropic patient. The practitioner must measure the deviation uncorrected at near and far fixation distances. Dry retinoscopy is then performed and the results are trial framed on the patient. Visual acuity is taken through the hyperopic correction. The cover test measurements are than repeated at both fixation distances with the retinoscopy results. Because additional plus is

TABLE 21.7 How to Determine Hyperoptic Correction for an Accommodative Esotropic Patient

1	Do a cover test measurement of strabismic deviation uncorrected at distance and near
2	Do dry retinoscopy
3	Do a trial framing of the dry retinoscopy results
4	Do a visual acuity and cover test measurement with the prescription
5	Do a trial framing with additional +2.00 D over dry retinoscopy findings
6	Do a visual acuity and cover test measurement with additional +2.00 D
7	Do a cycloplegic retinoscopy
8	Make the final prescription determination

often uncovered with cycloplegic retinoscopy, I recommend that +2.00 D of hyperopia is trial framed over the dry retinoscopy results. The visual acuity and cover test measures should be repeated through the additional hyperopia. This allows the examiner to calculate the AC:A ratio and determine if a bifocal prescription would be an adequate treatment option. Determining visual acuity through the additional hyperopia also reveals the maximal amount of plus tolerated by the patient (Table 21.7). See the case example below.

CASE EXAMPLE

- 3.5 year old patient
- Esotropia onset 3 months ago the mother notes right eye turns in when viewing close objects, greater frequency when tired
- Cover test (without prescription)
  - Near: 30Δ AE (T) intermittent, alternating esotropia
  - Distance: 15Δ AE (T) intermittent, alternating esotropia
- Low frequency deviation
- Dry retinoscopy: +3.00 D OD, OS (trial frame)
  - VA with +3.00 D: 20/20 OD, OS
  - CT with +3.00 D:10Δ E esophoria at near, ortho at distance
- Trial frame +2.00 D over dry retinoscopy (+5.00 D total)
  - VA: 20/30 distance, 20/20 near
  - Near CT with +2.00 add: 2Δ esophoria
- AC:A: 4:1 (8 ÷ 2)
- Cyclo retinoscopy: +5.50 sphere
- Prescription given:+5.00 sphere each eye (*oculus unitas*; OU)

The above case example illustrates the determination of the spectacle prescription in a fully accommodative esotropic patient. The cycloplegic retinoscopy findings (+5.50 D) did reveal additional plus when compared with the dry retinoscopy findings (+3.00 D). It is important to determine the patient's acuity and cover test measures through the cycloplegic retinoscopy before the installation of the cycloplegic medication. Our goal is to be certain that the final prescription allows the patients to have visual acuity that will keep them functional (20/30 is an adequate distance acuity for a 3.5 year old) and that the deviation is well controlled, allowing for the establishment of fusion with the spectacle prescription.

Prescribing a Bifocal for Accommodative Esotropia

The most difficult task at the onset of the diagnosis of accommodative esotropia is minimizing the strabismic angle and simultaneously maximizing the visual acuity. In regard to visual acuity, patients may have difficulty accepting the amount of hyperopia necessary to control the esotropia at all distances. If a residual deviation exists with the full amount of hyperopia or the patient cannot tolerate the full cycloplegic refraction, then a bifocal must be considered. Bifocal prescriptions are successful in patients with moderate to high AC:A ratios (19).

Several reasons exist to use a bifocal in the esotropic patient. The first may be to increase the plus acceptance of the patient. Many patients cannot accept the full cycloplegic prescription and maintain adequate distance visual acuity at the onset of treatment. A bifocal prescription allows the practitioner to maintain control of the deviation at near while creating the necessary distance visual acuity. The goal of bifocal use is to encourage relaxation of the accommodative system. This allows for an eventual increase of the hyperopic correction in single vision form as plus acceptance increases. Follow-up visits are suggested at 3-month intervals to check lens power changes.

A bifocal can also be used to eliminate or reduce a residual esotropia at near through the full cycloplegic prescription (20). Determination of the bifocal power for an accommodative esotropic patient should be based on the AC:A ratio. For example, if the patient's AC:A ratio is 4:1 with a 10-prism diopter intermittent esotropia at near with the full cycloplegic prescription, then a +2.00-D add would aim to reduce the deviation to a 2 prism diopter esophoria.

Many issues need to be considered in prescribing a bifocal segment in the pediatric population. In the younger, preschool population, consider prescribing in a manner that will enforce the ease of use of the bifocal. For the first bifocal prescription, the recommended segment height should be placed at the lower pupil margin. As the child matures, the segment height can be lowered to the lower lid margin. Proper frame selection will allow the bifocal segment to be functional. Preschool children should be given a flat top 35 segment, whereas the school-aged child can be given a flat top 28 segment. If cosmesis is an issue, a progressive addition lens (PAL) is an option for a young child (21). When using a PAL to control an esotropia at near, consider using the widest segment available, raising the segment height to the lower pupil and increasing the desired add power by at least +0.25 D.

Prescribing Relieving Prism in Accommodative Esotropia

Prism treatment for accommodative esotropia involves prescribing base-out prism for the patient that will decrease or eliminate the devi-

ation. In an accommodative esotropic patient with central fusion, relieving prism is an option to decrease the motor demand. Prism can be ground into spectacles for accommodative esotropic patients that show a mild-moderate residual deviation with their full cycloplegic correction (or maximal tolerated plus). Larger amounts of prism (>10Δ) can be prescribed as Fresnel membrane prisms to avoid lens thickness and weight. Some magnitude of the esotropia must be present at distance and near to prescribe prism. If the residual esotropia is only present at near, then a prism prescription is likely to create diplopia at distance. A bifocal is a better treatment option in this case. Relieving prism can be used in conjunction with a bifocal to control a residual esotropia.

Orthoptics in Accommodative Esotropia

Orthoptic training can be used to enhance motor fusion in those accommodative esotropic patients who have normal sensory fusion. Accommodative and ocular motor therapy can also be necessary tools as the child matures. All vision therapy procedures should be performed with the hyperopic spectacles.

Follow-up Care

Pediatric patients with a diagnosis of accommodative esotropia should be followed 3–4 weeks after the initiation of full-time spectacle correction. It often takes some time for an esotropia to respond to the hyperopia. This adaptation period to the spectacle prescription must be explained to the parents. Another very important education tool for parents includes the forewarning that the esotropia may present more often without the spectacles than noted before the glasses were dispensed. Pareats often perceive this phenomenon as the glasses "making the eye turn worse." It is important to educate the parents that the hyperopic correction gives the child clear and comfortable vision, which eliminates the need for excessive accommodation. Once the spectacles are removed, the child will initiate accommodation to see as clearly as the child did with the spectacles. This excessive accommodation can cause an increased frequency of the esotropia without the hyperopic spectacles. If the accommodative esotropia is controlled by spectacles, fusion is present, and no amblyopia exists, appropriate follow-up is every 9 to 12 months (22). In the case of an accommodative esotropia that is not well controlled by the hyperopic correction, the follow-up will be more frequent. It is important to work with the options of bifocal, prism, and vision therapy to control the residual deviation.

INTERMITTENT EXOTROPIA: TREATMENT OPTIONS

- Refractive error correction: patients with exotropia are sensitive to small degrees of refractive error, especially astigmatism
- Prism: excellent option to decrease frequency and magnitude of the exotropia
- Overcorrecting minus lens: therapy: stimulation of convergence with lenses may decrease the frequency or magnitude of the exotropia
- Orthoptic training: excellent option to improve vergence control
- Occlusion: for antisuppression measures
- Surgery: when angle is cosmetically apparent and cannot be controlled with spectacles, prism, or orthoptics

Nonsurgical treatment options are preferred in young, intermittent exotropic patients. The goal of these options is to decrease the frequency of the exotropia, thus increasing the amount of time that the child has bifoveal fixation. Intermittent exotropia is the most common form of childhood exotropia (23). The clinical characteristics of intermittent exotropia include an early age of onset and a sensitivity to clear, single retinal images. Manifestation of the deviation can include a higher frequency seen with fatigue and the child closing an eye to avoid diplopia (24). Differential diagnosis of an intermittent exotropia must consider the underlying organic cause, paresis, or history of trauma.

Refractive Error Correction in Intermittent Exotropia

The clear, single, retinal images produced with a proper refractive error correction can improve fusion and reduce or eliminate an exotropic deviation. Any effective degree of uncorrected my-opia, astigmatism, hyperopia, or anisometropia can be prescribed for the intermittent exotropic patient to elicit a higher frequency of fusion. A trial of the most appropriate corrective lenses is suggested to monitor any change in the magnitude and frequency of the exotropia (25).

Overcorrecting Minus Lens Therapy

Overcorrecting minus lens therapy is relevant when used with the appropriate patient and diagnosis. Many young patients presenting with an intermittent exotropia lack the maturity and cognitive abilities to participate in an orthoptic treatment program. The practitioner must now look to alternative methods that aim to control the exotropia and maintain bifoveal fixation for the young patient. Overcorrecting minus lens therapy can be viewed as a continuous form of vision therapy treatment in a young patient. The mechanism of action of this therapy technique is to enhance convergence by stimulating accommodation with the additional minus lens power.

The goal of overcorrecting minus lens therapy is to decrease the frequency of the strabismic deviation to allow the pediatric patient to maintain binocular vision for a higher percentage of the time. This treatment works with intermittent exotropic patients to stimulate accommodative convergence. Patients with high AC:A ratios will reveal qualitative changes in the magnitude of exotropia. Those with low to normal AC:A ratios may simply demonstrate a decrease in the frequency of the exotropia (even if magnitude remains unchanged) (26). Many practitioners fear the potential of this treatment to create myopia in an emmetropic or mildly hyperopic patient. Studies have shown that the trends toward myopia in intermittent exotropic patients treated with overcorrecting minus lens therapy are no different than that in those who are not treated with minus lenses (27).

The question often asked is how much overcorrecting minus is adequate to control the exotropia while minimizing the accommodative effects? Typically, -1.00 to -2.00 D of myopia is needed to implement overcorrecting minus lens therapy. For a patient who is already myopic, an additional -1.00 to -2.00 D is

TABLE 21.8 Overcorrecting Minus Lens Therapy

Clinical Findings
Young patient with intermittent exotropia
Deviation should be present ≥25% of the time
Therapy Considerations
Over minus patient by −1.00 D to −2.00 D
Consider addition of 4–6Δ base in prism split between the two eyes
Consider the addition of antisuppression occlusion treatment
Monitor for side effects (asthenopia, convergence excess)

TABLE 21.9 How to Determine the Overcorrecting Minus Lens Power Needed in Intermittent Exotropia X(T)

Step one	Do a UCT to determine the frequency of the X(T)
Step two	Do an ACT to determine magnitude of X(T)
Step three	Repeat UCT with −2.00 D lenses to determine how (−) lenses affect the frequency of the X(T)
Step four	Repeat ACT with −2.00 D lenses to determine how (−) lenses affect the magnitude of the X(T) and to determine the AC:A ratio

ACT, alternate cover test; UCT, unilateral cover test; AC:A, accommodative covergence/accommodation.

added. For a hyperopic patient, the cycloplegic refraction plus the additional minus making the spherical equivalent −1.00 to −2.00 D. should be prescribed. The practitioner should also consider the addition of a small amount of base-in prism (4–6Δ split between the two eyes) and antisuppression occlusion treatment in conjunction with overcorrecting minus lenses (28). As mentioned, the goal of the treatment is to prescribe the minimum minus lens power to constitute fusion. Once fusion is attained, the practitioner can reduce lens power and discontinue wear of the spectacles over time (Table 21.8).

Side effects of overcorrecting minus lens treatment are rare in young patients with strong accommodative systems. Practitioners should follow these patients closely (approximately every 3 months), monitoring for the onset of accommodative asthenopia, development of convergence excess, and the rate of myopic progression. The appropriate diagnostic testing must be done to determine if the patient (e.g., divergence excess exotropia) may need a bifocal in the overcorrecting minus lens prescription to control the deviation and aid in accommodation for near point work (24). Table 21.9 summarizes treatment of an intermittent exotropia with overcorrecting minus lens therapy.

Prescribing Relieving Prism in Intermittent Exotropia

Prism treatment for intermittent exotropia involves prescribing base-in prism for the patient that will decrease or eliminate the deviation. In a pediatric patient with exotropia, it is preferable to use prism as a relieving or demand-decreasing type of therapy. This passive therapy option will give the patient a stimulus for convergence. The goal of the prism prescription is to give the patient sufficient aid in convergence to place the exotropic deviation at a magnitude that can be compensated by the patient's convergence skills. In a pediatric patient, the practitioner may not be able to elicit accurate diagnostic values involving the patient's divergence and convergence amplitudes. If this is the case, it is suggested that the practitioner simply prescribe an amount of prism that will leave the patient with the desired 10 to 15 prism diopters of convergence demand. Larger amounts of prism (>10 prism diopters) may be prescribed as Fresnel membrane prisms to avoid lens thickness and weight. Relieving prism can be used in conjunction with orthoptics, overcorrecting minus lens therapy, or both to treat intermittent exotropia.

Part-time Occlusion Treatment for Intermittent Exotropia

Occlusion for intermittent exotropia is a passive form of treatment often used for exotropia in infants and toddlers. This is an excellent option when the early age of onset (≤4 years) of intermittent exotropia does not allow a child to participate in active forms of therapy. In addition, surgical treatment for intermittent exotropia is often reserved for a later age. The goal of occlusion therapy for exotropia is to limit binocular stimulation and eliminate the development of conditions leading to an anomalous sensory adaptation. The patching is aimed to reduce the development of suppression and anomalous correspondence when the exotropia manifests (25).

The occlusion regimen for intermittent exotropia is part time. Full-time occlusion has been known to deteriorate an intermittent exotropia to a constant exotropia (29). Determining which eye to patch is tailored to the fixation preference of the exotropic patient. For

TABLE 21.10 Occlusion Schedules for Intermittent Exotropia

Type	Antisuppression Treatment for Intermittent Exotropia						
Unilateral intermittent exotropia (X(T))	If LX(T), patch right eye (RE)			If RX(T), patch left eye (LE)			
	Day	Sun	Mon	Tues	Wed	Thur	Fri	Sat
	RE	4	4	4	4	4	4	4
	LE							

Type	Antisuppression Treatment for Intermittent Exotropia						
Alternating X(T): Equal frequency of right and left eye deviating	Patch RE 4 h day 1			Patch LE 4 h day 2			
	Alternate which eye is patched 7 d/wk						
	Day	Sun	Mon	Tues	Wed	Thur	Fri	Sat
	RE	4		4		4		4
	LE		4		4		4	

Type	Antisuppression Treatment for Intermittent Exotropia						
Alternating X(T): Right eye (RE) fixation preference	Patch RE 4 h days 1 and 2			Patch LE 4 h on day 3			
	Continue with this alternate patching schedule 7 d/wk						
	Day	Sun	Mon	Tues	Wed	Thur	Fri	Sat
	RE	4	4		4	4		4
	LE			4			4	

Type	Antisuppression Treatment for Intermittent Exotropia						
Alternating X(T): Left eye (LE) fixation preference	Patch RE 4 h day 3			Patch LE 4 h on days 1 and 2			
	Continue with this alternate patching schedule 7 d/wk						
	Day	Sun	Mon	Tues	Wed	Thur	Fri	Sat
	RE			4			4	
	LE	4	4		4	4		4

unilateral exotropia, occlusion is done on the dominant (nonstrabismic eye) to increase fixation and decrease suppression of the eye demonstrating the exotropia. If the exotropia is alternating, then the occlusion pattern will be alternated daily. If the alternating exotropic patient develops a strong fixation preference, a schedule is developed to occlude the eye with which fixation is preferred (exotropia seen less) more days per week than the eye that deviates more frequently. Approximately 4 hours of patching daily achieves the antisuppression goals of this therapy regimen (30). See Table 21.10 for a summary of occlusion schedules for intermittent exotropia. Occlusion is a form of antisuppression treatment in intermittent exotropia. It can be used in conjunction with overcorrecting minus lens therapy and a prism prescription to improve a patient's fusional ability.

Orthoptic Training/Vision Therapy in Intermittent Exotropia

Orthoptic training for intermittent exotropia is a viable option in a pediatric patient who is properly selected. The patient's age, maturity, and cognitive and developmental skills must allow for the successful implementation of vision therapy procedures. Intermittent exotropic patients who are well served with vision therapy, typically measure 20 to 25 or less prism diopters. The goal of orthoptic treatment in an intermittent exotropic patient is to improve fusional vergence ranges, eliminate suppression, and improve accommodation (31). Orthoptic training for intermittent exotropic patients is often enhanced by the use of relieving prism, overcorrecting minus lenses, and occlusion.

CASE EXAMPLE

- Intermittent exotropia involving a combination of treatments
  - Refractive error correction
  - Overcorrecting minus lenses
  - Prism
- History
  - 3 year old boy
  - Intermittent alternating exotropia for 1 year
  - Greater frequency in the morning, when tired, in sunlight
- Visual acuity (sc) Allen Pictures
  - 20/30 OD, OS distance and near
- Cover test (sc)
  - Distance: 45Δ AX (T) (95 %) frequency
- *Intermittent* alternating exotropia
  - Near: 35Δ AX (T)' (75%) frequency
    - *Intermittent* alternating exotropia
  - Stereopsis (sc)
    - (+) Forms Lang (random dot stereopsis)
  - Auto keratometry
    - 40.75/43.12 × 176
    - 41.00/43.87 × 019
  - Retinoscopy
    - +1.50 − 2.00 ×180
    - +1.50 −3.50 × 180

(continued)

- NCT (near cover test) and DCT (distance cover test): 40Δ AXT (alternating exotropia)
  - *Constant* alternating exotropia
    - Trial frame
- pl −2.00 ×180   20/20
- pl −3.50 ×180   20/20
  - NCT: 25Δ X' − exophoria
  - DCT: 40Δ AX(T)   (60%)
  - Intermittent alternating exotropia, lower frequency
    - Prescription given
- pl (plan) −2.00 × 180   20/20   5Δ base in
- pl (plan) −3.50 × 180   20/20   3Δ base in
  - Overcorrecting minus: by elimination of hyperopia
  - Prism to aid in convergence ability
  - Decreased frequency and magnitude of the deviation

Follow-up Care in Intermittent Exotropia

Pediatric patients with a diagnosis of intermittent exotropia should be followed one month after the initiation of any spectacle correction or occlusion treatment. At this visit the practitioner will evaluate the effectivity of the treatment in controlling the magnitude and frequency of the exotropia. This is done subjectively by a thorough case history regarding the awareness of the exotropia (cosmesis) by the parents. Objective testing will include stereopsis, sensory fusion and cover tests to determine the patient's fusional ability as well as the magnitude and frequency of the deviation. After finalizing the treatment plan three month follow-up visits are suggested for pediatric patients with intermittent exotropia.

TREATMENT OF VERTICAL STRABISMUS

Summary of Treatment Options

- Refractive error correction: as appropriate for vision and visual function
- Prism: effective for smaller vertical deviations (≤10 prism diopters)
- Orthoptic training: often effective when training of horizontal vergences is used in conjunction with a vertical prism prescription
- Occlusion: not applicable in most cases; amblyopia is rare.

- Surgery: common treatment option for larger vertical deviations or when nonsurgical treatments are ineffective.

Ninety percent of all vertical deviations can be attributed to paresis of the superior oblique muscle (32). The clinical presentation of the vertical strabismus is a hyperdeviation in the eye, with superior oblique palsy and a hypodeviation in the opposite eye. In the pediatric population, 29% to 66% of all superior oblique palsies have congenital etiology (33).

A superior oblique palsy in the pediatric population is typically benign, without the presence of underlying pathology. Pathologic causes to consider in the differential diagnosis include ischemia, neurologic disease, or demyelinating disease.

Other possible causes for vertical strabismus include a dissociated vertical deviation (DVD), Brown's syndrome, and an inferior oblique paresis. A dissociated vertical deviation is an upward elevation of either eye during periods of inattention or when fixation is disrupted (34). Clinically, it presents as a double hyperdeviation. Alternate cover testing on most vertical deviations reveals one eye as a hyperdeviation and the opposite eye as a hypodeviation. In a DVD, alternate cover testing reveals both eyes to be hyper (both eyes come down on an alternate cover test). A DVD is often associated with infantile esotropia, latent nystagmus, or inferior oblique overaction. Brown's syndrome is an anomaly that reveals a vertical deviation characterized by the inability to elevate an eye in adduction. No vertical deviation exists in primary gaze. An isolated inferior oblique paresis demonstrates a hypertropia of the affected eye in elevation on adduction only. Both Brown syndrome and an isolated inferior oblique paresis demonstrate a vertical deviation of the eye while adducting (35). The proper diagnosis between the two, and a true hypertropia is made by the presence of a hyperdeviation in primary gaze.

Treatment of vertical deviations has several goals. They include elimination of diplopia, improved fusion, and cosmesis. The cosmesis can present in the form of strabismus (one eye appears higher than the other) or a head tilt toward one shoulder. Patients with superior oblique palsies typically tilt their head to the opposite shoulder of the paretic muscle (e.g., with a right superior oblique palsy, the patient tilts the head to the left shoulder). Those with isolated inferior oblique palsies typically tilt their head to the same shoulder of the paretic muscle (e.g., with a right inferior oblique palsy, the patient tilts the head to the right shoulder). An anomalous head posture in a patient with vertical strabismus allows for the development and maintenance of binocularity. Therefore, the development of associated conditions such as amblyopia and anomalous correspondence are rare. Longstanding anomalous head postures (typically head tilts in vertical deviations) can cause muscular issues in the back and neck. Treatment of the vertical deviation by proper means often alleviates the postural issues.

Prescribing Relieving Prism for Vertical Strabismus

As with any strabismic deviation, the proper refractive error correction is the starting point of the treatment plan, when appropriate. Prism treatment for vertical strabismus involves prescribing vertical prism for the patient that will decrease or eliminate the deviation (base-down prism for a hypereye, base-up prism for a hypoeye). Deviations less than or equal to 10 prism diopters prism can be ground into spectacles. Greater amounts of prism (>10 prism diopters) can be prescribed as Fresnel membrane prisms to avoid lens thickness and weight. The goal of the prism prescription is to eliminate diplopia and any anomalous head posture as well as to improve fusional ability. In a pediatric patient, the practitioner may not be able to elicit accurate diagnostic values involving the patient's vertical vergence ranges. If this is the case, it is suggested that the practitioner simply prescribe an amount of prism that will leave the patient with the desired 2 to 4 prism diopters of vertical vergence demand. Relieving prism can be used in conjunction with orthoptics to treat a vertical strabismus.

Orthoptic Training/Vision Therapy for Vertical Strabismus

Orthoptic training for vertical strabismus is a viable option in a pediatric patient who is properly selected. The patient's age, maturity, and cognitive and developmental skills must allow for the successful implementation of vision therapy procedures. Cooper (36) developed an orthoptic plan that is well suited for treating vertical deviations. The emphasis of the training is on expanding the horizontal fusional ranges. The horizontal motor vergence system has a large fast and slow vergence component. Treatment of vertical motor vergence skills is thought to be less successful secondary to the lack of a large fast fusional vergence response system and the larger slow, adaptive component. Cooper's treatment of vertical deviations begins by prescribing the least amount of vertical prism that eliminates diplopia. Orthoptic training is than initiated with the goal of improving horizontal fusional vergences. As the process continues, the vertical prism prescription is reduced and additional horizontal fusional range extension is implemented. This process is repeated until reliance on prism is eliminated or the minimal amount of prism prescription is maintained.

Surgical Treatment of Vertical Deviations

A common treatment for large magnitude vertical deviations is strabismus surgery. When nonsurgical treatment options have been unsuccessful and the cosmesis of the vertical deviation or head posture is unacceptable, a surgical correction may be considered as a treatment option. It is important to educate the parents on success rates, risks, and complications of surgery.

The goal of a surgical correction in a pediatric patient with a vertical deviation is to reestablish alignment, eliminate diplopia, and improve stereopsis (37). Postsurgical follow-up visits for vertical deviations will include a measurement of the strabismic angle and visual acuity, and close monitoring of the resolving anomalous head posture.

SUMMARY

Strabismus is commonly seen in the pediatric population. Before initiating treatment, it is important to assess the clinical findings and determine the cause of the strabismic deviation. The treatment options for nonpathologic strabismus include orthoptics, occlusion, prism, spectacles, and surgery. Any underlying pathology must be addressed before treating the strabismus.

The most important thing to remember when treating strabismus in the pediatric population is to choose the treatment option that best fits the patient's diagnosis, maturity, cognitive level, and needs of the parent. It is suggested that written instructions, including the patient's diagnosis, follow-up visits, emergency contact information, and the specific treatment instructions are sent home with the parent.

As with any treatment modality, compliance is the greatest predictor of success. Proper education of the parent and patient ensures a higher rate of compliance. Education must include an explanation of the cause of the strabismus, the necessary treatment, and how the treatment works to manage the strabismus. Parents must also understand that strabismus is more responsive to treatment when diagnosed early. All of the treatment options presented emphasize the goal of the optometric profession—the early detection of childhood vision problems in order to decrease the negative effect on child development.

REFERENCES

1. Groffman S. Psychological aspects of strabismus and amblyopia—a review of the literature. J Am Optom Assoc 1978; 49:995–999.
2. Fletcher MC, Silverman SJ. Strabismus. Part 1: A summary of 1,110 consecutive cases. Am J Ophthalmol 1966;61(1):86–94.
3. www.eyemdlink.com/EyeProcedure.asp?EyeProcedure ID=59; accessed September 20, 2004.
4. Caloroso EE, Rouse MW. Clinical Management of Strabismus. Boston: Butterworth-Heinemann; 1993:149–150.
5. Weissberg E, Suckow M, Thorn F. Minimal angle horizontal strabismus detectable by lay observers. Optom Vis Sci 2004;81:505–509.
6. Scheiman M, Ciner E. Surgical success rates in acquired, comitant, partially accommodative and nonaccommodative esotropia. Journal of the American Optometric Association 1987;58:556–561.
7. Scheiman M, Ciner E, Gallaway M. Surgical success rates in infantile esotropia. Journal of the American Optometric Association 1989;60:22–31.
8. Cooper J, Medow N, Dibble C. Mortality rate in strabismus surgery. Journal of the American Optometric Association 1982;53:391–395.
9. Cotter SA. Clinical Uses of Prism: A Spectrum of Applications. St. Louis: Mosby; 1995:206.
10. Scheimann M, Wick B. Clinical Management of Binocular Vision. Philadelphia: Lippincott Williams & Wilkins; 2002:106.
11. Moore BD. Eyecare for Infants and Young Children. Boston: Butterworth-Heinemann; 1997:171–173.
12. Press L. Applied Concepts in Vision Therapy. St. Louis: Mosby; 1997:99–101.
13. Costenbader FD. Symposium: infantile esotropia, clinical characteristics and diagnosis. Am Orthopt J 1968;18:5.
14. Forbes, BJ, Khazaeni LM. Evaluation and management of infantile esotropia. Pediatric Case Review 2003;3(4):211–214.
15. Nordlow W. Age distribution of onset of esotropia. Br J Ophthalmol 1953;37:593–600.
16. Scheiman M, Ciner E, Gallaway M. Surgical success rates in infantile esotropia. Journal of the American Optometric Association 1989;60:22–31.
17. Coats DL, Avilla CW, Paysse EA, et al. Early-onset refractive accommodative esotropia. J AAPOS 1998;2(5):275–278.
18. Fawcett SL, Birch EE. Risk factors for abnormal binocular vision after successful alignment of accommodative esotropia. J AAPOS 2003;7(4):256–262.
19. Von Noorden GK, Morris J, Edelman P. Efficacy of bifocals in the treatment of accommodative esotropia. Am J Ophthalmol 1978;85(6):830–834.
20. Caloroso EE, Rouse MW. Clinical Management of Strabismus. Boston: Butterworth-Heinemann; 1993:79–81.
21. Smith JB. Progressive-addition lenses in the treatment of accommodative esotropia. Am J Ophthalmol 1985;99(1):56–62.
22. Raab EL. Follow-up monitoring of accommodative esotropia. J AAPOS 2001;5 (4):246–249.
23. Mahney BG, Huffaker RK. Common forms of childhood exotropia. Ophthalmology 2003;110(11):2093–2096.
24. Hutchinson AK. Intermittent exotropia [Review]. Ophthalmol Clin North Am 2001;14(3):399–406.
25. Coffey B, Wick B, Cotter S, et al. Treatment options in intermittent exotropia: a critical appraisal [Review]. Optom Vis Sci 1992;69(5):386–404.
26. Caltrider N, Jampolsky A. Overcorrecting minus lens therapy for treatment of intermittent exotropia. Ophthalmology 1983;90(10):1160–1165.
27. Rutstein RP, Marsh-Tootle W. Changes in refractive error for exotropes treated with overminus lenses. Optom Vis Sci 1989;66(8):487–491.
28. Kushner BJ. Does overcorrecting minus lens therapy for intermittent exotropia cause myopia? Arch Ophthalmol 1999;117(5):638–642.

29. Iacobucci I, Henderson JW. Occlusion in the Pre-operative Treatment of Exodeviations. Am Orthopt J 1965;15:42–47.

30. Freeman RS, Sherwin SJ. The use of part-time occlusion for early onset unilateral exotropia. *J Pediatr Ophthalmol Strabismus* 1989;26(2):94–96.

31. Singh V, Roy S, Sinha S. Role of orthoptic treatment in the management of intermittent exotropia. *Indian J Ophthalmol* 1992;40(3):83–85.

32. Bielschowsky A. Lectures on motor: anomalies. Hanover, NH, 1940, Dartmouth College.

33. Harris DJ, et al. Familial congenital superior oblique palsy. *Ophthalmology* 1986;93:88.

34. Braverman DE, Scott WE. Surgical correction of dissociated vertical deviations. *J Pediatr Ophthalmol* 1977;14(6):337–342.

35. Saldana KK, Rouse MW. Differential diagnosis of an isolated inferior oblique paresis vs. Brown's syndrome: a case report. *Journal of the American Optometric Association* 1993;64(5):353–358.

36. Cooper J Orthoptic treatment of vertical deviations. *Journal of the American Optometric Association* 1988;59:463–468.

37. Stavis MI, Niemann SJ. Medical and surgical treatment of vertical deviations. *Problems in Optometry* 1992;4(4):667–683.

22   Options in Amblyopia

Valerie M. Kattouf

Amblyopia is the most common cause of unilateral vision impairment in patients under 40 years of age. Early detection and proper compliance are strong predictors of successful treatment. The reports of the prevalence of amblyopia in the population vary from 1% to 5% (1). These varying percentages result from the different classifications of amblyopia as well as the age at which the diagnosis is made. In the pediatric population, the incidence of amblyopia is 2% (2). This chapter reviews the proper steps to the diagnosis of functional amblyopia in infants and preschoolers as well as the most successful treatment options that address the condition. The focus of this chapter is on unilateral amblyopia.

CLASSIFICATIONS OF AMBLYOPIA

To properly diagnose and treat amblyopia, the reduction in visual function detected must fall into the classifications discussed below.

Functional amblyopia is a unilateral (less frequently bilateral) condition in which the visual acuity is less than 20/20. No structural or pathologic anomalies exist and one or more of the following must occur *prior to 6 years of age* (3):

- Constant unilateral strabismus
- Amblyogenic anisometropia
- Amblyogenic bilateral isometropia
- Amblyogenic uni- or bilateral astigmatism
- Image degradation

The age of onset is critical to the diagnosis of amblyopia. This definition supports the importance of early detection and treatment.

DIAGNOSIS OF AMBLYOPIA IN PREVERBAL CHILDREN

As discussed in the visual acuity chapters (see Chapters 2 and 10), a number of methods are used to determine a quantitative visual acuity measurement in a preverbal child. Although often effective, many of these methods are unavailable to optometric practitioners in various modes of practice. The diagnosis of the *risk* of unilateral amblyopia is ultimately based on the presence of a potentially anisometropic refractive error or a constant unilateral strabismus. The risk for amblyopia is detected by monitoring qualitative fixation, reaction to occlusion, evaluation of the red reflex (with the Bruckner test), and refractive error of the right eye as compared with the left eye (Fig. 22.1).

STRABISMIC AMBLYOPIA

Strabismic amblyopia is defined as a unilateral decrease in visual acuity occurring with a constant, unilateral strabismus that onsets before 6 years of age (3). Intermittent and alternating strabismic deviations are rarely causes of amblyopia. The strabismic deviation must be present at distance and near. Strabismic amblyopia is most commonly seen with convergent

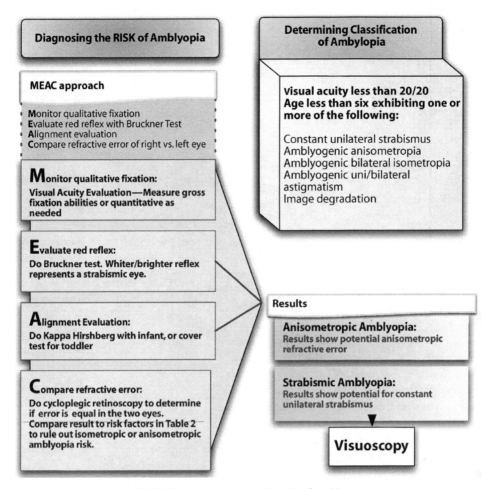

FIGURE 22.1. Diagnosing the risk of amblyopia.

strabismus (esotropia). Divergent strabismus is less likely to create amblyopia secondary to its intermittent nature. Patients with vertical deviations often develop anomalous head postures to afford binocularity and avoid amblyopia development (4). A high percentage of patients with constant, unilateral strabismus have amblyopia.

The development of strabismic amblyopia is secondary to the sensory adaptations made in response to the deviation. The initial deviation of the visual axis in the strabismic eye leads to diplopia and visual confusion. The strabismic deviation then causes the stimulation of noncorresponding retinal points, producing a *diplopic image*. In addition, a strabismic deviation causes the fovea of the deviated and nondeviated eyes to be directed at two different images, resulting in *visual confusion* (5). Dipolpia and confusion are important concepts in the development

of strabismic amblyopia. To avoid diplopia and confusion, the visual system suppresses the strabismic eye. The inhibition of the deviated eye results in cortical spatial changes and a secondary decrease in visual acuity, resulting in amblyopia. Understanding the mechanism causing the development of strabismic amblyopia aids in determining the appropriate treatment modality for each patient.

The Importance of Eccentric Fixation in Strabismic Amblyopia

Eccentric or monocular fixation is a condition that exists only in amblyopic patients. It is most common in strabismic amblyopia and rare in anisometropic amblyopia. It occurs when the amblyopic eye actively attempts to fixate with an off-foveal point under monocular

TABLE 22.1 Visual Acuity Findings in Relation to Retinal Eccentricity.

Eccentricity	Visual Acuity
Degrees/prism diopters	
1°/1.74Δ −2Δ	20/30
2°/3.48Δ 3–4Δ	20/40 to 20/50
3°/5.22Δ 5Δ	20/50 to 20/60

conditions (6). Eccentric fixation affects visual acuity, therefore it is important to be aware of it clinically. Testing for eccentric fixation can be completed successfully in a cooperative preschool patient. It is rarely (if ever) tested for in an infant, but should be evaluated as the amblyopic patient matures.

The fovea is the area of the retina with the highest cone density and largest cortical representation. In the amblyopic patient, the fovea remains the area of the retina with the highest visual resolution. Even in amblyopic patients, the best achievable visual acuity is at the fovea. Eccentric fixation with a nonfoveal point leads to a linear decrease in acuity the further fixation is from the fovea (7) (Table 22.1). The maximal magnitude of eccentric fixation observed clinically is 3 to 4 prism diopters from the fovea. Most esotropic patients exhibit nasal eccentric fixation and those who are exotropic exhibit temporal eccentric fixation. The cause of eccentric fixation is not completely known.

A Clinical Tool to Diagnose Eccentric Fixation

Visuoscopy is the most common clinical tool used to assess eccentric fixation (EF) in an amblyopic patient. The grid target on a direct ophthalmoscope is used to determine the presence of eccentric fixation, as well as its magnitude and direction. This procedure is most efficient when done with a dilated pupil (but can be performed on an undilated pupil). Visuoscopy *must* be done with the patient's eye not being tested occluded because eccentric fixation is a monocular condition.

In order to perform visuoscopy focus the grid target of the ophthalmoscope on the retina of the amblyopic eye while asking the patient to

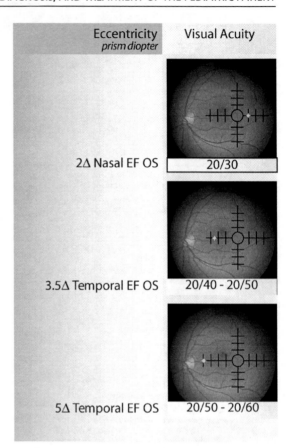

Eccentricity *prism diopter*	Visual Acuity
2Δ Nasal EF OS	20/30
3.5Δ Temporal EF OS	20/40 - 20/50
5Δ Temporal EF OS	20/50 - 20/60

FIGURE 22.2. Eccentric fixation.

view the center of the "bull's eye" target. Central fixation reveals the foveal reflex directly in the center of the grid. Eccentric fixation is represented by the foveal reflex located outside the center of the grid (Fig. 22.2). The examiner must identify the retinal location the patient is using to fixate. The direction of eccentric fixation is represented by where the grid lies in respect to the foveal reflex. Each mark on most ophthalmoscope target represents 1 prism diopter of eccentric fixation (8). In addition to determining the magnitude and direction of eccentric fixation, steadiness must also be addressed. Because of poor fixation abilities, most amblyopic patients demonstrate unsteady fixation. The steadiness of monocular fixation can also be evaluated with the visuoscopy technique. No matter what the location of monocular fixation, central or eccentric, the examiner must look for drifting away from the fixation point with saccadic movements to recover the fixation point (9).

Relevance of Eccentric Fixation Detection

The detection of eccentric fixation in strabismic amblyopia is crucial in determining the patient's prognosis and treatment plan. The presence of EF does not allow the practitioner to predict an outcome of 20/20 visual acuity in the patient with strabismic amblyopia. The information provided in Table 22.1 aids in predicting the best achievable visual acuity with full refractive error correction and occlusion treatment alone. It is not the scope of this chapter to discuss the treatment of eccentric fixation.

ECCENTRIC FIXATION

- A 4-year-old boy diagnosed with a 20Δ constant, left esotropia.
- No significant refractive error.
- Visual acuity OD 20/20, OS 20/200.
- Visuoscopy reveals central fixation OD, 3Δ nasal eccentric fixation OS.
- Occlusion therapy will be initiated.
- The best visual acuity predicted to parents with proper compliance will be approximately 20/40 to 20/50.

ANISOMETROPIC AMBLYOPIA

Anisometropic amblyopia is a unilateral decrease in visual acuity occurring with unequal, uncorrected refractive error that is present before 6 years of age (3). Anisometropic images differ in clarity, contrast, and size, causing a lack of visual stimulation to the eye with the greater significant refractive error. Strabismus is rare in the early stages of anisometropic amblyopia. If left undiagnosed and untreated, the eye with the higher refractive error may develop a strabismic deviation. The strabismic deviation usually presents intermittently and, without treatment, can become constant.

The degree of anisometropia needed to elicit unilateral amblyopia differs with each type of refractive error. The risk for hyperopic anisometropic amblyopia is produced with as little as a +1.50 D difference between the two eyes (e.g., +2.00 OD 20/20, +4.00 OS 20/80). The lesser hyperopic eye is used for fixation at all distances, whereas the more hyperopic eye receives an unclear retinal image, resulting in suppression (10). Myopic anisometropic amblyopia has a more liberal base for amblyopia development. Greater than 3 D difference between the two eyes must be present to produce the risk of anisometropic amblyopia. The need for a more substantial difference between the two eyes is because the eye with less myopia will receive visual stimulation at distance, whereas the eye with the higher degree of myopia will promote a clear image at a near fixation distance. The risk for astigmatic anisometropia is typically defined as greater than a 1.50 D difference in the cylinder component of the refraction. Against the rule astigmatism seems to be more sensitive to amblyopia development and requires longer treatment regimens with less improvement in visual acuity than with the rule astigmatism (11). Table 22.2 contains a summary of potentially amblyogenic refractive errors. Referencing these values

TABLE 22.2 Potentially Amblyogenic Refractive Errors

Refractive Error	Anisometropic
Hyperopia	±1.50 D
Myopia	≥3.00 D
Astigmatism	>1.50 D

will aid the practitioner in making proper decisions regarding prescribing and necessary follow-up care when examining infants and preschoolers.

Comparison of Strabismic and Anisometropic Amblyopia

Both strabismic and anisometropic amblyopia cause a unilateral decrease in visual acuity. Strabismic and anisometropic amblyopia create a range of vision loss across the entire visual acuity spectrum. Strabismic amblyopia tends to be a bit more difficult to treat secondary to the associated conditions that develop with a constant, unilateral strabismus (e.g., suppression, eccentric fixation). The average visual acuity measure in strabismic amblyopia is 20/74. The magnitude of the strabismus has no effect on the depth of the amblyopia. The average visual acuity measure in anisometropic amblyopia is 20/60. The higher the degree of anisometropia, typically, the more significant the decrease in visual acuity. A combined mechanism of strabismic and anisometropic amblyopia produces the most significant average visual decrease of 20/94 (12).

Summary of the Examination of an Infant or Toddler at Risk for Amblyopia

The examination of an infant or toddler focuses on the ability of the practitioner to rule out the presence of amblyogenic risk factors. To rule out the presence of amblyogenic risks, the following steps should be taken (Fig. 22.1)

1. Visual acuity evaluation: gross monocular fixation abilities or a quantitative measure as needed
2. Bruckner test: evaluate the quality or sameness of red reflex (a whiter or brighter reflex represents a strabismic eye)
3. Alignment evaluation: rule out strabismus; Kappa/Hirschberg for an infant, cover testing for a toddler
4. Cycloplegic retinoscopy: is the refractive error in the two eyes equal? Compare with amblyogenic risk factors in Table 22.2 to rule out risk of isometropic or anisometropic amblyopia.

AMBLYOPIA TREATMENT

The most important points to remember in the treatment of amblyopia are to keep all options open, make the proper diagnosis, and consider the needs of the patient and parent. Proper determination of the type of amblyopia and fixation status will allow for successful treatment as well as a fair and accurate prognosis. Factors affecting prognosis include age of onset of the amblyopia, age at which treatment is initiated, monocular fixation status, type of amblyopia, motivation, and compliance.

Refractive Correction

Treatment of amblyopia always begins with the most appropriate refractive correction. Many amblyopic patients are initially corrected with spectacles. All amblyopic patients are to be prescribed polycarbonate lenses for protection of the sound eye. Alternatives to spectacle prescriptions must be considered with various classifications of amblyopia.

Extended wear, high plus contact lenses are prescribed to aphakic infants with an amblyopia risk caused by the removal of congenital cataracts (13). Contact lens correction must be considered for anisometropic amblyopia to avoid aniseikonia (14), and is an excellent option for the high prescriptions in isometropic amblyopia.

Occlusion

Direct occlusion, via patching of the nonamblyopic eye, is the most common and widely used form of amblyopia treatment. The mechanism of action of direct occlusion is to stimulate the amblyopic eye while reducing the competition from the nonamblyopic eye. A variety of patches are used (elastic "pirate" patch, spectacle clips, adhesive bandage patch), which provide total occlusion and force fixation of the amblyopic eye. Other options (opaque filters, overplused contact lens or spectacles) provide partial occlusion by creating blur in the preferred eye, thus promoting fixation of the amblyopic eye (15). Opaque filters, pirate patches, and spectacle clips are less effective in the infant and toddler age group secondary to the unconscious tendency of the patient to *peek* around or over the spectacle occlusion device. Many practitioners are leery of contact lens occlusion for children. High plus contact lenses (often disposable) are excellent options for children with anisometropic amblyopia already wearing a contact lens for the eye with the higher prescription. The goal of the occlusion contact lens is to blur the better-seeing eye to create visual acuity less than that of the amblyopic eye. The blur of the nonamblyopic eye must force fixation to the amblyopic eye. An occlusion contact lens can be worn on a full-time, extended wear basis. Occlusion amblyopia is not a concern secondary to the light stimulation received while wearing a contact lens.

CONTACT LENS OCCLUSION

- 2-year-old boy.
- Prescription: $-1.00 - 2.00 \times 180$ OD (right eye)
  - $-14.00 - 2.00 \times 180$ OS (left eye)
- Prescribed: -10.00 D OS soft contact lens (SCL)
  - Disposable, extended wear contact lens
- Polycarbonate spectacles over CL: $-1.00 -2.00 \times 180$ OD
  - $-2.00 - 2.00 \times 180$ OS
- Occlusion device: $+10.00$ D SCL OD 8 hours daily

Compliance with prescribed occlusion schedules is the most critical issue for success in amblyopia treatment. Younger children are often more compliant than older children. Older children are often more resistant to occlusion secondary to a heightened awareness of the social and cosmetic concerns as well as the increased visual demands of their lives. A lack of compliance has led to the claim that amblyopia cannot be successfully treated after a certain age. A study by Wick et al. (16) reviewed the efficacy of occlusion therapy on compliant anisometropic amblyopia patients. The notable improvement of visual acuity in the amblyopic eye in patients ranging from 6 to 49 years of age determined that the treatment period for anisometropic amblyopia extends beyond the critical period of visual development (16). A 2001 study by Mintz-Hittner et al. (17) treated strabismic and anisometropic amblyopia patients ages 7 to 10 years successfully, given their compliance with occlusion. These studies conclude that compliance, not age, has the most significant effect on treatment success (17). That decreased compliance is synonymous with increased age of the patient supports the benefits of early detection and treatment of amblyopia in the infant and preschool population.

Occlusion Schedules

The practitioner is faced with many decisions when it comes to prescribing an occlusion schedule. The decision must be made whether to prescribe patching on a part-time versus full-time basis. This decision is based on factors including binocular vision status, age, and performance needs. Full-time occlusion gives the most rapid improvement in visual acuity. Children under the age of 5 years are at risk for developing occlusion amblyopia to the sound eye. This is a rare development in patients older than 5 years. Part-time occlusion is often prescribed to allow the child to perform the patching at home in a controlled environment so that school performance is not affected (18). Full-time occlusion is a rare form of treatment for children in school. Current studies are underway to determine the efficacy of full-time versus part-time patching in all age ranges. To avoid occlusion amblyopia secondary to full-time occlusion in children under 5 years of age, a schedule of alternate occlusion (direct and inverse) may be established.

The general rule is 1 day of patching of the nonamblyopic eye (direct occlusion) for every year of life countered with a day of patching of the amblyopic eye (inverse occlusion). For example, in a child 3 years of age, occlude the nonamblyopic eye for 3 days and the amblyopic eye for 1 day and repeat this cycle for the prescribed period of time.

Part-time, total occlusion has a benefit for the strabismic and anisometropic amblyopic patient. It does not eliminate the peripheral fusion of the patient on a full-time basis and, therefore, does not bear the risk of creating or worsening the strabismus in the amblyopic patient.

In determining the number of occlusion hours to prescribe for an infant or toddler, the depth of the visual acuity deficit must be considered, but it is often unknown. A minimum of 4 hours of patching per day is advised for the mildest amblyopia. Overestimating the number of patching hours achieved is recommended. As compliance is difficult, the number of occlusion hours achieved is typically less than what was suggested by the doctor.

Practical Issues of Patching

Active amblyopia therapy activities are recommended in conjunction with the passive occlusion treatment. The aim of these activities is to stimulate the fixational, oculomotor, accommodative systems, and gross motor activities and to minimize treatment time. For the infant and toddler, a home-based active vision therapy program can be initiated with the goal of in-office therapy as the maturity level is appropriate. A list of recommended activities is located in Fig. 22.3. It is suggested that a child be directed to perform about 30 minutes of active vision therapy during the prescribed direct occlusion time. Active vision therapy must be geared toward the individual patient's visual skill deficits. A program of weekly in-office treatment of accommodative, ocular motor, binocular vision, and visual perceptual skills may be implemented as acuity reaches the 20/70 range or as the patient's maturity allows (typically, age 5 to 6 years and up). Strabismic amblyopia therapy centers

on eye–hand coordination, ocular motility or fixation skills, and accommodative tasks. Anisometropic amblyopia therapy involves attention to antisuppression tasks, visual perceptual skills, and accommodation. The in-office therapy is supplemented with approximately 20 minutes of home-based therapy daily.

The success rates in occlusion therapy are almost solely based on compliance. To increase compliance, send the parents home with an instruction sheet that describes the condition of amblyopia, schedule of spectacle or contact lens wear, documentation of which eye should be patched, how many hours a day the patch should be worn, the active vision therapy activities that can be performed during occlusion time as well as how long these should be done, the brand names of the patches and where to purchase them, emergency contact number and their follow-up appointment date. See Fig. 22.4 for a sample instruction sheet for parents.

When visual acuity or visual function reaches desired levels, it is recommended to discontinue the occlusion treatment by tapering. If the occlusion schedule was 6 hours daily, recommendation is to decrease the number of hours per day during week 1 of the taper, aim to decrease the number of days per week during week 2 of the taper, decrease to an hour a day for 3 days of the week during week 3 of the taper, and so on. No scientific taper schedule exists, but the idea is to avoid the sudden end to the occlusion treatment. The loss of visual acuity gains in occlusion treatment are related to the depth of amblyopia at the onset as well as the age of the patient being treated. Stability of occlusion results should be achieved between the third and fourth year with increased maturity of the visual system (19). The goal of tapering the occlusion regime is to lesson the chance of visual acuity loss at any age.

FOLLOW-UP CARE FOR AMBLYOPIC PATIENTS

All types of amblyopic patients undergoing treatment should be followed on a 3- to 4-week basis. Each follow-up visit should include a review of compliance, a measure of visual acuity, and an assessment of binocularity. Patients reporting good compliance typically show

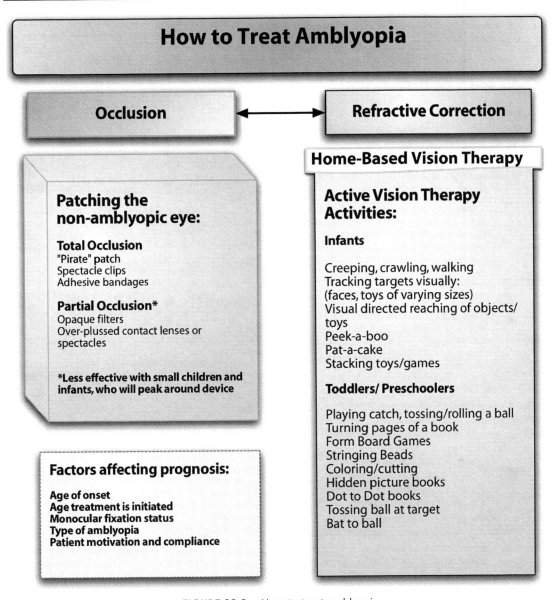

FIGURE 22.3. How to treat amblyopia.

improvement in the 4- to 6-week range. Occlusion schedules should include a minimum of 4 to 6 hours of patching daily for at least 2 months. Occlusion schedules can be tapered after the desired acuity level is reached, but should be continued at least 6 weeks after the last improvement was seen. After the desired visual acuity is achieved, the patient should be monitored every 2 to 3 months for regression. Depending on the stability achieved, 6 to 12 months of follow-up is required thereafter.

Penalization Therapy

To produce successful results with penalization therapy as a treatment for amblyopia, it is important to choose the patient appropriately. Variables to consider include clinical findings, patient age (in regard to visual function), dosage and administration schedules, patient and parent education, pharmacologic side effects, and follow-up care. The specifics of each of the above criteria are discussed below. Atropine penalization is an excellent treatment option for

Sample Instruction Sheet for Parents

Patching schedule

Day	S	M	T	W	Th	F	S
Right Eye	4hr				4hr		
Left Eye		6hr	6hr	6hr		6hr	6hr

Active vision therapy 30 minutes of patching hours:

☐ Peek-a-boo
☐ Stacking toys
☐ Creeping, crawling
☐ Pat-a-cake
☐ Reaching objects/ toys
☐ Tracking targets
☐ Playing catch
☐ Turning pages of a book
☐ Form Board Games

Definition of amblyopia:
Dimness of vision, especially when occurring in one eye without apparent physical defect or disease. Also called *lazy eye.*

Patch brands:

Follow up Appt._____
           mm/dd/yy

Doctor Name, Emergency contact info

FIGURE 22.4. Sample instruction sheet for parents.

patients who are not compliant with occlusion therapy.

As stated, failure of occlusion therapy often results from a lack of compliance. A recent amblyopia treatment study (ATS) by the Pediatric Eye Disease Investigator Group (PEDIG) revealed that results of atropine penalization and occlusion therapy are similar in regard to improvement of acuity in the amblyopic eye. Occlusion therapy results in more rapid progress initially, but the results produced by each treatment modality equalize at about 6 months of treatment. Atropine treatment was favored by parents surveyed in the study, which was thought to be because of the lack of the physical device in occlusion which produces an unfavorable cosmesis and often a lack of cooperation of the child. By choosing the appropriate patient for penalization therapy, the best results are achieved in patients with moderate to high hyperopia and moderate amblyopia (visual acuity of 20/100 or better) (20). The reasoning behind this is that the atropine prevents accommodation in the nonamblyopic eye and forces the amblyopic eye to be blurred at near distances. This mechanism of action works most effectively with hyperopic patients. The blur created at near forces the practitioner to consider the child's age in regard to the child's visual function needs. Part-time occlusion treatment

Atropine Penalization Checklist

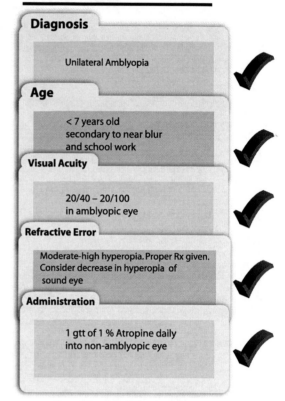

Diagnosis

Unilateral Amblyopia

Age

< 7 years old secondary to near blur and school work

Visual Acuity

20/40 – 20/100 in amblyopic eye

Refractive Error

Moderate-high hyperopia. Proper Rx given. Consider decrease in hyperopia of sound eye

Administration

1 gtt of 1 % Atropine daily into non-amblyopic eye

Do appropriate follow-up visits and evaluate acuity improvement

FIGURE 22.5. Atropine penalization checklist.

forces the child to view with the blurred amblyopic eye several hours per day and typically instructions are for use during nonschool hours. Atropine penalization produces a constant blur at near, which could have a negative impact on a child's school performance. Therefore, the age of 7 and under is considered ideal for this treatment modality. The downsides of the pharmacologic penalization include medication toxicity, constant blur, and the inability to perform visual tasks. An atropine penalization checklist is provided in Fig. 22.5.

To increase the effectiveness of pharmacologic penalization, the practitioner can consider cutting the hyperopic prescription in the sound eye or prescribing a plano prescription. This, in turn, increases the distances at which the amblyopic eye is fixating and blur is maintained in the sound eye (for near and distance fixation).

Atropine Administration Schedule

Day	S	M	T	W	Th	F	S
Right Eye	x	x	x	x	x	x	x
Left Eye							

Store away from children. Keep in original childproof container.

Possible Side Effects:
If you are sensitive to light (secondary to pupil dialation) wear sun-glasses or wide-brinned hat.

Ocular Side Effects (rare):
Allergic lid reactions, local irritation or redness, reverse amblyopia.

Systemic Side Effects (rare):
Dry skin and/or mouth, fever, increased heart rate, flushing, irritability

Follow up Appt. _____
mm/dd/yy

Doctor Name, Emergency contact info

FIGURE 22.6. Atropine administration schedule.

Protocol for pharmacologic penalization treatment involves installation of one drop of 1% atropine sulfate daily to the nonamblyopic eye. This dosage may seem excessive, but it is thought to be prescribed to ensure compliance versus the effect of the medication. New ATS studies are being developed to compare daily administration versus administration on weekends only. The frequency of installation can be reduced as acuity improvement is observed. The minimal installation is one drop of 1% atropine sulfate two times per week.

Provide written documentation to each patient and or parent leaving the practitioner's office with the diagnosis of amblyopia and treatment with atropine penalization with information regarding administration schedules, safety information, possible side effects, emergency contact numbers, and follow-up appointment dates (see Fig. 22.6).

At the onset of penalization therapy, it is important to record the patient's visual acuity in the atropinized and amblyopic eye at distance and near as a baseline measure.

It is important to closely monitor the progress of the patient as well as proper compliance and use of the pharmaceutical agent. The initial follow-up visit is to be scheduled 2 weeks after the initiation of treatment. The consecutive visits are scheduled every 3 to 4 weeks until the desired visual acuity improvement is reached. At each follow-up visit, monitor compliance and visual acuity in both eyes at distance and near. The sound eye must be monitored for reverse amblyopia. This side effect is rare and easily reversible. It typically resolves after the first 6 months of treatment, according to amblyopic treatment study (ATS). The follow-up visits at the conclusion of treatment should be at 1 month, initially, then 3 months and 6 months thereafter.

A comprehensive eye examination of the infant or toddler is the most important tool in the detection and treatment of amblyopia. Although research has shown that many amblyopic patients can be treated successfully at any age, identifying the condition early sets children up for a lifetime of maximizing their potential. Proper diagnosis and treatment of amblyopia includes understanding the proper classifications, determining the child's prognosis, and initiating treatment. Treatment options include correction of refractive error with spectacles, contact lenses, or both; occlusion therapy and atropine penalization. Amblyopia treatment requires the examiner to consider the needs of the patient and parent while making the proper diagnosis. Providing adequate education and instruction information to parents will result in the successful treatment of amblyopia.

REFERENCES

1. Dell W. The epidemiology of amblyopia. *Problems in Optometry* 1991;3(2):ix,197.
2. Flom MC, Bedell HE. Identifying amblyopia using associated conditions, acuity, and nonacuity features. *Am J Optom Physiol Opt* 1985; 153–60.
3. Ciuffreda KJ, Levi D, Selenow A. *Amblyopia: Basic Clinical Aspects.* Stoneham: Butterworth-Heinemann; 1991: 1–38.
4. Isenberg SJ, France TD. *Amblyopia: Eye in Infancy.* St. Louis: Mosby; 1994.
5. Von Noorden GK. *Binocular Vision and Ocular Motility: Theory and Management of Strabismus.* St. Louis: Mosby; 1990:200–207.
6. Rutstein RP, Daum KM. *Anomalies of Binocular Vision: Diagnosis and Management.* St. Louis: Mosby; 1998:3.
7. Kandel GL, Grattan PE, Bedell HE. Monocular fixation and acuity in amblyopic and normal eyes. *American Journal of Optometric and Physiologic Optics* 1977;54(9):598–608.
8. Caloroso EE, Rouse MW. *Clinical Management of Strabismus.* Stoneham: Butterworth-Heinemann; 1993: 24–25.

9. Garzia RP. Management of amblyopia in infants, toddlers and preschool children. *Problems in Optometry* 1990;2(3):438–458.

10. Caloroso EE, Rouse MW. *Clinical Management of Strabismus.* Stoneham: Butterworth-Heinemann; 1993:178.

11. Somer D, Budak K, Demirci S, et al. ATR. Astigmatism as a predicting factor for the outcome of amblyopia treatment. *Am J Ophthalmol* 2002;133(6):741–745.

12. Flom MC, Bedell HE. Identifying amblyopia using associated conditions, acuity, and nonacuity features. *Am J Optom Physiol Opt* 1985;62:153–160.

13. Garzia RP, Nicholson SN. Deprivation amblyopia. *Problems in Optometry* 1991;3(2):305–309.

14. Moore B. Contact lens therapy for amblyopia. *Problems in Optometry* 1991;3(2):366.

15. Caloroso EE, Rouse MW. *Clinical Management of Stra-bismus.* Stoneham: Butterworth-Heinemann; 1993:113–125.

16. Wick B, Wingard M, Cotter S, et al. Anisometropic amblyopia: is the patient ever too old to treat? *Optom Vis Sci* 1992;69:866–878.

17. Mintz-Hittner HA, Fernandez KM. Successful amblyopia therapy initiated after age 7 years: compliance cures. *Arch Ophthalmol* 2001;199:1226.

18. Cotter S. Conventional therapy for amblyopia. *Problems in Optometry* 1991;3:312–331.

19. Oster, JG, Simon JW, Jenkins P. When is it safe to stop patching? *Br J Ophthalmol* 1990;74(12):709–711.

20. Pediatric Eye Disease Investigator Group. A randomized trial of atropine vs patching for treatment of moderate amblyopia in children. *Arch Ophthalmol* 2002;120:268–278.

Vision Therapy for the Very Young Patient 23

Carl Gruning, David E. FitzGerald, and Robert H. Duckman

When an optometrist thinks of vision therapy, the patient is typically a school-aged child and, on occasion, an adult. In fact, many vision therapy (VT) clinics in schools of optometry are also known as *pediatric clinics.* Vision therapy has typically begun with first graders and older children. This is primarily because these children (a) might be able to attend; (b) may be able to follow directions, albeit minimally; (c) understand or know the alphabet, numbers, colors, shapes, and maybe even concepts of bigger, smaller, closer, and farther. Also, this age group has a considerably higher level of receptive and expressive language compared with the preschool child. The typical preschooler (and certainly the nonverbal infant or toddler) has limited or no concept of distinguishing such terms as single versus double, closer versus farther, 3-D or popping out, how many, and certainly not clear versus blurry.

So why should preschool vision therapy be part of any vision therapy practice?

- It is fun, albeit challenging!
- Results or outcomes are generally very good.
- Early intervention or remediation may be easier and less costly (i.e., an intermittent esotropia versus constant ET with anomalous retinal correspondence.
- Early application of lenses, prisms, and occlusion can be very successful.

- Lots of the work can be done by a well-trained therapist (i.e., Certified Optometric Vision Therapist).
- Who else offers these services? And if not offered, the void *will* be filled by others such as occupational therapists (OT) or physical therapists (PT) and educators.

The conditions most commonly treated, both in clinics and in private practice include

- Strabismus
  Intermittent esotropias (ET), exotropias (XT), divergence excesses (DE)
  Constant (noncongenital) ET, XT, or hypertropias (HT)
  Amblyopia
  Anisometropias
- Oculomotor or visuomotor dysfunction
  This category is composed of developmental delays and the exceptional population, including pervasive developmental delays (PDD), autism, Down syndrome, cerebral palsy, chromosomal disorders, and other neurologically based problems (1).

Referral sources usually are (a) OTs, (b) PTs, (c) nursery school teachers, (d) other doctors of optometry (ODs), (e) parents of children previously treated, and on rare occasions, (f) the child's pediatrician.

This chapter addresses activities that can be used for very young children to improve or enhance visual function. These activities will be grouped by category and will include objectives, step-by-step instructions for the parent, caregiver, or assistant and a list of necessary materials and resources and where to obtain them. Keep in mind the level of receptive (and expressive) language, as well as cognitive abilities of the preschool vision therapy patient. These factors can be vastly different from those of the school-aged child.

Additionally, duration of office- or clinic-based therapy sessions will often be significantly shorter than those for a child in second grade. Oftentimes, multiple brief encounters (10 minutes) may be necessary because of the limited attention span of the youngster. At times, it is better to work just with the parent or guardian and demonstrate the procedures for home use or practice before commencing with office-based treatments. Subsequent office visits can then be both progress evaluations to determine what has been accomplished and also to provide the parent or guardian with more advanced home therapy procedures.

PROCEDURES FOR AMBLYOPIA

The two most common causes of amblyopia encountered with the preschool population are anisometropic amblyopia and strabismic amblyopia (2). Other forms that might be encountered include (a) deprivation (congenital cataract), (b) nutritional, and (c) isoametropic amblyopia.

Until recently, patching regimens have included full-time direct occlusion of the nonamblyopic or nonstrabismic eye (3). This was done to treat the amblyopia, eliminate suppressions, and, in the case of strabismus, to reduce the chance for anomalous correspondence. More recent findings indicate that, for moderate amblyopia, full-time direct occlusion is not really necessary and that 2 to 3 hours per day of occlusion of the sound eye is adequate (4). Additionally, the use of atropine drops or ointment has been recommended in the sound eye in cases of poor compliance or cooperation with patching, or concern (parental) regarding

the cosmesis or stigma when wearing a patch (5). Recent studies of moderate amblyopia have shown that occlusion and pharmacologic penalization are equally effective (5). Additionally, weekend atropinization has yielded comparable acuity gains to full-time penalization (6). Lens-prescribing guidelines are covered in Chapter 20 of this text.

For maximal success in treating amblyopia, Krumholtz and FitzGerald (7) recommend the following three-part process:

1. Optimal spectacle prescription
2. Appropriate patching regimen
3. Active vision therapy

The following procedures are for both office- and home-based treatment and are done with total occlusion of the nonamblyopic eye. The method of feedback should be appropriate for the depth of amblyopia. In more severe cases, tactual methods should be used before visual feedback is used.

I. *FLASHLIGHT TRACKING:* This activity is done with two flashlights. The parent shines a light on a wall. The patient, with the other flashlight, shines its light on top of the parent's light. The parent then moves the light slowly, while the child keeps his or her light on top such that it always appears as if there is only one light. Having colored filters over the lights makes it easier for children to monitor their movements. Younger children may have manipulative issues with standard flashlights, so smaller ones are recommended.

II. *FLASHLIGHT TAG:* Again, this activity requires two flashlights. This time the parent shines a light on the wall, then quickly moves it to another spot. The child moves his or her light to "tag" the parent's light, such that there is one light viewed. To have the child search for the light, the parent should stand behind the child. When this activity is done as a binocular activity with anaglyphic glasses, younger children may have difficulty with accurately directing the flashlight. If so, the parent should be the cat (i.e., placing the light on top of the targeted light, the child's) and the child should be the mouse.

III. *PIE TIN ROTATIONS:* This activity is done with an aluminum pie tin and various sizes and weights balls (e.g., marbles, beads, ping-pong balls). The child places one of the balls in the pie tin. Holding the tin in both hands, the child rolls the ball around in the tin. The path of the ball must be followed by the child's eye accurately, without head movement. The child should note differences between different size and weight balls.

IV. *BROWNIE TIN ROTATIONS:* This activity is the same as pie tin, except a square or rectangular container is used, and the ball is to be kept along the sides, stopping briefly at each of the four corners.

V. *COLORING IN LETTERS:* Using letters large enough to be seen, have the child color in all the letters that have openings (e.g., A, B, D, O, P). Use colored pens or pencils so it is easier for the child to see. These activities should be guided by age and skill level. Larger pictures and crayons may be needed for the younger child, whereas the older preschooler may be able to have the demand increased by using a finer target (picture or letter) and a more sharpened pencil point. The parent can vary the demand by buying a regular coloring book and creating their own *number coloring book* by making lined sections within a picture.

VI. *SHOELACE SEWING:* Punch small holes in a piece of paper, cardboard, or felt. Using a shoelace, the child should thread the lace through the holes. If possible, have the child keep the lace from hitting the sides of the holes. The hole size should match the performance level, such that large holes may be used initially. As the performance improves, the holes and threading instrument can gradually be made smaller. Various size sewing needles and yarn and matching size holes are ideal for this technique.

VII. *STRINGING CHEERIOS* (or buttons, fruit loops): The child takes Cheerios or buttons and slips them, one by one onto a string with a knot at the end. Cheerio placing books, in which the child places Cheerios in designated areas of the book, are commercially available.

VIII. *TWEEZERS AND RICE:* Cover a cup with a piece of paper. Make a small hole on top to form an opening. Put some rice or beans on the table. Using the tweezers, the child must pick each piece up, one at a time, and place it in the opening without touching the sides of the opening. To make it more difficult, decrease the size of the opening through which the child must place the rice. If the child is too young to manipulate the tweezers, the child can use fingers. A pincer grip is preferred.

IX. *TOOTHPICK AND HOLE:* Make a hole in a piece of paper. The child must place a toothpick through the center of the hole, without touching the sides. To increase the level of difficulty, gradually make the hole smaller.

X. *SPEARING RAISINS:* Place raisins on the table. Using a toothpick, the child must spear the center of the raisins, one at a time. The child may be allowed to eat the raisins if parent has no objections.

XI. *SORTING SPRINKLES:* Buy a jar of assorted colored sprinkles and pour some onto a flat surface. Have the child then make piles of same colored sprinkles.

XII. *PENNIES IN A CUP:* Make a slot in a paper cup turned upside down. The child must place pennies through the slot, without touching the sides of the slot. Gradually make the slot narrower to increase the level of difficulty.

XIII. *MAZES:* "Homemade" or commercially available books that the child can trace through visually or with a marker.

XIV. *MICHIGAN SYMBOL TRACKING* (large to small): The child is to perform as directed, crossing out the consecutive letters in the alphabet, or picture sequences.

XV. *HIDDEN PICTURES:* Many workbooks with hidden pictures can be purchased. The child is to find the appropriate hidden pictures on the page. Once the picture is found, the child can color in the picture using an age-appropriate marker, crayon, or finely sharpened pencil.

XVI. *DOT TO DOT* with markers or felt-tipped pens: Make a series of dots or circles on the paper and ask the child to bring a colored felt-tipped pen down from a few inches away and put a dot in the center of the circle or on top of the dot. Simple dot patterns or the dot-to-dot games can also be used as techniques.

XVII. *CONNECT THE DOTS:* Many workbooks can be purchased, or patterns can be made, such that, by connecting the dots by consecutive numbers, will produce a picture. Once the picture is completed, the child is asked to carefully color it in. It is necessary for the child to have number and counting concepts to do this activity.

XVIII. *SCRUB THE LINE:* Make a series of zigzag lines on paper and ask the child to *scrub* them (i.e., continuously make lines back and forth over (and perpendicular to) the lines on the paper. The child should keep the point oscillating as rapidly as possible and make scrubs that are equal on either side of the drawn lines.

XIX. *FOLLOW THE PATH:* Make paths with two parallel lines (road) drawn closely together. The child is to draw a line inside the path with a different colored pencil or pen, trying not to hit the parallel lines. Reducing the road opening and increasing the number and sharpness of the curves can increase the demand. To make the task more interesting, for example, we have drawn a picture of an ice cream truck at the start and a picture of the child outside his or her house waiting for the delivery on the other end.

XX. *CUT OUTS:* Have the child cut out pictures from a coloring book, newspaper, or magazine, working on improvement of accuracy.

XXI. *PENNIES GAME* (Fig. 23.1): Get a few dozen pennies, some new and shiny and others old or worn so features of details on both sides are not easily seen. Have two paper or plastic cups. Place half the pennies with face up (face or man side) and half with face down (house side). Scatter randomly on a table. Ask child to rapidly sort pennies with face up into one cup and with faces down up into the other. Check for accuracy. Initially, all shiny pennies may be needed. As the child improves, all tarnished pennies can be used.

XXII. *STICKER TRACKING:* Obtain a half dozen tongue depressors or popsicle sticks. Purchase sheets of small stickers in a novelty toy or stationery store and affix a sticker on both sides of top and bottom. Holding the stick about 10 inches from child's face, ask the child to identify the sticker and follow it with the amblyopic eye. The stick can be rotated for a new picture and rotated 180° for two new pictures. Having a half dozen sticks will allow for 24 different stickers or pictures.

XXIII. *PUPPET SACCADES:* Obtain two or more different finger puppets. Separate them by 10 to 20 inches and call out the name of the puppet. The child must find it. Expect to see significant head movement with the preschool child.

XXIV. *CROSS-OUT ALL SAD FACES:* Using 8.5 × 11 inch sheets of a mixture of very small happy ☺ faces and sad ☹ faces, have the child circle, X out, or dot with felt marker all the sad faces. Size of faces can be enlarged for deep amblyopia and reduced as VA improves.

XXV. *LITE BRITE* (Toys "R" Us) and SPARKLE BRITE (Ohio Art or J. C. Penney catalog and online) using red and green glasses and just one color peg, seen by amblyopic eye (red sees red, green sees green).

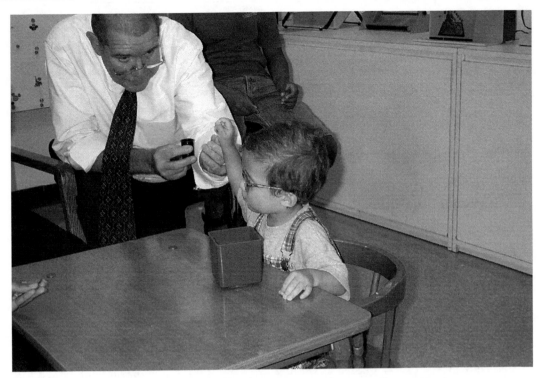

FIGURE 23.1. A small child plays the *Pennies Game* with his optometrist.

Once amblyopia becomes *shallow* (i.e., 20/40 or better), we can now commence with procedures without total occlusion but where both eyes are open and the target is seen only by the amblyopic eye. These procedures are known as monocular fixation in a binocular field (MFBF). These are often achieved via polarized targets and filters, or anaglyphic targets and filters. In MFBF, the *ground* is seen by both eyes and serves as a binocular lock. More advanced MFBF procedures will utilize two monocular targets, one seen by each eye. At this point in treatment, VAs need to be fairly equal and no deep suppressions present. Now, both red and green pegs and filters are used.

ANTISUPPRESSION/MFBF PROCEDURE

I. *LITE-BRITE*

Purpose

Antisuppression, monocular fixation in binocular field, eye–hand coordination, and monocular fixation amblyopia training.

Materials

Lite-Brite Game, red/clear or red/green filters

Procedure

For antisuppression, MFBF, and eye–hand coordination, Lite-Brite is used the same way as Sparkle Lights. Without the templates, Lite-Brite is a light box with holes for pegs to go into and, as such, can be used similarly to accomplish antisuppression training, MFBF, and eye–hand coordination, except the background is clear instead of black. As with Sparkle Lights, in the case of amblyopia, you can use red or clear filters with green pegs where the red filter goes over the nonamblyopic eye.

Using monocular fixation, patch the nonamblyopic eye. Place a Lite-Brite picture pattern onto the light box. Have the patient place the appropriate colored peg into each marked hole until the pattern is completed.

Resource Materials

Available at most toy stores, this product is from Milton Bradley Co.

Note: Remember that cancellation is opposite on the clear background than on the black background. On the clear background, the red peg will be seen by the eye with the green filter and vice versa. On the black background, the red peg will be seen by the eye with the red filter and vice versa.

II. *SPARKLE LIGHTS*

Purpose

Antisuppression training (use red and green pegs)

Monocular fixation in binocular field (use red, green and crystal pegs)

Eye–hand coordination and fine motor skills

Materials

Red and green (R/G) glasses, Sparkle Lights game

Procedure

Place R/G glasses on patient. Place R/G pegs on the board in patterns or randomly. Have patient touch all the pegs the child sees with one finger.

Place R/G glasses on patient. Place R/G pegs in a row. Have patient put a peg above or below *all* the pegs on the board.

Place R/G glasses on patient. Place R/G pegs in a pattern on the board (e.g., circle, square, line). Have the patient make the same pattern somewhere else on the board.

Place R/G glasses on patient. Place R/G pegs in a pattern on the board (e.g., circle, square, triangle). Have the patient make a matching outside border around your pattern.

Can also be done with red and clear filters with just green pegs for monocular fixation in a binocular field for amblyopia (red lens on the nonamblyopic eye).

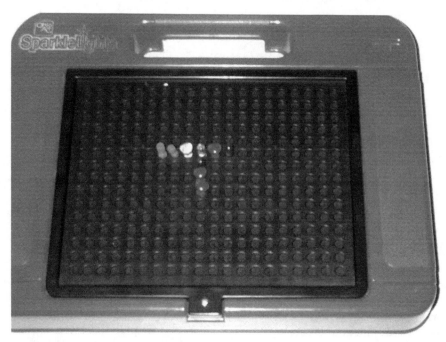

FIGURE 23.2. Sparkle Lights light box for the placement of red, green, and clear crystal pegs. (See color well.)

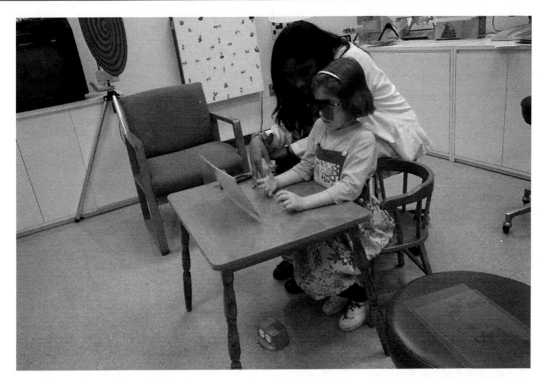

FIGURE 23.3. Child with red/green glasses interacting with anaglyphic stimulus for antisuppression training.

As above, adding clear pegs that can be seen by both eyes (Fig. 23.2).

Place R/G glasses on the patient. Place pegs that can only be seen with the normally suppressing eye (e.g., if the left eye is the suppressing eye and the green filter is on the left eye, use green pegs). Slowly introduce pegs seen by the normally fixating eye (red pegs) and have the patient try to keep all the pegs "on"/present. Instruct patient to touch each peg in an order (e.g., from right to left, from up to down).

All of the above utilize E/H components, but do not require the R/G filters for the eye-hand part.

Resource Materials

Manufactured by Ohio Art Company, Bryan, Ohio. Also sold at J. C. Penney and on the Internet.

Note: Best if done in dim or darkened room conditions. The advantage over Lite-Brite is that the black background is permanent and does not have to be replaced after each use. Lite-Brite pegs illuminate more brightly when used in Sparkle Lights box. Lite-Brite pegs are easier to insert and remove.

III. *ANAGLYPHIC MAZE GAMES*

Purpose

Antisuppression during a visuomotor activity

Materials

R/G glasses, white paper, black pen, and red color pencil (carmen red and vermillion red from Venus Company cancel well) (Fig. 23.3)

Procedure

Place the R/G glasses on the child. Have the child *walk* the red pencil through the black line maze from *Start* to *Finish*. Encourage the child to always stay inside the path. Have plenty of mazes available, ranging from very easy to complex. Ask the child to report if the maze disappears or goes away. In the case of an amblyopia, the red filter goes in front of the better eye and the green filter goes in front of the amblyopic eye. Good illumination should be used.

To increase difficulty, make the mazes narrower, longer, and more complex. Next, make the mazes with red pencil and the child "walks"/draws pencil (#2) through the red maze. Ask the child if anything disappears, "goes away."

IV. *THE HUNDREDS CHARTS WITH ANA-GLYPHIC OVERLAYS AND FILTERS*

Purpose

Antisuppression training

Amblyopia training

Saccadic fixations

Eye–hand coordination.

Materials

Hundred Charts are teaching tools to help children learn numbers from zero to one hundred. They are produced in various sizes and each can be presented in black on a white background or red on a white background, and R/G glasses. (Red cancels very well with red filters, therefore, the eye with the green filter will see the numbers).

Procedure

Place R/G filters on the child and place one of the charts at distance or at near. Point to a number and have child tell you what the number is. After several trials, reverse the position of the filters.

Using a green pencil or pen that cancels well, put green shapes around some of the red numbers. Call out a number and have the child tell you the shape OR have the child tell you all the numbers that are in squares, triangles, and so on.

Using a red filter over the normally fixating eye and transparent filter over the amblyopic eye, have child tell you which numbers you are pointing to OR cross out any number you call out.

Place the larger chart (red side) on the wall at a distance of about 7 to 10 feet and have the child read the numbers at the beginning and end of each line, second and next to the last number on each line, first and third number, and so on.

Place a clear piece of plastic over one side of the chart. Have the child draw circles around all the odd numbers or even numbers.

Resource Material

Available from Media Materials, Baltimore, MD.

V. *BEAD AND STRING GAMES*

Purpose

Can be used for antisuppression; monocular fixation in a binocular field; E/H coordination; and monocular acuity improvement for amblyopia.

Materials

Black string or black shoelace (about 2 feet long), assorted red, green, and black beads, which cancel appropriately through red or green filters, black felt (2- or 3-foot square piece needed).

Procedure

Place R/G filters on the patient. Have the child hold the string and tie a large enough knot at one end so that the beads will not fall off. Spread beads out on a piece of black felt and tell the child to look for the beads. The child should then pick up *ONE* bead at a time and put the end of the black string through the hole in the bead. The child should attend to both the string and the bead while doing this. If done accurately, have the child pull the string through so that the bead slides down the string. If done inaccurately, have the child start over on the same bead. Continue until all the beads are strung.

Resource Information

Red and green wooden beads are available through most arts and crafts stores.

Note: Be sure to check cancellation through the R/G filters. Full room illumination is necessary.

Variations

Make up different random bead configurations on several pieces of string. Place one of your configurations on a piece of black felt. Give the patient a black string and have the patient take beads from a box and string beads onto another string so that the patient's configuration matches yours so that when the two are laid next to each other they are exactly the same.

Take one of your prepared strings and lay it onto the black felt. Have the patient count how many red beads are on the string, how many green beads are on the string, and how many black beads are on the string. You can have the child touch each bead while counting.

Place red, green, and black beads randomly on the black felt. Have the child sort all of them into three piles of black, red, and green beads.

VI. *FLASHLIGHT TAG* while wearing red/green filters with one white light and one color filter; same color over amblyopic eye (projected light).

VII. *TV TRAINERS* using a red or green acetate filter over a TV screen and opposite color (green or red) in front of nonamblyopic eye.

VIII. *MONOCULAR ACCOMMODATIVE FACILITY* (rock) in a binocular field: Red Michigan symbol tracking with green filter on amblyopic eye; begin with ±1.00, gradually increase powers. Single spirangle or split spirangle with Polaroid's and ± flippers (or Bozo). Sherman rotator with anaglyphic discs, red/green filters and ± flippers.

IX. *BROCK POSTURE BOARD MAZES*

X. *RED-GREEN-BLACK BEAR GAMES*

Purpose

Antisuppression, monocular fixation in a binocular field, and eye–hand coordination.

Materials

R/G glasses; red, green, or black bears, large piece of black felt (good use for an old tangent screen)

Procedure

Spread out black felt on a flat surface. Place red and green bears on the felt randomly in two rows such that for each item in one row a matching item is in the other row (Fig. 23.4). Place R/G glasses on the patient. Have the patient take one item from the back row and place it in front of a matching item in the front row.

Place bears on black felt. Wearing R/G glasses, have the child count how many bears there are. Tell the child to touch each item while counting it and name the color.

Drape felt on a horizontal surface but also create folds so that there are a few "valleys." Place bears randomly (by color) on both the horizontal surface and in the valleys, trying to make some easy to see and others more difficult to see (partially behind a fold in the felt). Have the child localize the bears and identify the color of each one selected.

Resource Materials

The bears are available through A. C. Moore craft stores. This a chain of craft stores in the northeastern United States, but they sell on the Internet at *www.acmoore.com*

Note: This should be done in good illumination. Because the background is black, the red bears are seen through the red filter and the green bears are seen through the green filter.

Clinical Pearl: The difference in amblyopia treatment between prescribing and passive patching, versus active VT, is *hands on* (i.e., the tactile, kinesthetic, or proprioceptive feedback from either manual input or bimanual input seems to significantly improve acuity.

Clinical Pearl: Most monocular amblyopia procedures, besides addressing acuity improvement, also enhance or develop:

• Improved fixation (maintenance of fixation)
• Improved oculomotor skills (pursuits, saccades, and eye hand coordination)
• Greater accommodative accuracy, once accommodation "kicks in" (VA is 20/40 or better)

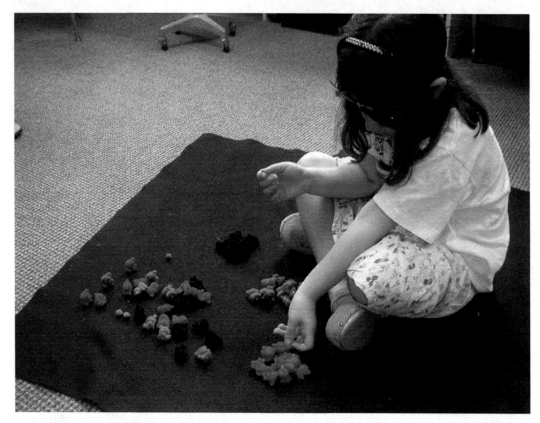

FIGURE 23.4. Red/green bears on black felt material for antisuppression training. (See color well.)

Once acuities are approximately equal and no deep suppressions exist (i.e., nonstrabismic amblyopic patients), it is critically important to establish and solidify binocularity and stereopsis to ensure no regressions or drop in acuity.

The following procedures are either MFBF where each eye sees a target via Polaroid or anaglyphic filters, or stereopsis is created via disparity with the same filters.

I. *LITE-BRITE* with red, green, and clear crystal pegs. In an ideal world, the crystal pegs are seen as yellowish or reddish-green.

II. *MAZES* with red plastic sheet, white paper with red pencil mazes, and penlight—using R/G filters. Here, red light is seen by red filter and red maze on white paper is seen by green filter. Complexity of mazes can go from simple to complex as the child's binocular coordination vision improves. This also develops or improves eye hand coordination.

III. *KEYSTONE ANAGLYPHIC FUSION GAMES* using anaglyphic 8.5 × 11 inch targets with pediatric appropriate pictures. Vergence demands vary from card to card and also within many of the cards. The clinician can determine whether the child appreciates float, localization, and parallax. Available from Keystone View—Reno, NV; Bernell Corp.—Meshawaka, IN.

IV. *KEYSTONE BASIC BINOCULAR TESTS.* Although designed to evaluate a number of binocular areas (e.g., posture, suppressions, stereo), these anaglyphic pictures are also excellent to use along with the fusion games. R/G filters are used to achieve the binocular response. Available: Keystone View—Reno, NV; Bernell Corp.—Meshawaka, IN.

V. *VECTOGRAMS* and Polaroid filters. These variable demand targets are excellent for young children and often easily elicit float, localization, and parallax. In addition, smooth vergence ranges of binocular vision can be measured at each session.

VI. *OPTOMATTER CARDS*

Purpose

Antisuppression training

Materials

OPTOMATTERS cards, R/G glasses

Procedure

Different cards, which are utilized in similar ways

- Card OPT/TFP: Four units per card with the largest on top and the smallest on the bottom. Each unit consists of three circles, one red, one green, and one clear. Each circle has a black line figure in it. If the child can maintain all three pictures on the top unit, move to the next smaller unit looking for suppression as you go from more peripheral to more central targets.

- Card OPT/OFP: Ten red geometrical figures with the largest on top getting smaller as you go down. Each red shape has a black line picture in it. The child looks at the top circle and names the picture and goes down to the more central targets. The green filter goes over the normally suppressing eye.

- CC1 and CC2: Antisuppression cards that can be viewed at any working distance. The child should see all figures on the card.

- Nonvariable OPT 1, 2, and 3: These are stereo fusion cards incorporating pictures of interest for young children. Targets are presented base-out (BO) and base-in (BI) on the same card in an anaglyphic format. Child can tell the therapist which objects are closer and which are further away. If the child is capable, localization in space is particularly useful.

- Variable OPT 1, 2, and 3: These are variable anaglyphic targets which can be made disparate to increase BO or BI demands. Each pair of slides presents a picture (fair, circus, or rope) with different version demands within it. During

disparateness, it is helpful to have the child localize parts of the picture.

Resource Materials

These cards are available through Stereo Optical Co., Chicago, IL; and also through OEP in Santa Ana, CA.

Note: You need good lighting for these cards, or you can mount them on a window so daylight comes through.

VII. *LOLLIPOP/SWIVEL PRISMS DIPLOPIA—RECOVERIES*

Swivel or lollipop prisms are loose prisms of varying power affixed to a plastic rod or small dowel or handle. Powers are available from as low as 2 prism diopters (p.d.) to as high as 25 p.d. When the handle is held vertically, BI or BO prism effect can be induced. When held horizontally, base-up (BU) or base-down (BD) prism effect can be achieved. For diplopia-recovery work, the beginning prismatic amount is determined by the least amount needed to create alternate fixation and vertical diplopia. This is achieved by using the swivel prism held horizontally that creates vertical diplopia. After diplopia is appreciated, the prism is removed and the child is encouraged to re-fuse the two images. With deep to moderate suppressors, R/G glasses and a light source in a darkened room would be a good starting point. The next sequence would be as above except in a fully lighted room. After that is achieved, the R/G filters can be removed to determine if diplopia can be appreciated. A darkened room might be needed first, and then with full illumination. As progress is noted, the vertical dissociating prism power can be reduced.

Swivel prisms are available from Bernell Corporation, Meshawaka, IN., Gulden Ophthalmics, Elkins Park, PA, and VTE Stresspoint, Milan Italy.

PROCEDURES FOR STRABISMUS

Because prescribing and patching regimens and surgical intervention have been mentioned earlier in Chapters 21 and 22, the emphasis in this section will be on those procedures for preschool strabismus.

An assumption is being made that whatever amblyopia existed before this aspect of treatment has been mostly resolved. Therefore, the population discussed here is comprised of constant alternating strabismic patients (ET, XT, HT) or intermittent strabismic patients. Obviously, the intermittent preschool strabismic is nearly always easier to work with and responds well to VT. I personally am not overly concerned with anomalous correspondence nor with eccentric fixation in the preschool patient, because these conditions rarely have an impact on outcomes of the children we work with and are not easily determined—at best! (8).

Regardless of the direction of the strabismus, early VT intervention should regularly include procedures to develop, enhance, or improve basic oculomotor skills, including direct fixation, pursuits, simple saccadic movements, and eye–hand coordination. The following activities are presented to aid the clinician helping the child develop improved oculomotor abilities.

I. *AN STAR PICTURE POINTING*

Purpose

Saccadic fixation and eye–hand coordination

Materials

Large AN Star with letters, numbers, or pictures at each star point

Procedure

Draw an AN Star pattern on a sheet of plain paper. At each point, place a figure appropriate for the child. Photocopy and laminate so these can be reused. Place on a wall within arm's reach of the child. Have the child move a finger from the ear to one specific point of the star. If successful, have the child bring the finger back to the ear and go to another point at your instruction.

As a variation and of increased difficulty, make up a sequence of pictures that appear on the AN Star on a separate page. Put this above or to the side of the star. Have the child then look at the row of pictures on the page with the random sequence, and one by one, in order, point to the pictures that match them on the star.

For an added cognitive component, code each picture with a symbol, such as a number or letter. Place these symbols on a sheet of paper in a random sequence. Then the child must look at the symbols on the sheet, decode what the symbol represents, and then point to the corresponding picture on the AN Star.

Resource Information

Any Clip Art program has sufficient numbers of pictures to generate the needed AN Stars and random sequences. AN Stars are also available from OEP @ *www.oep.org.*

II. *BEAD AND STRING GAMES*

III. *MONOCULAR/BINOCULAR LITE-BRITE* and *SPARKLE LIGHTS* (without red/green filters)

IV. *FLASHIGHT ACTIVITIES* without red/green filters

V. *BALL BUNTING*

Purpose

To improve the child's ability to maintain visual fixation, eye–hand coordination, and directional concepts

Materials

Sponge rubber ball attached to a string and suspended from ceiling; cardboard tubes (e.g., mailing tubes, gift wrap paper tubes, paper towel tubes); a 3-foot long wooden dowel stick (1 inch thick) (Fig. 23.5)

Procedure

Have the child face the ball, feet slightly apart, hands holding the tube raised to chest level. The ball is to be hung at mid-chest level. The child is instructed to gently bunt the ball forward without breaking the tube. When the ball returns, the ball is to be bunted forward again.

The child can be instructed to bunt the ball in different directions, but should try keep the ball under control at all times.

With different colored tapes around the dowel stick (at each end and in the

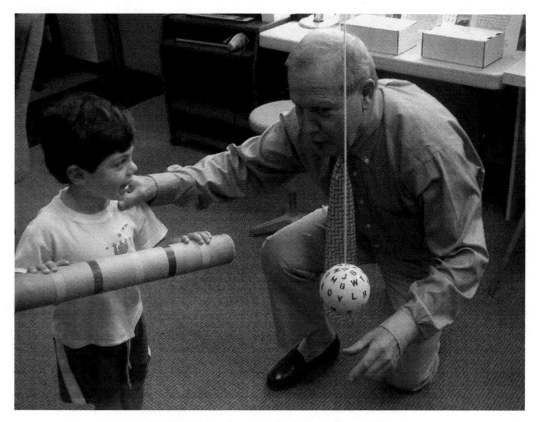

FIGURE 23.5. Preparing for ball bunting activity.

middle), have the child bunt the ball on the colored tapes consecutively or to verbal or visual commands.

Have the child call out the side of the stick (i.e., right, middle, or left) with which the child is bunting the ball while bunting it. This applies to the older child.

Numbers or letters can be printed on the ball (i.e., Marsden ball) and have the child call out a number or a letter that the child sees on the ball and bunt at that letter or number.

VI. *PING PONG POOL*

Purpose

To improve fixation and tracking monocularly, eye–hand coordination, and convergence.

Materials

Table, ping pong balls,

Mattel box cars, Brio trains, and cup or small box

Procedure

Have the child sit across a table from the therapist at one end of the table. Patch one of the eyes. The therapist then takes the ping pong ball and slowly rolls it toward the patient. Watching the ball the entire time, the patient must catch the ball in the cup as it falls off the edge of the table. Vary speed and trajectory.

Do the same as above, but with both eyes tracking the ball as it moves closer to the patient.

To maintain interest, other targets (e.g., box cars or trains) can be used.

Resource Information

Ping pong balls, trains, and boxcars are available at Toys "R" Us or other large toy stores.

VII. *BEAN BAG TOSS*

Purpose

To improve ocular motor and, convergence skills; and improve eye–hand coordination and gross motor skills

Materials

Beanbags and Nerf balls (or similar objects)

Procedure

Therapist and child sit on the floor. The therapist rolls the ball toward the child who has to visually track it and then catch it with two hands. This can be done monocularly or binocularly.

Child stands (unless handicapped) facing a pail or box placed on the floor at a distance of about 3 feet. The therapist hands the child a beanbag and asks the child to toss it so it gets into the box. If the child succeeds, the distance is changed and the child tries again. If the child misses, the beanbag is retrieved and the child tries again with the box at the same position.

Therapist and child sit on the floor. The therapist rolls the ball toward the child who has to visually track it binocularly as it approaches.

Place a beanbag on the floor. Have the child stand in front or behind it. Have the child jump over the beanbag without landing on it. If the child can do this, increase the distance between the child and the beanbag.

Resource Information

Beanbags and balls are available through craft or toy stores.

VIII. *BALLOON TOSS*

Purpose

To improve fixation and tracking skills and improve eye–hand coordination.

Materials

Thick rubber balloons (thicker rubber is safer for children because they are less likely to break)

Procedure

Blow up the balloon and tie a knot at the neck. The therapist and child stand facing each other. The examiner hits the balloon toward the child with both hands, a la volley ball. The child watches the balloon and, as it comes down toward the child, the child hits the balloon with both hands back toward the therapist.

Resource Information

Toys "R" Us

IX. *BUBBLE GAMES*

Purpose

To improve ocular motor skills and eye–hand coordination.

Materials

Bubble liquid, bubble wands of different sizes, or bubble blowing machine

Procedure

The therapist and child face each other; the therapist, using a wand dipped in the soap solution, blows a few bubbles toward the child. The child can then either break the bubbles while clapping two hands together, stamp on them with a foot as they fall to the floor, or catch them on a wand, one at a time, as they move through the air.

Resource Information

Bubbles and wands are available through most toy stores.

Suppressions

After acuities have been equalized and some degree of fixation skills have been developed, the next concern to address is suppressions, because very few preschool strabismic patients demonstrate frank diplopia. As discussed earlier in the amblyopia section, highly effective antisuppression can be achieved via MFBF techniques.

When the strabismus is primarily unilateral, procedures using only one target seen by the strabismic eye would be a starting point. With alternators and intermittent strabismic patients, procedures using two targets, one for each eye, can be used. This can be accomplished via anaglyphic or Polaroid filters or targets or vertical dissociation with 6Δ BU on one eye and 6Δ BD on the other. Numerous techniques using both means of MFBF have been described in the amblyopia section.

When acuities are close to equal and no deep suppressions exist, the next phase is development of binocularity and stereopsis. A need may exist at this point to use compensatory prisms, usually Fresnel Press Ons, as the amount often will be changed during the course of treatment.

Both Hirschberg and Krimsky tests, as well as the cover/uncover test using prism bars, can provide a starting point for what prism power is needed. Certainly, the least amount of prism that affects binocular responses would be the amount to use.

With esotropic patients having a significant accommodative component, extra plus lenses in clip-ons over the existing prescription may be indicated. Similarly, with divergence excess exotropic patients who seem to align with less plus, or a minus *add* on distance viewing, might well be a candidate for either a separate minus distance only prescription, or a minus distance prescription with an add to cancel the minus when doing near tasks. This use of a distance minus compensatory lens format will not be for long-term use, it is hoped. Significant literature suggests this minus distance overcorrection does not contribute to the development of myopia (9). Divergence excess patients who exhibit a high accommodative convergence:accommodation (AC:A) ratio, especially if esophoria is present at near, would most likely benefit from a plus add at near, often in a plano or plus add bifocal.

The use of binasal occluders with esotropic patients has also been recommended for several reasons, including possibly preventing anomalous retinal correspondence, and enhancing peripheral awareness or stimulation (10,11).

Whatever compensatory prismatic power, as well as plus for eso and minus for exo, the goal should be the reduction of magnitude and, eventually, elimination of whatever lens or prism format formerly served as a *crutch*.

POSSIBLE TREATMENT STRATEGIES

Numerous references indicate it is advised that therapy for esotropic patients begins at the centration point and move outward (8). Likewise, for a divergence excess patient who exhibits near alignment, treatment is often recommended to proceed from near to far (12). Conversely, an exotropia of the convergence insufficiency type might be best treated by working from far to nearpoint. These concepts are mechanistic or mechanical and follow long-standing orthoptic principles, (8) but do not necessarily have to be followed for success in treating preschool strabismic patients (8). Most therapy procedures can be applied to many of the strabismic patients you will be working with. Eso or exo categorizing here is not "etched in stone."

MORE PROCEDURES FOR STRABISMIC PATIENTS

I. For those with esotropia (ET), wide-angle monocular pursuits with puppets or stickers on tongue depressors, dangled cat bell on wire. Child is asked to follow target in different field of gazes.

  A. Although it is normal for a preschooler to track a target with much head movement (motor support or overflow), the child with ET should be encouraged to follow mainly with the eyes to emphasize eye position in an abducted field.

  B. As above, but emphasizing more in the adducted fields and question the child with exotropia (XT) regarding details in or on the target.

II. *NEAR-FAR FOCUSING SHIFTING* (Hart Charts with symbols or pictures). After any significant amblyopia has been eliminated, accommodative facility or flexibility procedures are most definitely indicated in all patients, regardless if the turn is in or out, or vertical. Modified Hart letter charts using symbols or pictures (e.g., Sponge Bob characters) can be easily made using Clip Art techniques. Color copiers (e.g., Kinko's) can be used, which can also shrink the pictures for near viewing and enlarge them for far viewing. These procedures are typically done monocularly to avoid diplopia or strabismus, typically ET with minus if done binocularly and XT with plus.

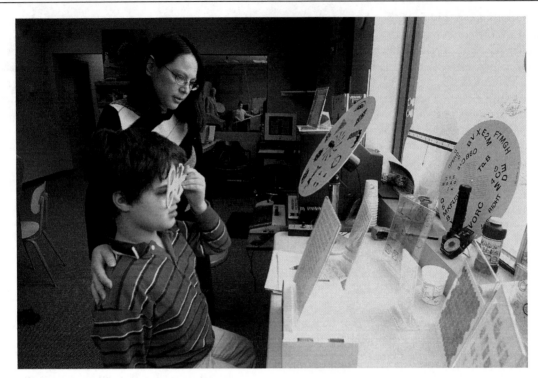

FIGURE 23.6. A child doing binocular accommodative rock with ± lens flippers.

III. *ACCOMMODATIVE ROCK FACILITY* using plus or minus lenses (Fig. 23.6). Monocular, and when indicated or possible, binocular rock can be achieved with young children using varying plus and minus lens powers in "Flipper" format. Pediatric picture charts or symbols usually work well. Both the lens powers and size of targets can readily change the demand on the patient. When working binocularly, if suppressions are suspected, anaglyphic targets can be used.

Resource Information

Plus minus flippers are available from Bernell Corp, Meshawaka, IN., and Optego, Thornhill, Ontario, Canada pediatric anaglyphic targets are available from the Red Green Toy Box, Santee, CA, or *redgreentoybox.com.*

IV. *POINTER AND STRAW*

Purpose

This procedure works well with both intermittent ET and intermittent XT or convergence insufficiency (CI). Plus and minus lenses, as well as training prisms, can be added. Expect fine motor control to be *shaky* with the younger children. It trains eye–hand coordination, use of the two eyes together for close work (convergence)

Materials

Straw, pointer (pick-up stick, uncooked spaghetti, pencil, pen)

Procedure

Have the child hold the pointer.

Sit directly in front of the child and hold the straw at child's eye level.

If child is using the right hand, use your right hand. Switch hands halfway through the exercise.

Have child line up the pointer with the straw. Then have child put the pointer *cleanly* into the straw as best possible.

Watch to see if there is any eye turn.

To Make It More Difficult

Have child hold the pointer above the straw 1 to 3 seconds before putting it in.

Move the straw closer and closer to the child. Stop if the child feels discomfort or sees double. Move the straw a little higher or off to the side, but not too far.

Hold the straw at different orientations: vertical, horizontal or diagonal.

Note: Do not face the opening of the straw toward the child.

V. BROCK STRING

This procedure works well with both intermittent ET and XT. Typically, a shorter string is needed and larger beads or targets should be employed. Often times, young children will deny physiologic diplopia. The child must know it is okay to see two (2) strings, although the child is holding one. As with the pointer and straw, plus and minus lenses and BO or BI and yoked prisms can be added. Older children might also respond when using anaglyphic filters, a white string (thicker than normal) and large red or green beads. A long black shoelace can be substituted for the white string.

A. BROCK STRING FIXATIONS: HOME TRAINING

Purpose

This training procedure teaches the use of both eyes at the same time and develops the ability to shift two-eyed vision from one point in space (near) to another point (far) easily and quickly without shutting off vision in one eye.

Procedure

Obtain a 6- to 8-foot long piece of string and thread two red and two green beads (or buttons) on it. Attach one end to a wall (e.g., light switch plate, bulletin board, doorknob) slightly below eye level. Have the patient wrap the other end of the string around the index finger and, standing in good posture, hold the string taut to the bridge of the nose. Keep both eyes open.

Start with two beads, one bead close to, or at the wall and one bead about 1 foot from the patient's nose (Fig. 23.7).

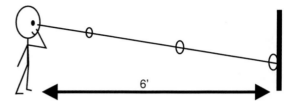

FIGURE 23.7. The Brock string set-up as shown with three beads. It can also be done with two beads as a simpler format.

Tell the patient to look at the far bead (closest to the wall). The patient should see two strings meeting at the far bead forming a "V." The near bead should appear doubled, and both strings should be the same height (Fig. 23.8).

Tell the patient, "if you see just one string, you are shutting off one eye" (right eye sees left string, left eye sees right string). If this happens, try blinking rapidly or "twanging" the string. Also, you can put on R/G glasses. If you put the red in front of the right eye and the green in front of the left eye, the right eye will see the left string which in now red, and the left eye will see the right string which is now green.

Now look at the near bead. It should become clear and single with both strings meeting at the bead and forming an "X" (the far bead should now be doubled) (Fig. 23.9).

The procedure is repeated, shifting from the far bead to the near bead; back and forth every 2→1 seconds. With improvement, have the patient move the near bead in closer to the eyes, to 10 inches, 8 inches, 6 inches,

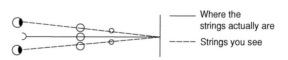

FIGURE 23.8. The figure shows what the normal response should be when the child fixates the far bead on a three-bead set-up.

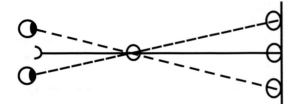

FIGURE 23.9. The figure shows what the normal response should be when the child fixates the near bead on a two-bead set-up.

4 inches, 2 inches. To make the task more difficult, add the other two beads in between. The two strings should cross or intersect at the bead where the patient is looking.

TIME: _____ minutes

Daily: two times per day_____. Three time per day_____

Glasses used: Yes No_____

VI. FUSION PROCEDURES

Many procedures are used in VT that lend themselves to preschool children and aid in developing or improving fusion and stereopsis, along with the spatial aspects (float, localization, parallax, Small *In*, Large *Out* (SILO).

Following is an overview; some of the procedures have been described earlier in this chapter.

A. Lite-Brite and Sparkle Brite using red, green, and crystal clear pegs with R/G filters: although not a fusion technique per se, good performance requires both eyes to function without suppression.

B. Carl's Cards: Have the child identify or label or find two cards, where one is seen by red filters and the other by the green filter.

C. Red, green, and black bears (A. C. Moore) on black felt. Again, not fusion but a good MFBF procedure with both eyes *controlled.*

D. Red/Green Sherman playing cards (Bernell/Keystone): same as Carl's cards but for the older preschooler.

E. Anaglyphic flashlight activities with R/G filters Technique

VII. *R/G FLASHLIGHT TAG*

Purpose

Antisuppression and ocular motor training.

Materials

Two flashlights (one with a green filter over the light and the other with a red filter), R/G glasses

Procedure

Have the child wear the R/G glasses. The child holds one of the flashlights and the trainer holds the other. In a large dim room, facing a white wall, the trainer puts the flashlight somewhere on the wall. The child is to place his/her light on top of the trainer's light as quickly and accurately as possible. With each *tag*, the trainer moves the light to another position on the wall.

Another variation is for the trainer to slowly move the light around on the wall while the child tries to stay right on top of the trainer's light.

Note: The child needs to be using both eyes to see both flashlights. If one of the lights disappears, have the child blink rapidly and try again. With younger children, this works better when the doctor places the light on the child's light, at which point the child must move his or her light again.

Because the anaglyphic filters can allow or encourage the child's visual system to manifest heterophoria, it is not unusual for the child to *see* the red light on top of (superimposed) the parent's green light, yet the two are not superimposed. This would be direct foveal projection where esophoria or esotropia would be crossed and exophoria or exotropia would be uncrossed.

Clinical Pearl: In any anaglyphic or vectographic procedure, and with MFBF procedures, intermittent suppressions can often be reduced or eliminated by having the child blink rapidly and or use a pointer or the touch or tactile system.

MORE STRABISMUS PROCEDURES

I. *KEYSTONE FUSION GAMES AND BASIC BINOCULAR TESTS.* As stated earlier, these are user friendly for the preschool child; they are portable and can be viewed at varying distances. The vergance demand on each target is fixed, but multiple targets are available, ranging from low vergance demand to moderate. Besides, R/G anaglyphic filters, flippers can also be used to confirm the child's responses as reversing the filters will reverse the BO or BI effect. Because the background is essentially white, the red filter sees the green ink and green filter sees the red. An older or more mature child might report the desired 3-D effect, but also be aware of a ghost image, which is flat on the paper.

OPTOMATTERS and Red Green Toybox offer similar anaglyphic targets, the latter with multiple eye–hand exercises.

II. *SWIVEL/LOLLIPOP PRISMS* (available from Bernell Corp., Gulden Corp., and Stress Point VT (Italy) Fusion recovery work can be changed with varying prismatic powers or demands, size of targets, and viewing distances.

Technique

Lollipop Prism Recoveries

Purpose

To improve the child's ability to make changes in vergence.

Materials

Lollipop prisms

Procedure

Find a good fixation target and hold it at about 16 inches. Tell the child to let you know if the target ever doubles. Place the prism in front of one of the child's eyes, first in the base-in position. Ask the child what he or she sees. If the child reports 1, swivel the prism 180° to the base-out position and again ask what the child sees. If the child is too young to report diplopia, watch carefully for changes in vergence. For example, if a 12-month-old looks at a target as a five base-in prism is put in front of the eye, you should see a divergence movement. This may be diffi-

cult to see, but when you take the prism away, a more rapid convergence should occur to resolve diplopia. If you put the prism in front of one eye and you see the child changing fixation between diplopic images, you know the child is not able to compensate for the prism value. Start with an appropriately difficult, but not doubling prism.

Resource Information

Bernell Corporation (Stick Prisms), Mishawaka, IN.

Additionally, diplopia recovery work can be done using vertical dissociating prisms (6 p.d. BU/BD), where the child should appreciate a doubled vertical image when the BU/BD prism is introduced. Depending on whether the deviation is exo or eso, the perceived doubling will be uncrossed or crossed. The desired goal is rapid fusional recovery when using BO/BI, and diplopia recovery when the prism creates vertical diplopia.

III. *VECTOGRAMS* (variable) and *ANAGLYPHS* (fixed or variable). Binocular or stereo responses are often best elicited when using stereo targets (versus first- and second-degree fusion targets). Vectograms and anaglyphic targets often can result in a desired binocular or stereo response. These targets (Bernell, Stereo Optical, OEP–OPTOMATTERS) can be viewed at different distances (near, intermediate, and distance). If the eyes are straight, effect stereopsis and the resultant spatial effects (SILO, float, localization, and possibly parallax).

VISION THERAPY FOR THE VERY YOUNG PATIENT

Procedures to improve vision in the very young patient include the following:

1. Eye–hand coordination
2. Visual tracking
3. Saccade eye movements

As mentioned earlier in this chapter, virtually all children in a preschool vision therapy program exhibit one or more problems in the following areas: acuity (amblyopia), binocularity (e.g. strabismus, binocular anomalies), accommodative dysfunction, (insufficiency or infacility), and deficits in oculomotor or visuomotor and visual perceptual areas, which often include lags or problems in balance and gross and fine motor control. Many of the children we see often exhibit deficits or problems in more than one of these areas. For instance, the young child with cerebral palsy is likely to have (a) atypical refractive *error*, (b) a greater likelihood of being strabismic (or binocular dysfunction), (c) more likely to have accommodative problems, and (d) oculomotor and visuomotor lags (1, 13).

This section will address the very young patient in vision therapy who is not amblyopic or strabismic, yet who exhibits problems in eye movement control or eye–hand coordination, and or visuomotor problems.

Differing philosophies abound, some espousing gross to fine (bottom up) and others fine to gross (top-down). Our opinion or preference is that, in most cases, basic issues such as balance (static or kinetic), bilateral integration, and bilateral reciprocity should be either initially addressed or be incorporated into the areas of oculomotor or eye–hand coordination, and visuomotor training procedures. Certainly, an occupational therapist familiar with this population could provide many of the basic motor (gross and fine) experiences and procedures.

Rather than separately list pursuits, saccades, eye–hand, and visuomotor procedures, we present a suggested sequence of activities.

I. *EYE-HAND PROCEDURES*

Technique

Sparkle Lights (use red, green and crystal pegs)

Purpose

Eye–hand coordination and improve fine motor skills.

Materials

Sparkle Lights game, R/G filters (optional)

Procedure

Place R/G glasses on patient. Place R/G pegs on the board in patterns or randomly. Have the patient touch all the pegs that the child sees with one finger.

Place R/G glasses on patient. Place R/G pegs in a row. Have patient put a peg above or below all the pegs on the board.

Place R/G glasses on patient. Place R/G pegs in a pattern on the board (e.g., circle, square line). Have the patient make the same pattern somewhere else on the board.

Place R/G glasses on patient. Place R/G pegs in a pattern on the board (e.g., circle, square, triangle). Have the patient make a matching outside border around your pattern.

This can also be done with red or clear filters with just green pegs for monocular fixation in a binocular field for amblyopia (red lens on the nonamblyopia eye).

As above, adding clear pegs that can be seen by both eyes. Place R/G glasses on the patient. Place pegs, which can only be seen with the normally suppressing eye (e.g., if the left eye is the suppressing eye and the green filter is on the left eye, use green pegs). Slowly introduce pegs seen by the normally fixating eye (red pegs) and have the patient try to keep all the pegs *on*. Patient is instructed to touch each peg in an order (e.g., from right to left, from up to down).

All of the above utilize eye–hand components but do not require the R/G filters.

Resource Materials

Manufactured by Ohio Art Company, Bryan, Ohio. Also sold at J.C. Penney for $14.99 and on the Internet.

Notes: 1. Best if done in dim or darkened room conditions. The advantage over Lite-Brite is that black background is permanent and does not have to be replaced after each use. Lite-Brite pegs illuminate more brightly when used in Sparkle Lights box. Lite-Brite pegs are easier to insert and remove.

Technique

Lite-Brite

Purpose

Antisuppression, monocular fixation in binocular field, eye–hand coordination, and monocular fixation amblyopia training.

Materials

Lite-Brite Game

Procedure

For antisuppression, MFBF, and eye–hand coordination, Lite-Brite is a light box with holes for pegs to go into and, as such, can be used to accomplish antisuppression training, MFBF, and eye–hand coordination, except the background is clear instead of black. As with Sparkle Lights, in the case of amblyopia, you may use red or clear filters with green pegs where the red filter goes over the nonamblyopia eye.

Using monocular fixation, put a patch on the nonamblyopic eye. Place a Lite-Brite picture pattern onto the light box. Have the patient place the appropriate colored peg into each marked hole until the pattern is completed.

Resource Materials

Available at most toy stores, this product is from Milton Bradley Co.

Note: Remember that cancellation is opposite on the clear background (projected) than on the white background. On the clear background, the red peg will be seen by the eye with the red filter and vice versa. On the white background, the red peg will be seen by the eye with the green filter and vice versa.

Technique

Monocular Line Tracing

Purpose

Improve eye–hand coordination, fine motor ability and visual fixation.

Materials

Patch, line drawings on sheets of paper

Procedure

Patch one eye. then, have the child slowly and accurately trace over the lines of the picture. Encourage the child to go slowly and accurately, and make the child aware of inaccuracies. Discourage impulsivity by making the child move slowly until accuracy improves. Repeat with the other eye and note any differences between the performance of each eye. Increase difficulty by using more complex pictures, pictures

with thinner lines, using a smaller writing utensil, adding verbal distractions during the task, and adding a time component so that the child can beat a previous *best time*.

Note: Be sure the child works at an appropriate working distance. Keep the child from getting too close.

Technique

Maze Games

Purpose

Antisuppression during a visuomotor activity and eye–hand coordination.

Materials

R/G glasses, white paper, black pen, and red color pencil (carmen red and vermillion red from Venus Company cancel well)

Procedure

Place the R/G glasses on the child. Have the child *walk* the red pencil through two parallel black line mazes from "Start" to "Finish." Encourage the child to always stay inside the path. Have plenty of mazes available, ranging from very easy to complex. Ask the child to report if the maze disappears or goes away. In the case of an amblyopia, the red filter goes in front of the better eye and the green filter goes in front of the amblyopic eye. Use good illumination.

To increase difficulty, make the mazes narrower, longer, and more complex and sinuous or curved.

Technique

Bead and String Games

Purpose

Antisuppression, monocular fixation in a binocular field, eye–hand coordination, and monocular acuity improvement for amblyopia.

Materials

Black string or shoelace (about 2 feet long), assorted red, green, and black beads, which cancel appropriately through R/G filters, and black felt background

Procedure

Place R/G filters on the patient. Have the child hold the string and tie a large enough knot at one end so that the beads will not fall off. Spread beads out on a piece of black felt and tell the child to look for the beads. The child should then pick up *ONE* bead at a time and put the end of the black string through the hole in the bead. The child should attend to both the string and the bead while doing this. If it is done accurately, have the child pull the string through so that the bead slides down the string.

If done inaccurately, have the child start over on the same bead. Continue until all the beads are strung.

Resource Information

Red and green wooden beads are available through most arts and crafts stores.

Notes: Be sure to check cancellation through the R/G filters. Full room illumination is necessary.

Variations

Make up different random bead configurations on several pieces of string. Place one of your configurations on a piece of black felt. Give the patient a black string and have the child take beads from a box and string beads onto his or her string so that the child's configuration matches yours so that when the two are laid next to each other they are exactly the same.

Take one of your prepared strings and lay it onto black felt. Have the patient count how many red beads are on the string and how many green beads are on the string; have the child touch each bead while counting.

Place red, green, and black beads randomly on the black felt. Have the child sort all of them into three piles of black, red, and green beads.

Technique

AN Star Picture Pointing

Purpose

Saccadic fixation and eye–hand coordination.

Materials

Large (8 1/2 × 11 inch) AN Star with letters, numbers, or pictures at each star point

Procedure

Draw an AN Star pattern on a sheet of plain paper. At each star point, place a figure ap-

propriate for the child. Photocopy and laminate so these can be reused. Place within arm's reach of the child. Have the child move a finger from his or her ear to one specific point of the star. If successful, have the child bring the finger back to the ear and go to another point at your instruction.

As a variation and of increased difficulty, make up a sequence of pictures that appears on the AN Star on a separate page. Put this above or to the side of the star. Have the child then look at the row of pictures on the page with the random sequence, and one by one, in order, point to the pictures that match them on the star.

For an added cognitive component, code each picture with a symbol (e.g., a number or letter). Place these symbols on a sheet of paper in a random sequence. Then, the child must look at the symbols on the sheet, decode what the symbol represents, and then point to the corresponding picture on the AN Star.

Resource Information

Any Clip Art program will provide you with sufficient numbers of pictures to generate the needed AN Stars, and random sequences.

Technique

Ball Bunting

Purpose

To improve the child's ocular motor abilities, eye–hand coordination, and directional concepts.

Materials

Sponge rubber ball attached to a string to be suspended from ceiling; cardboard tubes (e.g., mailing tubes, gift wrap paper tubes, paper towel tubes); and 3-foot long wooden dowel stick (1 inch thick)

Procedures

Have the child face the ball, feet slightly apart, hands holding the tube raised to chest level. The ball is to be hung at midchest level. The child is instructed to gently bunt the ball forward without breaking the tube. When the ball returns, the ball is to be bunted forward again.

The child can be instructed to bunt the ball in different directions, but must keep the ball under control at all times.

With different colored tapes around the tubes or dowel stick (at each end and in the middle), have the child bunt the ball on the colored tapes consecutively or to verbal or visual commands.

Have the child call out the side of the stick (i.e., right, middle, or left) that the child is bunting the ball while doing it.

Numbers or letters can be printed on the ball (e.g., Marsden ball) and have the child call out a number or a letter that the child sees on the ball and bunt at the letter or number.

Reference

Excellent Marsden balls are available from VTE/Stress Point Test (Italy) at *www.stresspointest.com.*

Technique

Bean Bag Toss or Ball Rolling

Purpose

Improve ocular motor skills, convergence skills; eye–hand coordination, and gross motor skills.

Materials

Bean bags and Nerf balls or similar objects

Procedure

Therapist and child sit on the floor. The therapist rolls the ball toward the child who has to visually track it and then catch it with two hands. This can be done monocularly or binocularly. This also can be done across a table top with child at one side or end and assistant at the other.

2. Child stands (unless handicapped) facing a pail or box placed on the floor at a distance of about 3 feet. The therapist hands the child a bean bag and asks the child to toss it so it gets into the box. If the child succeeds, the distance is changed and the child tries again. If the child misses, the bean bag is retrieved and the child tries again with the box at the same position.

Place a bean bag on the floor. Have the child stand in front or behind it. Have the child jump over the bean bag without landing on it.

If the child can do this, increase the distance between the child and the bean bag. Both feet should *depart and land* at the same time.

Resource Information

Bean bags and balls are available through craft or toy stores.

Technique

Picture Groffman Tracking

Purpose

Improve visual fixation and attention and "smooth" pursuit movement.

Materials

8.5 × 11 inch paper, colored inkpads, and rubber stamps of cartoon characters (e.g., Mickey Mouse, Pooh, Piglet, Donald Duck; see example page); or stickers

Procedure

Patch one eye and have the child follow the line from one figure on the top or left to its opposite on the bottom or right. Patterns can be as simple as straight lines from one to the other or as complex as very squiggly lines crossing over other lines many times. Making the angles at the crossings smaller increases the degree of difficulty. After a few minutes on one eye, switch the patch to the other eye and repeat the procedure. Then repeat with both eyes open.

Resource Information

Media Material, Baltimore, MD.

Technique

Three Card Monty

Purpose

To improve visual fixation, visual attention, and tracking skills.

Materials

Three paper cups turned upside down, one small *puff* ball, and eye patch

Procedure

This can be done monocularly or binocularly, but start with the monocular aspect first. Therefore, patch one of the eyes. Place the puff ball under one of the cups on a flat surface (e.g., a table) allowing the child to see where it is. Then slowly or quickly, depending on the child's abilities, move the cups around and position them in a new configuration. The child has to successfully show the examiner where the ball is. Repeat for a few minutes and then switch the patch to the other eye. Repeat the procedure. If indicated, repeat the procedure with both eyes open after the two monocular phases.

If the therapist chooses, this activity can be made even more involved by allowing the child to *bet* on each trial; you could start the child out with ten pennies and if the child gives a correct response, you give the child another penny. However, if the child responds incorrectly, the child has to give you a penny. It can also be played for pieces of candy (e.g., M&M's) or cookies, raisins, or Cheerios.

Resource Information

Paper cups can be obtained at any grocery store. The red and green puff balls are available through A.C. Moore craft stores, a chain of craft stores in northeastern United States, but they sell on the Internet at *www.acmoore.com.*

Technique

Driving to Cartoon Land

Purpose

To improve fixation and tracking, eye–hand coordination, and vergence skills.

Materials

Cartoon character rubber stamps, or stickers, paper, a small toy car, wedge, or lollipop prisms

Procedure

This can be done monocularly or binocularly. Draw a maze of paths leading from the center of the paper outward. At the end of each path, stamp a cartoon character's pictures. Give the child the small toy car and tell the child to drive from one character to another (e.g., from Winnie the Pooh to Eeyore) without hitting the sides of the road. The paths can be made as narrow or as wide as they need to be for the child to succeed. To work on vergence skills during this activity, interpose lollipop prisms in front of one of the child's eyes while the child is driving the car.

Resource Information

Cartoon character stamps can be obtained from Media Material, Baltimore, MD, or from most toy stores.

Technique

Ball Rolling

Purpose

To improve ocular tracking, eye–hand coordination, and visual attention.

Materials

Various sized balls with various sized containers (e.g., an empty food can, a small waste paper basket, an empty shoebox)

Procedure

Have the child sit at one end of a room. This activity can be done monocularly or binocularly. Place different containers in different positions and distances from the child. Give the child a ball and ask the child to try to roll it into the waste paper basket, for example. If the child succeeds, try a different ball in a different container. If the child misses, try the same target again. The child can start near the containers, but as accuracy improves, the distance of the container from the child should be increased.

Technique

Colored Hart-Like Charts for Saccadic Fixation

Purpose

To improve monocular and binocular saccadic fixation.

Materials

Colored pictures Hart charts (same as accommodation training targets)

Procedures

Place a large chart on the wall at a distance of about 10 feet. Have the child *read* the pictures monocularly or binocularly as follows:

1. In order, from left to right and top to bottom
2. In order, from top to bottom and left to right
3. In order, from bottom to top and right to left
4. First and last pictures on each row

5. Second and next to the last picture on each row
6. First and next to the last picture on each row

Resource Materials

Refer to sheet on accommodation or Hart charts

Technique

Wayne Saccadic Fixator

Purpose

To improve saccadic eye movements and eye–hand coordination.

Materials

Wayne Saccadic Fixator

Procedure

Have the child stand in front of the fixator (Fig. 23.10). Program one of the *predictable* patterns at first (not random pat-

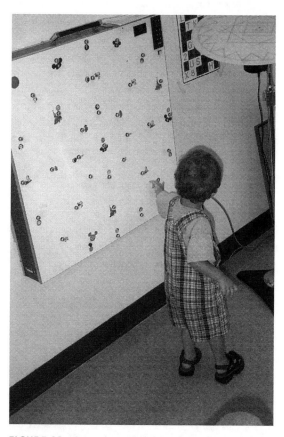

FIGURE 23.10. A young child attempting to follow the pattern of lights on the Wayne saccadic fixator.

terns at the beginning). Instruct the child to push the button that lights up as quickly as the child can and to keep going until the program stops. When the child is accustomed to the instrument and can do the predictable patterns with ease, introduce the random patterns. This activity may be done monocularly or binocularly. In cases of gaze restrictions, it is particularly useful to program the fixator so that the child is forced to look into the field of the affected muscle.

Resource Information

Wayne saccadic fixator is available through both Bernell Corp. or OEP Vision Catalog and Wayne Engineering.

Note: Young children love the fixator and will be motivated to do less fun activities with the promise of some time on it.

Technique

Flashlight Tracking

Purpose

To improve ocular motor tracking and eye–hand coordination.

Materials

Two regular flashlights with one or two colored filters

Procedure

Parent and child sit about 3 to 6 feet from a wall (preferably without anything on it). The child holds one of the flashlights and the parent holds the other. The flashlights should be color coded so that the child is aware of which of the flashlights is his or hers. The parent slowly moves the flashlight around the wall. The objective is for the child to keep his or her light directly on top of the parent's so that only one spot of light is seen on the wall. When the child *loses* the parent's light, the parent can stop and wait for the child to catch up. As the child gets better at the task, the speed of the parent's light can be increased or the patterns described on the wall can be made more complex and tortuous.

Ideally, the child should not move the head while tracking the parents light. Often, however, the child needs to do this at the beginning and should be allowed to do so. As skill at this task improves, the head should be stabilized. To help do this, place a small piece of cardboard (e.g., as from a laundered shirt) on the child's head and ask the child to balance it there during the activity. If it falls off, the child gets immediate feedback regarding head movement.

Resource Information

"Garrity" flashlights (available at Walmart) are light weight and focus the light well.

Technique

Ping Pong Pool

Purpose

To improve fixation and tracking monocularly and binocularly, eye–hand coordination, and convergence.

Materials

Ping pong balls, Mattel box cars, Brio trains, and cup or small box

Procedure

Have the child sit across a table with you at the other end of the table. Patch one of the eyes. Then take the ping pong ball and slowly roll it toward the patient. Watching the ball the entire time, the patient must catch the ball in the cup as it falls off the edge of the table. Vary speed and trajectory.

Do the same as above, but with both eyes tracking the ball as it moves closer to the patient.

To maintain interest, other targets can be used (e.g., box cars or trains).

Resource Information

Ping pong balls, trains, and box cars are available at Toys "R" Us or other large toy stores.

Note: The table top should be at stomach height of the child.

Technique

Magnet Mazes

Purpose

To improve tracking and fixation skills and eye–hand coordination.

Materials

Paper and pencil and several small magnets

Procedure

Draw a maze on a sheet of paper. Place one of the small magnets on top of the paper at the beginning of the maze. The child holds another magnet under the paper and, while moving that magnet, tries to move the magnet through the maze. As skill improves in this area, the lines should be made closer together. This can be done monocularly or binocularly.

Resource Information

Magnets are available at craft stores.

Technique

Balloon Toss

Purpose

To improve fixation and tracking skills and eye–hand coordination.

Materials

Thick rubber balloons (thicker rubber is safer for children because they are less likely to break)

Procedure

Blow up the balloon and tie a knot at the neck. Stand with the child facing you. Hit the balloon toward the child with both hands, a la volley ball. The child watches the balloon and as it comes down hits the balloon, with both hands, back toward you.

Resource Information

Toy stores, Toys "R" Us.

Technique

Bubble Games

Purpose

To improve ocular motor skills and eye–hand coordination.

Materials

Bubble liquid, bubble wands of different sizes, or bubble blowing machine

Procedure

Stand facing the child and using a wand dipped in the soap solution, blow a few bubbles toward the child. The child can then either break the bubbles while clapping two hands together, stamp on them with a foot as they fall to the floor, catch them on a wand, one at a time, as they move through the air, or break the bubble with one finger.

Resource Information

Bubbles and wands are available through most toy stores.

Technique

Pie Plate Rotations

Purpose

To improve visual tracking and eye–hand coordination.

Materials

A pie plate (9 inches or larger and preferably *NOT* glass) and a couple of marbles or ping pong ball

Procedure

The child places a marble or ball into the pie plate. The plate should be held in both hands. By moving the wrists while holding the plate, the child makes the marble move around the inside rim of the pie plate. As the marble moves around, the child has to keep fixating the marble or ball and follow its movement. If head movement is needed at the beginning, allow it. As the skill improves, the head should be stabilized.

To increase difficulty, change the object that moves around to spheres of differing size and material (e.g., a wooden circular bead, ping-pong ball, larger and smaller marbles). Note carefully the child's ability to control the movement of the different objects and the child's tracking ability.

ADDITIONAL GROSS MOTOR AND EYE–HAND COORDINATION PROCEDURES

I. *WALKING RAIL/BALANCE BEAM:* Home Training

Purpose

To improve body balance, eye–foot coordination, eye fixation, and eye movement control.

Materials

Balance beam (1 × 5 inches or 1 × 6 inches × 8 feet piece of common pine. As progress evolves, beam can be changed to an 8 foot 2 × 4 inch beam. Sand edges and surface to avoid splinter, Traction or grit tape can be applied to enhance performance. Also, an eye patch, and fixation charts (e.g., letters, pictures, symbols).

Procedure

In bare feet or wearing socks, the patient walks the beam forward toe-to-heel, first looking at feet, later fixating on eye chart.

Repeat going backward; toe-to-heel, first looking at the feet then at the fixation target.

The child calls aloud, in sequence, the letters or pictures on the fixation charts, going left to right, then right to left, and top to bottom.

A metronome can be used to vary speeds or beats, taking each step with a beat.

Procedures should be done, right eye only, left only, and finally both eyes.

Training lenses can be used by office—you will be advised.

The above procedures can be repeated by raising beam off floor with small 1 × 5 or 1 × 6 or 2 × 4 blocks a few inches in length. This increases the difficulty or demand level. Similarly, a bean bag or paper cup can be balanced on top of the head and questions and answers can be added.

With Rx _____   Without Rx _____
     Duration:_____ min
     _____ 1 × day
     _____ 2 × day

II. *ANGELS IN THE SNOW*

Purpose

Laterality

Materials

Marsden ball, metronome.

Method

Have the child lie with back on the floor, arms along the side the body, and heels touching. As you touch or call out one or more of the child's limbs, the child moves them out and away from the body.

Observations

Limbs are not to move off the floor, the child is to drag them across the floor. Limbs are to reach the end positions at the same time. End position for arms is over the head. End position for legs is spread out as far as possible.

Level 1

- Touch the arm or leg you want the child to move. The child calls out what he or she is doing and moves the limb.
- Repeat, but point to the limb to be moved. Do not touch it.

Level 2

- Have the child move two limbs so that they arrive at the extreme outward position at the same time. For example, both arms over the head, right arm and right leg, or right arm and left leg.

Level 3

- Set metronome at about 40 beats per minute. Use any arm and leg combination. The limbs are to be moved by a certain number of beats, usually starting with four. They are both to arrive at their extreme position at the end of four beats and start their return and arrive at their original position by the end of another four beats.
- Decrease to eight beats, and increase to every 2 beats.

Level 4

- With this activity you will use a Marsden ball. This is a ball about the size of a tennis ball, hanging from the ceiling about 3 feet over the child's chest. The child is to lie under the Marsden ball. Swing the ball in a head to foot direction. Tell the child that when the ball is up toward the child's head, put the right arm and right leg out and when it is at the child's feet, put the left arm and left leg out and bring the right arm and right leg back at the starting position.
- Vary the direction of ball and limbs to be moved. For example, swing the ball left to right. When it is at the child's right, both arms go over the head. When it is at the

child's left, both legs go out and the arms come back to the side. Vary combinations.

Level 5

- Set metronome to about 40 beats per minute. Use any leg and arm combination. Tell the child that the limbs are to be moved to a certain number of beats. They are to arrive at their extreme positions at the end of the required number of beats, and return to their original position at the required number of beats. Vary the number of beats per limb. For example, arms over the head in four beats and legs out in eight beats. Use any limb and beat combination.

REFERENCES

1. Maino D, ed. *Diagnosis and Management of Special Populations.* St. Louis: Mosby; 1995:143, 159.
2. Ciuffreda KJ, Levi DM, Selenow A. *Amblyopia: Basic and Clinical Aspects.* Boston: Butterworth-Heinemann; 1991:15–17.
3. Ciuffreda KJ, Levi DM, Selenow A. *Amblyopia: Basic and Clinical Aspects.* Boston: Butterworth-Heinemann; 1991:411.
4. The Pediatric Eye Disease Investigator Group. A randomized trial of patching regimens for treatment of moderate amblyopia in children. *Arch Ophthalmol* 2003;121:603–611.
5. The Pediatric Eye Disease Investigator Group. A randomized trial of atropine vs. patching for treatment of moderate amblyopia in children. *Arch Ophthalmol* 2002;120:268–278.
6. The Pediatric Eye Disease Investigator Group. A randomized trial of atropine regimens for treatment of moderate amblyopia in children (ATS4). *Ophthalmology* 2004;111:2076–2085.
7. FitzGerald DE, Krumholtz I. Maintenance of improvement gains in refractive amblyopia: a comparison of treatment modalities. *Optometry* 2002;73:153–159.
8. Press L, ed. *Applied Concepts in Vision Therapy.* Boston: Mosby, 1997:100, 203.
9. Rutstein RP, Marsh-Tootle W, London R. Changes in refractive error for exotropes treated with overminus lenses. *Optom Vis Sci* 1989;66:487–491.
10. Cox J. Binasal occlusion in vision therapy. Lenses, Occluders and Filters. Optometric Extension Program (OEP). 1996;38(1):56–61.
11. Greenwald I. Effective strabismus therapy. Optometric Extension Program Foundation, 1979:117.
12. Cooper J, Medow N. Intermittent exotropia—basic and divergence excess type. *Binoc Vis Eye Muscle Surg Q* 1993;8(3):201–203.
13. Duckman R. The incidence of visual anomalies in a population of cerebral palsied children. *Journal of the American Optometric Association* 1979; 50:1013–1016.

PART 4

Normal and Abnormal Development

Development of a Normal Child

24

Robert H. Duckman and David A. Maze

A very important component of a pediatric patient's case history is the child's developmental history. Optometric students and clinicians should always ask the parents about developmental patterns of the child. A comprehensive knowledge of this process is crucial in rendering appropriate optometric care to young patients. Understanding normal developmental sequences can help with clinical decision making (including appropriate referrals) for a slowly developing child.

The study of child development focuses on changes that involve behavioral reorganizations and qualitative differences from one age to the next (1). Many theories have been perpetuated over many decades to explain motor development, cognitive development, and emotional development. All of the theories state that changes taking place will follow a lawful and logical sequence; they are cumulative and become more complex as the child ages (1,2).

The term *normal development* pertains to typical changes that are shared by almost all children over time (3). These changes may not take place at the same time in all children, but most researchers recognize that there are average ages at which various milestones are reached.

Two early views have been influential in the study of child development. The English philosopher, John Locke, and French philosopher, Jean Jacques Rousseau, formulated their theories in the 17th and 18th, centuries respectively. Locke felt that children developed into what they are as a function of their environment. Rousseau thought that human development unfolds naturally as long as society allows it. The latter theory appealed to child development researchers who stressed a general developmental pattern that nearly all children share. Perhaps one of the best known of these researchers was Arnold Gesell.

Arnold Gesell conducted research in the 1920s and 1930s at Yale University. His studiesc focused on children's physical development and acquisition of motor skills. Gesell felt that patterns unfold naturally with maturation. Gesell studied and recorded changes in children from birth to 10 years of age. He felt that all children pass through universal stages in life and that motor development is the foundation for all mental life (4).

Out of the many researched child development theories, the two major theories involve cognitive development. The information-processing theory views the human brain as a computer. Developmentalists who take this perspective are concerned with changes in a maturing child's memory and problem-solving skills (5,6). One of the most well-known human development theorists, Jean Piaget, developed his theory based on normative cognitive development. He felt that children not only know less, but also have a different qualitative knowledge than adults. Piaget's theories, although not accepted by everyone, are still the most embraced and researched philosophies on child development.

Theories that pertain more to social and emotional rather than cognitive development are social learning theory, psychoanalytic theory, and Bowlby's adaptational theory (3). Social learning theory views development as a gradual and cumulative process focusing on behavior. That is, children learn by understanding the consequences of their own actions and learning from the consequences of others' behavior. Freud's psychoanalytic theory purports that abnormal behavior results from an inadequate expression of innate drives. Erickson broadened this to a psychosocial theory. Bowlby's adaptational theory integrates social, emotional, and cognitive aspects of development.

Of the numerous theories relating to child development, each focuses on different aspects of that development. Currently there is no universally accepted theory in the field of development psychology. Findings in this area can sometimes be interpreted in different ways. Most theories fall between two beliefs—either an infant is naive at birth and learns from the environment or the brain develops in a predetermined, preprogrammed manner (7). As a clinician trying to understand normal child development, this can be a confusing concept. However, considering development to be a combination of "pre-wiring" and environmental learning may be helpful in understanding normal child development.

NORMAL PREGNANCY

One important group of questions to ask while evaluating a pediatric patient's optometric case history concerns the pregnancy and birth process. While normal pregnancy and birth generally lead to normal development, abnormal pregnancy and birth often lead to abnormal development. From the moment of conception all the way through the delivery process many events occur that can have a large impact on the development of a child.

Conception

Conception takes place when a sperm penetrates the woman's egg cell, or ovum. For this to happen, a series of events must take place. The egg cell will ripen in a woman's ovary in about 28 days. When this ovum is ready for fertilization, it is released from the ovary to the fallopian tube. The egg passes through the fallopian tube down to the uterus. This passage takes place over several days, and the process is called *ovulation.* If the ovum is not penetrated by a sperm cell within the first day, it will disintegrate when it reaches the uterus. If, however, sexual intercourse takes place at the proper time, the egg meets potentially millions of sperm. When one of these sperm penetrates the ovum, a single-celled organism called a *zygote* is created, and conception has taken place (8). If two eggs are fertilized by two separate sperm, the result is dizygotic, or fraternal, twins. If, however, a single fertilized egg splits into two separate units early on, monozygotic, or identical, twins result.

Prenatal Development

Germinal Period: Conception Through Week 2

The germinal period begins the moment after conception. The zygote remains a single cell and pushes its way down the fallopian tubes. The process of *mitosis,* or cell division, takes place and the parent cell divides into two. The chromosomes in the original cell duplicate themselves. In a normal zygote, 46 chromosomes should be present: 23 from the sperm and 23 from the egg.

These cells continue to divide until the cells become a clustered, hollow, ball-like structure called a *blastocyst.* Usually around the sixth day, the blastocyst makes contact with the wall of the uterus. The lining has already become rich with blood in order to nourish the egg. The end of this stage is usually about 14 days, and the blastocyst becomes fully embedded in the uterine wall (8).

Embryonic Period: Weeks 3 Through 8

At weeks 3 through 8, the zygote becomes firmly implanted into the uterine wall, and becomes known as the *embryo.* This is a time of rapid cell division and differentiation. It is at this time that the process called *organogenesis* (when cells develop into organs and body structures) takes place (8).

The embryo has an intricate support system that is composed of three major parts: the placenta, the umbilical cord, and the amniotic sac. The placenta is tissue that forms from uterine cells and part of the blastocyst. Blood vessels are linked from the placenta to the embryo by the umbilical cord. Nutrients, oxygen, waste products, and carbon dioxide are transferred to and away from the embryo by these blood vessels. The transfer of these materials occurs through cell membranes in the placenta with the uterine lining. This creates two separate blood supplies; the mother's blood supply is separate from that of the embryo. Oxygen, carbon monoxide, and other small molecules can pass through the cell membranes, but blood cells cannot because they are too large. The membranes offer some protection against large molecules (e.g., most bacteria). They do not offer protection against smaller molecules such as viruses, alcohol, or many other chemicals.

The fluid-filled sac surrounding the embryo is called the *amniotic sac.* This sac provides a closed, protective environment for the embryo to develop. By acting as a cushion, it prevents harm or damage from bumping and shaking. This sac also acts to minimize any temperature changes when the mother is exposed to warmer and colder environments.

During the third week of this process, the first week of the embryonic period, the organism becomes oval with an indentation. The indentation will become the mouth and digestive tract. At the end of this week, the cells have differentiated into three major tissue types: endoderm, mesoderm, and ectoderm. The *endoderm* will develop into internal organs such as the stomach, liver, lungs, and so on. The *mesoderm* will become muscles, skeleton, and blood. The *ectoderm* will form the sensory organs, including the central nervous system and the skin.

Embryonic induction is a process of tissue interaction that shapes various organs and parts of the body (9). An example of this is when the lens forms based on the interaction of the ectoderm with the mesoderm.

By the end of the third week, the central nervous system has started to form and the eyes can be seen. In the fourth week, the heart and the digestive tract start to appear. By the end of the embryonic period, the fingers, toes, and bones are developing. This time period is very important as the critical period for organ development and differentiation takes place (8). The unborn child is vulnerable at this stage, but the mother may not realize that she is pregnant at this time. It becomes important for women to take care of their health if pregnancy is suspected because substance abuse or improper nutrition can lead to embryo damage.

The Fetal Period: Week 9 to Birth

The fetal period is an important one in which organs are now refined (8). This is when the skin becomes developed; the eyebrows and eyelashes grow; and, in the seventh month, the testes in males usually descend into the scrotum. The fetus grows in length dramatically from about 1 inch at 8 weeks to 12 inches at 24 weeks. The weight of the organism increases from 1 ounce at 12 weeks to 3 pounds at 28 weeks (1). The refinement and growth during this time frame becomes very important.

During this stage, the fetus becomes responsive to stimuli. After 10 weeks, the fetus flexes if any part of its body parts is touched. At about 18 weeks, the response given to body part stimulation becomes very specific. For example, touching the foot will produce a leg withdrawal at this time. At 7 months of age, the fetus may suck its thumb or hand. The eyes are now able to open and close because the lids have separated (8).

BIRTH

Normal Birth

The normal duration of gestation is 40 weeks. Infants have a good chance of survival if born in the seventh month and later (9). The fetus moves into a head-down position as it prepares for its journey down the birth canal. (Any posture other than this will cause birth complications and put the child at risk.) As the fetus changes position, the uterus responds by contracting; this process helps move the infant along.

There are three stages of labor. The first stage involves regular contractions that are

TABLE 24.1 Apgar Scores

Criterion	Score		
	0	1	2
Heart rate	Absent	<100	>100
Respiratory effort	Absent	Weak cry	Strong cry
Muscle tone	Limp	Flexion	Active movement
Color	Blue or pale	Body pink, extremities blue	Pink
Reflex irritability	No response	Motion	Cry; grimace and cough or sneeze

15 to 20 minutes apart. They become more frequent and stronger as labor progresses. The second stage is the crowning of the infant's head. The head pushes its way from the cervix into the vagina. The contractions at this stage are much closer together—usually 1 minute apart. The final stage begins when the baby is born. The uterus continues to contract *after* the baby is delivered; this is so the placenta and other membranes can be expunged from the mother.

After the birth, it is common practice to evaluate the condition of the infant. Virginia Apgar created a system by which the baby can be assessed shortly after birth. The Apgar score is determined by rating the muscle tone, heart rate, reflexes, respiration, and color, each on a scale of 0 to 2. The Apgar scores are routinely assessed at 1 minute and at 5 minutes after birth (Table 24.1) (10). If an infant receives a score of 7 at the 5-minute scoring, the infant is considered to not be at risk. Lower scores usually indicate immediate medical attention is needed. Most infants score 7 or higher (11), with the maximal score being 10.

Average birth weight is 7.5 lb (~3400 g), and the average length is 18 in (45.7 cm). The average newborn's skull has become distorted after childbirth. The infant is usually bald, except possible thin hair in areas such as the neck, ears, and back. The infant's breathing pattern is sporadic and filled with a fluidlike sound (9). Most newborns are unable to physically regulate body temperature because sweat glands are not developed nor is the ability to shiver. The newborn can have a striking appearance and is a very delicate entity.

Abnormal Birth

With advances in technology, viability of the fetus in premature births, even premature babies with extremely low birthweights, is becoming increasingly more likely (12). More than half of babies born after just 24 weeks of gestation can survive. Any infant born before 35 weeks is considered premature. Classification of low birthweight (LBW), 2500 to 1500 g (5.5 to 3.3 lb), very low birthweight (VLBW), 1499 to 1000 g (3.4 to 2.2 lb), and extremely low birthweight (ELBW), less than 1000 g (<2.2 lb), often accurately reflects how *at risk* the child is for developmental anomalies. The lower the birthweight, the greater the risk for developmental delays or disabilities in the premature baby (13). If an infant weighs less than 700 g (1.5 lb), it has a very low chance for survival. These infants often have a high incidence of neurologic problems, lung ailments, and other physical problems when they do survive.

Caesarean section deliveries are performed when significant fetal distress is encountered during the delivery process. When a vaginal delivery is not perceived as going well, or if an abnormal heart rate is detected, a caesarean section birth may be elected. No evidence exists which indicates that a caesarean section delivery increases mortality in infants or even damages the nervous system (3). Frequently, for a host of different reasons, the obstetrician will opt for a caesarean section ahead of time and the delivery will be planned for a specific date.

REFLEXES

Infant reflexes disappear as the baby grows older. Most of these built-in reactions should not persist into childhood. Reflexes can be broken down into *survival* reflexes and *nonsurvival* reflexes. An example of a survival reflex is the sucking reflex: When an object is inserted into the child's mouth, the child will begin sucking. This reflex turns into a voluntary one after about 2 months. This is important biologically because if a nipple is presented to the infant, the infant must instinctively begin to feed. Another survival reflex is that of the rooting reflex. If an infant's cheek is lightly stroked, the child will turn its head toward the cheek and open its mouth.

Reflexes may also be present that have no survival value. One such example is the Babinski reflex, in which the infant will fan the toes outward if the foot is stroked near the heel. This reflex should disappear by the age of 1 year. The grasping reflex is also a nonsurvival reflex. The infant will curl the fingers when pressure is placed on its palm. This can weaken by 3 months, but after this point the infant may develop a voluntary grasp (14).

Reflexes are seen as lower brain center activities (15). Because voluntary activities require higher brain center function, the transfer of reflexes to voluntary action may be related to the development of cerebral cortex neurons (15). The control from primitive reflexes to voluntary muscle control is attained through myelinization of the cerebral cortex. (16).

MOTOR DEVELOPMENT

Physical growth is important for normal motor development. Two areas important to motor control in young children are large, gross muscle control and small, or fine, muscle control. For a child to develop motor abilities, it becomes important for muscles to develop. Large muscles develop before small muscles develop.

Infant motor control can be limited by physical development. Physical development should be rapid within the first year (1,2). By 2 months, the reflexes begin to disappear. The baby at this time can move his or her entire body, begin to raise the head while lying on the abdomen, and may begin to hold the head up for a few moments while sitting up.

By 3 months, the primitive reflexes should have disappeared. During this time period, when the infant's reflexes disappear and voluntary control is gained, the baby may not move arms and legs as much. Around this time, the baby can raise the head and can hold it up in the sitting position. When supporting the self on forearms while lying on the abdomen, the infant can coordinate arm and leg movements on both sides. At 3 months, the grasp reflex may also have disappeared. The infant, however, is not yet able to pick things up.

The infant at 5 months is now beginning to roll over from the stomach onto the back. The infant's body is now firm and the infant can raise its head from a lying position. This is the beginning of the time period during which the child can now support its own weight. The child may now start to reach for objects. The grasp at this point is down with the palms and is very imprecise (16).

Between 5 and 8 months, the child will eventually be able to sit without any support. During this time frame, the baby learns how to roll from the back to the stomach. The child will also develop the ability to creep by 7 months of age. The infant now will grasp things with the base of the thumb and the little finger.

From 8 to 10 months, the infant becomes very active. During this time, the baby learns to crawl. This process begins near the 9-month mark and usually in the beginning crawling is done backward. Most infants at this time crawl with contralateral extremities. For example, the left arm and the right leg are in synchrony; however, about one quarter of infants do not have this coordinated skill (11). By 10 months, infants can also stand up on their own while holding onto nearby furniture. The child at this time may also be able to walk a few steps while holding onto furniture (cruising). The hand grip changes as the forefinger becomes a more important part of the grip, which allows for more accuracy when attempting to pick up smaller objects.

At 11 months of age, infants may start to stand on their own and begin to take first steps.

If an adult holds both hands, the infant will start to walk at this age. By 12 months, the infant will walk with one hand being held, and tries to do this autonomously. The infant will be able to lean down from this upright position to pick things up. Some children at this age may even be able to kick a ball. The child at this age will practice the precision of releasing an object (16). The grip at around 1 year may be accurate enough to fit objects into small openings. Infants become very entertained when games are devised to test this ability.

Shortly after a year, infants can walk by themselves. This should normally be in place by the age of 15 months. Around 15 months of age, the infant can kneel and stand up, despite having some moments of unsteady balance. The child should be able to crawl up stairs, and may begin to start walking up stairs. This is the age at which the infant likes to throw objects and learns to be precise when releasing them. Infants at this age can also hold onto a spoon and turn pages in a book. They can build a tower that is two cubes high, and put a block into a hole of a specific shape and size.

Between 15 months and 2 years, the infant begins to climb up and down stairs, especially if a hand is held. This is the time frame in which children can walk backward, begin to jump, and are able to pull objects behind themselves. They will be able to throw a ball more efficiently as well. Children begin to eat by themselves at this age, being able to manipulate a spoon and hold a cup with two hands. The child may begin to scribble on paper, but does not attempt to "make" anything.

At 2 years of age, the infant will now walk up and down steps unaided; both feet, however, will be put on each step. The child will be able to run faster and in circles, and will be able to kick a ball, jump, and bend over to pick things up. The child will have the ability to open and shut doors. They will be able to dress themselves to a limited capacity, and put on their shoes. The child at 2 years of age can build a tower of 1-in wooden cubes up to seven blocks high (16).

At 3 years of age, the child begins to climb stairs like an adult. Jumping skills become better because the child can do it with one leg. The child now walks like an adult with contralateral arm and leg moving together. The child now has fine motor abilities sufficient to correctly manipulate zippers and buttons. Shoes can be put on properly and, between 3 and 4 years of age, the child should be able to tie shoelaces. At 3 years of age, the child should be able to draw a circle and build a tower as high as 10 blocks (16).

Children continue to refine motor skills after 3 years of age. If an appropriate foundation is developed in these motor tasks, higher-level activities may be possible. By the time the child begins school, the child should have fine motor control sufficient to manipulate a pencil and paper for drawing and coloring tasks. Most children have unconsciously chosen a dominant hand by the age of 2 years (7).

By 5 years of age, a child should be able to copy a circle, cross, square, and triangle. Between ages 3 and 6 years, a mature pencil grip will develop in most children (17).

Individual motor skills start to vary after the age of 6. Some children will have an ability to play instruments and others will not. Some will have excellent abilities during sports activities. General trends become less applicable after 6 years because individuals vary in the refinement of motor skills.

COGNITIVE DEVELOPMENT

Thinking skills that become common to all normal infants and how children acquire knowledge to understand the world is the study of cognitive abilities (18). Cognitive development progresses in an orderly and predictable manner. The child must be an active participant in his or her own cognitive development. Children learn *causality* early on—meaning understanding that an action can produce an effect. Infants learn that doing one thing may allow them to do another (or an understanding of means and ends). Children's cognitive abilities have limitations as well. Infants begin life and learn through their own actions primarily, or experience, not by thinking about them. This limitation changes with time, but early on infant cognitive ability has limitations. These themes remain constant in the development of cognitive abilities. Piaget's perspective has helped create a framework that can be used to understand concepts in this area of development.

Piaget's theory uses stages to describe development in children. His theories are based on the idea that children will pass through these stages in order. Indeed, the child *must* pass through them in order, and each stage prepares the child for the next. An important concept of his theory is that the *timing* is not as important as the *sequence*. Piaget developed four stages: sensorimotor, preoperational, concrete operational, and the formal operational period (19).

Sensorimotor Period

The first of these periods, the sensorimotor period, lasts from birth until about 2 years of age. These years are shaped by immediate experiences. That is, the child's thinking is limited to direct actions or experiences. Piaget subdivided this period into six specific stages.

Stage one of the sensorimotor period takes place within the first month. The infant's capabilities are limited to the reflexes, which are genetically programmed. Piaget felt that during this time frame no new behavior emerges. At this point, children do not define themselves as something different from other objects.

The second stage of the sensorimotor period involves a circular reaction. A *circular reaction* is when a behavior produces an event, initially by chance, and is then repeated. An example of this phenomenon is when one pushes on the eye to create diplopia, then repeatedly does this because it may be interesting initially. This is defined as a *primary circular reaction* because it involves one's own body. Piaget felt that thumb sucking is also an example of this. As a child moves hands and arms randomly, the thumb comes in contact with the mouth. The young baby, according to Piaget, will pull the thumb out and attempt to repeat the initial action (19). This stage usually lasts from 1 to 4 months. The child during this stage displays curiosity and reaches the end of this stage when new behaviors result from intrinsic motivation.

Piaget's third stage of the sensorimotor period involves *secondary circular reactions*. These relate to the effects behavior has on external objects. The baby will repeat behavior to understand the consequences. A pairing of a behavior and a sensory consequence often occurs. An example of this is when an infant throws a cup or utensil on the floor repeatedly—much to the dismay of the parents. Piaget felt this stage took place approximately from 4 until 10 months.

The fourth stage is called the *coordination of schemes*. This stage involves goal-oriented be-

havior and is seen in children from the age of 10 months until about 1 year. The child will do something in order to accomplish something else. This becomes an important stage, as the child now develops the ability to anticipate future consequences. The child also begins to learn to imitate actions, including ones that the child seldom will perform spontaneously.

Tertiary circular reactions, or reactions that involve experimentation, are encountered in the fifth stage of Piaget's sensorimotor period. Now, the infant discovers cause-and-effect relationships. Infants at this stage actively explore new objects to try to discover ways to use these objects. This stage will last until approximately 18 months of age.

The final stage of the period involves the beginnings of symbolic thought. Usually lasting until 2 years of age, this stage is a significant transitional period. One major theme described by Piaget in this stage is the concept of *delayed imitation.* The child at this point will imitate an action without a direct model. The child also develops the concept of symbolic relationships, leading to the ability to think about problem solving without physically doing anything. A *memory* is created to be contemplated and stored for a later time.

Preoperational Stage

The second period defined by Piaget lasts from 2 until about 7 years of age. The concept of creating symbols for things becomes consistent. At this stage, the child learns that language can be used to represent something. During this period, the child also learns the concepts of time and space. The child now will learn the concept of conservation. *Conservation* is the understanding that amount remains the same despite a spatial transformation. This becomes important when a child learns mathematics. An experiment that Piaget used to demonstrate conservation involved the concept of conservation of liquid volume and is known as the *beaker experiments.* Piaget presented children two glasses that were equal in size and shape and filled them with equal amounts of water. When the children were asked which glass had more water, most of them stated that they had the same amount. He then poured the water from one of the glasses into a third glass that was shaped shorter and wider than the original two glasses. He did this *while* the child watched. Piaget then asked the children which glass had more water, the original one or the shorter and wider one. The children in the preoperations period of development, or transitional period, often took long periods of time to answer and, depending on where they were within the period, answered correctly if they acquired the understanding or incorrectly if they had not.

Concrete Operations

Piaget's stage-three children have developed a mature concept of conservation. When presented with the beaker experiment, these children answered correctly with confidence. This stage begins around the age of 7 and continues to about 11 years of age. The idea of concrete operations also allows for children to understand reversibility, or how the effects of a transformation can be undone. In the example of the water in the glass, the child may simply just pour the water back into the original glass. Previous to this stage, children view the world from a very ego-centered perspective. Piaget felt that during this period the child learns the concept of decentering. Children will gain an ability to see things from a different perspective than their own.

Formal Operations

In adolescent years, children begin to develop an ability to use abstract reasoning and formal logic, according to Piaget. He called this the *formal operations stage*. School children can use logic when relating to concrete things; however, adolescents can think about hypothetical situations. The adolescent can understand various outcomes and consequences to actions.

Piaget felt that cognition develops when an *adaptation* can be made—when a behavior is modified to meet challenges. This allows children to pass through these stages.

Piaget's theories on cognitive development have not gone unchallenged. Some critics believe that skills develop at earlier ages than those Piaget reported or that some children develop in a different order than his stages (20). Nonetheless, Piaget created a framework in which cognitive development can be understood, and his influence in this area still has yet to be matched by any other researcher.

EMOTIONAL AND SOCIAL DEVELOPMENT

The development of emotion is usually first seen in the creation of a relationship with caregivers, usually parents. These bonds help create the first social interactions and set the groundwork for emotional stability. The infant must develop a social partnership with caregivers and be engaged by voices and faces. As the infant ages, the infant must react to others and then must learn *how* to react to others. A toddler must then learn to acquire the rules and values of society. Socialization becomes important to further build emotional relationships with others and the toddler must learn to become independent from parents as well. After preschool, many years are then spent on developing adultlike abilities. With these abilities, children experience all that is included emotionally with success, failure, and self worth.

Emotional and social development vary in individual children. These differences among children may be caused by differences in environments or differences in each baby's inborn temperament. Some psychologists feel that infants are born with certain social dispositions if raised in a responsive caregiving environment (21,22). Infants have natural responses to caregivers and caregivers need to be responsive to these reactions and provide appropriate stimulation (23). For example, to have any social development, the infant must learn to recognize faces. This process begins to develop around 3 months of age. By the age of 4 to 5 months, infants smile at specific faces and will stop smiling at strangers. During the second half of the first year, the infant begins to develop some sense of self (24). This is when the baby will develop attachments to caregivers.

The development of emotions, or a state of feeling, is seen in infants by 3 months of age. Emotional responses can be immediate and are in response to a meaning or event at the present time (25). An infant will give a variety of emotional responses to new experiences, such as meeting strangers. Infants at this age may show fear, distress, or joy. By the age of 10 months, the infant begins to regulate these patterns. The infant will learn to cope with emotions such as not crying immediately around strangers. Toward the end of the first year, the baby will also begin to signal to caregivers or gesture at them. These infants will create bonds to caregivers with repeated interactions. This attachment will help create a feeling of security with this person when something is seen as a threat. The attachment will be strongest to the person with whom the infant has the most interaction.

Harlow and Harlow studied this sense of attachment in rhesus monkeys (26). In an infamous study, they raised monkeys with two surrogate "mothers." One mother was made of bare wire, yet had a bottle to feed from, and the other was made of terry cloth. The infant monkeys developed an attachment to the cloth mother (not the bare wire surrogates) and, when distressed, the monkeys would run to this one. The study demonstrated that infant monkeys do not develop attachments to mothers simply because they feed them. This thought process may be applied to humans—the idea that humans develop attachments merely because mothers feed them seems unreasonable. Infant attachments become important for future development of the child.

Physical contact becomes important for normal emotional development. Children differ in the amount of contact desired (27). Mistrust patterns can develop during this time. This mistrust can develop from ignoring the crying child, or yelling at the crying infant.

A toddler begins to acquire self-reliance. The child moves toward developing an understanding of the rules and values of society (28). Initially, children are concerned with the responses and expectations of their parents. As children grow, they begin to incorporate these standards into themselves. This process begins before the age of 2, but continues for many years. The demands imposed on children change with time. Children learn to walk as well as develop language and become very exploratory. The child is expected to learn the importance of the word "no." By the age of 5, most children do many things for themselves; they are able to control impulses and have a sense of what is appropriate behavior and what is not.

Two ideas exist about how social development takes place as the child ages. One theory states that the child begins as an impulsive

individual and society will redirect their behaviors. Another theory is that the child wants to comply with parents' wishes and social values are innate (27).

The toddler also develops new emotions and changes take place in relation to existing emotions. Toddlers begin to control emotions better. Separation anxiety still persists, but the toddler begins to control the feelings associated with this. Things that were disorganizing or immobilizing before (e.g., a loud noise) are now handled more appropriately. The child at this age begins to differentiate self and others. This awareness allows the child to express more to his or her caregivers. Defiance may be noted at this age as the child begins to demonstrate independent will. Shame emerges during this age range (29). Other emotions involved with an idea of self develop also. These emotions have been called *secondary emotions*, because they are separate from the primary emotions of fear, anger, surprise, and joy (30).

All of these changes that take place emotionally and socially become important for development. Personality development is rooted in this time period, and individual children make adaptations now. The child responds differently than previously and differently from other children (31). These differences are based on the self-reliance of toddlers.

During early childhood, peer relationships develop, self-control continues to develop, children begin to explore adult roles, and a greater independence is exhibited. In early childhood, the child's work begins to expand, especially with school attendance. Children learn the roles of sexes at this age and gender-role development becomes an integral part of social and emotional development during early childhood.

Peer interaction becomes important to young children. They begin to develop friendships at this age based on their own efforts (32). Children begin to act differently around those they view as friends and those they do not view as friends. Children begin to judge each other and reject other children (33). These interactions with other peers become important for learning. Children at this age learn the concept of fairness, cooperation, and reciprocity (34).

Emotional changes during the early school years are dependent on and interrelated to cognitive and social ones. The child learns to understand his or her emotions during this time period and begins to evaluate how he or she feels. After the age of 4, children learn to understand that emotional influences are not only things that happen, but also involve expectations (35). At this age, children continue to learn to regulate emotional expression. Frustration is tolerated increasingly during this time frame. The child learns to control frustration in relation to a delay in gratification. At this age, the flexibility to control impulses also increases. The concept of internal standards of right and wrong develop. The child will comply with a parent's wishes even if the parent is not present (36). Along with this concept, the child begins to feel genuine guilt and pride. This is different than the shame experienced earlier. As a child becomes independent, there arises an emotional conflict in reliance on others. The child still needs help from adults when doing tasks, but strives for independence. The feelings of self-worth evolve at this point and confidence in ability is increased.

Aggression is developed during early toddlerhood and continues to change as the child grows. The child learns concepts of self that influence the way a young child interprets how peers should act. During preschool years, one child will show aggression for no other reason than to cause distress in another (37). During preschool and early elementary school, aggression is used as a way of getting something (37).

Empathy toward others and altruistic behaviors are noted initially during early childhood (38). These develop as the child learns to understand the perspective of others and also has the capacity to respond to the needs of others. The development of these concepts seems to follow the same course as aggression (38).

Identity conflict becomes important at this age. The child explores questions of sexual identity and the importance of it. The child begins to explore the interaction with others and how they are important. These feelings will persist throughout childhood, but become important when the child is young.

Critical social and emotional development takes place from the ages of 6 to 12 years. The child begins to understand the feelings associated with success. In the middle of this age range, the child develops a sense of competence and an ability to initiate activities. Children expand their social world and loyal friendships are built on trust and support. Groups are formed and peer relationships become integral to development (39).

Social interaction becomes a significant aspect in the lives of children. Peer groups become very important and almost rival family in importance (40) as the child learns the equality of peers. From 6 to 12, the child learns to form loyal friendships. The complexity of a friendship is understood by the time the child becomes a teenager (40). Concepts of trust and loyalty begin to form in relation to nonfamily members. Peer group formation and networks become important. The sense of being part of a group becomes understood at this age. A sense of equality among these groups begins. Children learn to share with each other, and among friends. (40). Usually, children maintain gender boundaries before high school is reached (41). Elementary school children interact with members of the opposite sex, but this usually does not come in the context of peer groups.

Emotional development at this age is still undergoing rapid growth. Guilt and pride as concepts continue to become more understood in these children (42). Emotional experiences are dependent on many things, including expectations. Children begin to mask emotions during this age range as well. A concept of self in relationship to internal emotions becomes well developed. Children also have an understanding of who they are in relationship to people around them. These two concepts of self help form emotional stability in the normal child.

Normal social and emotional development in the child can vary in individual children. As with most areas of child development, however, normal trends are observed. As the child goes from infancy to adolescence, concepts of self, independence, and friendship change dramatically. Concepts developed early help build a foundation for normal development later on. Many reasons may exist why a child does not develop according to a normal emotional pattern. Depression in children is the most common cause of abnormal emotional development and can have a significant impact later in adulthood (43). The relationship between cognitive, social, and emotional development becomes more important as the child ages. Normal developmental patterns are important in all of these areas if a child is to develop self-esteem.

LANGUAGE DEVELOPMENT

Language is defined as communication of thoughts and feelings through a system of arbitrary signals, such as voice, gestures, and written symbols. Language is not necessarily defined as simply speech. For example, when a parrot imitates a word, it is just mimicking the sound, in the absence of language. Normal language acquisition in humans, however, does depend on the ability to hear. Language can be broken down into five major subsystems: phonology, semantics, morphology, syntax, and pragmatics. *Phonology* is the sounds used in language. *Semantics* are the meaning of the words used. *Morphology* is the system in which one combines small language units called *morphemes*. *Syntax* is how words are organized into sentences (44). The rules that govern the use of the language are *pragmatics* (45). For one to fully grasp a language, it becomes important to learn all five subsystems.

This process of language acquisition is a development of two processes: reception and expression. As an infant attends to sounds, the infant learns to recognize them (7). This process of hearing different sounds has been shown to be developed even shortly after birth (46).

At around 4 months, infants pay obvious attention to nearby sounds that have meaning to them (e.g., familiar voices) (7). At this age, the child attempts to vocalize when involved in a face-to-face interaction. The child is noted at this age to babble and will cry loudly when hungry or bothered. This early level of communication becomes very important when the child is hungry or thirsty. Parents often can recognize the different crying sounds of their own infant so that the needs of their child can be met expediently (47).

At 7 months, the child is able to respond to emotional overtones in the speech patterns of known adults. The baby still babbles but does so in long strings of syllables while varying pitch. The infant will combine vowel sounds

with single consonant sounds during this time period. Now, when in a face-to-face setting, the infant will try to imitate the adult's playful vocalizations (48).

At a little over a year, infants will recognize their own names and those of family members. They are able to also recognize words for common activities. It is important for the child to understand language at this time. The ability to produce language is preceded by the process of understanding (49). Around this time, single words are used correctly and consistently. The words at this point are not imitative, but occur spontaneously, but only in a situational context.

At 21 months, the child is correctly responding to spoken communications. The vocabulary has now potentially reached the 50-word mark (7). Usually, children begin to combine two words or three to form a meaningful sentence. The sentences will contain a pivot word, which does not have to be a noun, but with which other words can be associated (50).

The 3-year-old child begins to understand the meanings of words and variations in semantics. The vocabulary of these children is enlarging very rapidly. Sentences can be formed of three to five words. At the age of 3, the child has nearly 900 words in his or her vocabulary (51).

Around the age of 5, the child is able to understand the language for most situations, if the vocabulary used is that which reflects the child's experiences. Speech becomes intelligible even to strangers. The child can narrate long stories, but may have some articulation problems with such letters or combinations as s, f, and th (7). The child's vocabulary at this point is about 1500 words (51).

Developmentally normal 7-year-old children have a complete understanding of home, school, and social situations. Spoken language is fluent and elaborate conversations can be had. If, at this age, the child does not have the ability to read or write, that child will develop a strong interest in learning to do so.

Language acquisition and development are closely linked to cognitive development. Various theories explain how the child acquires the necessary skills to build a usable vocabulary in spoken or written form (49). Although a universal understanding regarding the acquisition of language may not exist, several milestones should be monitored in language development.

CONCLUSION

Normal child development encompasses many areas. It becomes important for all practitioners in any profession to understand the developmental tract. The interaction between cognition, emotion, social development, and language skills is relatively complex. The inhibition or delay in just one of these areas might have a significant impact on the others. An understanding of what is to be expected and what deviates from this can help practitioners appropriately manage their young patients.

REFERENCES

1. Glick J. Werner's relevance for contemporary developmental psychology. *Dev Psychol* 1992;28:558–565.
2. Kitchener RF. Developmental explanations. *Review of Metaphysics* 1983;36: 791–817.
3. Sroufe AL, Cooper RG, DeHart GB. The nature of development. In: *Child Development: Its Nature and Course.* New York: McGraw Hill, 1996, 3rd Edition, pp 4–34.
4. Gesell A, Amatruda CS. *Developmental Diagnosis: Normal and Abnormal Child Development.* New York: Hoeber, 1941.
5. Kail R. Development of processing speed in childhood and adolescence. In: Reese W, ed. *Advances in Child Development and Behavior.* San Diego: Academic Press; 1991:58–64.
6. Siegler RS. *Children's Thinking: What Develops?* Lawrence Erlbaum Associates, Inc., Hillsdale, New Jersey, 2nd Edition, 1978; pp.15–16.
7. Holt KS. *Child Development: Diagnosis and Assessment.* London: Butterworth-Heinemann, 1991.
8. Larsen WJ. *Human Embryology.* New York: Churchill Livingstone, 1993.
9. Oski FA, DeAngelis CD, Feigin RD, et al., eds. *Principles and Practice of Pediatrics,* 2nd ed. Philadelphia: JB Lippincott, 1994.
10. Apgar V, Holaday DA, James LS, et al. Evaluation of the newborn infant—second report. *J AMA* 1958;168:1985–1988.
11. Cratty BJ. *Perceptual and Motor Development in Infants and Children.* Englewood Cliffs, NJ: Prentice Hall, 1979.
12. Lorenz JM. Management decisions in extremely premature infants. *Semin Neonatol* 2003;8:475–482.
13. Gage TB. Classification of births by birth weight and gestational age: an application of the multivariate mixture models. *Ann Hum Biol* 2003;30:589–604.
14. Cliften R, Muir DW, Ashmead DH, et al. Is visually guided reaching in early infancy a myth? *Child Dev* 1993:64;1099–1110.
15. Zelazo PR. The development of walking: new findings and old assumptions. *J Mot Behav* 1983;15:99–137.
16. Gassier J. *A Guide to the Psycho-motor Development of the Child.* New York: Churchill Livingstone, 1984.
17. Schneck CM, Henderson A. Descriptive analysis of the developmental progression of grip position for pencil and crayon control in non-dysfunctional children. *Am J Occup Ther* 1990;44:893–900.
18. Piaget J. *The Construction of Reality in the Child.* New York: Basic Books, 1952.
19. Piaget J. Piaget's theory. In: Mussen PH, ed. *Carmichael's Manual of Child Psychology* New York: Wiley, 1970.
20. Case R. *Intellectual Development: Birth to Adulthood.* New York: Academic Press, 1985.
21. Fogel A. *Developing Through Relationships.* Chicago: University of Chicago Press, 1993.
22. Ainsworth M, Blehar MC, Waters E, et al. *Patterns of Attachment.* Cambridge: Harvard University Press, 1973.
23. Schore AN. *Affect Regulation and the Origin of the Self: The Neurobiology of Emotional Development.* Hillsdale, NJ: Erlbaum, 1994.
24. Emde RN. The infant's relationship experience: development and affective aspects. In: Sameroff A, Emide R, eds. *Relationship Disturbances in Early Childhood.* New York: Basic Books; 1989:33–51.
25. Sroufe LA. *Emotional Development: The Organization of Emotional Life in the Early Years.* New York: Cambridge University Press, 1995.
26. Harlow HF, Harlow MK. Learning to love. *Am Scientist* 1966;54:244–272.
27. Ainsworth M, Bell S, Stayton D. Infant-mother attachment and social development: Socialization as a product of reciprocal responsiveness to signals. In: Richards M, ed. *The Integration of the Child into a Social World.* Cambridge, UK: Cambridge University Press, 1974.
28. Maccoby EE. The role of parents in the socialization of children: an historical overview. *Dev Psychol* 1992;28:1006–10017.
29. Erikson EH. *Childhood and Society,* 2nd ed. New York: Norton, 1963
30. Lewis M. The self in self-conscious emotions. Commentary on Stripek et al. *Monogr Soc Res Child Dev* 1992;57:85–95.
31. Mahler M, Pine R, Bergman A. *The Psychological Birth of the Human Infant.* New York: Basic Books, 1975.
32. Gottman J. How children become friends. *Monogr Soc Res Child Dev* 1983; (3 Serial No 201):43
33. Rubin K, LeMare L, Losllis S. Social withdrawal in childhood: development pathways to peer rejection. In: Asher S, Coie J, eds. *Peer Rejection in Childhood.* 1990. Cambridge, UK: Cambridge University Press; 1990:217–249.
34. Hartup WW. Peer relations. In: Mussen P, Hetherington EM, eds. *Manual of Child Psychology,* 4th ed. New York: Wiley, 1983.
35. Harris PL. The child's understanding of emotion: development change and the family environment. *J Child Psychol Psychiatry* 1994;35:3–28.
36. Kopp CB, Krakow JB, Baughn BE. The antecedents of self-regulation in young handicapped children. In: Perlmutter M, ed. *Minnesota Symposia on Child Psychology.* Hillsdale, NJ: Erlbaum, 1984;17:93–128.
37. Hartup W, Laursen B Conflict and context in peer relations. In: Hart C, ed. *Children on Playgrounds: Research Perspective and Applications.* Ithaca, NY: State University of New York Press, 1993.
38. Zahn-Waxler C, Radke-Yarrow M, Wagner E, et al. Development of concerns for others. *Dev Psychol* 1992;28:126–136.
39. Kestenbaum R, Farber E, Sroufe LA. Individual differences in empathy among preschoolers: concurrent

and predictive validity. In: Eisenberg N, ed. *Empathy and Related Emotional Responses: No 44. New Directions for Child Development.* San Francisco: Jossey-Bass; 1989: 51–56.

40. Hartup W. Social relationships and their developmental significance. *Am Psychol* 1992;44:120–126.
41. Thorne B. Girls and boys together, but mostly apart: gender arrangements in elementary schools. In: Hartup W, Rubin Z, eds. *Relationships and Development.* Hillsdale, NJ: Erlbaum, 1986.
42. Ferguson T, Stegge H, Damhuis I. Children's understanding of guilt and shame. *Child Dev* 1991;62:827–839.
43. Toolan JM. Therapy of depressed and suicidal children. *Am J Psychother* 1978;32:243–251.
44. http://dictionary.reference.com.
45. Vigliocco G, Vinson DP, Lewis W, et al. Representing the meanings of object and action words: the featural and unitary semantic space hypothesis. *Cognit Psychol* 2004;48:422–488.
46. MacFarlane A. What a baby knows. *Human Nature* 1978;32:74–81.
47. Morsback G, Bunting C. Maternal recognition of their neonates cries. *Dev Med Child Neurol* 1979;21:178–185.
48. Saslkind NJ, Ambron SR. *Child Development.* New York: CBS College Publishing, 1987.
49. Cron M. Overview of normal child development. In: Schieman MM, Rouse MW, eds. *Optometric Management of Learning-related Vision Problems.* St. Louis: Mosby, 1994.
50. Braine MDS. The ontogeny of English phrase structure: the first phase. *Language* 1963;39:1–13.
51. Duffy JK, Irwin JV *Speech and Hearing Hurdles.* Columbus, Ohio: School Service, 1951.

25

Visual Concerns in the Child with Special Needs

Barry Kran, Stacy Lyons, and Melissa Suckow

This chapter was written to familiarize the reader with many of the issues related to the care of children who are visually or multiply impaired. This chapter explores the common causes of significant vision impairment and the typically associated medical conditions in children in the United States. It also includes discussions of other professionals involved in the care of this population; adaptations to the examination process; and recommendations, including the functional and educational considerations that are significant for this population.

Estimates indicate that in 2005 of the 73.6 million children from 0 to 17 years of age in the United States, 13.5 million of these children (18.34%) will have some type of vision problem (1,2). The Metropolitan Atlanta Developmental Disabilities Surveillance Program (MADDSP), a 10-year longitudinal study of individuals aged 3 to 10 years, determined that between 1991 and 1993, 68% of the visually impaired individuals also had one or more developmental disability. These disabilities included mental retardation, cerebral palsy, hearing loss, and epilepsy. Furthermore, individuals with more severe levels of vision impairment are more likely to have at least one additional disability (3). Mervis et al. (3) determined visual impairment (VI) etiology and onset during the pre-, peri-, and postnatal periods. They found that prenatal causes accounted for 43% of the children; 38% of which causes were genetic. Perinatal causes were found in 27% of the children and postnatal

causes were rare. Isolated VI was more common prenatally and multiple disabilities were more commonly associated with perinatal and postnatal issues. More severe vision loss was also associated with peri- or postnatal causes (3). The MADDSP survey has estimated the prevalence of vision impairment to be 0.09% in children 3 to 10 years of age (4).

CAUSES OF VISION IMPAIRMENT IN CHILDREN IN THE UNITED STATES

In the United States, the "Babies Count: The National Registry for Children with Visual Impairments, Birth to Three" years was conducted by American Printing House for the Blind, Inc. from January 2000 through March 2004. Data were obtained by vision educators at participating agencies with specialized early intervention programs. Fourteen states reported data during the survey period with data collected on 1533 children. Preliminary data presented by Deborah Hatton and Burt Boyer at the 2004 biennial international conference of the Association for Education and Rehabilitation of the Blind and Visually Impaired revealed the following:

- Most prevalent visual conditions
  - Cortical visual impairment (24%)
  - Retinopathy of prematurity (17%)
  - Optic nerve hypoplasia (9%)
  - Albinism (6%)
  - Retinal disorders (5%)

- Amount of vision
  - 40% legally blind
  - 25% not legally blind
  - 35% unknown
- Most prevalent disabling conditions
  - Syndromes associated with cognitive disabilities (19%)
  - Brain trauma or damage associated with cognitive disabilities (16%)
  - Cerebral palsy (15%)
  - Developmental delay (14%)
  - Deafness or hard of hearing (9%)
- Most prevalent health or medical conditions
  - Orthopedic impairments (23%)
  - Feeding problems (18%)
  - Technology dependent (12%)
  - Seizures (5%)
  - Respiratory problems (5%)

Cortical (Cerebral) Vision Impairment

Cortical visual impairment (CVI) and retinopathy of prematurity (ROP) are examples of vision loss secondary to perinatal factors. Retinal dystrophies and albinism are examples of vision loss associated with heredity. An example of a condition of unknown etiology that has an associated hearing impairment as well as numerous other issues is CHARGE, an acronym that stands for coloboma, heart defects, atresia of the choanae, retarded growth and development, genital and urinary anomalies, and ear abnormalities.

Studies have found CVI along with ROP to be the leading causes of vision impairment in children from developed countries (5). CVI is associated with many causes, including hydrocephalus, cerebral vascular accidents, meningitis or encephalitis, hypoglycemia, seizures, neurodegenerative disorders, and trauma whether accidental or nonaccidental. The most common cause of CVI in children is perinatal hypoxic-ischemia and subsequent blood hypoperfusion of the brain (6). As a result of a loss of oxygen to the brain, various biochemical changes occur that ultimately have deleterious effects within various areas of the brain. Broadly speaking, there are two groups of infants with very different structural changes.

With affected premature infants, magnetic resonance imaging (MRI) reveals changes to the periventricular white matter. Because the corticospinal tracts also run through this area of the brain, spastic diplegia can be involved. Spastic diplegia is the most common neurologic impairment found in this population, affecting approximately 5% to 15% (7). VI is evident in as many as 70% of the premature infants with spastic diplegia (8).

The parts of the brain more commonly affected in term infants, as reported with the use of MRI, are the frontal and parieto-occipital areas. One study found that, in general, premature individuals had poorer vision at initial visit and had less improvement in vision over time compared with term individuals (5). Further, a much higher percentage was seen of premature individuals with strabismus, ocular motor apraxia or gaze palsy, and nystagmus compared with the term population with CVI.

Thus, CVI is a heterogeneous condition associated with other medical issues and, as a result, visual outcomes will not be uniform. Because of the concomitant medical issues, it is not unusual to see variability within an individual over a series of office visits (which mirrors what parents or care givers will note). Individuals with CVI commonly have vision equal to or worse than 20/60 or may be limited to light perception only (5). Eye care practitioners are hesitant to diagnosis CVI early on because it may initially be confused with the less devastating diagnosis of delayed visual maturation. With delayed visual maturation, visual behaviors are approaching normal levels over the first 6 or so months of life. CVI, on the other hand, typically does not show rapidly improving visual skills during this time frame. CVI is diagnosed when a child has poor or no visual response to visual stimuli and yet has normal pupillary reactions and an otherwise normal eye examination. The child's eye movements are usually full, but fixation is not typically maintained. Strabismus, nystagmus, abnormal eye movements, and optic nerve atrophy have been reported to occur in patients with CVI (9). Currently, MRI, along with appropriate serial testing by the eye care provider, provides the basis for the diagnosis (10,11). Multicenter studies that follow children from birth on and include neuroimaging, electrophysiologic testing, such as visually evoked potentials (VEP), as well as a range of visual function tests (e.g., visual acuity, visual field, contrast sensitivity, response to color and motion) are necessary to further elaborate a more precise natural history of this condition.

Behavioral findings associated with CVI can include poor visually guided behaviors, poor fixation, and delayed visual reaction to stimuli. Visual function and visual attention appear to be quite variable. A light source tends to be a high interest target when evaluating a child with CVI (12). Brightly colored, high-contrast toys are also motivational. Children with CVI also tend to respond better to targets that are kinetic rather than stationary. Many children with CVI also tend to use their peripheral vision more effectively than their central vision, appearing as if they are looking away from the target. Therefore, when an object is presented, often times a child with CVI may turn away as they reach for it (6,13).

Some children with CVI seem to show improvement in their visual status. Most children with CVI, however, will not regain normal vision. In a retrospective study by Huo et al. (14), 170 patients with CVI were followed for an average length of 5.9 years. At the onset of the study, the patient was assigned a descriptive level of functioning where level 1 indicated light perception and level 5 was reliable visual acuity not better than 20/50. At the conclusion of the study, 40% of the patients improved by one level of vision, 38% showed no improvement, 14% improved by two levels, 5% improved by three levels, and 1% had improved four levels of vision. 2.1% experienced a decrease in visual functioning. In this study, no correlation was found between the cause of the CVI and prognosis; however, the earlier the child's condition was diagnosed, the greater the improvement of visual functioning (14).

Mechanisms behind this recovery have been hypothesized to be attributed to the neural plasticity that exists in normal infants as a function of visual maturation and to some extent this process still functions in children with CVI (5). The mechanism behind this recovery process needs to be elucidated.

Vision educators have developed a couple of approaches to stimulating the development of vision in young children; however, none have

been rigorously studied. From a visual rehabilitation point of view, studies still need to be done to confirm or elaborate the most effective intervention(s) for CVI. It would be anticipated that the child would be involved in an early intervention program and would be receiving services from vision educators, among others.

Retinopathy of Prematurity

Retinopathy of prematurity (ROP), which is covered in Chapter 13, is a retinal vascular condition that adversely affects the developing retina. If left untreated, it could lead to total blindness because the retina will ultimately detach from the posterior surface of the globe of the eye. Historically, it was termed *retrolental fibroplasia* with the first outbreak occurring in the mid 1940s through the mid 1950s as neonatal care was in its infancy. Incubators at the time used 100% oxygen and it was ultimately determined that reducing the level of oxygen dramatically decreased the prevalence of this condition. As our ability to care for the spectrum of premature infants has improved, this visually threatening condition has increased. It is believed that 5% to 18% of childhood blindness in developed countries is caused by ROP in extremely low birthweight (ELBW) (<1000 g; <2.2 lb) infants (15). Numerous multicenter clinical trials have been conducted to determine levels of risk and standard of care with respect to identification, follow-up, and surgical intervention.

Studies looking at the natural history of the disease show that the earliest sign of ROP appears at approximately 31 to 33 weeks postmenstruation. The disease then progresses over the next 2 to 5 weeks (16). Threshold disease, the risk of attaining an unfavorable outcome, peaks at approximately 37 weeks postmenstruation (17). In the 1980s, the International Classification of Retinopathy of Prematurity was developed describing the diseases severity by stage, location by zones, extent by clock hours of retinal involvement, and the presence of plus disease (dilation and tortuosity of the retinal vasculature at the posterior pole). Plus disease is often a sign of advancing disease (18).

The staging marks the progressive advancement of the retinal disease. Stage 1 is characterized as a demarcation line between vascularized central retina and avascularized peripheral retina. Stage 2 includes an intraretinal ridge between vascularized central retina and peripheral retina. Stage 3 adds a ridge with extraretinal fibrovascular proliferation. In stage 4 is, partial retinal detachment (foveal or nonfoveal) occurs, and in stage 5 is a total retinal detachment.

The area of the retina affected by ROP is divided into three zones. Zone 1 (area centered on the optic disc and extends from the disc to twice the distance between the disc and the macula) is most centrally located, and ROP develops in this zone in those eyes in which the retina is most underdeveloped. Disease in zone 1 is more severe compared with disease limited to zone 2 (a ring, concentric to zone 1, which extends to the edge of the peripheral retina) or zone 3 (the remaining crescent area of the peripheral retina) (18).

Stages 1 and 2 do not usually require treatment, because of spontaneous regression of the disease process. Some infants who have developed stages 3, 4, 5, ROP tend to require treatment. The treatment is usually performed either by laser or cryotherapy. The studies investigating surgical intervention of cryotherapy and laser therapy found both treatments to be safe and efficacious (19,20). Today, however, laser therapy is more commonly used now than cryotherapy because of various advances in both hardware and surgical protocol of infants with stage 3 ROP who require treatment. Most of the infants who require laser or cryotherapy develop threshold disease between 32 and 42 weeks post-conceptual age (PCA).

Timing is one of the most important factors in the successful treatment of ROP, because the disease can advance very quickly and delay in treatment often reduces the chances of success. Stage 4 ROP is characterized by a partial retinal detachment. Treatment modalities consist of cryotherapy or scleral buckle. Stage 5 ROP is characterized by total retinal detachment and is described as a dense white scar behind the lens with the detached retina adherent to the fibrous scar tissue. When the disease is particularly aggressive, an open-sky vitrectomy is necessary in which as much retina as possible is surgically attached with the replacement of the vitreous and removal of the lens. The visual prognosis with these patients is guarded. In some cases, a low level of functional vision will remain. These patients are at a high risk for the development of glaucoma (21). If the treatment is monocular, then protective eyewear is indicated.

Other ocular manifestations that can occur with infants with ROP include moderate to severe myopia, strabismus, cataracts, glaucoma, nystagmus, and corneal problems (22).

Further research is needed to understand the underlying mechanism in order to eradicate this condition. Clinical guidelines ensuring screening protocols that identify at-risk infants for ROP have been instituted. These guidelines recommend two dilated fundus examinations for at-risk infants weighing less than 1500 g (3.3 lb) at birth or born with less than 28 weeks' of gestation in addition to those at-risk infants who weigh less than 1500 to 2000 g (3.3–4.4 lb) at birth (23). Follow-up evaluations and early treatment have made a tremendous difference in reducing blindness secondary to low birthweight. With the survival of extremely premature infants increasing, screening guidelines for these infants may need to be revisited (24). Long-term care and follow-up are necessary because some are still at risk for retinal detachment, vision impairment, strabismus, and high levels of myopia.

Optic Nerve Hypolasia

Bilateral optic nerve hypoplasia (ONH) is more commonly found than unilateral optic nerve hypoplasia. With optic nerve hypoplasia, the discs present very small with the vasculature appearing large relative to the disc. Surrounding the disc is a white circumpapillary ring of sclera also known as a *double ring sign.*

Acuity levels or impact on the visual field based on the size of the disc is very difficult to predict. Vision can range from relatively normal to no light perception. The effect on the visual field may be varied in presentation as well from a generalized defect in both central and peripheral fields to subtle peripheral scotoma. ONH is a stable condition in which visual function does not deteriorate with time.

Weiss and Kelly (25) found that they were able to predict ultimate acuity by developing a formula based on the size of the optic nerve,

VEP, and preferential looking acuity results (25). In some cases, especially when monocular, there is an associated amblyopia requiring treatment (26).

This anomaly is congenital and can be associated with the following ocular findings: extremely poor acuity, sluggish pupillary reactions, nystagmus, and strabismus, in particular, or visual field defect (27,28). No predilection is seen for gender, race, or socioeconomic group (29). Numerous contributory factors exist, including environmental, such as maternal diabetes; maternal alcohol abuse; maternal infection (e.g., cytomegalovirus, syphilis, rubella); maternal use of antiepileptic drugs; and young maternal age (27,30). Although most patients with ONH have no associated systemic abnormalities, ONH can be a factor in clinical syndromes such as septo-optic dysplasia, tumor within the anterior visual system, and significant brain maldevelopment (26,29).

Systemic findings can include associated brain disorders (e.g., an absence of the septum pellucidum), failure to thrive possibly secondary to endocrine issues (e.g., growth hormone deficiency, hypoglycemia, and hypothyroidism) (28).

Depending on the severity of the child's visual impairment or developmental delay, it would be anticipated that the child would benefit from an early intervention program and would be receiving services from an orientation and mobility specialist as well as a teacher of the visually impaired to aid in visual function.

Albinism

Albinism is the most common genetic condition causing VI in the United States. Melanin is a pigment found in skin, hair, and the eyes (31). Defects in approximately 12 genes have been identified as being responsible for the various types of albinism because they relate to the synthesis or stabilization of melanin, integrity of the melanosome membrane, and the development of the melanosome itself (32). Genetic testing is now the accepted method of appropriate identification of the form of albinism rather than the unreliable and inexact hair bulb test. This heterogeneous condition is typically associated with decreased vision, nystag-

mus, decreased contrast sensitivity, photophobia, and foveal hypoplasia, and iris transillumination is the hallmark sign of albinism. Delayed visual maturation is not uncommon. Many infants with albinism may appear to have minimal vision early on but will improve over the first year of life.

Ocular albinism is primarily an X-linked recessive disorder with prevalence among men of 1 of 50,000 (33,34). Men with sex-linked recessive albinism may have slightly lighter skin and hair color than their family members do, but will exhibit a subtle iris transillumination and foveal hypoplasia (34). Many patients exhibit nystagmus, pupillary hippus, photophobia, strabismus, moderate to high degrees of hyperopia, or astigmatism, and abnormal accommodation. Acuity can range between 20/50 and 20/200.

Oculocutaneous albinism (OCA), an autosomal recessive disorder, is caused by defective tyrosinase activity. It is found in 1 of 20,000 people (35). OCA1 is a result of absent or greatly reduced tyrosinase activity, an enzyme involved in the synthesis of melanin. OCA1, the more severe form, is characterized by a complete absence of melanin pigment of the skin, hair, and eyes, whereas OCA2 typically has a better prognosis because pigmentation may develop as the patient ages.

OCA1a is caused by the completely inactive enzyme, and most mutations result in the inability to produce melanin pigment throughout the patient's life. Its gene is located at 11q14–21 (36). OCA1a is the classic tyrosinase-negative form of OCA. A typical individual is born with pinkish-colored skin, white hair, blue-gray irises, and a prominent red reflex. Also, typical are decreased visual acuity in the range of approximately 20/100 to 20/300, photophobia, transillumination, nystagmus, foveal hypoplasia, the misrouting of optic nerve fibers, strabismus and moderate to high degrees of hyperopia or astigmatism (37). With this type of albinism, pigmentation in the hair, skin, and eyes do not change as the patient ages.

OCA1b is characterized by reduced activity of the tyrosinase enzyme. Despite this, however, small levels of pigment can be produced and can accumulate over time. Clinical manifestations usually reveal white skin and hair, and blue eyes at birth. However, pigment may be acquired with time. A patient's hair, for example, may turn to a light or golden blonde, or the skin may acquire a tan as well as freckles. The ocular findings of transillumination and foveal hypoplasia with OCA1b still persist.

Patients with OCA2 may accumulate pigment with age because the tyrosinase gene is normal and the enzyme is present and functional. The gene responsible for OCA2 is on chromosome 15q11.2–q12 (36). Clinical manifestations of these patients may include pigmented hair as well as skin, including pigmented birthmarks. Over time, OCA2 albinos may have an increase in pigmentation in the skin, hair, and eyes. Irides can be blue or become a light brown, with time. The red reflex may decrease as pigment develops. Photophobia and nystagmus are usually less severe. Visual acuity is also impaired.

Corrective lenses, low vision aids, and the involvement of a teacher of the visually impaired, as well as potentially an orientation and mobility specialist, should be recommended. The National Organization for Albinism and Hypopigmentation (NOAH) is an excellent resource for information about albinism as well as resources for support of patients and families.

Charge Association

A condition that represents not only deafblindness, but has several of the common associated medical conditions listed above is CHARGE. It is a condition whose incidence is approximately 1 in 12,000 to 15,000 births (38). No gender or race predilection is found and the cause is unknown. In 1981, Pagon et al. (39) first described this condition based on six clinical characteristics. Most cases of CHARGE syndrome occur sporadically. Differential diagnosis from other chromosomal abnormalities including cat's eye, trisomy 13,22, VACTERL (vertebral, anal, cardiac, tracheal, esophageal, renal, limb), and Joubert syndromes (40).

A definitive diagnosis of CHARGE association has been revised to include at least three major anomalous defects or at least two major and three minor anomalous defects (41). Individuals with CHARGE association, therefore, will have some, but not all of the anomalies described below. Coloboma, heart defects,

retarded growth, and development and ear anomalies have been noted to present in about 80% of diagnosed cases (42).

Coloboma

The major ocular feature in CHARGE association is coloboma with an approximate 80% to 90% penetrance (42,43). Colobomas are usually bilateral, with chorioretinal colobomas the most common and iris colobomas being less common (42).

In normal fetal eyes, during the invagination of the optic vesicle in the embryo, a groove remains open at the inferior portion with the formation the optic cup, permitting the paraxial mesoderm to go through, which later forms the hyaloid system. At 5 weeks, the fissure begins to close centrally, continuing anteriorly and posteriorly. The complete closure of optic fissure occurs at 6 weeks of gestation. When the embryonic fissure does not completely close anteriorly, however, it can leave a small notch on the lid, a missing area of iris (typically inferior nasally), and an incomplete closing of the retina, usually inferior but adjacent to the optic nerve (39). Incomplete closure posteriorly will result in an optic nerve coloboma. Significant visual field loss, typically superior, tends to accompany the coloboma. Patients have reported photophobia. This may result because the exposed sclera reflects too much of the incident light rather than having the normal retinal pigmented epithelium present to absorb the extraneous light. Bilateral or unilateral microphthalmos occurs in 50% of patients. Also present may be optic nerve hypoplasia; unilateral persistent hyperplastic primary vitreous; strabismus; nystagmus, which may be horizontal, vertical, or rotary; ptosis; and cataracts, in association with retinal detachment. Visual maturation can be delayed, but visual function is usually not affected when the macula and optic nerve are not involved (42,44).

Heart Defects

Congenital heart defects reported in patients with CHARGE association are varied. These heart defects have been report to be predominately right-sided (45). The most common defects are atrial and ventricular septal defects, tetralogy of Fallot, patent ductus arteriosus, and pulmonary stenosis (39,40,43,46).

Atresia of the Choane

Atresia of the choane (blocked nasal breathing passages) is typically bilateral. It is caused by membranous or bony obstruction of the posterior nasal choanae. Although it has been included in the diagnostic criterion, its incidence is minimal (40,45,46).

Retardation of Growth and Development

The severity of retarded growth and development varies individually. Neurologic issues (e.g., facial palsy, microcephaly, hyperrefexia, feeding difficulty, and ventriculomegaly) have been reported. Other abnormalities include cleft palates, skeletal abnormalities, tracheoesophageal fistula, and esophageal atresia (45,46).

Genital and Urinary Anomalies

Genital hypoplasia, urinary tract anomalies, or both are present in more than 70% of cases. Delayed maturation of the secondary sexual characteristics is present in both males and females. Micropenis and cryptorchidism (failure of one or both testes to move into the scrotum) are common in male patients and labial hypoplasia in females (45,46).

Ear Abnormalities and Hearing Loss

At least 90% of the patients have external ear anomalies and hearing impairment (43,46). Both the conductive and sensorineural components are reported types of hearing loss. Conductive hearing loss results from both middle ear effusion and ossicular malformations and sensorineural hearing loss from abnormalities of the cochlear or semicircular canals (40,45,46). Obviously, early identification of the relative strengths of vision and hearing are important to determine the appropriate communication systems to implement. Sign is often one component of the communication system (47).

MEDICAL AND EDUCATIONAL TEAMS

Children with special needs are a heterogeneous population with a spectrum of visual and medical issues. Although many aspects of the care of infants, toddlers, and children have been well laid out in this text, additional considerations must be addressed regarding adequate and appropriate care for this more involved population. Many receive pediatric ophthalmologic care at major tertiary care centers, but too often functional aspects of their visual development and needs are not addressed during these medically oriented visits.

Our special needs patients variably rely on their vision for information about their environment. Some children will use their vision differently, depending on the task at hand. Some may use their vision to locate their parent in the room, but may choose to turn off their visual cues when trying to locate a toy held in front of them. Some may use their vision superbly in familiar environments, but may become overwhelmed with new environments and attempt to eliminate visual cues. Others may use their vision when given the proper motivation, but not use visual cues appropriately when working on their own. Because much of this information is typically observed by the classroom teacher or other professionals working with the child more frequently, it is often difficult for an eye doctor to be aware of these particular situations.

Ideally, two teams of individuals are involved in the care of children with visual and other impairments: the medical team and the educational team. Optometrists are often an important bridge between these teams because they attempt to explain the functional vision implications of the vision impairment, provide recommendations for the educational team to explore, and recommend low vision devices and assistive technology, as needed. The members of the medical team might include the following: developmental pediatrician, geneticist, audiologist, neurologist, pediatric ophthalmologist, retinologist, pediatric glaucoma specialist, endocrinologist, cardiologist, gastroenterologist, and an optometrist. The educational team might include the following: psychologist, speech and language specialist and other communication specialists, occupational therapists, physical therapists, teachers of the visually impaired, orientation and mobility specialists, special education teacher, adaptative physical education teacher, and assistive technology professionals. No hard line exists between these teams; some medical institutions have extensive ancillary services and some school systems or early intervention agencies have either a constricted or broader array of professionals associated with them. Although the reader may be familiar with many of these professionals, several require further explanation..

Teachers of the visually impaired (TVI) are university trained, certified teachers who have pursued additional coursework to meet the educational needs of children who are visually impaired to those who are totally blind. TVI may work in a public or private school system or at a school for the blind. It is not uncommon for a TVI to be dually certified in orientation and mobility as well.

Orientation and mobility (O&M) specialists have completed an accredited university program with a master's degree or national certification to teach orientation and mobility. O&M specialists teach the concepts, skills, and techniques necessary for a person with a visual impairment to travel safely and efficiently in any environment under all conditions and situations. O&M specialists work with clients of all ages and may work in public or private schools, state commissions, agencies for the blind or residential rehabilitation agencies, or may privately contract with individual school systems.

Occupational Therapists (OT) are university trained professionals whose education "includes the study of human growth and development with specific emphasis on the social, emotional, and physiological effects of illness and injury" (48). Although active in a variety of settings, OT provide training for preschool and school-aged children with disabilities in the following areas: social skills; self-help skills, including behavior modification for acute sensory stimulation issues; prevocational skills; access to curricular and extracurricular activities; and training of caregivers and others who work with this population.

A *certified low vision therapist* (CLVT) can be a TVI, O&M, rehabilitation therapist, or an OT who works within an interdisciplinary professional relationship with other vision and vision rehabilitation professionals. LVTs are nationally certified and must demonstrate knowledge in functional implications of eye pathologies, in-terpretation of clinical reports, preclinical functional assessments, optics and the visual system, optical devices, human development, therapeutic intervention, psychosocial aspects of visual impairment, and driving. LVT may work in a vision rehabilitation clinic or privately contract with individuals or agencies.

Physical therapists (PT) are university trained professionals whose qualifications are rapidly changing to post–baccalaureate-degree programs. PT pass a national examination and are state licensed. They may receive advanced certification in the following areas: orthopedics, neurology, cardiopulmonary, pediatric, geriatrics, or sports physical therapy. At the school-based settings where we practice, PT help provide therapies that maximize the physical skills of the broad array of multiply handicapped students.

Assistive technologists (AT) are professionals with extensive knowledge of the numerous hardware and software applications available for the entire spectrum of individuals with disabilities. They can be involved in evaluation, training, or both. Some AT work strictly with computer-based technologies (e.g., text to voice, modified interfaces, including modified keyboards, braille interfaces). Others focus on solutions for many other aspects of the individual's life, ranging from mobility options (e.g., modified automobiles, custom wheelchairs, ramps) to electronic vocalization equipment and adaptive switches for individuals whose use of limbs or vision may be impaired. These solutions, however, are rarely found under one roof, which makes it difficult for parents and school systems to determine the best integrated solutions. Sometimes the term *adaptive* is used instead of *assistive*. Often, *adaptive technologists* concentrate on issues of mobility, adaptations to home, school, or office, and other non–computer-based solutions.

The Evaluative Model

An effective method of collecting and synthesizing optometric and educational information is to utilize a transdisciplinary approach during the evaluation. The transdisciplinary approach to ocular examination requires that an optometrist or ophthalmologist, a vision teacher, CLVT, or O&M instructor, and a classroom teacher be present for the examination (49,50). At the very least, the team should include an eye care specialist, the vision educator, and the caregiver. This allows for parts of the functional vision evaluation to be conducted in conjunction with the clinical vision examination. Also, better communication occurs between these specialists, benefiting the child, the parents, and all others involved in care. A unified report will provide more information than the two separate reports would. The TVI may need to spend additional time with the child in the child's normal environments, but should have a better sense of what to look for in each particular instance. The presence of a child's classroom educator or aide can be very valuable to address specific issues that they have. Possible modifications for better visual learning can be demonstrated to the teacher. If the child is already receiving services, then it is important for interested members of the TEAM to attend the examination.

Because it is not always possible to have a TVI, O&M instructor, or classroom teacher present for the examination; it is beneficial to receive and review their reports before the evaluation. This allows the examiner to answer any questions they may have about the child's vision as well as a more complete picture of the child's needs before the onset of the evaluation.

The Modified Clinical Evaluation

The examination should be scheduled during the child's most responsive time of day. A child who is missing a nap for the eye examination will not be as responsive as one who is more awake. If the parents or care giver do not volunteer whether the child is having a "good day" or a "bad day" before the onset of the examination, it should be one of the first questions asked and noted because it can have a direct impact on the quality of the findings from the evaluation. The array of clinical findings for an individual, depending on mood, general alertness, or overall health that day can provide significant insight to the potential variation of visual function of the patient outside of the examination room. Understanding this will be critical when providing recommendations for the parents and educators with respect to print size, complexity of visual space, and so on.

When charting, never note that the patient was uncooperative for a specific test; instead, note that it was unable to be assessed. This is a small but important point in understanding how to relate to the patient and their families. It is not the *patient's* responsibility to cooperate, but rather it is the *doctor's* task to create an effective environment where the patient feels comfortable and safe to cooperate! It is this principle, in fact, that guides the examination process. Furthermore, these observations are crucial to the recommendation section of the report. For example, if the patient was most visual in a quiet and visually simplified environment (with room lights off except for the area of interest), this should be noted along with the data obtained. It should also be used in the recommendation section as evidence for the need to create a visually simplified environment for the child.

To provide an environment conducive to a high level of patient cooperation, neither the doctor (staff) nor the examination room should be cold and medical. Children with special needs often see many doctors and they tend to be quite nervous when they arrive and may shut down if they feel that they are in a sterile medical environment. Doctors should not be in *uniform*. A large examination room with plenty of space for the patient to initially roam is ideal. Having the ability to use that space with adaptations for the particular child is critical for a successful visit.

1. **Background Information**
   Ideally, the following areas should be reviewed before the examination to allow the examiner to prepare appropriately. An information packet is sent to the patient when the appointment is scheduled. This information should be returned to the office ahead of the appointment. Be sure to leave time to look over this information before the examination. Information that can be obtained before the examination includes a medical history, including medical diagnosis, any past visual diagnosis, medications used, mobility of the patient, how the patient currently uses vision, and the major concerns that the parents or guardians hope to have answered.

Knowing the medical and visual diagnosis of the patient in advance allows you to look up any new information in the field, as well as educate yourself on the disease. Importantly, this preparation helps to focus your thoughts for how to set up the examination room as well as to establish a priority list of tests and findings to obtain, which can be modified through additional history and interaction with the patient and those who accompany the patient.

2. **History**

A thorough, goal-oriented case history is essential to a comprehensive ocular examination. If the patient is currently attending school, an educational history is also important. The case history has been covered in Chapter 9; however, be certain to explore sensitivities or allergies to drops or latex (52). Somewhat unique elements under "Educational History" for this population include the following:

- Does the child have an individualized education program or individualized family service plan? (See Appendix.)
- Has the child had a community-based functional vision assessment or a learning media assessment? (See *Collaborating with Vision Educators* in this chapter.)
- What type of communication does the patient currently use (verbal, sign language, communication board, gestures, other)?
- What is the mobility of the patient (walks without assistance, walker, wheelchair, sighted guide, long cane, immobile, other)?
- What is the primary learning media (braille, regular print, enlarged print, tape or auditory, tangible symbols, other)?
- What other professionals are involved in patient care (TVI, rehabilitation teacher, physical therapy, orientation and mobility, occupational therapy, speech or language, other)?
- How much time per week is the child working with each professional?
- What is being done to transition the child from early intervention to preschool programs; high school to future residential, vocational, or post secondary educational settings?

3. **Observation**

Much information can be gathered from simply observing the child, which begins as you observe the patient in the waiting room. Note how the patient interacts with the parents and how the patient seems to respond to others in the area. If there are toys in the waiting area, notice how the child reacts to them, if at all. To develop rapport with the child, it is important to engage some appropriate level of communication with the child. For some, this may be just simple initial eye contact either before or after introducing yourself to the parent or care giver. Others who are quite shy (or extremely nervous) demonstrate by hiding behind their mother as you attempt to shake their hand and they may need a few extra minutes of free play time in the examination room before you begin the examination. Keep in mind that tone of voice, speed of physical movement, and body language can have an impact on rapport throughout the examination.

Once you have greeted the patient, observe how the child enters the examination room. Is the child able to walk on his or her own, with the aid of a cane, walker, and so on? When entering the examination room, note how the child reacts to the new environment. Does the child scan the entire room at once, or does the child simply look at a small section at first? Note how the child adjusts to the new surroundings. Is the child anxious to explore and play with any toys present? Does the child cling to the mother while exploring the room?

4. **Examination Modifications**

Not only is it necessary to modify the environment of the examination room, but it is often necessary to modify the typical examination sequence to obtain as much information as possible before the patient becomes too fatigued or unresponsive. Thus, acuities are often tested with both eyes open before occluding an eye. (Binocular acuity was not used because the incidence of strabismus or functional monocular status is so high, the use of that term would confuse parents and educators.) Attempts to occlude an eye should be made, but if it appears that the patient will simply not tolerate it, try again at another point in the evaluation. The practitioner must constantly weigh the need to acquire a piece of information against the *cost* of it as it relates to maintaining rapport with the patient. Once acuity is obtained, the other essential data should be collected. As time and cooperation allow, less essential (but important) information can be obtained. For children who are tactile defensive, it may be more appropriate to perform all testing that does not require direct contact with the child first. If you begin the examination by invading their space, they may not respond for the duration of the visit. For example, after performing visual acuity with both eyes open, obtain other noninvasive procedures (e/g/ motilities, gross alignment measurement via Hirschberg test, or modified confrontation visual field assessment with both eyes open). Modeling or explaining each technique before performing it is extremely helpful in gaining trust and cooperation from the patient.

Modifications can also be necessary to position the patient comfortably. It is important to remember that individuals with physical handicaps have difficulty controlling their movements and changing positions. Therefore, finding supportive, comfortable positions for them will enhance their ability to adequately use their vision (53). A patient who cannot sit correctly in the examination chair may need other options (51). Typically, a parent holding the child on the lap is an adequate solution. Even this is sometimes not enough to keep children calm or have them visually engaged. Parents can be helpful in providing information about posture and visual engagement. It is not uncommon to find young cerebral palsy (CP) patients to be more engaged visually when in a supine position rather than in the parent's lap. Use whatever position the patient finds comfortable and which keeps the patient most at ease. Bean bag chairs can be extremely useful for children who are unable to sit in the examination chair because it forms to the child's body, thereby providing support and comfort. Bean bag chairs have been used in dentistry to aid in examinations in children with cerebral palsy (54). Additionally, some patients who are quite active, such as those with sensory integration dysfunction, respond well to deep pressure stimulation. A weighted blanket placed on these patients can sometimes result in a dramatic decrease in movement and a significant increase in visual attention and cooperation (55).

Just as lighting is an important aspect of a child's normal environments, it may also need to be modified to help the child attend to different tasks during the examination. For children who are easily distracted, it helps to have lighting focused on the target that you are asking them to look at, keeping the rest of the room dim. This will help keep their focus where you want it. If the child tends to stare at lights, all lights directly above the child should be extinguished.

5. **Visual Acuity**

Choose a visual acuity test and paradigm that is appropriate for the functional level of the patient (Fig. 25.1). For example, if the patient is able to perform matching tasks (with a minimum of two of the four symbols), LEA symbols, Patti Pics, or HOTV may be appropriate tests to utilize. If the child communicates solely by gestures, however, resolution acuity with a forced-choice preferential looking (FPL) technique will be a better method. Knowledge of the patients' developmental age may help with this decision (51). Specific visual acuity techniques were discussed in Chapter 10.

It is important to remember that response time is often slower in children with special needs than in the general population. Often, they will know what they see, but need extra time to process it into an ocular motor, verbal, or tactile response.

If the patient is high functioning, monocular visual acuities are attempted

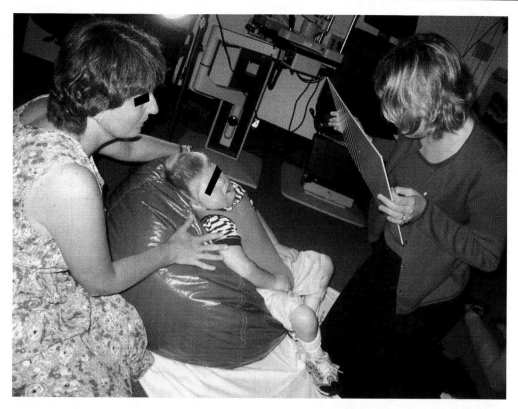

FIGURE 25.1. Alternate positioning; Teller acuity testing—bean bag chair. Based on feedback from his teachers, this patient needed to be positioned in this manner to provide the best posture and comfort to engage him visually.

first. If there is an issue of tactile defensiveness, or a concern that the child may tire quickly during the examination, initially opt to assess acuities with both eyes open (51). A patch or occluding glasses can be tried later in the examination, once the child is more comfortable with the examiner. Be creative with methods used for occlusion in tactile defensive children. For example, a child's hood (from a winter coat), favorite stuffed toy, or blanket may be the most acceptable occluder. Many patients are aware of which is the better-seeing eye and can be masterful in their ability to use it, despite being behind the occluder. Practitioners have favorite stories about this and ours is the case where the young boy needed to have his preferred eye covered by three adhesive patches that were spread out to ensure that the acuity obtained was from the weaker eye.

If the doctor has been unable to assess acuity via FPL techniques, consider other methods of assessing visual acuity such as optokinetic nystagmus (OKN), vestibular-ocular reflex (VOR), and light perception, and light localization (projection). Both the OKN and VOR techniques test the integrity of lower visual pathways. They measure involuntary eye movements in response to movements of the patient's head or of the visual stimulus (56,57). The OKN drum contains black and white stripes and, when rotated, should elicit a slow pursuit movement in the direction of the rotation of the drum followed by a fast saccade in the opposite direction. If this response is not present, however, it does not necessarily indicate that the optokinetic response is absent because appropriate attention and accommodation are necessary for an appropriate response. The VOR is tested by the examiner spinning the child several times in one direction. While spinning, the child should begin to show a nystagmoid response. When the spinning is ceased, the nystagmus should continue for one to two beats, and then stop. Sustained nystagmus is typically a sign of very poor vision or an abnormal optokinetic pathway. Light perception and localization should be tested with a large, bright light source. One caveat is that individuals who are visually impaired may have other senses that are particularly acute. Therefore, be sure that the patient is not responding to the heat generated by the light source or by the sound of the light source being turned on or off. Finally, be sure that the patient is not using echolocation to determine where the light source is in the room by either the sound of the switch or by your voice.

With patients who have complex medical or developmental issues, it is sometimes difficult to know if you have reached their visual acuity threshold versus fatigue or cooperation with the task. One way to differentiate this is to have the patient return in 1 to 3 months for a focused visit to explore acuity. After several unsuccessful visits (or sooner depending upon the doctor's comfort and other medical issues) to determine a standard behavioral (resolution or grating) acuity, however, the practitioner should refer to a center where VEP can be performed (56). Although the results are not an absolute predictor of acuity potential, findings of the patient's visual acuity can serve a few functions. First, it gives a sense of the relative integrity of the central visual pathway. Second, if performed serially, it can track visual development or visual loss over time. If it plateaus or decreases over time, it is a strong negative predictor of visual potential. Finally, change in the VEP usually mirrors change in observed visual behaviors or behavioral acuity measurement. Care should be taken in the interpretation of the VEP results as they can sometimes reflect better visual acuity than the child will show with standard acuity techniques, such as preferential looking (58).

As low vision practitioners are well aware, oftentimes a significant difference is seen between visual function and functional vision. It is important to keep this potential in mind as information is being acquired as well as when providing recommendations. For example, when measuring acuity, note head, eye, and body position and whether it changes as threshold approaches, as well as the last measure that seemed easy for the patient. Aside from formal testing, observation of the patient throughout the examination (and in combination with the findings of others and input from the parents) can help to provide a functional vision profile. Further testing and observation may be necessary by the doctor as well as by the vision educators.

If a child will not perform preferential looking tasks, but is able to locate a Cheerio held 3 feet away, this should be noted in the chart. The size of the object that is viewed can be measured and a rough visual acuity estimate determined. Functional vision, such as that elicited in this example, can be measured with toys, food, individuals, or any object the child is interested in observing. Take care to measure the size of the object as well as the distance at which it was observed. Assessment of functional vision requires assessing vision in different positions in the patient's visual field as well as with varying degrees of contrast. Can the patient find a favorite brown stuffed animal on a brown background, or is more contrast needed for them to find the object? Will the patient be able to locate the stuffed animal if it is presented in different locations in the patient's visual field? One can have parents and educators note these observations and report back at the follow-up visit. For higher functioning children, threshold visual acuity of 20/50 may not correlate with a print size that they can comfortably read for extended periods of time. It is important that the teacher of the visually impaired or classroom teacher know that this acuity is the child's lower limit, and material should be presented at least a few sizes larger than this for optimal performance.

6. **Refraction**

The incidence of refractive error is significantly higher in individuals with fragile X syndrome, Down syndrome, cerebral palsy, hydrocephalus, and other syndromes than it is in the general population (59–66). A thorough refraction, therefore, is necessary to assess the possible need for optical correction. Retinoscopy is performed with a retinoscopy rack, or loose lenses. Loose lenses are less invasive, and are often the better choice. An appropriate distance target that keeps that patient's attention should be used. It is often difficult, however, to get the child to maintain fixation at distance. For this reason, cycloplegic refraction is important. Also, several disabilities (e.g., cerebral palsy and Down syndrome) are associated with fluctuations in accommodation (66–68). For these patients, cycloplegic refractions are always recommended. Autorefractors are often difficult to use in children with special needs. These children have difficulty putting their chin in an autorefractor and maintaining focus on the image in the machine. Handheld autorefractors (e.g., Suresight), which do not come in contact with the child, can be used easily in young children and, therefore, with this population as well (69).

Subjective refraction can be performed with loose lenses or a trial frame, if permitted by the patient. Even if a typical subjective refraction cannot be performed, it is still beneficial to perform a trial of any prospective glasses prescriptions to have some knowledge of the patient's response to them.

7. **Visual Field Testing**

Visual fields are an essential part of the examination of children with special needs. If part of the visual field is missing, adjustments may be made for the mobility and education of the child. A child who has a right hemianopsia needs to learn appropriate scanning skills that would be effective for mobility as well as for numerous tasks such as found in the classroom.

As needs change, additional training may be necessary. Appropriate seating in the classroom would also be necessary to be sure that most of the instructional space is easily accessible to the student. Such necessary adjustments would not be known without adequate visual field testing.

Parents may note that their child bumps into objects; even in familiar environments, and find it puzzling when the assessment of the visual field does not reveal a defect. This is a classic example of the difference between visual function and functional vision. When assessing fields via modified strategies, it is sometimes noted that when the central target is extremely interesting, awareness of the periphery seems to diminish; resulting in a functionally constricted field. Thus, the apparent dichotomy may be explained by the impact of the task rather than an organic defect.

Confrontational visual field testing can easily be done using a small object. Typically, we use a 1.5 inch high contrast target suspended from a stiff wire, which is brought from behind the patient. One individual sits in front of the child to maintain the child's attention while another examiner stands behind the child and presents the target into different visual field positions. The moving object should be kept about 13 inches from the patient (70). Nonverbal children will move their eyes to look at the target when it enters their field of vision. The target should be presented several times in each quadrant. It is essential that the child maintains fixation on the individual in front before the object is presented into the child's visual field. Often, after the first few measurements, the child will search for the toy. This behavior should be noted by the examiner watching the child's eyes, and the area of the field should be retested. For children who do not respond to the above target, a lighted target of approximately the same size is used (71). The room lights are dimmed for this. If a field defect is found with the above method, it is often beneficial to perform more standardized testing.

Automated perimetry is difficult to perform on individuals with multiple handicaps. Even for the mildly impaired, it is sometimes difficult to keep the patient's head *properly positioned* inside the perimetry bowl for an extended period of time. Recent studies of frequency doubling perimetry in children have found that those under the age of 8 to 9 years have many fixation errors on this test, making it unreliable (74,75). Furthermore, 78.6% of normal children aged 4 to 8 years had abnormal visual field results with frequency doubling perimetry. Goldman visual fields are easier to perform because the patient can take breaks as necessary. It also allows for the modification of the number of points the patient is shown. Other perimetry devices with LED lights that the patient does not have to sit in are also effective, although hard to obtain as few companies supply them (72,73).

8. **Pupillary Responses**
Pupillary responses should be recorded (56). Any medications that can affect pupil size or reaction must be addressed as well. We typically use a transilluminator to assess pupils; however, in individuals with extremely reduced acuity, it is sometimes necessary to use a brighter light source. To that end, the binocular indirect ophthalmoscope with the rheostat at maximum is an excellent alternative. Thus, note the response to light and the source used, if atypical. Any nonphysiologic difference in pupil size or afferent pupillary defect requires referral to a neurologist, unless the patient is already being monitored.

9. **Ocular Alignment**
The incidence of strabismus and amblyopia is higher in special needs individuals than in the general population (59–62,65–66). Therefore, care must be taken when examining ocular alignment. Ocular alignment should be measured with the following techniques.
  • Cover test: The cover test is the gold standard for evaluating the presence and size of strabismus and phorias. As with young children, this test can be performed with

a small sticker or toy rather than a letter, as indicated for adults. Take care, however, to make sure that the item of fixation is as small and as close to the child's visual acuity threshold as possible.
  • Hirschberg and Krimsky test: If the patient will not tolerate the occlusion of an eye for the cover test, the Hirschberg technique can be performed to monitor ocular alignment (51). The angle of deviation can then be measured with a prism over the fixing eye (Krimsky test) if the child will allow it.
  • Stereopsis tests: When possible, random dot stereotests (e.g., random dot E or the stereosmile test) should be performed (76,77) (Fig. 25.2). A recent study has shown that the stereosmile test is slightly more sensitive than the randot E test in detecting strabismus, amblyopia, and high refractive error in children ages 3 to 5 years; however, this difference was not statistically significant (78). If the child will not wear the polarized glasses required for the above testing, either the Stereo Optical Random Dot Butterfly, Lang, or the Frisby Stereotest can be used (79–81).

10. **Accommodation**
Accommodative dysfunction is common in individuals with special needs. Approximately 42% of patients with cerebral palsy have an abnormal accommodative response (67). Occasionally, the accommodative response in individuals with cerebral palsy is completely absent (82). Up to 80% of children with Down syndrome have been shown to have reduced accommodation (68). For these reasons, accommodative function should be evaluated during the examination.

When possible, a variety of tests that measure the patient's accommodative amplitude, facility, and response should be utilized. The amplitude of accommodation is typically measured by the push-up method or the minus lens to blur test. Because of the need for subjective responses, however, this will not be possible for more severely challenged children. Accommodative facility is tested using

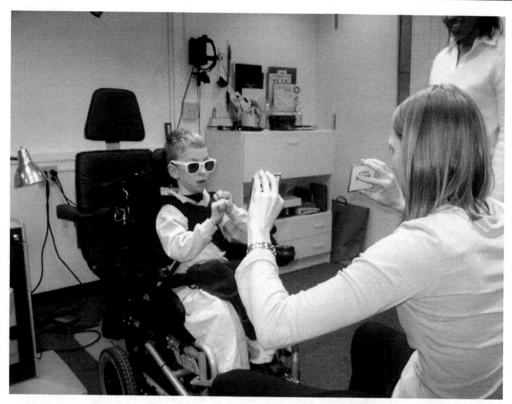

FIGURE 25.2. Random Dot E testing. This boy with cerebral palsy is being asked to locate the card that has the Random Dot Stereogram E rather than just the random dot background alone.

plus and minus lens flippers. This test also requires subjective responses. Dynamic retinoscopy allows measurement of the lag or lead of the accommodative response, with little subjective reply needed and minimal invasion of patient space.

11. **Contrast Sensitivity**

Knowledge of a child's contrast sensitivity can be extremely important. Children with Down syndrome, in particular, have been noted to have decreased contrast sensitivity (83,84). Decreased contrast sensitivity can influence the child during daily activities such as walking up and down stairs and recognizing the faces of caregivers (51). Commercially available contrast sensitivity tests for children include the Hiding Heidi Low Contrast "Face" test, the Visitech CSF gratings, and the Lea low-contrast symbols. Hiding Heidi and Visitech tests are a preferential looking task, whereas the Lea low-contrast symbols require the child to match or name the symbols (85–87).

Functional contrast sensitivity can also be assessed. This information is easier for the parents and educators of the child to translate into daily living tasks. To test functional contrast sensitivity, several objects (e.g., color chips) are presented. One object of each color would be presented on a black background and one on a light or white background. Individuals with poor contrast awareness may fail to locate the dark green chip on the black background or the yellow chip on the light background. Another technique often used is placing Cheerios on a light and dark background. Children with decreased contrast sensitivity will eat all of the Cheerios on the dark background (high contrast), but not notice the cereal located on the lighter (low contrast) background. If the child is found to have decreased functional contrast sensitivity, modifications such as placing food on a contrasting plate and marking edges of stairs with a high contrast color may aid them in daily activities.

12. **Ocular Motility**

Ocular motilities are an essential part of any ocular examination and are covered in detail in Chapter 16. In special populations, however, they can also provide valuable information to parents and educators. For example, a child with nystagmus and a null point may function best when information is presented in a manner that will maximize the utilization of the null posture. A child with a nerve palsy, abduction, or adduction deficit may not be able to adequately scan with their eyes to read information across a page. Therefore, they may need to be taught cues for how to locate the beginning of a paragraph or how to move their head instead of their eyes to find the end of the paragraph. Motilities can be tested with toys, lights, or with a familiar face moving in all necessary positions of gaze (51).

13. **Color Vision**

Assessment of color vision in special populations is important for several reasons. Primarily, many early educational tasks (e.g., matching) require color discrimination (88). Some tasks of self-care (e.g., currency discrimination in some countries) require ability to distinguish colors. Color is often used as part of communication materials. For example, Mayer-Johnson symbols, which can be produced in various sizes, can include numerous colors as well. Thus, for these symbols and other educational materials, visual acuity and color discrimination are important factors that should be understood by the educational team (89). Color discrimination can also be important in certain vocations. An individual who is not able to distinguish red and green would be less likely to be trained for a vocation where sorting objects by color is necessary.

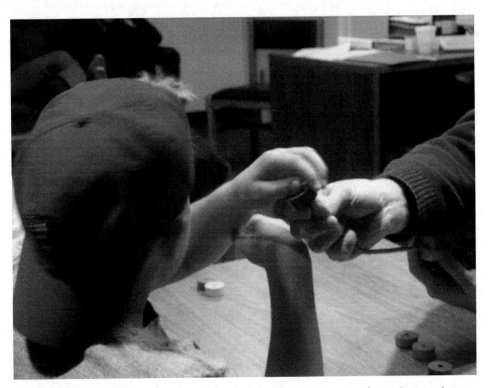

FIGURE 25.3. Caterpillar test. This game, which has three discs each of six colors can be used to assess color awareness, hand–eye coordination in different positions of gaze, scanning skills, and peripheral awareness. Various levels of complexity can be used, depending on the skill level of the patient. (See color well.)

Many of the commercially available color vision tests, including the Ishihara, may be difficult for special needs children to comprehend (90). Often, they are unable to discriminate the numbers on the plate, and have difficulty tracing the required lines. The Waggoner Color Vision Testing Made Easy test, however, appears to be easily understood by this population. Typically, we ask that the child to locate the circle on each page. The Pease-Allen Color test (PACT) preferential looking plates are also used frequently for these children (91).

If this task proves too difficult for the patient, such as having a possible figure-ground issue with the Waggoner, a color matching task can be done. Color matching can also be attempted if the child has a known contrast sensitivity deficit. Color matching typically begins with highly saturated colors. A beads-on-a-string is a technique that is often used (Fig. 25.3). Colored beads approximately 1 inch in diameter are placed on a high contrast background. The beads are placed directly in front of the patient as well as to the left and right of the patient. For color matching, the child is told to locate all beads of a certain color first, and place them on the string. If the child does not know colors, a bead is held up to demonstrate the proper color. This task allows us to observe children's color matching skills, as well as how they scan their visual field. Children who pick up all of the central beads first, and then move their gaze to right or left, are not properly scanning the environment. Once the child locates a bead, the child is asked to place it on the string. Typically, the examiner holds the string, which can be moved into different positions of the child's visual field. This allows us to monitor the alignment of the child in different positions of gaze as well as to assess the use of visually guided versus tactile placement of the bead on the string.

Individuals with decreased contrast sensitivity may be unable to distinguish differences in less saturated colors. If this is a concern for vocational or other

reasons, the Precision PV 16 test can be used. This test is similar to the D15 test, except that the chips are significantly larger and there are pairs of each chip.

14. Ocular Health
The gold standard assessment of ocular health includes the slit lamp for external health, the binocular indirect ophthalmoscope for internal examination under dilation, and Goldman tonometry for intraocular pressures (Fig. 25.4). Two handheld devices useful with this population for assessment of intraocular pressure are the Perkins tonometer and the Tonopen. The Tonopen is typically not used in individuals with spina bifida because of their possible sensitivity to latex (52).

Because ocular health anomalies are common in special populations, dilated

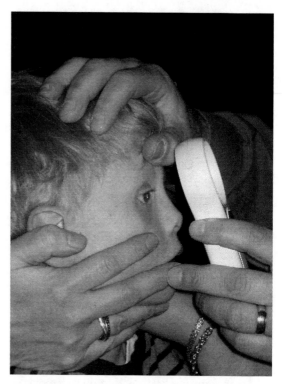

FIGURE 25.4. Alternative means of assessing anterior ocular health. For this young boy with Dubowitz syndrome being gently held by his mother, a 4× illuminated handheld magnifier was used to assess the health of his anterior ocular health. Using people familiar to the patient when examining individuals with disabilities, is often critical for a successful visit.

examination is important. If retinal problems are suspected and the child will not cooperate with a thorough examination, examination under anesthesia may be necessary. Often times this procedure is scheduled at a time when another procedure needs to be performed under anesthesia as well. Although this takes significant lead time and organization, it minimizes the need for multiple anesthesia procedures.

15. **Recommendations**

Once the practitioner has collected and assimilated the information gathered during the examination, the difficult task of synthesizing the findings with other medical and educational information to produce recommendations that are useful for the parent and others involved with the care of the child begins. The practitioner must leave time for this discussion with those who brought the patient. although one attempts to address all of the concerns at the time of the office visit, it is not unusual to think of other recommendations as the report is being prepared. Therefore, it is wise to inform those present that, based on further reflection, the recommendations in the report may differ from the initial impression. If significant changes ensue, you may wish to communicate directly with the caregiver in advance of sending the report.

Reports can be structured as follows: (a) first, the chief concerns are noted, including feedback from the parents, educators, caregivers, and whenever possible, directly from the patient; (b) a comprehensive history, which includes a review of ocular history, medical history, current medications, allergies, and educational or support services; (c) findings; and (d) summary and recommendations.

An expeditious approach to these reports is to attempt to compose them in such a manner that is understandable by other medical professionals, educators, and most importantly, the parents. It is vital to make the connection between the visual system findings and their implications in the classroom, home, or the vocational setting. Because we are not educa-

tors, however, care must be made not to prescribe timeframes for treatments or overstep our bounds in general. One of the most important aspects of the vision examination is follow up of the recommendations. It is imperative, therefore, that the report be sent in a timely manner and that the recommendations are clear and specific so that they are easier for teachers and parents to carry out. The following outline highlights much of what should be contained in this section.

1. Visual System
   - If glasses are prescribed, provide information on how and when they should be used.
   - Many of these children are tactile defensive, especially on their face and head and, therefore, a desensitization program will need to be instituted. This can be coordinated by the vision professional and OT

2. Ocular Health Status
   - Binocular status and accommodative status
   - Visual prognosis (both short and long term)
   - Presence of any color vision or visual field defects
   - If low vision devices are recommended, address the purpose of the device and how or when it should be used. Also include recommendations regarding additional training by vision educators.

3. Medical and Other Referrals
   - If, after several visits, sufficient health or refractive data cannot be obtained, consider referral to a pediatric ophthalmologist who might then need to perform an examination under anesthesia.
   - Other members of the medical team may need to be consulted
   - Follow-up schedule with your office

4. Educational
   - It is important to let educators and physicians know exactly what size targets these children can see. Understand that the acuity found is the child's threshold acuity and that the child will probably be more comfortable with items a few sizes larger

than this. If crowding will be a problem for a child, note this as well.

- Note impact of visual field defect so that parents and educators can adjust accordingly.
- If contrast is an issue for the child, suggest increasing the contrast between background and the object of interest. For example, primary colors should be used when possible. A favorite blue toy might be best presented against a yellow background.
- Note any decrease in tracking ability.
- Include information regarding proper lighting, if appropriate.
- Examples of modifications that may aid these children in school include reduced visual clutter, improved lighting and glare control, use of high contrast materials, large print, possible braille instruction, and reduced use of overheads and chalkboards, unless the student has the information on a paper in front of them.
- Recommendation of a Community Based Functional Vision Assessment with or without a Learning Media Assessment with sensory channel assessment. (Refer to the following discussion.)

Collaborating with Vision Educators

Based on the evaluation, the doctor will recommend that the appropriate vision educator(s) perform an evaluation and initiate services. As eye care providers, we support the need of most children with a visual disability for a Community Based Functional Vision Assessment. This assessment (depending on the age of the child) is typically conducted by the early intervention team or school district, and can be performed by a qualified TVI or an O&M instructor (53,70,92). For this assessment children are observed in their natural environments, at several different times of day, with a variety of visual challenges that they encounter in their daily routine. Recommendations are made to enhance vision or modify tasks for success. Lighting, types of print materials, and availability of low vision aids are all taken into consideration for the functional vision assessment. The child is most often assessed through observation, with

formal testing left for the eye care professionals. If the community-based visual assessment is conducted before the eye examination, visual acuity and a few other basic examination procedures may be performed. This visual assessment should be performed again any time the child's routine changes significantly or the child is introduced to a new environment. For example, if a child with a seizure disorder has a change in medication, after a period of adjustment, a new functional visual assessment should be performed. Seizure medications can make a child more attentive because of less seizure activity, or they can make a child less attentive because of side effects of the medications. Also, if a child is entering preschool, an assessment should be conducted in the new classroom so that modifications can be made for the child as soon as possible.

The teacher of the visually impaired can also conduct a learning media assessment for visually impaired children so that proper learning environments can be prepared for the child (93). The assessment will evaluate the sensory channels by which the child most efficiently learns and try to identify the most appropriate learning strategies for the patient. A learning media assessment includes both general learning media (e.g., pictures or written material) and instructional methods for teaching the child (e.g., demonstrations, prompting, and modeling). Also, appropriate tools for learning to read and write may be assessed. Often the learning media assessment may need to be refocused for children with multiple handicaps. These children may benefit from more functional learning media, which can support community-based instruction.

Vision educators are involved in the delivery of services, either directly or consultatively. Direct services can include teaching appropriate mobility skills with a cane, the implementation of the use of a line guide, or training the student in the use of a low vision device. Consultation can include meeting with the classroom teacher on a regular basis to help with numerous items such as seating, how and where to present information (with a field defect), appropriate visual materials (crowded or not, use of a line guide), and environmental modifications. Beyond these and other practical issues, the vision educator may need to work extensively with the teacher and the patient's classmates to provide for the student's needs in a manner that is inclusive and not disruptive to the classroom. If optical or nonoptical aids are to be used in the classroom—during a class activity, for example—the vision educator either consults with or assists the classroom teacher. Finally, vision educators may pick up additional issues during their evaluation that will warrant a referral to the school PT or OT.

BRAILLE ISSUES

Although eye doctors may be able to conclude, for a specific patient, that vision will not be an effective sense for learning, it is *not* their role to recommend braille. Eye doctors do not have sufficient knowledge of the strengths of the child's other senses to prescribe this option over other possible options. With knowledge of the eye doctor's findings, a qualified teacher of the visually impaired should be consulted for a specialized evaluation.

Even straightforward cases (e.g., an individual with congenital blindness without other obvious issues) should be evaluated. If the individual's tactile skills are poor, then braille may not initially be recommended and an aural approach to learning along with pre-braille activities might be instituted. Further, the decision and timing to switch to braille is often not clear cut and should involve the caregiver and the vision educators. For example, a very young person with Stargardt's disease, who still has good vision, should continue to learn to read visually for as long as possible so that the choice is open to continue to use print as the primary literacy media. As vision declines, the patient may only use print functionally (for price tags, travel, spotting) and develop other forms of educational literacy via audition (books on tape) or tactile means (braille). This decision becomes even more complex with individuals who have a retinal degeneration in the retinitis pigmentosa (RP) family of conditions because of the presence of associated developmental issues, problems with fine motor coordination (Bardet-Biedl syndrome), or hearing (Usher's syndrome). In theses cases, it is clear that a significant loss of peripheral and central vision will have occurred over the childhood years.

Two exceptional vision educators have formalized the concept of a learning media assessment where sensory channels are explored (93). On completion of this evaluation, recommendations are made to the form(s) of literacy (visual, tactile, auditory) that will be most appropriate for learning or functional purposes for the present as well as keeping an eye on future needs. For example, it is relatively common for our young patients to be learning via audition as well as visually and also receiving pre-braille activities to develop the tactile discrimination necessary to learn braille. Given the cognitive level of the child, the transition to learning braille, however, may be more accelerated. (As vision decreases, reading speed, even with aids, will eventually become slower than the reading rate with braille.)

Thus, when the doctor believes that the level of vision may not be sufficient for success in the classroom, recommendation for a learning media assessment should be done that includes a sensory channel analysis to determine the appropriate sensory channels for leaning. This recommendation is crucial because parents often need the advocacy of a doctor to pursue this step. If that analysis shows that the tactile channel is the strongest, braille may be aggressively pursued. If, however, the auditory channel is superior, auditory literacy will be pursued and braille may be introduced over time. Importantly, however, this is a decision made after a thorough evaluation by a teacher of the visually impaired in consultation with the parents and the rest of the educational team.

Some fascinating recent work has looked at the acquisition of braille skills in individuals with simulated low vision and where the changes are occurring in the brain via fMRI. It was shown that the area of the brain with the greatest activity during the learning of braille was the visual cortex (94)! This result needs to be contemplated seriously as a part of this discussion because it could be argued that if a patient still has a good level of acuity and is learning visually, to interpose braille at this point may impede the acquisition of both. Research over the next few years should help to clarify this issue.

OTHER COMMUNICATION SYSTEMS

For some individuals with disabilities, the best forms of communication may be sign language, the use of symbol cards or tangible symbols. For some patients, the development of a communication system centers on allowing expression of choice, assistance with scheduling activities, or otherwise expressing their needs.

- Sign language
- Mayer Johnson Symbols (Fig. 25.5)
  - These are standard symbols that can be made in various sizes and colors or remain in black and white. Often, the determination of appropriate size (e.g., 2″ × 2″), use of color, or area of presentation is the purpose for the visit. Occasionally, some patients have a book with pages filled with small symbols (1″× 1″) and will flip through the organized book to find the appropriate symbol to express

themselves. Many others will have a limited vocabulary centered on activities of daily living (ADL) or choices at mealtime. They may also have symbols for their daily academic or vocational activities.
  - With digital cameras and photo editing software becoming more accessible, it is no longer unusual to see actual pictures being used as part of this system of communication.
  - Some deaf and blind patients use both Mayer Johnson symbols and sign language to communicate.
- Tangible Symbols
  - Some patients are seen for whom the best form of communication is with a limited number of representative three-dimensional tactile symbols that represent an ADL, place, or a choice for the patient.

Input from the caregiver and child, our care, and the efforts of the other members of the

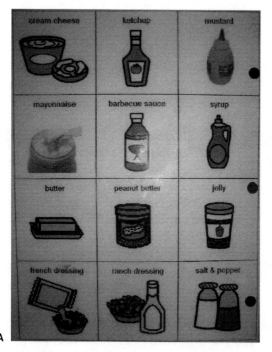

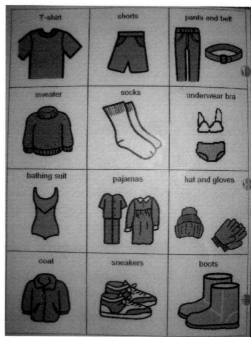

A

B

FIGURE 25.5. Mayer-Johnson symbols. These symbols are often used for expressive communication and for previewing (e.g., a schedule of events for a day). They can be just black and white or have color as shown in the color well. Depending on the student's level of acuity and visual processing, the pictures can be larger and much fewer shown at a given time. Placement within the child's visual field is sometimes critical for awareness.

medical team and educational team that ultimately provides students with the best training and tools available to access the environment and maximize their ability to participate in society.

SUMMARY

A chapter cannot be a comprehensive treatise regarding all of the issues involved in the care of this complex patient population. We have provided highlights of the common causes of vision impairment in American children, an overview of the numerous professionals involved, ideas for examination modification, composition of the report, and the need for collaboration for the optimal care of patients who are visually or multiply impaired. Working with this population is difficult, fascinating, rewarding, and humbling. We hope that you are stimulated to identify the practitioners in your community who are passionate about caring for this population and that some of you will become more actively involved in this area of practice.

APPENDIX

Educational and Accessibility Laws; Implications for Care

The following is an extremely condensed version of the accessibility and education laws that affect individuals with disabilities in public settings. This legislation has established mechanisms for students to receive vision services from birth through age 21. Transition points exist where repeat evaluations are particularly useful and it is at these times, as well as between, that optometric evaluations and recommendations can have a meaningful impact for individuals with visual and other disabilities. These timeframes are intervention programs (birth through 2 years); preschool programs (3–5 years); school age (5–21 years), and the switch from an IFSP (Individualized Family Service Plan) to an IEP (Individualized Educational Plan), which occurs at age 3, are important because, through our reports, we can advocate for necessary services that could become part of the family and educational plan. It is rare to see an

infant or a toddler with a significant visual impairment that is not already in an early intervention program. Sometimes, however, the child is so involved medically that the parents are first addressing the child's visual needs at 1 year of age or beyond. It is in these circumstances that recommending an evaluation by a teacher of the visually impaired and, if necessary, an orientation and mobility specialist to confirm or embellish our observations and recommendations and to aid with device training, specifically addressing recommendations as they pertain to seating and environmental modifications as well as assessing the child's academic, functional, and adaptive goals as they relate to the educational plan (1).

Section 504 *PL 93-112* Rehabilitation Act of 1973 (2,3)
- First "Civil Rights" law for Americans with disabilities.
- Any program that receives federal finding must comply.
  This includes early intervention programs as well as public preschools and K-12 schools.
- Disabilities are broadly defined.
  With respect to vision impairment, individuals who may not qualify under state definition for a broad array of services can get some services under this program.
- School or agency must provide *appropriate* services in the least restrictive environment that are *comparable* to those of the nondisabled.
- Evaluation and plan are provided under this law.
- Plan does *not* have to be written and effort to comply is all that is required.

Education for All Handicapped Children and Individuals with Disabilities Education Act (IDEA) *PL 94-152 (S.6) 1975, PL 99-457 1986, PL 101-476 1990 & reauthorized in 1997 and H.R.1350 2004 (2,3,4,5)*
- Clearly articulates the evaluative, planning, and delivery of educational services to individuals with disabilities.
  Federally funded educational programs must comply.

- Each state has developed its own statutes pursuant to these laws.
- The tenets of IDEA are provided for students in a maximal age range of birth through 21 years.
- Process and documentation to meet a child's needs are broken into two age groups
   - Birth through 2 years: **IFSP** (Individualized Family Service Plan)
      - Recognizes that services may be necessary for family members as well as the disabled child. Such services can include learning to sign or read braille or support services for the parents or siblings to deal with the significant changes in their lives.
- Age 3 through 21 years: **IEP** (Individualized Educational Plan)
- IFSP or IEP
   - IDEA requires a comprehensive evaluation and written treatment plan.
      - Short-term and long-term goals and steps to achieve them are delineated.
      - Plans are developed collaboratively and a process for conflict resolution is outlined.
      - The vision service providers are
- Teachers of the visually impaired
- Orientation and mobility specialists
- Frequency of service delivery is spelled out in the IFSP or IEP.
   - Some services these individuals could provide are
- Evaluative
- Community-based functional vision assessment
   - Observation of child in familiar and unfamiliar environments (e.g., school, home, playground)
- Assessment of vision level, fullness of visual fields, usefulness of vision for learning, mobility
   - Placement of child in classroom as it relates to the myriad of rooms or places in a room where learning may occur
   - Assessment of the child's utilization of aids or spectacles (if any)
   - Learning media assessment (including assessment of learning channels)
- Critical for quantifying utilization of vision and other senses for learning

- A *critical* tool for determining if braille should be taught
   - Direct service
   - Mobility training
   - Device training
   - Scanning training
   - Improvement of visual attention and hand–eye coordination
   - ADL (activities of daily lving) training (either directly or through consultation with other team members)
- Consultative
   - As discussed in Chapter 24, other professionals (e.g., OT, assistive technologist as well as the classroom teacher), as part of the educational team, could be involved with some aspects of vision.
   - Services could include helping the classroom teacher understand the vision issues with the student, how best to present information to the child, seating, other accommodations; when the student should use aids, spectacles, or other devices; providing sensitivity training for the teacher(s) or students who will interact with the student; environmental modifications to the facility (indoors and out); and other factors, as needed.
   - The educational team (along with the parent or guardian) will meet on a regular basis throughout the year to monitor the child's progress with the plan, implement changes as needed, and thoroughly re-evaluate in a prescribed timeframe (every 3 years in Massachusetts) or sooner should significant issues develop
- High stakes testing required via 1997 reauthorization, even for those with disabilities
   - Issues
- Level of mastery of curriculum is beyond the attainment of a significant number of disabled individuals.
- What is essential curriculum for individuals with disabilities? Expanded core curriculum (ECC) developed by the National Agenda for the Education of Children and Youths with Visual Impairments, Including those with Multiple Disabilities as a response to '97 IDEA Reauthorization and is still applicable with NCLB.

ECC covers issues for disabled in the following areas: compensatory or functional academic skills, including communication modes, orientation, and mobility; social interaction, recreation and leisure, and career skills; assistive technology; and visual efficiency skills.

- HR1350 Part C: Infants and Toddlers with Disabilities Sec 632 (4) Early Intervention Services (F) lists 12 qualified personnel to provide services, including those of ophthalmologists and optometrists as well as pediatricians and other physicians

The American with Disabilities Act (ADA) 1990 (2)

- As it relates to individuals with vision impairment

  Access to materials otherwise denied via voice output devices, use of braille on signage, and text enlargement in public settings (e.g., state and federal office buildings, amusement parks, museums, historical sites)

No Child Left Behind Act (NCLB) 2001 (6)

- As it relates to individuals with disabilities

  Reiterates need for high stakes testing in the areas of mathematics and science.

  Students with significant cognitive impairments can utilize specially designed alternative assessments.

  Federal government will increase spending for special education (but decrease total spending for education in general).

  Does not acknowledge that high stakes testing is not appropriate for everyone.

Resources for Information on Children with Visual and Other Impairments

Texts

Cassidy S, Allanson J. *Management of Genetic Syndromes*, 2nd ed. Hoboken, NJ: Wiley & Sons, 2005

Hartnett M, ed. *Pediatric Retina*. Philadelphia: Lippincott Williams & Wilkins, 2005

Holbrook MC, ed. *Children with Visual Impairments: A Parent's Guide*. Bethesda, MD: Woodbine House Inc., 1996.

Johnson GJ, Minassian DC, Weale RA, et al., eds. *The Epidemiology of Eye Disease*, 2nd ed. London: Arnold Publishers, 2003.

Manio DM, ed. *Diagnosis and Management of Special Populations*. St. Louis: Mosby-Yearbook, 1995 (now available through the Optometric Extension Program).

Taylor D, Hoyt C. *Paediatric Ophthalmology and Strabismus*, 3rd ed. Philadelphia: WB Saunders, 2004.

Websites

www.AFB.org: Excellent site for exploring vision educators' resources (texts, journals, position papers) and excellent listing of resources for patients.

www.tsbvi.edu: Excellent search engine and repository of information for patients with visual impairment and their families.

www.e-advisor.us: A collaboration of The Children's Hospital of Boston and the Perkins School for the Blind, this site provides information for doctors, teachers, and parents and includes an e-collaborative of New England organizations that are involved in the care of children with vision impairment.

REFERENCES

1. Federal Interagency Forum on Child and Family Statistics. America's Children in Brief: Key National Indicators of Well-Being, July 2004. Available at http://www.childstats.gov. Link to Table POP1 Child population: Number of children under age 18 in the United States by age, 1950–2002 and projected 2003 through 2020. Available at http://www.childstats.gov/ac2004/tables/pop1.asp. Accessed December 2004.
2. Ferebee A. Childhood Vision: Public Challenges and Opportunities, A policy Brief. The Center for Health and Health Care in Schools. November 2004. Available at http://www.healthinschools.org/sh/visionfinal.pdf. Accessed December 2004
3. Mervis CA, Yeargin-Allsopp M, Winter S, et al. Aetiology of childhood vision impairment, Metropolitan Atlanta, 1991–1993. *Paediatric and Perinatal Epidemiology* 2000;14:70–77.
4. National Center on Birth Defects and Developmental Disabilities. Metropolitan Atlanta Developmental Disabilities Surveillance Program. Available at http://www.cdc.gov/ncbddd/dd/ddsurv.htm.Accessed December 18, 2004.
5. Hoyt CS. Visual function in the brain damaged child. *Eye* 2003;17:369–384.
6. Dutton G, Jacobson L. Cerebral visual impairment in children. *Semin Neonatol* 2001;6:477–485.
7. Weisglas-Kuper N, Baerts W, Fetter W. Minor neurological dysfunction and quality of movement in relation to neonatal cerebral damage and subsequent development. *Dev Med Child Neurol* 1994;36:727–735.
8. Pinto-Martin JA, Dobson V, Cnaan A, et al. Vision outcome at 2 years in a low birth weight population. *Pediatr Neurol* 1996;14:281–287.

9. Afshari MA, Afshari NA, Fulton AB. Cortical visual impairment in infants and children. *Int Ophthalmol Clin* 2001;41:159–169.

10. Good WV, Jan JE, DeSa L, et al. Cortical visual impairment in children. *Surv Ophthalmol* 1994;38:351–361.

11. Good WV, Jan JE, Burden SK, et al. Recent advances in cortical visual impairment. *Dev Med Child Neurol* 2001; 43:56–60.

12. Jan JE, Gronveld M, Sykanda AM. Light-gazing by visually impaired children. *Dev Med Child Neurol* 1990;32:755.

13. Baker-Nobles L, Rutherford A. Understanding cortical visual impairment in children. *Am J Occup Ther* 1995;49:899–903.

14. Huo R, Burden SK, Hoyt CS, et al. Chronic cortical visual impairment in children: aetiology, prognosis, and associated neurological deficits. *Br J Ophthalmol* 1999;83:670–675.

15. Gilbert C, Rahi JS, Quinn GE. Visual impairment and blindness in children. In: Johnson GC, Minassian DC, Weale RA, et al., eds. *The Epidemiology of Eye Disease*, 2nd ed. London: Arnold Publishers; 2003:275.

16. Cryotherapy for Retinopathy of Prematurity Cooperative Group. Incidence and early course of retinopathy of prematurity. *Ophthalmology* 1991;98:1628–1640.

17. Gilbert C, Rahi JS, Quinn GE. Visual impairment and blindness in children. In: Johnson GC, Minassian DC, Weale RA, et al., eds. *The Epidemiology of Eye Disease*. 2nd ed. London: Arnold Publishers; 2003:276.

18. The Committee for the Classification of Retinopathy of Prematurity: An international classification of retinopathy of prematurity. *Arch Ophthalmol* 1984;102:1130–1134.

19. Cryotherapy for Retinopathy of Prematurity Cooperative Group. Multicenter trial of cryotherapy for retinopathy of prematurity. *Arch Ophthalmol* 1989;106: 471–479.

20. Cryotherapy for Retinopathy of Prematurity Cooperative Group. Multicenter trial of cryotherapy for retinopathy of prematurity: three-month outcome. *Arch Ophthalmol* 1990;108:195–204.

21. Quinn GE, Dobson V, Barr CC et al. Visual acuity of eyes alter vitrectomy for ROP: follow-up at 5.5 years. *Ophthalmology* 1996;103:595–600.

22. Robinson R, O'Keefe M. Follow-up study on premature infants with and without retinopathy of prematurity. *Br J Ophthalmol* 1993;77:91–94.

23. A joint statement of the American Academy of Pediatrics, the American Association for Pediatric Ophthalmology and Strabismus, and the American Academy of Ophthalmology Screening examination of premature infants for retinopathy of prematurity. *Pediatrics* 1997;100:273–274.

24. Subhani M, Combs A, Weber P, et al. Screening guidelines for retinopathy of prematurity: the need for revision in extremely low birth weight infants. *Pediatrics* 2001;107:656–659.

25. Weiss AH, Kelly JP. Acuity, ophthalmoscopy, and visually evoked potentials in the prediction of visual outcome in infants with bilateral optic nerve hypoplasia. *J AAPOS* 2003;7:108–115.

26. Lim SA, Siatkowski RM; Pediatric Neuro-Ophthalmology. *Curr Opin Ophthalmol* 2004;15: 437–43.

27. Marsh-Tootle WL, Alexander LJ. Congenital optic nerve hypoplasia. *Optom Vis Sci* 1994;71:174–181.

28. Taylor D, Stout A. Optic nerve: congenital abnormalities. In: Taylor D, ed. *Paediatric Ophthalmology*, 2nd ed. Oxford: Blackwell Science Ltd; 1997:660–700.

29. Tait PE. Optic nerve hypoplasia: a review of the literature. *Journal of Vision Impairment and Blindness* 1989;83: 207–211.

30. Tornqvist K, Ericsson A, Kallen B. Optic nerve hypoplasia. *Acta Ophthalmol Scand* 2002;80:300–304.

31. Young TL. Ophthalmic genetics/inherited eye disease. *Curr Opin Ophthalmol* 2003;14:296–303.

32. Marble M. Albinism, lysosomal storage diseases and other metabolic conditions. In: Hartnett ME, ed. *Pediatric Retina*. Philadelphia: Lippincott Williams & Wilkins; 2005:77–94.

33. Shen B, Samaraweera P, Rosenberg B, et al. Ocular albinism type 1: more than meets the eye. *Pigment Cell Res* 2001;14:243–248.

34. Lyle WM, Sangster JOS, Williams TD. Albinism: an update and review of the literature. *Journal of the American Optometric Association* 1997;68(4):623–645.

35. Moore BD, ed. *Eye Care for Infants & Young Children*. Boston: Butterworth-Heinemann; 1997:213.

36. Okulicz J, Shah R, Schwartz R, et al. Oculocutaneous albinism. *J Eur Acad Dermatol Venereol* 2003;17:251–256.

37. Day S, Narita A. The uveal tract. In: Taylor D, ed. *Paediatric Ophthalmology*, 2nd ed. Oxford: Blackwell Science Ltd; 1997:410–444.

38. CHARGE Syndrome Foundation. CHARGE syndrome. 1998. Available at http://www.kumc.edu/gec/charge.html. Accessed December 2004.

39. Pagon RA, Graham JM, Zonana J, et al. Congenital heart disease and choanal atresia with multiple anomalies. *J Pediatr* 1981;99:223–227.

40. Davenport SL, Hefner MA, Mitchell JA. The spectrum of clinical features in CHARGE syndrome. *Clin Genet* 1986;29:298–310.

41. Mitchell JA, Davenport SLH, Hefner MA, et al. Use of an expert system to test diagnostic criteria in CHARGE syndrome. *J Med Syst* 1985;9:425–436.

42. Russell-Eggitt IM, Blake KD, Taylor DS, et al. The eye in the CHARGE association. *Br J Ophthalmol* 1990;74: 421–426.

43. Lalani SR, Safiullah AM, Fernback SD, et al. Toward a genetic etiology of CHARGE syndrome. I: A systematic scan for submicroscopic deletions. *Am J Med Genet* 2003;118A:260–266.

44. Chestler RJ, France TD. Ocular Findings in CHARGE Syndrome. *Ophthalmology* 1988;95:1613–1619.

45. Byoung-Sun A, Yeul OS. Clinical Characteristics of CHARGE Syndrome. *Korean J Ophthalmol* 1998;12: 130–134.

46. Blake KD, Davenport SL, Hall BD; et al. CHARGE Association: an update and review for the primary pediatrician. *Clin Pediatr* 1998;37:159–173.

47. Jones TW, Dunne MT. The CHARGE Association: implications for teachers. *Am Ann Deaf* 1988;133: 36–39.

48. American Occupational Therapist Association. About occupational therapy practitioners. Available at www.aota.org/featured/area6/index.asp. Accessed December 2004.

49. Lueck AH. *Functional Vision: A Practitioner's Guide to Evaluation and Intervention*. New York: AFB Press; 2004: 6–9.

50. Bishop VE. *Teaching Visually Impaired Children*, 3rd ed. Springfield, IL: Thomas Books; 2004:203–204.

51. Appel S, Ciner E, Graboyes M. Developing comprehensive vision care for multiply impaired children. *Practical Optometry* 1997;8:225–234.

52. Bernardini R, Novembre E, Lombardi E, et al. Risk factors for latex allergy in patients with spina bifida and latex sensitization. *Clin Exp Allergy* 1999;29:681–686.

53. Erin JN, Paul B. Functional vision assessment and instruction of children and youths in academic programs. In: Corn AL, Koenig AJ, eds. *Foundations of Low Vision: Clinical and Functional Perspectives*. New York: AFB Press; 1996:185–220.

54. Cramer JJ, Wright SA. The bean bag chair and the pedodontic patient with cerebral palsy. *Dental Hygiene (Chic)* 1975;49:167–168.

55. Olson LJ, Moulton HJ. Occupational therapists' reported experiences using weighted vests with children with specific developmental disorders. *Occup Ther Int* 2004;11:52–66.

56. Orel-Bixler D. Clinical vision assessments for infants. In: Chen D, ed. *Essential Elements in Early Intervention: Visual Impairment and Multiple Disabilities*. New York: AFB Press; 1999:107–156

57. Harris C. Other eye movement disorders. In: Taylor D, ed. *Paediatric Ophthalmology*, 2nd ed. Oxford: Blackwell Science Ltd; 1997:897–924.

58. Orel-Bixler D, Haegerstrom-Portnoy G, Hall A. Visual assessment of the multiply handicapped patient. *Optom Vis Sci* 1989;66:530–536

59. Maino DM, Maino JH, Maino SA. Mental retardation syndromes with associated ocular defects. *Journal of the American Optometric Association* 199;61:707– 716.

60. Van Splunder J, Stilma JS, Evenhuis HM. Visual performance in specific syndromes associated with intellectual disability. *Eur J Ophthalmol* 2003;13:566–574.

61. Van Splunder J, Stilma JS, Bernsen RM, et al. Prevalence of ocular diagnoses found on screening 1539 adults with intellectual disabilities. *Ophthalmology* 2004;111:1457–1463.

62. Tsiaras WG, Pueschel S, Keller C, et al. Amblyopia and visual acuity in children with Down's syndrome. *Br J Ophthalmol* 1999;83:1112–1114.

63. Sobrado P, Suatez J, Garcia-Sanchez FA, et al. Refractive errors in children with cerebral palsy, psychomotor retardation, and other non-cerebral palsy neuromotor disabilities. *Dev Med Child Neurol* 1999;41:396–403.

64. Castane M, Peris E, Sanchez E. ocular dysfunction associated with mental handicap. *Ophthalmic Physiol Opt* 1995;15:489–492.

65. Woodhouse JM, Adler PM, Duignan A. Ocular and visual defects amongst people with intellectual disabilities participating in Special Olympics. *Ophthalmic Physiol Opt* 2003;23:221–232.

66. Cregg M, Woodhouse JM, Pakemon VH, et al. Accommodation and refractive error in children with Down syndrome: cross-sectional and longitudinal studies. *Invest Ophthalmol Vis Sci* 2001;42:55–63.

67. Leat SJ. Reduced accommodation in children with cerebral palsy. *Ophthalmic Physiol Opt* 1996;16:385–390.

68. Woodhouse JM, Meades JS, Leat SJ, et al. Reduced accommodation in children with Down syndrome. *Invest Ophthalmol Vis Sci* 1993;34:2382–2387.

69. Steele G, Ireland D, Block S. Cycloplegic autorefraction results in pre-school children using the Nikon Retinomax Plus and the Welch Allyn SureSight. *Optom Vis Sci* 2003;80:573–577.

70. Topor I. Functional Vision Assessments and Early Interventions. In: *Essential Elements in Early Intervention: Visual Impairment and Multiple Disabilities*. Chen D, ed. New York: AFB Press, 1999; Ch. 5.

71. Bailey IL. Optometric care for the multihandicapped child. *Practical Optometry* 1994;5:158–166.

72. Mayer DL, Fulton AB, Cummings MF. Visual fields on infants assessed with a new perimetric technique. *Invest Ophthalmol Vis Sci* 1988;29:452–459.

73. Dobson V, Brown AM, Harvey EM, et al. Visual field extent in children 3.5–30 months of age tested with a double-arc LED perimeter. *Vision Res* 1998;38:2743–2760.

74. Blumenthal EZ, Haddad A, Horani A, et al. The reliability of frequency-doubling perimetry in young children. *Ophthalmology* 2004;111:435–439.

75. Becker K, Semes L. The reliability of frequency-doubling perimetry in young children. *Optometry* 2003; 74:173–179.

76. Schmidt PP. Vision screening with the RDE stereotest in pediatric populations. *Optom Vis Sci* 1994;71:273–281.

77. Ruttum MS, Bence SM, Alcorn D. Stereopsis testing in a preschool vision screening program. *J Pediatr Ophthalmol Strabismus* 1986;23(6):298–302.

78. Schmidt PP, Maguire MG, Moore B, et al. Vision in Preschoolers Study Group. Testability of preschoolers on stereotests used to screen vision disorders. *Optom Vis Sci* 2003;80(11):753–757.

79. Broadbent H, Westall C. An evaluation of techniques for measuring stereopsis in infants and young children. *Ophthalmic Physiol Opt* 1990;10(1):3–7.

80. Brown S, Weih L, Mukesh N, et al. Assessment of adult stereopsis using the Lang 1 Stereotest: a pilot study. *Binocul Vis Strabismus Q* 2001;16:91–98.

81. Schmidt PP, Kulp MT. Detecting ocular and visual anomalies in a vision screening setting using the Lang stereotest. *Journal of the American Optometric Association* 1994;65:725–731.

82. Duckman RH. Accommodation in cerebral palsy: function and remediation. *Journal of the American Optometric Association* 1984;55:281–283.

83. Courage ML, Adams RJ, Hall EJ. Contrast sensitivity in infants and children with Down syndrome. *Vision Res* 1997;37:1545–1555.

84. John FM, Bromham NR, Woodhouse JM, et al. Spatial vision deficits in infants and children with Down syndrome. *Invest Ophthalmol Vis Sci* 2004;45:1566–1572.

85. Chen AH, Mohamed D. New paediatric contrast test: Hiding Heidi low-contrast 'face' test. *Clin Experiment Ophthalmol* 2003;31(5):430–434.

86. Leat SJ, Wegmann D. Clinical testing of contrast sensitivity in children: age-related norms and validity. *Optom Vis Sci* 2004;81(4):245–254.

87. Richman JE, Lyons S. A forced choice procedure for evaluation of contrast sensitivity function in preschool children. *Journal of the American Optometric Association* 1994;65(12):859–864.

88. Cotter SA, Lee DY, French AL. Evalution of a new color vision test: "Color Vision Testing Made Easy." *Optom Vis Sci* 1999;76:631–636.

89. Mayer Johnson R. *The Picture Communication Symbols Book*. Solana Beach, CA: Mayer-Johnson Co.;1985.

90. Erickson GB, Block SS. Testability of a color vision screening test in a population with mental retardation. *Journal of the American Optometric Association* 1999;70:758–763.

91. Pease PL, Allen J. A new test for screening color vision: concurrent validity and utility. *Am J Optom Physiol Opt* 1988;65:729–738.

92. Goodman SA, Wittenstein SH. *Collaborative Assessment: Working with Students Who are Blind or Visually Impaired, Including Those with Additional Disabilities.* New York: AFB Press; 2003;83–87.

93. Koenig AJ, Holbrook MC. *Learning Media Assessment of Students with Visual Impairments,* 2nd ed. Lubbock, TX: Texas School for the Blind and Visually Impaired; 1995

94. Kauffman T, Théoret H, Pascual-Leone A. Braille character discrimination in blindfolded human subjects. *Neuroreport* 2002;13:572–574.

Educational and Accessibility Laws References

1. Brasher B, Holbrook MC. Early intervention and special education. In: Holbrook MC, ed. *Children with Visual Impairments: A Parents Guide.* Woodbine House Inc; 1996: pgs for chpt 8.

2. Blackman K, Smith TEC Legal issues. In: Holbrook MC, ed. *Children with Visual Impairments: A Parents Guide.* Woodbine House Inc, 1996: pgs for chpt 9.

3. Maine Parents Association. *504/IDEA Fact Sheet.* Available at http://www.mpf.org/SPIN/FAQ%20SHEET/504IDEA.html. Accessed December 2004.

4. AFB National Agenda for the Education of Children and Youths with Visual Impairments, Including Those with Multiple Disabilities. Goal 8: Expanded Core Curriculum. Available at http://www.afb.org/Section.asp?SectionID=56&DocumentID=2467. Accessed December 2004.

5. HR 1350 Part C. Available at http://thomas.loc.gov/cgi-bin/query/F?c108:7./temp/~c108Mw8vg3:e310083. Accessed December 2004.

6. No Child Left Behind Act. Available at http://www.ed.gov/print/nclb/overview/intor/execsumm.html. Accessed December 2004.

Index

Note: Page numbers followed by *t* indicate table; those followed by *f* indicate figure.